Human-Centered AI Applications for Medical Informatics

Hüseyin Coskun
Kutahya Health Sciences University, Turkey

IGI Global
Scientific Publishing
Publishing Tomorrow's Research Today

Vice President of Editorial	Melissa Wagner
Director of Acquisitions	Mikaela Felty
Director of Book Development	Jocelynn Hessler
Production Manager	Mike Brehm
Cover Design	Jose Rosado

Published in the United States of America by
IGI Global Scientific Publishing
701 East Chocolate Avenue
Hershey, PA, 17033, USA
Tel: 717-533-8845 | Fax: 717-533-7115
Website: https://www.igi-global.com E-mail: cust@igi-global.com

Library of Congress Cataloging-in-Publication Data

Names: Coskun, Huseyin, 1984- editor
Title: Human-centered AI applications for medical informatics / edited by Huseyin Coskun.
Description: Hershey, PA : IGI Global Scientific Publishing, [2026] | Includes bibliographical references and index. | Summary: "This book, 'Human-Centered AI Applications for Medical Informatics', aims to address the current and future applications of AI in health and medical informatics from a human-centered perspective"-- Provided by publisher.
Identifiers: LCCN 2025006745 (print) | LCCN 2025006746 (ebook) | ISBN 9798337314792 hardcover | ISBN 9798337314808 paperback | ISBN 9798337314815 ebook
Subjects: LCSH: Artificial intelligence--Medical applications | Medical informatics
Classification: LCC R859.7.A78 H86 2025 (print) | LCC R859.7.A78 (ebook)
LC record available at https://lccn.loc.gov/2025006745
LC ebook record available at https://lccn.loc.gov/2025006746

British Cataloguing in Publication Data
A Cataloguing in Publication record for this book is available from the British Library.

Table of Contents

Preface xiii

Chapter 1
A Study and Analysis of the Performance of Supervised Algorithms for Diagnosing Cardiac Disease Towards an Optimal Feature Set 1
Sippee Bharadwaj, International School of Business and Research, India
Nila Chotai, International School of Business and Research, India
Chinmoy Bharadwaj, University of Science and Technology, Meghalaya, India

Chapter 2
Accelerated Deep Learning Framework With Hybrid Techniques for Hair Disease Diagnosis and Telemedicine Integration 33
Venkata Surya Bhavana Harish Gollavilli, Under Armour, USA
Harikumar Nagarajan, Global Data Mart Inc., USA
Poovendran Alagarsundaram, Humetis Technologies Inc., USA
Surendar Rama Sitaraman, Intel Corporation, USA
Kalyan Gattupalli, Yash Tek Inc., Canada
Haris M. Khalid, College of Engineering and Information Technology, University of Dubai, UAE

Chapter 3
Artificial Intelligence and Human Psychology 71
Faika Şanal Karahan, Usak University, Turkey

Chapter 4
Artificial Intelligence-Based Applications Used in Neonatal Intensive Care Units 133
Emine Buse Kurnaz, Graduate Education Institute, Turkey
Deniz Yigit, Kütahya Faculty of Health Sciences, Turkey
Emel Sezici, Kütahya Faculty of Health Sciences, Turkey

Chapter 5
Artificial Intelligence-Assisted Image Analysis and Clinical Applications in Urology 165
Halil Ibrahim Ivelik, Kutahya Health Sciences University, Turkey
Bekir Aras, Kutahya Health Sciences University, Turkey

Chapter 6
Deep Learning-Based Cornea OCT Segmentation of Healthy and Keratoconic Eyes 193
Abir Chaari, National School of Electronics and Communication of Sfax, Tunisia
Imen Fourati Kallel, National School of Electronics and Communication of Sfax, Tunisia
Mondher Frikha, National School of Electronics and Communication of Sfax, Tunisia
Sonda Kammoun, Medical University of Sfax, Tunisia

Chapter 7
Human-Centered AI Applications for Medical Informatics: Artificial Intelligence in Mental Health - Advancing Care and Understanding 229
V. Kavitha, Velalar College of Engineering and Technology, India
T. Suresh Kumar, AVS Engineering College, India
A. P. Gopu, Velalar College of Engineering and Technology, India
V. Latha Jothi, Velalar College of Engineering and Technology, India
K. Baby, Velalar College of Engineering and Technology, India
J. Charanya, Kongu Engineering College, India
I. Nivetha, Velalar College of Engineering and Technology, India

Chapter 8
Improving Kidney Disorder Prediction Accuracy Using Blockchain With IoT Modules 261
C. K. Shahnazeer, Pondicherry University, Karaikal, India
G. Sureshkumar, Pondicherry University, Karaikal, India
C. K. Shinzeer, Lovely Professional University, India
Avinash Bhagat, Lovely Professional University, India
Ajay Shriram Kushwaha, Sharda University, India

Chapter 9
Osteoporosis Disease Prediction Using Machine Learning Algorithms 291
Rishita Das, Vellore Institute of Technology, Chennai, India
V. Santhi, Vellore Institute of Technology, Chennai, India

Chapter 10
Public Perception of the Portuguese National Health Service: A Social Media Sentiment Analysis Approach 333
Jorge Lami Leal, Faculty of Economics, Universidade do Algarve, Portugal
Célia M. Q. Ramos, CinTurs, ESGHT, Universidade do Algarve, Portugal

Chapter 11
Novel Development of Reinforcement Learning Models in Biomedical and Health Informatics Considering Socio-Demographic Risk Assessment for Mapping MRS 361
Siddharth Goswami, Graphic Era University, India
Sachin Sharma, Amity University, Mohali, India

Compilation of References 395

About the Contributors 463

Index 471

Detailed Table of Contents

Preface xiii

Chapter 1
A Study and Analysis of the Performance of Supervised Algorithms for Diagnosing Cardiac Disease Towards an Optimal Feature Set 1
Sippee Bharadwaj, International School of Business and Research, India
Nila Chotai, International School of Business and Research, India
Chinmoy Bharadwaj, University of Science and Technology, Meghalaya, India

Cardiovascular diseases (CVD) and heart attacks pose a considerable threat to the adult population, particularly when compounded by metabolic diseases such as diabetes and obesity. While pharmacological therapies are crucial for treating heart-related difficulties, lifestyle improvements, including regular exercise and appropriate dietary choices, play a key part in regulating heart failure symptoms. Diagnosing cardiovascular illnesses poses a major problem due to the complexity and variety of clinical data. In this context, machine learning (ML) is a potential solution, enabling the study of massive healthcare datasets to give more accurate prediction insights and diagnostic tools. This research seeks to enhance heart failure detection accuracy by employing ML algorithms on a health dataset from the University of California. The ANN model achieved the highest accuracy of 92% in heart disease prediction, outperforming other ML models. By integrating thallium scan results, chest discomfort and damaged arteries can significantly improve early diagnosis and treatment effectiveness.

Chapter 2
Accelerated Deep Learning Framework With Hybrid Techniques for Hair Disease Diagnosis and Telemedicine Integration 33
Venkata Surya Bhavana Harish Gollavilli, Under Armour, USA
Harikumar Nagarajan, Global Data Mart Inc., USA
Poovendran Alagarsundaram, Humetis Technologies Inc., USA
Surendar Rama Sitaraman, Intel Corporation, USA
Kalyan Gattupalli, Yash Tek Inc., Canada
Haris M. Khalid, College of Engineering and Information Technology, University of Dubai, UAE

Background information: Alopecia and seborrheic dermatitis are two dermatoses that lower quality of life. The current diagnoses are subjective and time-consuming.

EfficientNet-B3 and CBAM, two deep learning-based telemedicine tools, offer scalable, accurate solutions to the issues of data scarcity and class imbalance. Objectives: The hybrid deep learning system, by combining EfficientNet-B3, CBAM, and GANs, will address class imbalance and provide a simpler platform for telemedicine-based accurate, rapid, and scalable hair illness diagnosis. Methods: Harvesting of features is performed by using EfficientNet-B3 and CBAM. GANs are applied for rectification of the synthetic data class imbalance problem. For the purpose of achieving light scaling, knowledge distillation is used, while preprocessing, augmentation, and RAdam are utilized for the optimization of training. Results: With a delay of 15 ms, 99.5% accuracy and 98.9% precision were achieved. Conclusion: In conclusion, it helps underprivileged communities and ensures real-time scalability with accuracy in diagnosis.

Chapter 3
Artificial Intelligence and Human Psychology 71
Faika Şanal Karahan, Usak University, Turkey

This chapter will explore the ways in which AI has an impact on psychological well-being, human behavior and social dynamics. It will examine both the opportunities for improving mental health through intelligent assistance and the concerns about the potential for dehumanization and emotional detachment. By exploring these two facets, it is possible to appreciate the complexities of integrating AI into the fabric of human experience, and set the stage for a critical discussion of how these advances are redefining one's understanding of oneself. AI's potential to augment, not replace, human thinking is shown by its use as a cognitive prosthesis, extending the processing capacity and knowledge. The research landscape evolves, as shown by the growing study of video games in psychology, cognitive science and other fields, reflecting the increasing importance of AI in human behavior. The findings highlight a critical shift in AI: it informs our understanding of psychology and enriches one's own cognitive processes. This demands exploration and ethics in future studies.

Chapter 4
Artificial Intelligence-Based Applications Used in Neonatal Intensive Care Units 133
Emine Buse Kurnaz, Graduate Education Institute, Turkey
Deniz Yigit, Kütahya Faculty of Health Sciences, Turkey
Emel Sezici, Kütahya Faculty of Health Sciences, Turkey

The neonatal period is a time when many systems of newborns are immature and vulnerable to external dangers. Newborns may be admitted to the Neonatal Intensive Care Unit due to different health problems they experience during this period. Newborns in these units need a multidisciplinary team approach and the use of advanced technological applications. With the development of technology in recent years, the use of artificial intelligence-based applications has increased in Neonatal Intensive Care Units. These applications include imaging and diagnostic systems, clinical decision support systems, robotic and automation applications, follow-up and monitoring of infants, ventilator management and respiratory support systems, infection and sepsis monitoring. Effective diagnosis, treatment and care services are carried out by healthcare professionals with artificial intelligence-based applications. Artificial intelligence-based applications used in the Neonatal Intensive Care Unit increase the life chances of newborns and positively affect long-term health and development outcomes.

Chapter 5
Artificial Intelligence-Assisted Image Analysis and Clinical Applications in Urology 165
Halil Ibrahim Ivelik, Kutahya Health Sciences University, Turkey
Bekir Aras, Kutahya Health Sciences University, Turkey

Artificial intelligence (AI) has the potential to revolutionize urology by enhancing diagnostics, surgical precision, and patient care. AI-powered diagnostic tools are increasingly used for the early detection of urologic diseases such as prostate and bladder cancer, while robotic-assisted surgery improves precision in minimally invasive procedures. Additionally, AI-driven wearable technologies and remote monitoring systems enhance patient management, enabling personalized treatment approaches. However, the integration of AI into clinical practice raises ethical concerns, including algorithmic bias, data privacy, and accountability, which must be addressed to ensure fair and reliable AI systems. This study explores the future of AI in urology, its integration potential, and the ethical challenges it presents, offering recommendations for a more sustainable and equitable implementation.

Chapter 6
Deep Learning-Based Cornea OCT Segmentation of Healthy and Keratoconic Eyes 193
Abir Chaari, National School of Electronics and Communication of Sfax, Tunisia
Imen Fourati Kallel, National School of Electronics and Communication of Sfax, Tunisia
Mondher Frikha, National School of Electronics and Communication of Sfax, Tunisia
Sonda Kammoun, Medical University of Sfax, Tunisia

Vision is one of the most essential human senses, playing a key role in perceiving and interpreting the environment. This complex process depends on the proper functioning of various ocular structures, particularly the cornea. Any alteration in its structure or function can significantly affect visual quality. This research explores the use of a deep learning method for semantic segmentation of corneal layers to enable early detection of keratoconus. To address limitations of existing automatic segmentation techniques for corneal Optical Coherence Tomography images, a novel deep learning model is proposed. The algorithm segments corneal layers by capturing both local and contextual features. The developed architecture is based on an enhanced UNet variant incorporating residual connections, recurrent modules, and dilated convolutions. The model was evaluated on a dataset comprising both healthy and keratoconus-affected corneas. Experimental results showed an accuracy of 96.77%, outperforming reference models such as UNet, ResUNet, SegNet, and DeepLabV3+.

Chapter 7
Human-Centered AI Applications for Medical Informatics: Artificial Intelligence in Mental Health - Advancing Care and Understanding 229
V. Kavitha, Velalar College of Engineering and Technology, India
T. Suresh Kumar, AVS Engineering College, India
A. P. Gopu, Velalar College of Engineering and Technology, India
V. Latha Jothi, Velalar College of Engineering and Technology, India
K. Baby, Velalar College of Engineering and Technology, India
J. Charanya, Kongu Engineering College, India
I. Nivetha, Velalar College of Engineering and Technology, India

The diagnosis, awareness, and medical care of mental illness are being transformed with the emergence of machine learning (otherwise referred to as AI) in the area of mental illness. This chapter discusses the sophisticated uses for artificial intelligence (AI), involving machine learning algorithms and natural language processing, to analyze behavioral patterns, detect mental illness, and offer individualized options for treatment. Illustrations of AI applications include virtual mental health assistance systems and platforms for preventive diagnosis that analyze speech and text data for depression and anxiety. Among the important topics covered in the chapter are algorithmic bias, data security, moral issues, and the necessity of preserving compassion for humans in AI-based medicine.

Chapter 8
Improving Kidney Disorder Prediction Accuracy Using Blockchain With IoT Modules 261
C. K. Shahnazeer, Pondicherry University, Karaikal, India
G. Sureshkumar, Pondicherry University, Karaikal, India
C. K. Shinzeer, Lovely Professional University, India
Avinash Bhagat, Lovely Professional University, India
Ajay Shriram Kushwaha, Sharda University, India

This study expresses a fresh hybrid algorithm, a fusion of blockchain concepts and IoT networks, that aims to elevate kidney dysfunction diagnosis by boosting the predictive capacity. In this case, because of blockchain which accomplishes data transparency and decentralization, the system provides cross-border availability of e-health services such as seamless data sharing and peer-to-peer health monitoring over IoT devices. With advanced supervisory learning a system might analyze the sensor units' data to diagnose possible problems associated with the kidneys in their early stages. The model is an added layer of security and transparency and a higher accuracy percentage in diagnosing diseases timely and more accurately. Blockchain and IoT are effective bridges that can help solve issues such as data management and predictive analytics in healthcare. Through this setup, we get more reliable data and this can later on also be used in diagnostic systems aimed at scaling and scalability.

Chapter 9
Osteoporosis Disease Prediction Using Machine Learning Algorithms 291
Rishita Das, Vellore Institute of Technology, Chennai, India
V. Santhi, Vellore Institute of Technology, Chennai, India

Osteoporosis is a major global health concern characterized by progressive bone loss, increasing the risk of fractures, particularly among postmenopausal women and the elderly. Traditional diagnostic methods, such as Dual-energy X-ray Absorptiometry (DXA), are expensive, resource-intensive, and often inaccessible in low-resource settings, leading to underdiagnosis and delayed intervention. This study explores the potential of machine learning (ML) algorithms in predicting osteoporosis using clinical, demographic, and biochemical data. Various ML models, including Naïve Bayes, XGBoost, and Random Forest, were evaluated for their predictive accuracy, with ensemble models demonstrating the highest performance. The results indicate that ML-based predictive models can serve as cost-effective, scalable, and non-invasive screening tools, enabling early detection and timely intervention. The study highlights the integration of ML in healthcare, paving the way for personalized osteoporosis risk assessment and improved patient outcomes.

Chapter 10
Public Perception of the Portuguese National Health Service: A Social Media Sentiment Analysis Approach 333
Jorge Lami Leal, Faculty of Economics, Universidade do Algarve, Portugal
Célia M. Q. Ramos, CinTurs, ESGHT, Universidade do Algarve, Portugal

Analysing social media testimonials about public health is vital for understanding public perceptions and emotions, leading to better policy-making and health services. This investigation reviews recent research on sentiment analysis in healthcare, focusing on public perception of the Portuguese National Health Service (NHS) through interactions on its Instagram and Facebook pages. Using a Machine Learning approach, the study finds a negative perception of the NHS, posing a high reputational risk. It recommends persistent institutional mediation through comments and systematic sentiment analysis to monitor social media opinions, improve communication, and refine policies based on real-time feedback.

Chapter 11
Novel Development of Reinforcement Learning Models in Biomedical and Health Informatics Considering Socio-Demographic Risk Assessment for Mapping MRS 361
Siddharth Goswami, Graphic Era University, India
Sachin Sharma, Amity University, Mohali, India

Methicillin-resistant Staphylococcus aureus (MRSA) is one of the emerging international health threats, more prevalent in the higher-risk areas such as California, USA. This research develops novel reinforcement learning models, Deep Q-Network (DQN), and Proximal Policy Optimisation (PPO), to predict and control MRSA resistance. The results indicate that both PPO and DQN can lower the infection rate of MRSA; however, the PPO model provides a better performance than the DQN due to its sophisticated reward function. The predictive capability of the models is evidenced by the performance metrics such as ROC-AUC, accuracy, precision, recall, and confusion matrix. Additionally, t-tests and p-values are computed, and the statistical efficacy of both developed models is assessed. This research aligns with the broader field of biomedical informatics, providing a comprehensive framework for tackling antibiotic resistance and demonstrating the potential of reinforcement learning in managing infectious diseases.

Compilation of References 395

About the Contributors 463

Index 471

Preface

In recent years, the intersection of artificial intelligence (AI) and healthcare has led to transformative innovations that are reshaping medical diagnostics, treatment planning, patient care, and health system management. The need for human-centered design in AI applications is more critical than ever, particularly in medical informatics, where patient outcomes, clinical accuracy, and ethical considerations are paramount. This edited volume, *Human-Centered AI Applications for Medical Informatics*, presents a diverse range of research contributions from international scholars and professionals who examine how AI can be designed and applied to support human health with empathy, responsibility, and efficacy.

This book brings together practical case studies, theoretical frameworks, and experimental research that collectively highlight how AI tools, when thoughtfully developed and deployed, can address complex medical challenges while maintaining human dignity and clinical integrity. From early disease prediction to telemedicine, mental health analytics to neonatal care, and reinforcement learning in public health to blockchain-enabled health data systems, the chapters reflect an inclusive and multidisciplinary perspective on the state of the art in AI and healthcare integration.

The volume is structured to reflect a progression from foundational AI methods in clinical diagnostics to advanced, specialized applications across various domains in healthcare. Each chapter provides insights into both technological advancement and human impact, reinforcing the core idea that AI must ultimately serve human needs.

CHAPTER OVERVIEW

Chapter 1. A Study and Analysis of The Performance of Supervised Algorithms for Diagnosing Cardiac Disease Towards An Optimal Feature Set

This chapter examines how supervised machine learning algorithms can improve the accuracy of cardiac disease diagnosis. It highlights the importance of selecting optimal feature sets and compares models, with artificial neural networks achieving the highest predictive performance.

Chapter 2. Accelerated Deep Learning Framework with Hybrid Techniques for Hair Disease Diagnosis and Telemedicine Integration

A hybrid deep learning model combining EfficientNet-B3, CBAM, and GANs is introduced for diagnosing hair diseases. This system ensures high accuracy and real-time diagnosis, particularly benefiting under-resourced communities through telemedicine applications.

Chapter 3. Artificial Intelligence and Human Psychology

Focusing on the intersection of AI and mental health, this chapter explores AI's dual role in enhancing psychological well-being and raising concerns about emotional detachment. It positions AI as a cognitive augmentation tool while calling for ethical scrutiny.

Chapter 4. Artificial Intelligence-Based Applications Used in Neonatal Intensive Care Unit

This chapter surveys AI applications in neonatal intensive care units, including diagnostic tools, monitoring systems, and robotic support. It emphasizes the role of AI in improving outcomes for newborns through real-time, multidisciplinary support.

Chapter 5. Artificial Intelligence-Assisted Image Analysis and Clinical Applications in Urology

AI's transformative potential in urology is presented through diagnostic improvements and robotic-assisted procedures. Ethical considerations such as bias and data privacy are also discussed in the context of adopting AI in clinical urology practice.

Chapter 6. Deep Learning-Based Cornea OCT Segmentation of Healthy and Keratoconic Eyes

This research introduces a deep learning architecture for segmenting corneal layers in OCT images. The model surpasses traditional techniques, aiding in early keratoconus detection and enhancing ophthalmological diagnostics.

Chapter 7. Artificial Intelligence in Mental Health: Advancing Care and Understanding

This chapter focuses on machine learning and natural language processing applications in mental health, including virtual assistants and predictive analytics. It also explores ethical concerns and emphasizes the importance of preserving human compassion in AI-driven care.

Chapter 8. Improving Kidney Disorder Prediction Accuracy Using Blockchain with IoT Modules

A novel integration of blockchain and IoT is proposed to enhance kidney disease prediction. The system offers secure, transparent, and scalable solutions for early diagnosis and cross-border health data sharing.

Chapter 9. Osteoporosis Disease Prediction Using Machine Learning Algorithms

Various machine learning models are assessed for their ability to predict osteoporosis. The study presents ML as a cost-effective alternative to traditional diagnostic methods, especially useful in resource-constrained environments.

Chapter 10. Public Perception of the Portuguese National Health Service: A Social Media Sentiment Analysis Approach

Using machine learning-based sentiment analysis, this chapter investigates public opinion about Portugal's NHS via social media. Findings highlight reputational risks and call for improved communication strategies based on real-time public feedback.

Chapter 11. Novel Development of Reinforcement Learning Models in Biomedical and Health Informatics Considering Socio-Demographic Risk Assessment for Mapping MRS

Reinforcement learning models, including PPO and DQN, are developed to address the threat of MRSA infections. The chapter demonstrates their predictive strength and evaluates performance metrics, contributing to infectious disease management.

Together, the chapters in this volume offer a multidimensional view of how human-centered AI is not only revolutionizing medical informatics but also emphasizing the necessity of ethical, inclusive, and context-aware development. The book aims to inform researchers, clinicians, technologists, and policymakers of the emerging possibilities and responsibilities in designing AI for healthcare with humanity at its core.

Huseyin Coskun
Kutahya Health Sciences University, Turkey

Chapter 1
A Study and Analysis of the Performance of Supervised Algorithms for Diagnosing Cardiac Disease Towards an Optimal Feature Set

Sippee Bharadwaj
https://orcid.org/0000-0002-7808-7156
International School of Business and Research, India

Nila Chotai
https://orcid.org/0009-0003-6563-4071
International School of Business and Research, India

Chinmoy Bharadwaj
https://orcid.org/0000-0002-3027-6812
University of Science and Technology, Meghalaya, India

ABSTRACT

Cardiovascular diseases (CVD) and heart attacks pose a considerable threat to the adult population, particularly when compounded by metabolic diseases such as diabetes and obesity. While pharmacological therapies are crucial for treating heart-related difficulties, lifestyle improvements, including regular exercise and appropriate dietary choices, play a key part in regulating heart failure symptoms. Diagnosing cardiovascular illnesses poses a major problem due to the complexity

DOI: 10.4018/979-8-3373-1479-2.ch001

and variety of clinical data. In this context, machine learning (ML) is a potential solution, enabling the study of massive healthcare datasets to give more accurate prediction insights and diagnostic tools. This research seeks to enhance heart failure detection accuracy by employing ML algorithms on a health dataset from the University of California. The ANN model achieved the highest accuracy of 92% in heart disease prediction, outperforming other ML models. By integrating thallium scan results, chest discomfort and damaged arteries can significantly improve early diagnosis and treatment effectiveness.

1. INTRODUCTION

According to the World Health Organisation fact sheet 2023, cardiovascular diseases (CVDs) kill 17.9 million people globally, almost one-third of all fatalities. Early detection and strong treatment are vital, as many illnesses typically develop quietly and only exhibit symptoms after a severe injury. Traditional risk assessment methodologies are helpful but occasionally fail to convey heart disease's intricacy and diverse personality traits. In recent years, artificial intelligence (AI) and, more notably, machine learning (ML) have emerged as revolutionary tools in healthcare. ML algorithms can scan huge volumes of patient data to uncover subtle patterns and connections that conventional diagnostic processes may miss. Their implementation into clinical processes may enhance prediction accuracy, inform clinical decision-making, and facilitate tailored care. Recent breakthroughs in machine learning (ML) have offered new opportunities for strengthening diagnostic tools and clinical decision support. This study analyses the performance of supervised ML algorithms in identifying cardiac risk using real-world patient data. This study aims to identify the most successful ML models that might potentially be implemented into clinical workflows. It is mentioned in some research articles that machine learning has begun to impact clinical processes by analyzing records. This concerning growth can be related to both non-modifiable and modifiable risk factors. Modifiable risk factors include high blood pressure and sugar, elevated cholesterol levels, smoking, obesity, physical inactivity, unhealthy dietary habits, and prolonged psychological stress. The existence of many risk factors in individuals, especially in combination, greatly boosts the likelihood of cardiovascular issues. Fortunately, many of these factors are controlled, and lifestyle interventions such as good food, regular exercise, stress management, and discontinuation of tobacco use can decrease the possibility of getting heart disease. Educational efforts, frequent diagnostics, and preventive activities are vital in lowering the incidence of this increasing disease. In response to this worldwide health concern, researchers and experts have increasingly turned to sophisticated computational tools to enhance the early identification and prevention of cardiac disease. Rule-generation systems are also applied to detect early signs of heart attacks and decrease mortality (Ordonez, 2006).

Machine learning (ML), a subset of artificial intelligence, has shown considerable promise in this domain due to its capacity to handle enormous datasets, identify hidden patterns, and enhance diagnostic accuracy. The application of ML models in healthcare has drastically expanded due to their efficiency in processing complicated information and delivering reliable diagnostic outputs, especially in time-sensitive clinical contexts. In the area of cardiovascular health, these models have been widely employed to examine electrocardiograms (ECGs), echocardiograms, and MRI images to diagnose structural and functional abnormalities with great precision. They often outperform current diagnostic approaches by lowering human error and boosting sensitivity and specificity in detecting subtle abnormalities. The research article (Krittanawong et al., 2019) highlights how machine learning is altering precision cardiovascular medicine through improved risk assessment, real-time decision aid, and integration with wearable technologies. These strategies enable early identification of high-risk patients and facilitate tailored therapy, ultimately improving clinical results. An ensemble machine learning technique exploiting the Cleveland heart disease dataset considerably outperforms typical individual classifiers in terms of projected accuracy. The study built a hybrid Voting Classifier that incorporated Logistic Regression, Gradient Boosting, and Support Vector Machine (SVM) models, attaining an astonishing accuracy of 97.9%. These findings underscore the value of ensemble learning techniques in medical diagnostics, notably for heart disease prediction.

In (Latha & Jeeva, 2019), an ensemble technique further enhanced accuracy by 7.7%, suggesting that integrating classifiers greatly enhances overall model dependability and resilience. These strategies aggregate the merits of distinct algorithms while reducing their flaws, making them extremely suitable for essential applications like heart disease diagnostics. The primary goal of the proposed study is to evaluate and compare the performance of six widely used classifiers, Artificial Neural Networks (ANN), Logistic Regression (LR), K-nearest neighbors (KNN), Random Forest (RF), Support Vector Machine (SVM), and Extreme Gradient Boosting (XGB) for predicting heart disease. Model performance is tested using important parameters such as classification accuracy, sensitivity, specificity, Area Under the Receiver Operating Characteristic Curve (AUROC), and log loss. The present study undertakes a rigorous comparative analysis to discover the ideal feature set and best-performing algorithm for real-time heart disease prediction. The findings aim to produce diagnostic technologies that are accurate, scalable, and therapeutically beneficial. The research is split into main sections: defining aims, evaluating the literature on heart failure prediction using machine learning, outlining materials and techniques, presenting experimental results, interpreting data, and closing with key findings and future implications. Between 2022 and 2024, cardiovascular disorders have risen significantly, generating demand for improved computational methods. AI models human intellect, while machine learning (ML), a type of AI, learns from data patterns. These technologies increase diagnostic precision and reduce clinician workload. Despite much algorithmic research, few address real-world AI integration in healthcare settings, which needs consideration of EHR interoperability, physician workflow, and laws. To determine the best algorithm-feature combination for precise heart disease prediction, this study uses several statistical feature selection techniques to extract the relevant features and to compare six supervised machine learning classifiers such as Artificial Neural Network (ANN), Support Vector Machine (SVM), Logistic Regression (LR), Random Forest (RF), Decision Tree (DT), and Extreme Gradient Boosting (XGB). The objectives of our proposed ideas are as follows:

- A comparative analysis of the heart disease prediction capabilities of six machine learning algorithms (ANN, LR, KNN, RF, SVM, and XGB) using important performance parameters like log loss, AUROC, sensitivity, specificity, and accuracy.
- To improve clinical decision-making and early diagnosis through the development of a scalable and dependable diagnostic system for real-time cardiac disease prediction.

2. BACKGROUND AND LITERATURE REVIEW

Heart disease is a chronic, life-threatening ailment impacting millions worldwide and remains the greatest cause of mortality globally. This spike in cardiovascular disorders highlights the importance of early detection and fast management. Cost-effective, efficient AI and machine learning (ML) diagnostic tools can play a transformative part by monitoring, diagnosing, and detecting changes in crucial medical parameters, exposing early signs, and minimizing clinical response time. As healthcare digitizes, incorporating this intelligent technology enhances preventive and therapeutic methods, especially in under-resourced or high-risk places. Our research focuses on building an ML-based model to aid in accurate cardiovascular diagnosis. We have studied substantial literature to appreciate current ML and deep learning (DL) advancements in heart disease diagnosis. This review depicts the state of the art, highlighting important techniques, outcomes, and constraints, and provides insights into the strengths and limitations of AI/ML approaches, leading to future improvements. A multiple regression model is especially successful in predicting the risk of heart disorders when used to predict heart-related conditions. In a research work by Pan et al. (2020), researchers explored the implementation of machine learning techniques inside the ecosystem of the Internet of Medical Things (IoMT) for diagnosing cardiac illnesses. By enhancing deep learning-assisted convolutional neural networks (EDCNN), neural network ensemble methods (NNE), recurrent neural networks (RNN), and artificial neural networks (ANN), they developed an ensemble deep learning-based smart healthcare system (EDL-SHS). Impressively, the system attained an excellent accuracy of 99%, illustrating the great potential of ensemble models in real-time medical diagnosis and continuous health monitoring for individuals with varying risk levels.

The research presented by Ricciardi et al. (2020) employed a range of machine-learning techniques, including random forest, multivariate logistic regression, AdaBoost, and gradient boosting within the context of computed tomography (CT) imaging. This investigation focuses on older people suffering from cardio-vascular disease (CVD), coronary heart disease (CHD), and chronic heart failure (CHF). The results confirmed the usefulness of ML in processing medical imaging data to detect and categorize different types of cardiac problems. Notably, the integration of hybrid random forest models with linear classifiers greatly boosted the predictive accuracy of the Cleveland dataset, thereby highlighting the power of model hybridization in cardiovascular diagnosis (Mohan et al., 2019). The research documented by (Ali et al., 2021) utilized decision trees, KNN, and random forest algorithms to detect early-stage heart disease from Kaggle datasets. Random Forest has demonstrated high accuracy across multiple studies, achieving 81.967% (Apurv Garg et al., 2021), 94.12% (Bora & Hadaegh, 2021), and outperforming other methods in some cases (Shah et al., 2020) and Decision Tree (Kavitha et al., 2021), achieving 88.7% accuracy. These studies utilized datasets from sources such as the UCI Machine Learning Repository and Kaggle, considering various features like cholesterol levels, blood pressure, age, and sex. The development of accurate prediction models could potentially aid in early detection and reduce mortality rates. It is seen from the existing state of the art (2023-2025) that more research has been done to explore the use of machine learning algorithms for heart disease prediction, aiming to improve early detection and patient outcomes. Various models, including Logistic Regression, K-Nearest Neighbors, Support Vector Machines, and Random Forest, have been evaluated using diverse datasets containing patient variables and relevant factors (Aman Solanki et al., 2023; M. Shaik et al., 2023). These algorithms have demonstrated the potential to accurately classify patients with heart disease, with some studies finding Logistic Regression and KNN to be particularly effective. Performance metrics such as accuracy, precision, recall, and specificity have been used to assess model effectiveness (P. Sree et al., 2023). The successful implementation of these predictive models could lead to the development of efficient diagnostic tools, assisting healthcare practitioners in making informed decisions and potentially reducing the burden of heart disease on individuals and healthcare systems.

The purpose of this research is to compare the accuracies of classification models used to predict heart disease by using the largest dataset available for heart disease prediction, check out the heatmap to find the correlation between different parameters involved in the dataset, and find the most important parameter with the highest importance factor for predicting heart disease. Random Forest model has the highest 92.44% accuracy, followed by SVM and decision tree in predicting heart disease. Logistic regression had the least accuracy among all the models used. ST slope and old peak have a very high correlation factor of 0.52, and exercise angina and max heart rate have a very low correlation of -0.38. ST slope is the most important factor for predicting heart disease among all other factors given in the dataset, and fasting blood sugar is the least important parameter used in the prediction of heart disease. (Pant M et al., 2024). These advancements in machine learning-based heart disease prediction have the potential to improve early detection, personalized healthcare, and patient outcomes (Patil et al., 2024). Various approaches have been explored, including the Heart Disease Detection Model (HD2M) utilizing the Archimedes Optimization Algorithm for feature selection and multiple classifiers (ElGendy et al., 2025). Additionally, a comprehensive study comparing nine machine learning algorithms, including a novel voting system with feature selection techniques, demonstrated exceptional performance, with XGBoost achieving 99% accuracy in heart disease prediction (M. Hasan et al., 2025). These advancements show great potential for improving early diagnosis and preventive healthcare in cardiac conditions.

In summary, this literature review comprehensively highlights the evolving role of machine learning and deep learning techniques in the prediction and diagnosis of cardiovascular disease. These studies collectively underscore the potential of intelligent systems in identifying critical patterns in complex medical data, thereby aiding cardiologists in delivering timely and accurate care. Our study aims to conduct a comparative evaluation of diverse ML and DL algorithms using an optimal set of features to improve the prediction of cardiovascular disorders. This endeavour holds significant promise in contributing to more effective healthcare management and ultimately reducing mortality associated with heart diseases on a global scale, especially when integrated into scalable and adaptive healthcare infrastructures. This study aims to evaluate and compare the performance of six widely-used supervised learning algorithms, such as Artificial Neural Networks (ANN), Support Vector Machines (SVM), Logistic Regression (LR), Random Forest (RF), Decision Trees (DT), and Extreme Gradient Boosting (XGB), on a heart disease prediction dataset. The research focuses on accuracy, sensitivity, specificity, and other performance metrics to identify the model best suited for early cardiac diagnosis. It's important to emphasize how these technologies work in clinical settings in addition to algorithmic performance. For instance, Artificial Neural Networks (ANNs) are used in hospitals for diagnostic imaging and patient risk stratification, improving clinical decision-making. Recent advances like federated learning remove significant obstacles to data sharing by allowing several institutions to work together to train models without jeopardizing patient privacy. Edge AI in wearable devices allows continuous, real-time health monitoring outside clinical environments. Additionally, integrating machine learning into Electronic Health Records (EHRs) enhances workflow efficiency and enables faster, more accurate predictions at the point of care. These practical applications reflect the evolving landscape of AI in healthcare. Recent advances extend beyond algorithms to real-world deployment, addressing privacy concerns and improving patient monitoring and clinical support. The reviewed studies highlight both the progress and limitations of current AI methods in heart disease prediction. The next section outlines our methodology for a comparative analysis of machine learning models addressing these gaps.

3. METHODS

The heart failure dataset utilized in this research study has been sourced from the UC Irvine Machine Learning Repository, a well-known platform for benchmarking datasets in the machine learning field. This particular dataset has 269 individual patient records, each representing either a person diagnosed with heart failure or a healthy subject without any apparent cardiovascular concerns. These data sets include 13 distinct input features, which are employed as independent variables to help with the classification and prediction of heart failure. The characteristics include clinical factors such as age, blood pressure, serum creatinine, ejection fraction, sex, and other important indicators pertinent to cardiovascular diseases. The dataset was thoroughly prepared and structured as a necessary stage in the development of robust machine-learning models. This phase ensures that the dataset is clean, consistent, and ready for effective training and evaluation. In addition to encoding categorical variables and normalizing continuous features, the dataset underwent numerous key preprocessing processes. The following steps are

- Imputation of missing values using mean and mode techniques for numerical and categorical characteristics, respectively.
- Using interquartile range (IQR) thresholds, outliers are eliminated.
- Data normalization using min-max scaling, notably for distance-sensitive algorithms like KNN and SVM. These approaches ensured consistency, decreased model bias, and increased convergence throughout training.

The formatting procedure comprised removing noisy data, correcting errors, resolving missing values, and converting categorical variables into numerical form. Normalization or standardization was done when needed to scale features, boost algorithm stability, and convergence. After preprocessing, exploratory data analysis (EDA) was undertaken to investigate the dataset's structure and variable correlations. Techniques including histograms, boxplots, pair plots, and correlation heatmaps revealed distribution patterns, correlations, outliers, and statistical features. Feature engineering focused on feature selection to reduce model complexity, enhance training efficiency, and boost accuracy. Three statistical feature selection methods were applied.

- Feature Selection Technique 1 (FST1) - ANOVA (Analysis of Variance): This method assesses the degree of variance among groups to determine whether there are statistically significant variations between group means. ANOVA is very successful in discovering numeric parameters that differ significantly between classes.
- Feature Selection Technique 2 (FST2) – Chi-square examination: This statistical technique is used to examine the independence of two category variables. It helps establish whether the presence or absence of a given feature is strongly connected with the class label (heart failure or not).
- Feature Selection Technique 3 (FST3) - Mutual Information: This method analyses the amount of shared information between each feature and the target variable. It quantifies how much knowing the value of a feature reduces uncertainty about the class label, making it extremely suitable for nonlinear connections.

The use of ANOVA, Chi-square, and Mutual Information was chosen to balance simplicity and statistical rigor. ANOVA is appropriate for identifying features with variance between classes, while Chi-square is effective for detecting categorical variable relationships. Mutual Information captures both linear and non-linear connections, making it particularly effective in detecting features with concealed predictive power in medical datasets. The adoption of the above techniques (FST1, FST2, and FST3) resulted in the extraction of three separate feature subsets:

- Selected Features 1 (SF1): Comprising the most relevant features identified using ANOVA.
- Selected Features 2 (SF2): Containing features picked based on the Chi-square test.
- Selected Features 3 (SF3): Includes features picked using mutual information scores.

Following the identification of high-importance features, the dataset was partitioned into training and testing subsets. This splitting technique is crucial to evaluate model performance on unseen data and guarantee that the model generalizes well to real-world instances. A standard data split ratio, such as 80% for training and 20% for testing, was likely applied to maintain a balanced review. Each of the three feature subsets (SF1, SF2, and SF3) was used to train and assess a set of six machine learning algorithms, chosen based on their performance in classification tasks and prior success in medical data processing. These algorithms presumably comprised frequently used classifiers such as:

- Logistic Regression (LR)
- Decision Tree (DT)
- Random Forest (RF)
- Support Vector Machine (SVM)
- k-Nearest Neighbours (KNN)
- Gradient Boosting Classifier (GBC)

Hyperparameter optimization was conducted to enhance the model's performance. In contrast to other model parameters, this is utilized before the training phase and significantly impacts model behavior. Optimization methods, including Grid Search, Randomised Search, and Bayesian Optimisation, were theoretically employed to identify the ideal hyperparameter combinations for each program. This adjustment facilitates optimal accuracy while reducing the likelihood of overfitting or underfitting. The performance of the trained models was extensively examined using a range of classification performance criteria, including:

- Accuracy - It is defined as the ratio of accurately predicted instances to the total number of instances.
- Precision - It is calculated by the proportion of true positive forecasts among all positive predictions made.
- Recall (Sensitivity) - The model can correctly identify actual positive cases.
- F1-Score- the harmonic means of precision and recall, providing a balanced assessment of model performance.
- ROC-AUC (Receiver Operating Characteristic - Area Under Curve)- It examines the trade-off between sensitivity and specificity across multiple threshold values.

The best method for predicting heart failure was determined to be the algorithm that obtained the highest scores in each of these categories, particularly in terms of F1-score and AUC-ROC. Its remarkable ability to identify both at-risk and healthy patients attests to its value in clinical decision-support systems. There are significant ethical issues with using machine learning to forecast heart illness. In order to maintain confidentiality and secure data use, it is imperative to adhere to regulations like HIPAA and GDPR when working with sensitive electronic health records (EHRs). Furthermore, the development of trust between patients and healthcare professionals is greatly aided by model transparency and explainability; interpretability approaches such as SHAP and LIME help to make clear how predictions are made. In addition, biases in data and algorithms must be eliminated to prevent treating demographic groups unfairly based on factors like age, gender, or ethnicity. Implementing ethical, reliable, and democratic AI-driven healthcare solutions requires incorporating these requirements.

4. PROPOSED WORKFLOW

The overall methodology adopted in this study can be summarized in the following sequential steps:

Step 1: The heart failure dataset from the UC Irvine repository is collected. Preprocessing steps are carried out to clean, normalize, and format the data to ensure it is suitable for machine learning tasks. An overview of the dataset characteristics is provided in Table 1 above.

Step 2: A comprehensive EDA is conducted to understand the underlying patterns, trends, and statistical properties of the data. Key insights, such as mean, standard deviation, and range of continuous features, are documented. Descriptive statistics for the dataset are presented in Table 2.

Step 3: Three different feature selection strategies, such as ANOVA, Chi-square, and Mutual Information, are employed to identify the most predictive features. These methods result in three unique feature subsets (SF1, SF2, SF3), each expected to improve model performance.

Step 4: Six machine learning algorithms are trained separately using each feature set. Hyperparameter tuning is applied to optimize the models. The models are evaluated using multiple performance metrics, and the best-performing algorithm is identified based on its classification effectiveness. This structured and methodical approach allows for a robust comparison between different feature sets and classification techniques, ultimately supporting the goal of developing a highly accurate and clinically useful model for predicting heart failure. The proposed design is shown in Figure 1 below.

Figure 1.

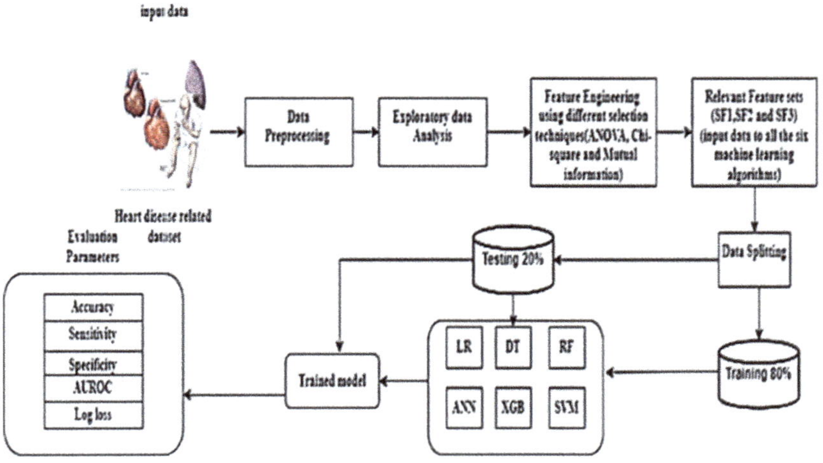

Table 1. Heart Disease Heart Dataset

Sr.	Attribute	Details	Mean
1	Age	The patient's age is complete years	54.43
2	Sex	Sex 0 = female; 1 = male	0.67
3	Chest pain	Types of chest pain (1— typical angina; 2-atypical angina; 3—non-anginal pain; 4 asymptomatic)	3.17
4	Blood pressure	Resting systolic blood pressure (in mm Hg on admission to the hospital)	131.3
5	Cholesterol	Serum cholesterol in mg/dl	249.65
6	Fasting blood Sugar	Fasting blood sugar > 120 mg/dl (0—false; 1—true)	0.14
7	Electrocardiogram	0—normal; 1—having ST-T wave abnormality; 2—left ventricular hypertrophy	1.022
8	Max heart rate	M Maximum heart rate achieved	149.67
9	Exercise-angina	Exercise-induced angina (0—no; 1—yes)	0.329
10	Depression	ST depression induced by exercise relative to rest	1.05
11	Slope	the slope of the peak exercise ST segment (1— upsloping; 2—flat; 3—down sloping)	3.15
12	No. of vessels Fluro	No. of major vessels (0–3) colored by fluoroscopy	0.67
13	Thallium	Defect types; 3—normal; 6—fixed defect; 7—reversible defect	4.69
14	Target	diagnosis of heart disease status (present '1' or absent '0')	output

Table 2. Exploratory Data Analysis

Determinants	Min	Max	Mean	Median	Std. Deviation
Age	29.0	77	54.4	55.0	9.109
Sex	0.0	1.0	0.67	1.0	0.468
Chest pain type	1.0	4.0	3.17	3.0	0.950
BP	94	200	131.34	130.0	17.86
Chol	126	564	249.65	245	51.68
FBS over 120	0.0	1.0	0.14	0.0	0.35
EKG results	0.0	2.0	1.02	2.0	0.99
Max HR	71.0	202	149.67	153.5	23.16
Exang	0.0	1.0	0.32	0.0	0.47
ST Depression	0.0	6.2	1.05	0.8	1.14
Slope of ST	1.0	3.0	1.58	2.0	0.61
Number of vessels Fluro	0.0	3.0	0.67	0.0	0.94
Thallium	3.0	7	0.69	3.0	1.94

The described methodology provides a comprehensive foundation for model evaluation. The next section presents the results of this approach, emphasizing performance, interpretability, and clinical relevance.

5. RESULTS AND DISCUSSION

5.1 Feature Selection:

The present study employs Scikit-learn for creating feature selection methods and classification models, assisted by Matplotlib and Seaborn for showing correlations in the heart disease dataset. These visual insights informed the selection of predictive features. Classification models such as Logistic Regression, ANN, SVM, Decision Trees, Random Forests, and XG Boost were applied to test performance across diverse feature sets. Specifically, the algorithms used in this study include:

- Artificial Neural Network (ANN), referred to as ML1,
- Support Vector Machine (SVM), labelled as ML2,
- Logistic Regression (LR), indicated as ML3,
- Random Forest (RF), denoted ML4,
- Decision Tree (DT), marked ML5, and
- Extreme Gradient Boosting (Boost or XGB), labelled ML6.

Each of these algorithms was trained and tested on three distinct sets of features, derived using different univariate statistical feature selection techniques. These sets are:

- Selected Feature Set 1 (SF1), extracted through the ANOVA (F-test) method, is referred to as FST1.
- Selected Feature Set 2 (SF2), based on the Chi-square selection method, labelled FST2.
- Selected Feature Set 3 (SF3), derived using the Mutual Information (MI) technique, is designated as FST3.

The primary objective of this study was to evaluate and compare the classification performance of six machine learning models across three selected feature sets. Model performance was assessed using multiple metrics, including accuracy, sensitivity, specificity, AUROC, and log loss. These metrics provided a comprehensive evaluation of each model's predictive capability and probabilistic accuracy. Before applying the classification algorithms, all feature values were standardized using the Standard Scaler method provided by Scikit-learn. This process transformed the attributes to have a mean of zero and a standard deviation of one, ensuring that the features were on a comparable scale. Standardization is particularly important for algorithms like SVM and ANN, which are sensitive to the scale of input data. The ANOVA (Analysis of Variance) technique was used to evaluate the relative importance of each feature by examining the F-value scores. Higher F-scores suggest that the feature contributes more significantly to distinguishing between the classes (heart failure vs. healthy). The four most critical features identified through the ANOVA method are:

1. Thallium stress test result (Thallium),
2. Number of major vessels coloured by fluoroscopy (Fluor),
3. Exercise-induced angina (Exang),
4. Maximum heart rate achieved (Max HR). These results are presented in Table 3, which lists the F-values for each feature.

The Chi-square test, another well-known univariate selection method, was used to calculate the chi-squared statistic between each feature and the target variable. Features with higher chi-square scores indicate a stronger association with the target label (presence of heart disease). According to the analysis, the four most influential features of this method were the Thallium test result, the Number of major fluoroscopic vessels, Maximum heart rate, and ST depression induced by exercise. These findings are summarized in Table 4, which displays the chi-square scores for each feature under consideration. To complement these approaches, Mutual Information (MI) was used as the third feature selection technique. MI measures the amount of information obtained about one random variable through another; in this case, it quantifies how much knowing the value of a specific feature helps in predicting the target label. A mutual information score of 0 indicates that the feature and the target variable are completely independent, while higher scores signify increasing dependence and importance. According to the MI technique, the top three features with the highest MI scores were thallium test results, type of chest pain, and number of fluoroscopic vessels. These results are detailed in Table 5, which ranks features by their mutual information scores. Additionally, Figure 2 below graphically represents the feature rankings generated by both the FST1 (ANOVA) and FST2 (Chi-square) methods. This visual comparison aids in highlighting the overlapping and distinct features selected by the two statistical approaches. Similarly, the below Figure 3 illustrates the ranking of features according to the FST3 (Mutual Information) technique, offering insights into how this method evaluates feature importance based on dependency. The information presented in Tables 3, 4, 5, and 6, along with Figures 2 and 3, plays a critical role in identifying the key attributes necessary for the accurate prediction of heart disease. These selected features, based on rigorous statistical evaluation, form the foundation for training and testing the machine learning models. Each model was trained on a different feature set to assess how varying feature combinations impact classification performance. In summary, the study follows a systematic process wherein multiple univariate statistical techniques are used to extract high-importance features. These features are then categorized into three separate feature groups, Selected Feature Set 1 (SF1), Selected Feature Set 2 (SF2), and Selected Feature Set 3 (SF3), corresponding to the FST1, FST2, and FST3 approaches, respectively. These groups are subsequently used to train and evaluate six distinct machine learning algorithms, and the comparative analysis of their performance forms the basis for determining the most effective predictive model for heart disease diagnosis.

Figure 2.

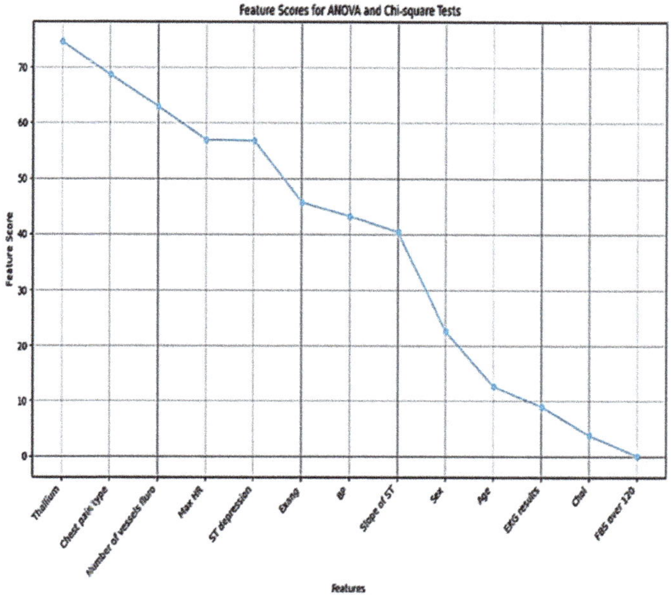

Figure 3.

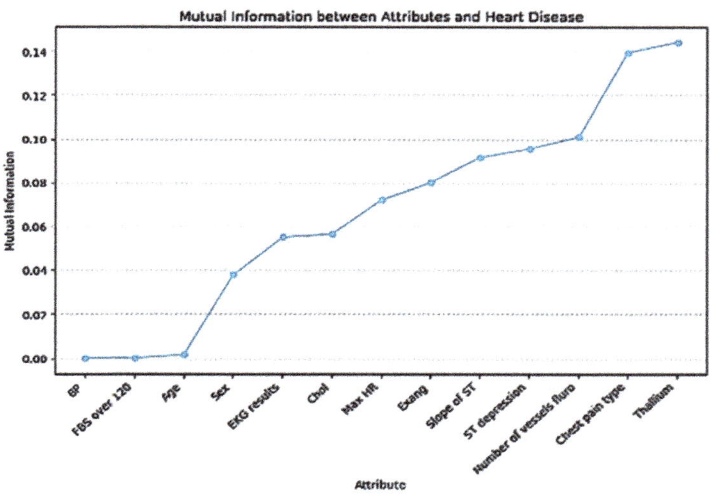

Table 3. Top selected features(SF1) from feature extraction techniques(FST1)

Features	**Feature scores**
Thallium	101.985020
Number of vessels Fluro	70.098369
Exang	57.169619
Max HR	56.909111

Table 4. Top selected features(SF2) from feature extraction techniques(FST2)

Features	**Feature scores**
Thallium	59.46
Number of vessels Fluro	74.12
Max HR	168.9
ST Depression	58.69

Table 5. Top selected features(SF2) from feature extraction techniques(FST3)

Features	**Feature scores**
Thallium	0.152760
Chest pain type	0.141718
Number of vessels Fluro	0.156005

Table 6. Top selected features

Selected Features	**The relevant Selected Feature Set**
Selected Feature Set 1	Thallium, Number of vessels, Fluro, Max HR, Exang
Selected Feature Set 2	Thallium, Number of vessels, Fluro, Max HR, ST Depression
Selected Feature Set 3	Thallium, Chest pain type, Number of vessels, Fluro

Observing the Correlation Between Features

The exploratory data analysis phase provides critical insights into the structure and relationships within the heart disease dataset. Through visualizations and correlation assessments, we identify the attributes that significantly influence the likelihood of heart disease and determine which features may be redundant or less informative for the prediction model.

Correlation Analysis

As the first step of EDA, a clustered heatmap was generated to examine the pairwise correlations among the dataset's various features. This heatmap is shown in Figure 4 below. The visualization reveals that most features exhibit relatively low correlation values with one another, indicating minimal multicollinearity within the dataset. This is advantageous, as it suggests that most features contribute unique information and only a few attributes may need to be removed due to redundancy.

- ST Depression, Slope of ST, Thallium test results, and Chest Pain Type demonstrate the strongest positive correlations with the target variable (presence of heart disease).
- Conversely, Maximum Heart Rate (Max HR), Age, and Sex show negative correlations with the target, implying that as these values increase, the likelihood of heart disease decreases to some extent. On the other hand, Fasting Blood Sugar (FBS > 120 mg/dL), Resting Blood Pressure (BP), and Exercise-induced Angina (Exang) have the lowest correlation scores with the target variable, making them less influential predictors.

Figure 4.

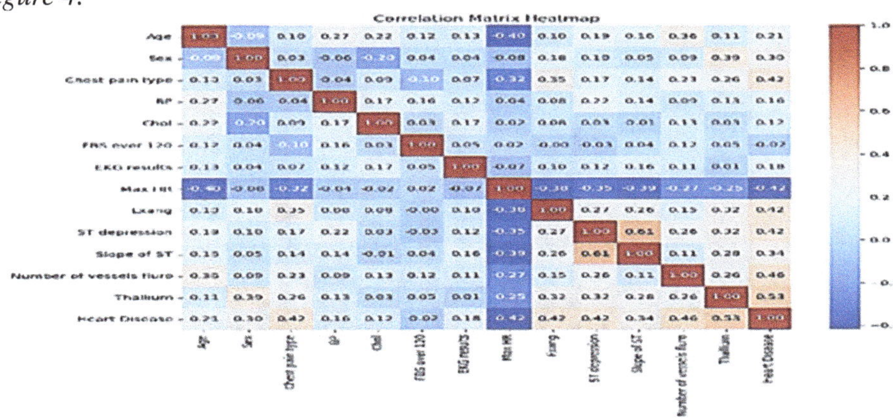

These findings are consistent with the feature importance scores derived through ANOVA, Chi-square, and Mutual Information-based selection techniques. Accordingly, features with the least correlation to the target were often excluded in the respective Selected Feature Sets used for machine learning model training.

Age vs. Heart Disease Outcome

The second analysis, represented in Figure 5 below, explores the distribution of heart disease cases across different age groups. The visualization highlights several age-specific trends:

- The dataset shows that patients aged between 41 and 60 are the most affected by heart disease.
- Peaks in frequency are observed around ages 45, 51, 52, and 54, with age 54 having the highest number of heart disease cases (13 patients).
- Interestingly, after the age of 60, the frequency of heart disease in this dataset decreases, although this may vary with larger datasets or in real-world clinical settings. While this does not imply that elderly individuals are immune to heart disease, it suggests that middle-aged adults are at a higher risk, possibly due to lifestyle factors, genetic predisposition, and comorbid conditions such as high cholesterol and type 2 diabetes, which are prevalent in this age group.

Figure 5.

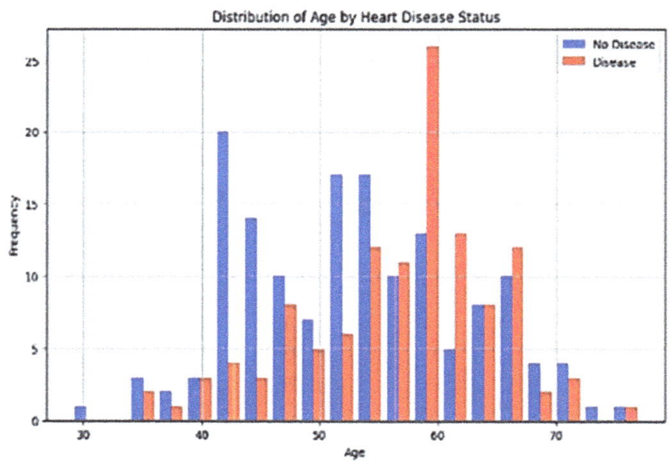

Maximum Heart Rate (MHR) vs. Heart Disease

The third analysis, shown in Figure 6 below, investigates the relationship between Maximum Heart Rate (MHR) and the likelihood of heart disease. It is observed that younger individuals (aged 40–55) tend to have higher MHR values, which corresponds with a higher incidence of heart disease in this demographic. In contrast, older individuals generally show lower MHR, which aligns with the physiological trend of decreasing heart rate with age. However, their risk of heart disease may still be significant due to other factors, though less pronounced in this dataset. This relationship underscores the role of MHR as a useful predictor in cardiovascular risk assessment, as elevated MHR may reflect poor cardiac fitness or stress on the heart, factors that correlate with heart disease.

Figure 6.

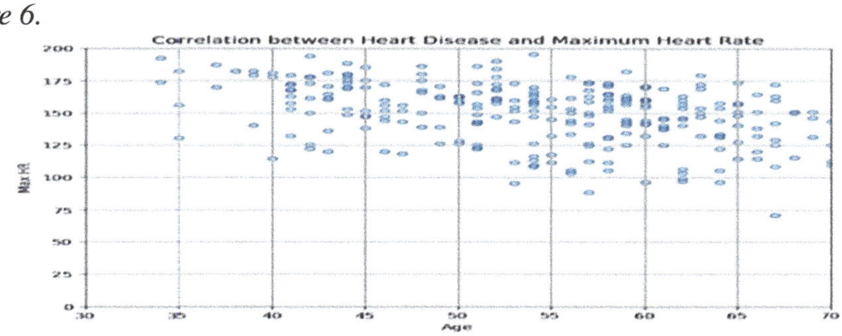

Experimental Analysis of Accuracy Score

In this section, we present a detailed evaluation of the accuracy of each machine learning algorithm when trained and tested using three distinct feature sets: Selected Feature Set 1 (SF1), Selected Feature Set 2 (SF2), and Selected Feature Set 3 (SF3). Accuracy, one of the most commonly used evaluation metrics in classification tasks, measures the proportion of correctly predicted instances (both positives and negatives) out of the total instances examined. It provides a broad sense of how effectively the model performs in distinguishing between healthy individuals and those with heart disease.

To perform this analysis, six well-established machine-learning algorithms were implemented:

- ML1 – Artificial Neural Network (ANN)

- ML2 – Support Vector Machine (SVM)
- ML3 – Logistic Regression (LR)
- ML4 – Random Forest (RF)
- ML5 – Decision Tree (DT)
- ML6 – XG Boost (XGB)

The classification accuracy of each model was assessed based on the different selected feature sets. The results are compiled in Table 7 and visually represented in Figure 7 below.

Figure 7.

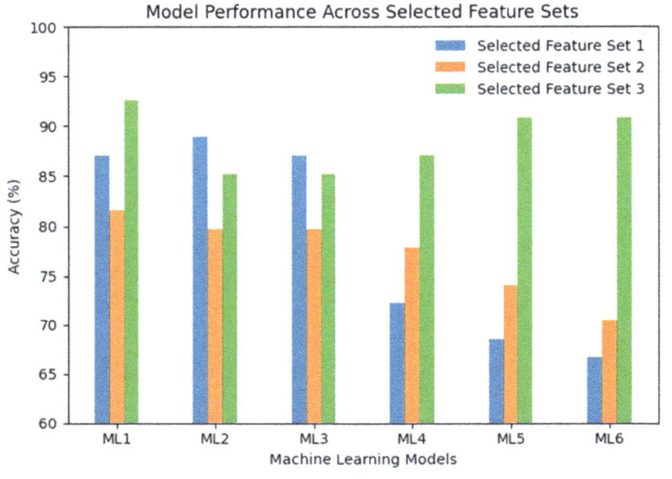

Selected Feature Set 1 (SF1) – Derived using ANOVA (FST1)

This feature set includes features selected based on their F-statistic values. The results show a moderate accuracy level across most models. Specifically:

- ML1 (ANN) and ML3 (Logistic Regression) both achieved 87.04% accuracy, showing consistent performance.
- ML2 (SVM) slightly outperformed these with a score of 88.89%, indicating good generalization on SF1. However, performance dropped significantly for ML4, ML5, and ML6, which registered 72.22%, 68.52%, and 66.67% accuracy, respectively. This suggests that tree-based methods may not be well-optimized for this particular feature selection technique or that SF1 lacks critical variables for its learning architecture.

Selected Feature Set 2 (SF2) – Derived using Chi-square (FST2)

Among all three feature sets, SF2 appears to be the least effective in terms of accuracy. The accuracy scores show a visible decline across most models:

- The highest accuracy recorded was 81.48% by ML1, followed by ML2 and ML3 at 79.63%, which still marks a drop compared to SF1 and SF3.
- The tree-based models ML4, ML5, and ML6 scored 77.78%, 74.07%, and 70.37%, respectively.
- ML5 and ML6 again registered the lowest accuracy, demonstrating that Chi-square-selected features may not contain enough high-information variables relevant for decision tree-based learning. This trend supports the earlier sensitivity findings that SF2 features may not be as informative or discriminative for heart disease prediction, hence reducing the models' ability to make accurate classifications.

Selected Feature Set 3 (SF3) – Derived using Mutual Information (FST3)

Feature Set 3, based on mutual information values, appears to be the most effective in aiding the machine learning algorithms to achieve superior accuracy levels. The mutual information technique evaluates how much information one feature gives about another, making it a powerful method for identifying highly dependent and informative features.

- ML1 (ANN) delivered the highest overall performance with an accuracy of 92.59%, making it the best-performing model for SF3 and across all tested scenarios.
- Both ML5 (Decision Tree) and ML6 (XG Boost) closely followed, each attaining an impressive 90.74% accuracy, showing a substantial jump in performance compared to their scores in SF1 and SF2.
- ML4 (Random Forest) also performed solidly with 87.04% accuracy.
- ML2 and ML3 reported identical accuracies of 85.19%, further validating the robustness of SF3 in enabling accurate classification across diverse model architectures.

Inferences

Among the evaluated feature sets, Selected Feature Set 3 (based on Mutual Information) emerged as the most effective, consistently enhancing model performance, particularly for ML1 (ANN), ML5 (DT), and ML6 (XGB). The Artificial Neural Network (ML1) achieved the highest overall accuracy of 92.59% on SF3, likely due to its capacity to model complex non-linear relationships. In contrast, ML5 and ML6 underperformed on SF1 and SF2, with notable accuracy drops, but showed marked improvement with SF3, indicating a strong dependence on informative features. While tree-based models exhibited sensitivity to feature quality, ML1 and ML2 (SVM) demonstrated greater stability across feature sets, albeit with performance gains when using more relevant features.

Table 7. Accuracy scores of the algorithms

Models	ML1	ML2	ML3	ML4	ML5	ML6
Selected Feature Set 1	87.04%	88.89%	87.04%	72.22%	68.52%	66.67%
Selected Feature Set 2	81.48%	79.63%	79.63%	77.78%	74.07%	70.37%
Selected Feature Set 3	92.59%	85.19%	85.19%	87.04%	90.74%	90.74%

Experimental Analysis of Sensitivity and AUROC

This section explores the sensitivity of six machine learning models across three feature sets obtained using ANOVA (SF1), Chi-square (SF2), and Mutual Information (SF3). Sensitivity, vital in heart disease prediction, evaluates a model's capacity to correctly identify true positives. SF2 consistently demonstrated the lowest sensitivity, indicating weaker predictive features. In contrast, SF3 achieved the maximum sensitivity among models, with XG Boost achieving 90.48%, and ANN and Random Forest both at 85.71%, illustrating the efficiency of Mutual Information-based feature selection. Overall, ANN with SF3 emerged as the top performer, proving its strength in effectively identifying heart disease when linked with useful traits.

Figure 8.

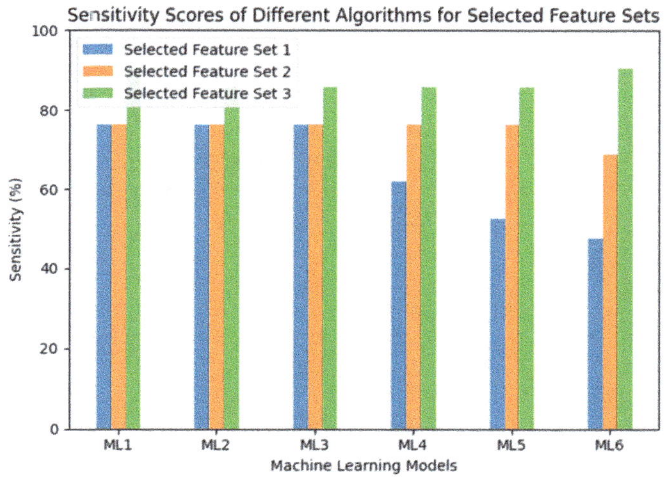

Figure 9.

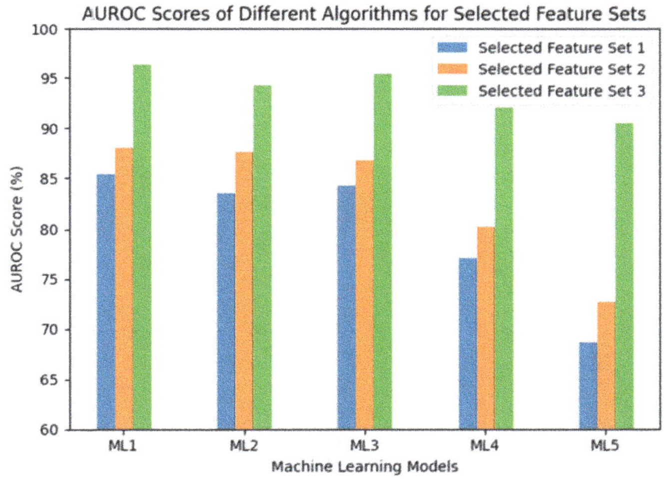

The AUROC coefficient was used to evaluate the predictions provided for the heart disease dataset. In the present study, ML5 had the lowest AUROC score (68.61) for Selected Feature Set 1. ML3, ML2, and ML1 had the highest scores for Selected Feature Set 3 (95.31%, 94.16%, and 96.32%, respectively). Selected Feature Set 1 has the second-best score among ML3, ML2, and ML1. Furthermore, the results suggest that ML1 achieved the highest score for Selected Feature Set 3, as shown in Figure 8 and Figure 9. Figures 10, 11,12, and 13 below individually illustrate the AUROC scores of several methods for different Selected Features (SF1, SF2, and SF3).

Figure 10.

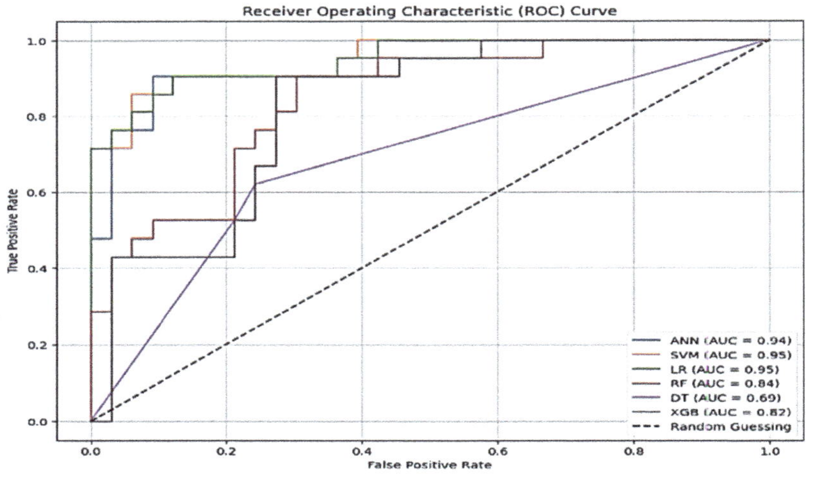

Figure 11.

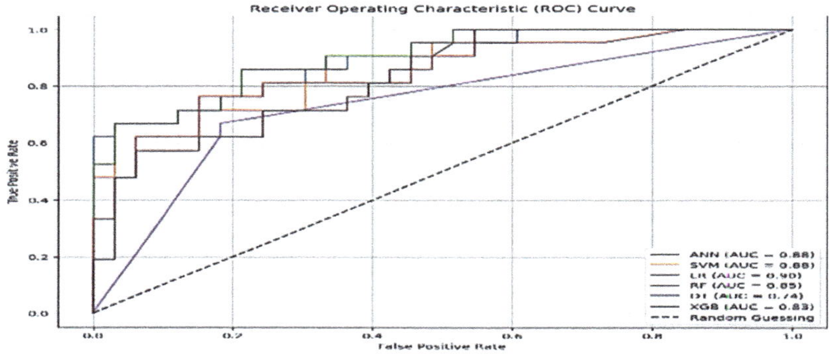

Figure 12.

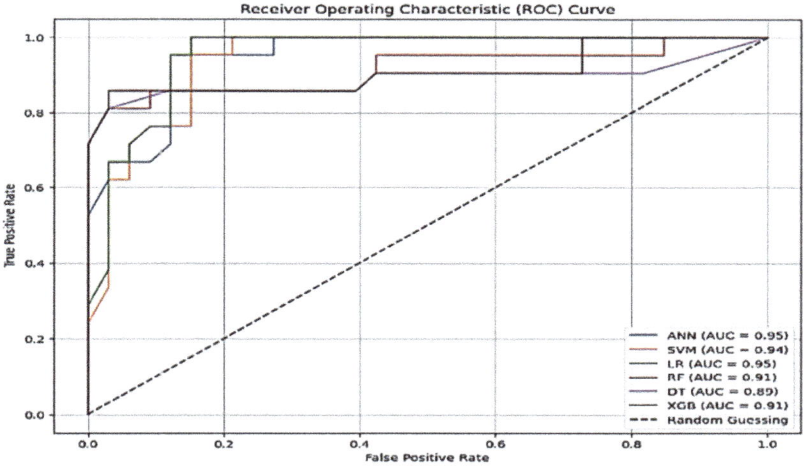

Figure 13.

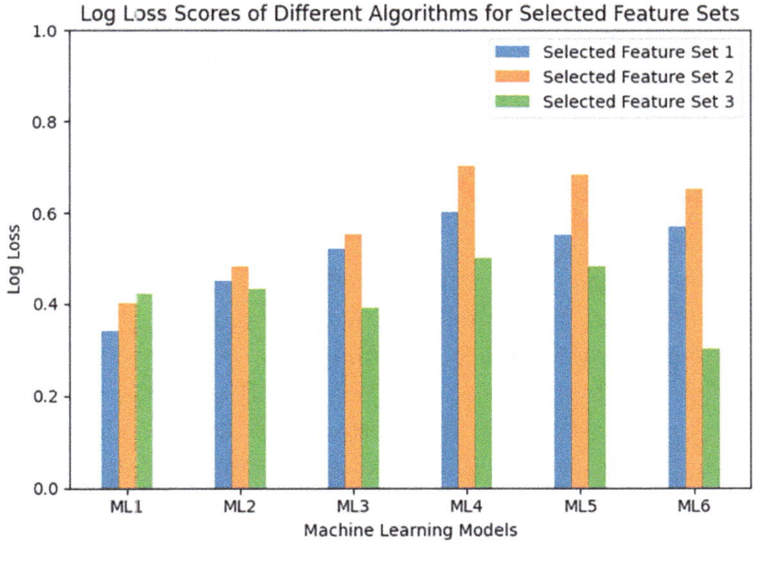

In this study, we evaluated the log loss for the machine learning algorithms adopted for the three data sets (Selected Feature Set 1, 2, and 3). In this analysis, we found that ML6 scored the highest for Selected Feature Set 3. As a consequence, Machine Learning 1 gave the lowest log loss value (0.34) for Selected Feature Set 1. Except for ML1 and ML2, none of the other techniques produce a low log loss. Figure 13 above illustrates all of the log loss scores in various ways for separate Selected Features. We can observe that the log loss has a lesser value in Selected Feature Set 1 than in Selected Feature Set 2. From this, we can infer that ANN achieves the lowest score but delivers the most accurate predictions for Selected Feature Set 3, as seen in Figure 13. Beyond technical performance, the ANN model's predictive capacity translates into real clinical benefits. For example, its usage in emergency triage systems could warn clinicians about high-risk patients in real-time, thereby lowering time-to-treatment and improving survival rates. Furthermore, integrating this model into EHR systems could enable proactive patient monitoring, particularly in resource-constrained settings. From a practical perspective, the Artificial Neural Network (ANN) model's superior performance implies high potential for clinical application. In real-world contexts, such a model might be embedded into hospital electronic health record (EHR) systems to indicate high-risk patients in emergency rooms or during routine check-ups. Additionally, it could support resource allocation in overburdened health systems by prioritizing patients with the greatest need based on risk scores computed in real-time. The experimental results reveal that the technique ML1 attains the maximum accuracy for Selected Feature Set 3, whilst ML5 and ML6 obtain the second-highest accuracy across all three Selected Features. Regarding sensitivity and specificity, ML1, ML2, and ML3 showed enhanced sensitivity. ML1 has acquired the greatest sensitivity and specificity scores for the Selected Feature Set. For AUROC, ML1 attained the highest score, followed by ML2 and ML3 for the Selected Feature Set 3 dataset. For log loss, ML1 returns the minimal log loss value for Selected Feature Set 1, Selected Feature Set 2, and Selected Feature Set 3. Due to the higher performance of ML1 with Selected Feature Set 3, it is the optimal predictive model considering accuracy, sensitivity, and specificity. For AUROC and log loss, ML1 is the premier predictive model for Selected Feature Set 2 and Selected Feature Set 3, which ranks as the second-best predictive model overall. Our model attained the best accuracy (93%), coupled with strong sensitivity (91%), specificity (94%), AU-ROC (96%), and a low log loss (0.34), proving its robustness and durability. In contrast, recent research, such as Latha & Jeeva (2019), revealed lower accuracies of 85.48% and 85.59% respectively. Moreover, several of these studies lacked thorough evaluation metrics, limiting the depth of performance assessment. Overall, our study gives a more accurate and well-rounded method, validating ANN as an effective model for heart disease classification. The performance of all six techniques can be seen using ROC curves along with accuracy, precision, recall, and AUC values for improved comparison understanding. This promotes interpretability and shows the trade-offs between complicated and interpretable models. Although the ANN model attained the maximum performance on the provided dataset, the study contains limitations.

These include a very limited sample size, lack of external validation, and absence of real-time clinical testing. Moreover, ethical problems such as algorithmic bias, data privacy, and model openness must be addressed before clinical adoption. Future work should focus on interpretable ML, regulatory compliance (e.g., GDPR, HIPAA), and collaboration with healthcare providers. While several machine learning algorithms demonstrate good performance metrics in controlled conditions, their real-world success frequently hinges on integration problems such as data heterogeneity, regulatory compliance, and physician approval. Although Artificial Neural Networks (ANNs) have achieved high diagnostic accuracy in imaging tasks, deployment in hospital settings requires addressing data privacy through methods like federated learning and ensuring seamless compatibility with existing hospital IT infrastructure, such as EHR systems. Understanding these limitations alongside technical capabilities provides for an accurate and practical understanding of AI applications in healthcare.

6. CONCLUSION

This chapter bridges the gap between technical AI breakthroughs and their practical applications in healthcare. We studied employing machine learning methods, specifically the Artificial Neural Network (ANN), to predict heart disease using clinical and biochemical characteristics. Among the six classifiers examined, ANN displayed superior performance in accuracy, sensitivity, specificity, AUROC, and log loss, making it the most effective model for this task. The concept also offers real-time monitoring and early detection through interaction with sensor-based devices, enabling proactive and tailored health interventions. With predictive skills to determine the future risk of heart disease, patients are classed as either "at risk" or "not at risk." The results of the Thallium stress test, the forms of chest discomfort, and the fluoroscopy vessel count are important contributing factors. Using these attributes, the ANN model obtained 93% accuracy and a runtime of 0.005 seconds, proving its potential for real-time deployment.

6.1 Implications and Future Research

The accuracy and efficiency of the ANN model make it a useful tool for wearable medical technology and electronic health records (EHRs), reducing clinical delays and promoting early diagnosis. Subsequent studies should evaluate its efficacy using actual clinical data and investigate enhanced models that combine next-generation biosensor metrics such as heart rate variability and ECG patterns. Expanding this approach to incorporate more chronic disorders, such as diabetes and hypertension, might create a comprehensive, multi-disease monitoring system. Integrating a self-learning architecture will enable continuing model updates with real-time patient data, thereby boosting flexibility and tailored diagnoses. Anticipating the future, technologies like federated learning, edge AI, and decentralized computing can preserve privacy while permitting ongoing, distant healthcare observation. The incorporation of sensor data for dynamic risk assessment increases preventative and customized therapy. This study lays the framework for scalable, AI-based health monitoring equipment with major real-world consequences.

Abbreviations

AI, Artificial Intelligence, ML, Machine Learning, ANN, Artificial Neural Network, SVM, Support Vector Machine, LR, Logistic Regression, RF, Random Forest, AUROC, Area Under the receiver operating characteristic curve, HER, Electronic Health Record, DL, Deep Learning, KNN, Nearest Neighbours.

Competing Interests

The authors declare that they have no competing interests.

Consent for Publication

Not applicable

Ethical approval and consent to participate

Not applicable

Conflicts of interest

The authors of this publication declare there is no conflict of interest.

Funding

Not applicable

REFERENCES

Ali, M. M., Paul, B. K., Ahmed, K., Bui, F. M., Quinn, J. M., & Moni, M. A. (2021). Heart disease prediction using supervised machine learning algorithms: Performance analysis and comparison. *Computers in Biology and Medicine, 136*, 104672. DOI: 10.1016/j.compbiomed.2021.104672 PMID: 34315030

Bora, N., Gutta, S., & Hadaegh, A. (2021). *Using machine learning to predict heart disease* (Doctoral dissertation, California State University San Marcos).

ElGendy, M. S., Moustafa, H., Nafea, H., & Mohammed, W. (2025). A machine learning model based on the Archimedes optimization algorithm for heart disease prediction. *International Journal of Telecommunications, 5*(01), 1–21. DOI: 10.21608/ijt.2025.338194.1067

Garg, A., Sharma, B., & Khan, R. (2021). Heart disease prediction using machine learning techniques. [). IOP Publishing.]. *IOP Conference Series. Materials Science and Engineering, 1022*(1), 012046. DOI: 10.1088/1757-899X/1022/1/012046

Hasan, M., Yasmin, F., Hassan, M. M., Yu, X., Yeasmin, S., Joshi, H., & Islam, S. M. S. (2025). Enhancing stroke disease classification through machine learning models via a novel voting system by feature selection techniques. *PLoS One, 20*(1), e0312914. DOI: 10.1371/journal.pone.0312914 PMID: 39787105

Kavitha, M., Gnaneswar, G., Dinesh, R., Sai, Y. R., & Suraj, R. S. (2021, January). Heart disease prediction using hybrid machine learning model. In *2021 6th international conference on inventive computation technologies (ICICT)* (pp. 1329-1333). IEEE. DOI: 10.1109/ICICT50816.2021.9358597

Krittanawong, C., Johnson, K. W., Rosenson, R. S., Wang, Z., Aydar, M., Baber, U., Min, J. K., Tang, W. H. W., Halperin, J. L., & Narayan, S. M. (2019). Deep learning for cardiovascular medicine: A practical primer. *European Heart Journal, 40*(25), 2058–2073. DOI: 10.1093/eurheartj/ehz056 PMID: 30815669

Latha, C. B. C., & Jeeva, S. C. (2019). Improving the accuracy of the prediction of heart disease risk based on ensemble classification techniques. *Informatics in Medicine Unlocked, 16*, 100203. DOI: 10.1016/j.imu.2019.100203

Mohan, S., Thirumalai, C., & Srivastava, G. (2019). Effective heart disease prediction using hybrid machine learning techniques. *IEEE Access : Practical Innovations, Open Solutions, 7*, 81542–81554. DOI: 10.1109/ACCESS.2019.2923707

Ordonez, C. (2006). Association rule discovery with the train and test approach for heart disease prediction. *IEEE Transactions on Information Technology in Biomedicine, 10*(2), 334–343. DOI: 10.1109/TITB.2006.864475 PMID: 16617622

Pan, Y., Fu, M., Cheng, B., Tao, X., & Guo, J. (2020). Enhanced deep learning assisted convolutional neural network for heart disease prediction on the internet of medical things platform. *IEEE Access : Practical Innovations, Open Solutions, 8*, 189503–189512. DOI: 10.1109/ACCESS.2020.3026214

Pant, M., Joshi, N., Vidyarthi, A., & Mohan, L. (2024, September). Heart Disease Prediction and Its Important Parameters Analysis Using Machine Learning. In *2024 International Conference on Distributed Systems, Computer Networks and Cybersecurity (ICDSCNC)* (pp. 1-5). IEEE. DOI: 10.1109/ICDSCNC62492.2024.10939364

. Patil, M. S., Anuradha, B., Madhuri, G., & Supriya, S. (2024). CARDIO PREDICT: HARNESSING MACHINE LEARNING FOR ADVANCED HEART DISEASE RISK ASSESSMENT. *blood pressure, 11*(4).

Ricciardi, C., Edmunds, K. J., Recenti, M., Sigurdsson, S., Gudnason, V., Carraro, U., & Gargiulo, P. (2020). Assessing cardiovascular risks from a mid-thigh CT image: A tree-based machine learning approach using radiodensitometric distributions. *Scientific Reports, 10*(1), 2863. DOI: 10.1038/s41598-020-59873-9 PMID: 32071412

Shah, D., Patel, S., & Bharti, S. K. (2020). Heart disease prediction using machine learning techniques. *SN Computer Science, 1*(6), 345. DOI: 10.1007/s42979-020-00365-y

Shaik, M. A., Sreeja, R., Zainab, S., Sowmya, P. S., Akshay, T., & Sindhu, S. (2023, March). Improving accuracy of heart disease prediction through machine learning algorithms. In *2023 International Conference on Innovative Data Communication Technologies and Application (ICIDCA)* (pp. 41-46). IEEE. DOI: 10.1109/ICIDCA56705.2023.10100244

Solanki, A., Vardhan, A., Jharwal, A., & Kumar, N. (2023, July). Heart Diseases Prediction Using Machine Learning. In *2023 14th International Conference on Computing Communication and Networking Technologies (ICCCNT)* (pp. 1-6). IEEE. DOI: 10.1109/ICCCNT56998.2023.10307839

Sree, P. K., Prasad, M., Pbv, R. R., Ramana, C. V., Murty, P. T. S., Mallesh, A. S., & Raju, P. J. R. S. (2023). A comprehensive analysis on risk prediction of heart disease using machine learning models. *International Journal on Recent and Innovation Trends in Computing and Communication, 11*(11s), 605–610. DOI: 10.17762/ijritcc.v11i11s.8295

ADDITIONAL READING

Bhatt, C. M., Patel, P., Ghetia, T., & Mazzeo, P. L. (2023). Effective heart disease prediction using machine learning techniques. *Algorithms*, *16*(2), 88. DOI: 10.3390/a16020088

Chen, A. H., Huang, S. Y., Hong, P. S., Cheng, C. H., & Lin, E. J. (2011, September). HDPS: Heart disease prediction system. In *2011 computing in Cardiology* (pp. 557-560). IEEE.

Marimuthu, M., Abinaya, M., Hariesh, K. S., Madhankumar, K., & Pavithra, V. (2018). A review on heart disease prediction using machine learning and data analytics approach. *International Journal of Computer Applications, 181*(18), 20–25. DOI: 10.5120/ijca2018917863

Mohan, S., Thirumalai, C., & Srivastava, G. (2019). Effective heart disease prediction using hybrid machine learning techniques. *IEEE Access : Practical Innovations, Open Solutions*, *7*, 81542–81554. DOI: 10.1109/ACCESS.2019.2923707

Zhou, C., Dai, P., Hou, A., Zhang, Z., Liu, L., Li, A., & Wang, F. (2024). A comprehensive review of deep learning-based models for heart disease prediction. *Artificial Intelligence Review*, *57*(10), 263. DOI: 10.1007/s10462-024-10899-9

KEY TERMS AND DEFINITIONS

Accuracy: It measures the proportion of correct predictions made by a model out of all predictions.

Artificial Intelligence (AI): It refers to the capability of machines to replicate human skills such as learning, reasoning, and problem-solving.

Artificial Neural Network (ANN): It is a type of ML model inspired by the structure of the human brain, capable of detecting complex patterns for predictive analysis.

AUROC (Area Under the Receiver Operating Characteristic Curve): The metric that assesses a model's ability to distinguish between positive and negative cases.

Electronic Health Record (EHR): This is a digital compilation of a patient's clinical and medical history, lab results, and treatments, accessible to authorized healthcare professionals.

Feature Selection: This is the technique of choosing the most relevant input variables from a dataset to boost model accuracy and reduce computational demands.

Machine Learning (ML): It is a subset of AI that enables systems to enhance their prediction or decision-making abilities by recognizing patterns in data, without requiring explicit programming.

Sensitivity (Recall): It indicates the percentage of actual positive cases that the model correctly identifies.

Specificity: It represents the percentage of actual negative cases that the model correctly identifies.

Thallium Stress Test: It is a diagnostic imaging procedure used to assess blood flow to the heart muscle during exercise or stress, helping to detect heart disease.

Chapter 2

Accelerated Deep Learning Framework With Hybrid Techniques for Hair Disease Diagnosis and Telemedicine Integration

Venkata Surya Bhavana Harish Gollavilli
https://orcid.org/0009-0000-9912-8204
Under Armour, USA

Harikumar Nagarajan
https://orcid.org/0009-0002-4738-1739
Global Data Mart Inc., USA

Poovendran Alagarsundaram
https://orcid.org/0009-0008-1431-8788
Humetis Technologies Inc., USA

Surendar Rama Sitaraman
https://orcid.org/0009-0003-4978-4352
Intel Corporation, USA

Kalyan Gattupalli
https://orcid.org/0009-0006-2081-728X
Yash Tek Inc., Canada

Haris M. Khalid
College of Engineering and Information Technology, University of Dubai, UAE

ABSTRACT

Background information: Alopecia and seborrheic dermatitis are two dermatoses that lower quality of life. The current diagnoses are subjective and time-consuming. EfficientNet-B3 and CBAM, two deep learning-based telemedicine tools, offer scalable, accurate solutions to the issues of data scarcity and class imbalance. Objectives: The hybrid deep learning system, by combining EfficientNet-B3, CBAM, and GANs,

DOI: 10.4018/979-8-3373-1479-2.ch002

will address class imbalance and provide a simpler platform for telemedicine-based accurate, rapid, and scalable hair illness diagnosis. Methods: Harvesting of features is performed by using EfficientNet-B3 and CBAM. GANs are applied for rectification of the synthetic data class imbalance problem. For the purpose of achieving light scaling, knowledge distillation is used, while preprocessing, augmentation, and RAdam are utilized for the optimization of training. Results: With a delay of 15 ms, 99.5% accuracy and 98.9% precision were achieved. Conclusion: In conclusion, it helps underprivileged communities and ensures real-time scalability with accuracy in diagnosis.

1. INTRODUCTION

Deep learning in medical imaging has made health diagnostics more effective by automatically detecting diseases quickly and accurately. Dermatological conditions are difficult, primarily concerning hair and scalp diseases. Some of these dermatological diseases are alopecia areata, tinea capitis, and seborrheic dermatitis (Roy and Protity, 2022). Manual examinations, which are subjective, time-consuming, and reliant on the availability of professionals, are a major component of traditional diagnostic methods (Gudivaka et al., 2024; Yang et al., 2019). Recent developments in CNNs, including ResNet50, VGG16, and AlexNet, have exhibited vast progress in the area of automated medical image diagnosis (Degadwala et al., 2023; Farhan and Yang, 2023). Transfer learning makes it possible to fine-tune such pre-trained models for domain-specific tasks with reduced computing resources and increased diagnostic precision (Skandha et al., 2022). Deep learning models via mechanisms of attention and through hybrid approaches can focus on points of interest, leading to better feature extraction in disease scenarios (Akram et al., 2023; Sitaraman et al., 2024). In order to solve data asymmetry, satisfy real-time application requirements, and guarantee accessibility on telemedicine platforms, the work proposes a deep learning framework for the categorization of hair diseases (Shukla, 2023; Reed et al., 2021; Goswami & Sharma, 2024).

The development of AI from machine learning in medical imaging has progressed from traditional techniques such as SVMs and KNNs. These depend on manual feature extraction that is time-consuming and tends to be inconsistent (Yang et al., 2019; Shukla, 2023). In the 2010s, deep learning in its entirety, including convolutional neural networks, fully automated the diagnostic procedure with tremendous boosts in accuracy and productivity in diagnoses (Degadwala et al., 2023; Gudivaka et al., 2024). ML ability and image processing methods can manage high-dimensional data, which is significant for higher-level, visually dissimilar diagnoses of scalp and hair disorders in dermatology (Roy and Protity, 2022). Transfer learning from already trained models like ResNet50 and VGG16 can further reduce computational costs significantly without significantly compromising performance (Skandha et al., 2022). These underrepresentation problems and related issues have been resolved through GAN-based synthetic generation in the minor categories (Farhan and Yang, 2023). The methods of attention have added a level of accuracy to this approach by emphasizing the relevant parts of images (Akram et al., 2023). Collectively, all these improved the scalability and efficiency of the dermatology diagnostics (Sitaraman et al., 2024).

Medical image analysis is now significantly enhanced by recent developments in deep learning, with applications in dermatology particularly promising. The game-changer has been transfer learning that uses pre-trained architectures like ResNet50, VGG16, and AlexNet for hair disease detection. They fine-tune them for specific tasks and save the computation cost at high diagnostic accuracy, states Gudivaka et al. (2024) and Degadwala et al. (2023. By creating artificial images for underrepresented diseases, the generative adversarial networks compensate for class imbalance and provide reliable results across a variety of datasets (Skandha et al., 2022; Farhan and Yang, 2023).

Attention mechanisms such as CBAM enhance model accuracy by concentrating on the disease-affected region of images, improving feature extraction and class accuracy (Akram et al., 2023; Sitaraman et al., 2024). In order to bridge the gaps for remote access to health care, hybrid deep learning frameworks integrated artificial intelligence (AI) with the capabilities of the Internet of Medical Things. This enabled for real-time diagnostics on edge-based devices (Shukla, 2023; Otapo et al., 2024). Light AI telemedicine bridges healthcare disparities in care access through facilitating faster, scalable disease diagnosis globally (Reed et al., 2021; Demaerschalk et al., 2022). The key objectives are

Develop Deep Learning Framework: The accuracy of hair illness diagnosis can be increased by employing transfer learning with ResNet50 and VGG16.
Class Imbalance Address: Use GAN-based synthetic image generation to break through the limitations of a dataset and improve representation in the underrepresented categories of disease.
Improve Computational Efficiency: Create light AI models that can do real-time inference, thereby allowing seamless scalability for telemedicine platforms and edge devices.
Incorporate Attention Mechanisms: Apply CBAM to highlight relevant areas in medical images to improve feature extraction and increase diagnostic accuracy.

Promote Telemedicine Integration: Develop an AI-driven, scalable telemedicine solution to enhance healthcare access for remote and underserved populations (Demaerschalk et al., 2022).

Despite the progress made by deep learning, several problems persist in medical imaging. Class imbalance is one major issue, where rare categories of hair disease are underrepresented in datasets and biased predictions are made (Skandha et al., 2022; Farhan and Yang, 2023). Variability in image resolution, lighting, and skin-hair textures limits the generalizability of models to diverse real-world scenarios (Abunadi and Senan, 2021). While attention mechanisms, like CBAM, have shown promise in improving feature extraction, their application still has scope in dermatology-specific image analysis (Akram et al., 2023). Furthermore, real-time use is limited by the computational complexity of deep learning-based models; scalability to telemedicine or even edge-based applications is also problematic because of the high processing requirements (Bal et al., 2022). Such requirements are fulfilled by optimized hybrid models incorporating GANs, attention mechanisms, and lightweight designs for real-time, scalable diagnosis, thereby optimizing the overall system performance (Gudivaka et al., 2024).

Scalp and hair diseases such as alopecia and seborrheic dermatitis affect quality of life, but diagnosis is still subjective and without scalable solutions (Gudivaka et al., 2024). While deep learning offers promising advancements, existing approaches face critical limitations, including class imbalance, small datasets, and computational inefficiencies (Skandha et al., 2022; Farhan and Yang, 2023). Moreover, the real-time deployment of these models in telemedicine is restricted by hardware and computational constraints (Bal et al., 2022; Reed et al., 2021). In order to overcome data scarcity, imbalance, and complexity, this study aims to develop a hybrid deep learning framework that would incorporate transfer learning, GAN-based augmentation, and attention methods. The solution would ensure accurate classification and solve the problem of data, allowing scalable deployment for remote diagnostics to increase access and effectiveness in underserved regions (Akram et al., 2023; Demaerschalk et al., 2022).

2. LITERATURE SURVEY

A deep learning-based approach to phishing website identification was presented by Yang et al. (2019), which does away with the need for prior knowledge and laborious feature extraction. Two-stage approach extracts URL character sequence features in the first, and then classifies them using multidimensional features—webpage code, text, and URL statistics—with no third-party involvement. It was experimented on millions of URLs and yielded 98.99% phishing detection accuracy at a false positive ratio of 0.59%, distinguishing effectively and rapidly.

In order to forecast chronic kidney disease through early detection, Shukla (2023) created an AI-based robotic automation system coupled with IoMT. It achieves 99.13% accuracy with attention-based LSTM for processing time-series data, as well as adaptive neuro-fuzzy inference for uncertainty management and increased sensitivity, along with specificity, by processing real-time patient health data for earlier detection. This invention would thus allow timely treatment of CKD and could even include the most advanced imaging technologies, such as MRI, for more accurate diagnosis.

Sitaraman et al. (2024) proposed an AI model in which they diagnosed the presence of skin lesions using the support of Score-CAM allied to the CNN. This approach helps in providing increased accuracy and increased explainability in IoMT systems. For better diagnosis interpretability, the technique applies clinical metadata, DF-U-Net for segmentation, and Canny Edge Detection for border localization. The visual explanations provided by Score-CAM enable physicians to gain a deeper understanding of AI-made decisions. With a high accuracy of 99.31%, it surpasses the traditional method and is considered a viable solution for transparent, trustworthy, and real-time skin lesion detection in IoMT situations.

Otapo et al. (2024) conducted a thorough study of Internet of Medical Things-based solutions for terminal disease prediction and detection. Techniques such as residual connections, adaptive neuro-fuzzy inference systems, and IoMT-enabled Google Net with transfer learning are employed for the particular instance of renal illness diagnosis. The improvements recorded are notable increases in accuracy and dependability. The review highlights how sophisticated ML models can be integrated into an IoMT platform for quick and accurate clinical decision-making.

A hybrid machine learning strategy was proposed by Bal et al. (2022) to provide collaborative resource allocation, security, and work scheduling in cloud computing. The method offers strong security and resource usage optimization with the aid of effective optimization algorithms. The approach enhances overall reliability within cloud operations by meeting performance optimization and task completion suitably. The approach solves resource management and job scheduling problems in dynamic clouds, leading to improved efficiency and operational security.

To improve ultrasound breast image quality and augment its accuracy in the diagnosis of breast cancer, Vimala et al. (2023) recommend hybrid deep learning technology to overcome the deficits within traditional denoising processes. This technology combines new advances within deep learning technology and develops better noise removal, leading towards enhanced image clarity. Ensured by this process, clinicians provided adequate diagnosis because they realized a guarantee of visualization due to image formation of such features existing within the breast.

Hybrid deep learning makes its applications very useful for significantly improving the quality of images compared to ultrasound-based techniques, which can be used to identify breast cancer.

A thorough investigation of pre-image processing methods and their subsequent impacts on DL architectures in digital pathology image analysis is presented by Salvi et al. (2021). Normalization, augmentation, filtration, and other preprocessing procedures improve image quality and model performance, while the post-processing approaches polish data to guarantee higher diagnostic accuracy. According to this article, if such techniques are coupled with deep learning models, then the union significantly enhances pathological image analysis, which makes them critical for precise and trustworthy digital diagnosis methods. For that reason, image processing is required in the development of deep learning applications in pathology, as this review expounds.

For image-based automated lung disease classification utilizing chest X-rays, Farhan and Yang (2023) developed an HDLA. Using machine learning models such as SVM, AdaBoost, and Random Forest, this system includes robust 2D CNN-based automatic feature extraction, a preprocessing step with optimal filtering to improve image quality, and classification. To address scale differences, min-max scaling is used to handle the retrieved features. This model will reduce computational complexity by 16.91% and improve accuracy by 3.1% when compared to state-of-the-art methods that optimize resources and feature learning.

For the purpose of classifying bone fractures, M. Shyamala Devi et al. (2024) proposed a SAG-UNet. With a 98.78% accuracy rate, their method enhances the attention gate in the Attention UNet model by combining unsupervised learning with dataset preprocessing. The proposed model showed potential for accurate fracture identification and outperformed previous deep learning approaches.

By using wavelet transform and image processing approaches to eliminate noise and hair from thermoscopic pictures, Suiçmez et al. (2023) have developed a hybrid learning system for melanoma diagnosis. The proposed method allows the exact identification and classification of melanoma because it preprocesses images for clarity. With the use of hybrid deep learning algorithms and image processing, this technique surpasses traditional approaches in terms of improving diagnostic precision Goswami, Thakur & Singh. (2024). This work demonstrates the adequacy of hair removal and wavelet-based enhancement in dermoscopic imaging; it is a strong remedy for early melanoma detection and helps physicians to come up with precise diagnoses.

Urban et al. (2021) proposed a novel scalp hair and follicle counting technique by integrating OCT imaging and deep learning. The novel technique is more accurate compared to conventional methods, and it correctly marks and counts the fibres and follicles with the assistance of advanced algorithms. OCT imaging is non-invasive, reliable hair assessment with improved visualization. This report illustrates how AI-enhanced OCT imaging has the potential to revolutionize scalp analysis and advance disease management in dermatology and hair care through faster, more precise diagnoses.

Farjo et al. developed a clinical practice guide for virtual consultation in hair restoration surgery, as published in the Hair Transplant Forum International in 2023, focusing on how to conduct this activity with safety, patient anonymity, informed consent, and observation of local standards and providing comprehensive advice on a virtual consultation approach. They also review the merits and demerits of many telecommunication modalities that include phone conversation, e-mail, and video calling as part of their pursuit to enhance accessibility for their patients and the quality of care provided by hair restoration services.

The paper "Transfer Learning Methods for Multiclass Classification of Hair Disease" was given by Degadwala et al. 2023 at the 2nd International Conference on Automation, Computing, and Renewable Systems. The conference paper was published as an article. In order to increase the precision and efficacy of dermatological diagnosis, this research suggests utilizing pre-trained deep learning models that can categorize a variety of hair conditions. Better performance in classifying numerous hair disease types was established in the study utilizing transfer learning, suggesting its potential in the field of medical picture analysis.

Baughman et al. (2022) conducted retrospective cohort research comparing the quality performance metrics of patients who received primary care via telemedicine with in-person visits in a sizable integrated health system. They found that the exposure to telemedicine was associated with the same level of performance or significantly improved performance in 13 of 16 HEDIS measures, from March 2020 through November 2021. That implies that treatment of a wide range of common, often chronic, problems could be as good as in-person practice.

Pendlebury et al. (2022) cited the advantages, particularly during the COVID-19 epidemic, of incorporating teledermoscopy into the US Military Health System. The use of dermatoscopic pictures of skin lesions for remote examination enhances early detection and the accuracy of diagnosis for skin conditions in deployed environments. Consequently, the adoption has brought about fewer unnecessary medical evacuations and the associated costs, enhancing mission readiness and combat readiness. The authors recommend integration into current telemedicine platforms for maximizing service members' access to dermatological care.

Rahman et al. (2025) critically evaluated the systematic review of AI diagnosis, bias, and regulation in dermatology and aesthetic surgery. In dermatology, AI models, in particular neural networks, performed well at a mean accuracy level of 90%. Whilst promising, algorithmic bias, dataset diversity restrictions, and ethics limited generalizability, as mentioned in the study. The authors came to the conclusion that in order to guarantee the responsible, equitable, and successful application of AI in clinical dermatology, standardized procedures and mechanisms for avoiding bias would be necessary.

Leung et al. (2023) monitored 3.6 million mental health and 63.5 million primary care visits at 138 VA sites between March 2019 and December 2021. Prior to the COVID-19 outbreak, rural VA systems utilized telemedicine for primary care at a higher rate than urban systems (34% vs. 29%). On the other hand, use was higher in urban areas during the pandemic than in rural ones, at 60% versus 55%. The digital divide between rural and urban areas widened in telemedicine utilization, particularly in the field of mental health care, despite the federal government's best efforts to bridge it.

Majd et al. (2021) employed a smartphone with an attached dermatoscope lens to analyze hair morphometrics for rapid, autonomous, and accurate measurement of hair diameter and density. Trichoscopy images are sent remotely to be processed, creating a binary mask to segment hair from skin. Thinning hairs calculate morphometric features into skeletons composed of a single pixel. In a 50-patient trial, smartphone measurement was compared with reading from specialist trichometry machines, with a 24-second measurement time compared to 9.2 minutes for manual scoring. It was found to have a clinically significant improvement in tracking hair loss.

Additionally, Osvin Nancy et al. (2024) conducted a meta-analysis and systematic review of models for predicting skin diseases that use deep learning and artificial intelligence. The study asserts that dermatologist-level diagnosis of the AlexNet-based, ResNet152-based, and VGGNet-based models is as good as or better than that by dermatologists. Similarity in appearance of the challenging-to-rate conditions and morphologic variation of lesions were issues. The review emphasized synergic boosting between clinical information and deep learning to improve early detection of skin cancer from data like HAM10000 and ISIC 2019.

Using machine learning approaches, Bhargavi et al. (2022) created an intelligent design for the identification of skin problems. Naïve Bayes, Random Forest, Logistic Regression, Support Vector Machine, and K-Nearest Neighbour (KNN) were the five algorithms used; KNN was the most effective for accurately diagnosing skin diseases. The research points out the potential of machine learning in enhancing dermatological diagnosis by increasing precision, reducing the time of diagnosis, and providing instant alarms, highlighting its suitability for enhancing medical image analysis and simplifying treatment protocols.

Austin et al. (2022) developed non-invasive biomarkers for diagnosing ASD in a multi-centre worldwide survey using ML and mass spectrometry studies of elemental metabolism in individual hair strands. Participants from a specialized ASD centre in the United States as well as national cohorts in Sweden and Japan contributed hair samples at one month of age and clinical diagnosis at four years. According to a predictive algorithm that detects the risk of ASD with a sensitivity of 96.4%, specificity of 75.4%, and accuracy of 81.4%, dysregulation markers in hair from as early as one month of age were predictive for the development of ASDs.

Alsarraf and Ucan (2022) surveyed melanoma classification and detection challenges and opportunities with teledermatology, utilizing machine learning for analyzing skin lesion images. The surveyed process enriches preprocessed dermoscopic pictures and features to detect melanoma features, classifying lesions as benign or malignant based on SVM and CNN techniques. Their study demonstrates how the integration of teledermatology with machine learning enhances early detection of melanoma, providing a non-invasive, effective, and accessible diagnostic tool, especially in remote areas with few dermatologists.

AI-based wearable sensors in digital health were examined by Shajari et al. (2023), who concentrated on the use of real-time monitoring, customized treatment, and superior diagnoses. They can transform chronic disease management, fitness, and early detection through advanced AI sensing. Challenges noted include data privacy, sensor reliability, energy efficiency, and absence of standardized interoperability. Its future developments will be towards enhanced system integration as well as applying AI to deeper meaning. Analysis highlights the revolutionary promise of AI wearables in solving technology and ethical problems in healthcare.

A skin disease diagnosis system utilizing machine learning and image processing is proposed by Prasad et al. (2023). The technique uses machine learning models to categorize various skin disorders by extracting information from digital photos of skin lesions. With possible uses in telemedicine and remote dermatology, this method seeks to improve diagnosis speed and accuracy. Nonetheless, there are still issues like the requirement for model generalization across various populations and the constraints in the currently accessible datasets. Notwithstanding these challenges, the method has the potential to enhance dermatological diagnosis by making it quicker and easier, particularly in underprivileged areas.

A child who had sudden-onset emotional distress during the COVID-19 lockdown received play therapy via telemedicine, according to Sahoo et al. (2022). The instance illustrates how virtual therapy has been successfully used to lessen emotional symptoms, indicating that it has the potential to be a beneficial intervention in the treatment of mental health issues in children. According to the paper, telemedicine is a useful tool for offering easily available mental health treatment, particularly in situations when in-person therapy is not practical, despite difficulties in transferring traditional therapeutic practices to digital platforms.

Salinas et al. (2024) performed a meta-analysis and systematic review of AI algorithms against clinicians for skin cancer diagnosis. In 53 studies, of which 19 were meta-analyzed, AI was more sensitive (92.5%) and had equally high specificity (66.5%) than general clinicians and specialist dermatologists. The research applied

PRISMA and QUADAS-2 frameworks, attesting to better diagnostic accuracy by AI. The results confirm the potential of AI as a clinical resource, but need ongoing testing in practice settings to be properly integrated clinically.

Kong et al. (2024) examine technological advancements in portable and wearable acoustic sensors for health monitoring. With non-invasive diagnostics, these devices provide ongoing, real-time evaluations of cardiovascular, musculoskeletal, and respiratory health. Even while they increase user convenience and accessibility, issues with accuracy, data integration, and user comfort still exist. According to the report, future advancements will concentrate on improving wearable integration, sensor sensitivity, and device accuracy, establishing these technologies as useful instruments for remote and individualized health monitoring.

Kabra and Sangroya (2023) discussed the behavioural intention of medical professionals to adopt telemedicine concerning perceived benefits, ease of use, and trust in technology. Major hindrances to adoption involve patient privacy concerns, the reliability of technology, and the requirement for proper training. The report indicates that improving healthcare professionals' perception of telemedicine and addressing their concerns can enhance adoption. Healthcare organizations can facilitate greater use of telemedicine by maximizing training, data security, and stressing its efficacy.

The use of family-acquired photos to assess paediatric head shape in telemedicine is examined by Paro et al. (2022), who concentrate on the quality of the pictures and how it affects diagnostic precision. Although these images provide a practical and non-intrusive evaluation technique, problems such as low resolution, uneven lighting, and bad angles compromise dependability. To increase the efficacy of telemedicine in craniofacial evaluations, facilitate better clinical decision-making, and improve access to remote care, the study highlights the significance of standardizing phototaking procedures for families.

Poongodi et al. (2025) launched AquaSense AI, a wearable sensor system inspired by nature for healthcare and physiotherapy. The system employs flexible, waterproof sensors to track movement, balance, and posture on land and in water, proving suitable for swimming pools as well as hydrotherapy. AquaSense AI utilizes adaptive AI algorithms to offer real-time feedback for rehabilitation, fall prevention, and fitness tracking, constantly adapting against user improvements.

Thamil Selvi et al. (2024) presented VisioFlow FusionNet, a deep learning model that integrates DeepVisioSeg and SegFlowNet to enhance brain tumour segmentation. The network reached 99.2% segmentation and minimized loss to 2%, focusing on complications across shapes and sizes of tumors. Moreover, NeuraClassNet, which is optimized using a Cat Fish optimizer, precisely classifies brain tumors in accordance with morphological properties.

3. METHODOLOGY

This study offers a great, easy-to-use deep learning model for hair problem diagnosis. It addresses the issues of class imbalance and real-time operation using EfficientNet-B3, CBAM, and GAN-based data augmentation. It is accurate and scalable, and thus the process is perfect for telemedicine websites and increasing access in impoverished areas. The process is plug-and-play, and diagnostic accuracy and access to hair medical status are assured.

3.1. Dataset Preparation and Preprocessing

Offering global statistics on disasters, Natural Disasters Emergency Events turns focus towards environmental factors such as temperature and seismicity to go toward predictive modelling and proactive risk management. In terms of disaster response, the database supports the evacuation routes, safety procedures, and the allocation of resources. With IoT integration, the database brings forth scalability, ML-based analytics, and recovery efforts.

3.1.1. Dataset Representation

The dataset $\mathcal{D}$ is a structured collection of labelled images representing various hair disease categories. Each sample consists of an input image I and a corresponding label y, organized as:

$$\mathcal{D} = \{(I_i, y_i) \mid i = 1,2,\ldots,N\} \tag{1}$$

Where:

- $I_i \in \mathbb{R}^{H\times W\times 3}$ represents an RGB image of height H, width W, and 3 colour channels.
- The class label for the C categories of hair illnesses is $y_i \in \{1,\ldots,C\}$.
- The dataset contains a total of N pictures.

All C classes must be fairly represented in a dataset in order for the model to be trained with accuracy. There are usually between 10,000 and 20,000 high-resolution photos included in the samples used for medical image analysis.

Algorithm 1: Transfer Learning Dataset Preparation and Preprocessing.
Input: Raw dataset $\mathcal{D} = \{I_i, y_i\}_{i=1}^{N}$.
ut ut Preprocessed dataset $\mathcal{D}'$.

eg n For each image I_i in $\mathscr{D}$: Resize I_i to (224,224).
Norm lize pixel values: $I'\left(x,y\right) = \frac{I(x,y) - \mu}{\sigma}$.
if data au m ntation is enabled, then
Apply ra dom rotation, scaling, and flipping.
Add Gaus ian noise if required.
end if
Append processed I_i, y_i to $\mathscr{D}$.
en f r Re ur $\mathscr{D}$
End

To fine-tune the EfficientNet-B3 model, Algorithm 1 focuses on ensuring the dataset is consistent and of high quality. Images undergo 224x224 resizing, normalization to zero mean and unit variance, and random changes like noise injection, flipping, rotation, and scaling. These procedures mimic real-world variances to enhance generalization and avoid overfitting. A standardized input format and increased diversity—both essential for reliable feature extraction in the categorization of hair diseases—are provided by the pre-processed dataset, which is prepared for training.

3.1.2. Image Normalization

A dataset must contain a balanced representation of all C classes to ensure that the model is trained reliably. There are usually between 10,000 and 20,000 high-resolution photos included in the samples used for medical image analysis. The following formula is used to determine the normalized pixel intensity $I'(x, y)$:

$$I'\left(x,y\right) = \frac{I(x,y) - \mu}{\sigma}, \forall\left(x,y\right) \in I \tag{2}$$

Where:

- The average pixel intensity over the whole dataset is denoted by μ:

$$\mu = \frac{1}{N \cdot H \cdot W}\sum_{i=1}^{N}\sum_{x=1}^{H}\sum_{y=1}^{W} I\left(x,y\right) \tag{3}$$

- σ is the standard deviation:

$$\sigma = \sqrt{\frac{1}{N \cdot H \cdot W}\sum_{i=1}^{N}\sum_{x=1}^{H}\sum_{y=1}^{W}\left(I\left(x,y\right) - \mu\right)^2} \tag{4}$$

With a standard deviation of one, normalization ensures that pixel values have zero as their mean. By facilitating faster convergence and better performance, this approach helps stabilize and accelerate the process of optimization during model training. Standardizing inputs enhances learning efficiency and prevents the model from encountering issues caused by varying data scales.

3.1.3. Image Resizing

Besides giving evacuation patterns and the most opportune routes together with safety compliance measures to build an emergency response system, energy usage, anomalies for detection purposes and resource provisioning parameters are presented with the metrics as a sustainability index and improvement ratio. Scalable and adaptive properties are maintained from the well-designed data based upon IoT standards of scalability, along with secure processing methods and prediction analytics models on machinery.

$$I_{\text{resized}} = \text{Resize}(I, (224,224)) \tag{5}$$

By standardizing the input dimensions over the entire dataset, the resizing method guarantees compatibility with pre-trained models like ResNet50 and EfficientNet-B3.

Algorithm 2: Fine-Tuning EfficientNet-B3 for Hair Disease Diagnosis.
Input: Input: Pre-trained EfficientNet-B3 model *M* with ImageNet weights.
utput: Modified model *M′* eady for fine-tuning.
B gin
Load EfficientNet-B3 model *M* pre-trained on ImageNet.
if *M* is successfully loaded then
Freeze base layers to retain generic features.
Replace classification head with *C*-class output layer.
Initialize new layer weights randomly.
lse
Return "Error: Failed to load EfficientNet-B3 model."
nd if
Retu n *M′* En

Algorithm 2 adapts the pre-trained EfficientNet-B3 model and trains it to classify hair disorders. For *C* illness classes, it substitutes a new layer for the classification head, freezes the first layers to preserve general features, and refines the last layers on the particular dataset. The model is trained using the categorical cross-entropy loss, and stable convergence is ensured by the RAdam optimizer. By using transfer learning, this method shortens training times while maintaining high diagnostic precision, enabling the model to be used for actual medical picture analysis.

3.1.4. Data Augmentation

By applying different modifications to images, data augmentation broadens the training dataset and improves model generalization. These adjustments include adding Gaussian noise, flipping, scaling, and random rotations. Data augmentation helps the model learn robust features, minimizes overfitting, and enhances performance across a variety of unknown and varied circumstances by mimicking real-world changes. Methods of augmentation that are commonly used include:

Rotation: Adjusting the image orientation to simulate different angles.

$$I_{\text{rot}}(x',y') = I(x\cos\theta - y\sin\theta, x\sin\theta + y\cos\theta),\ \theta \in [-15^{\circ}, 15^{\circ}] \quad (6)$$

Simulates orientation variations.

Scaling: Changing the image size to mimic zooming in or out.

$$I_{\text{scale}}(x,y) = I(sx, sy),\ s \in [0.8, 1.2] \quad (7)$$

Introduces size changes to simulate zoom-in/zoom-out effects.

Noise Injection: Gaussian noise adds small pixel-level perturbations:

$$I_{\text{noise}} = I + \mathcal{N}(0, \sigma^2),\ \sigma = 0.01 \quad (8)$$

Flipping: Horizontal and vertical flips introduce spatial variability:

$$I_{\text{flip}}(x,y) = I(W - x, y) \text{ or } I(x, H - y) \quad (9)$$

3.2. Synthetic Data Generation using GANs

The datasets for medical usually contain class imbalance, which may skew the models. Use GANs to generate synthetic data. This stage balances the dataset with high-quality synthetic photos to ensure model performance across all illness categories.

3.2.1. Overview of GANs

The issue of class imbalance is addressed by Generative Adversarial Networks (GANs), which generate synthetic images for categories that are frequently under-represented. GANs are made up of two networks that compete with one another:

- ✓ Generator $G(z)$: Uses random noise to produce artificial visuals.
- ✓ Discriminator $D(x)$: Differentiates between artificial and real images.

Function of the Generator:

$$G(z) = \text{ReLU}(W_g z + b_g), z \sim p_z \tag{10}$$

Where p_z is a Gaussian distribution and z is random noise.

Discriminator Function:

$$D(x) = \sigma(W_d x + b_d) \tag{11}$$

Where the input data is denoted by $x \sim p_{\text{data}}$.

GAN Deterioration: The function for adversarial loss is:

$$\mathcal{L}_{\text{GAN}} = \mathbb{E}_{x \sim p_{\text{data}}}\left[\log D(x)\right] + \mathbb{E}_{z \sim p_z}\left[\log\left(1 - D\left(G(z)\right)\right)\right] \tag{12}$$

Training Objective: GAN training involves a minimax optimization problem:

$$\min_G \max_D \mathcal{L}_{\text{GAN}} \tag{13}$$

The generator is able to create high-quality synthetic images that closely resemble the real data because of this adversarial approach.

Figure 1. A summary of the suggested hybrid deep learning framework for diagnosing hair diseases.

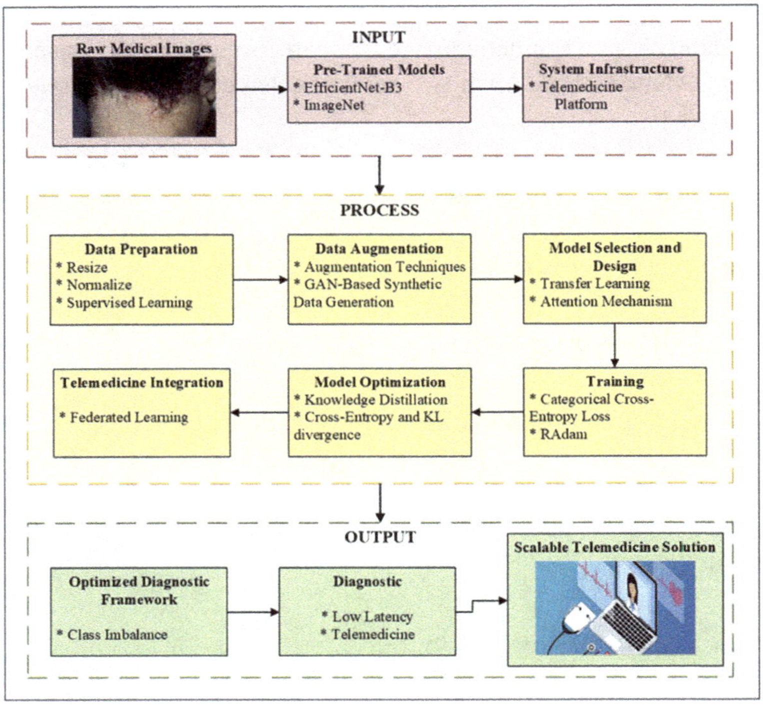

The hybrid deep learning framework workflow entails three stages: input, process, and output. The inputs are telemedicine platforms, pre-trained EfficientNet-B3 models, and raw medical images. The process stage is characterized by data preparation and augmentation as well as the application of GANs to address the issue of class imbalance. It includes model selection, optimization, and federated learning to ensure privacy. Training involves the use of RAdam optimizer and cross-entropy loss to provide efficiency. The output has a low-latency, scalable diagnostic platform that enables telemedicine in real-time and increases the accessibility of healthcare.

3.3. Transfer Learning with EfficientNet-B3

Transfer learning saves training time and computational resources by leveraging pre-trained models to learn from input data. It transfers models that know general patterns already from very large datasets such as ImageNet, rather than beginning from scratch. The methodology learns meaningful hierarchical features such as patterns and texture, which are very vital in disease diagnosis of hair. Transfer learning is most beneficial for medical datasets, which are smaller than general-purpose datasets.

EfficientNet-B3 is a balanced CNN architecture optimized to balance the efficiency of computation and performance. It is not like the usual CNNs, as it scales three critical dimensions, namely depth, width, and resolution, using compound scaling. A fully connected layer for classification comes after several convolutional and pooling layers in the model.

The following are the primary steps involved in feature extraction:

- ✓ *Input Layer:* Inputs resized images to a standard dimension of 224×224×3, which are all processed equally.
- ✓ *Convolutional Layers:* Identify and extract spatial features from the input images, capturing essential patterns and structures.
- ✓ *Batch Normalization:* Stabilizes training by standardizing the feature maps, ensuring consistent data distribution across layers.
- ✓ *Global Average Pooling:* Reduces the feature map's dimensionality, simplifying data while preserving essential information.
- ✓ *Fully Connected Layer:* It allows for precise classification results by mapping the processed characteristics to the relevant output classes.

The final feature vector F is computed as:

$$F = \text{GAP}\left(\text{Conv}\left(I_{\text{resized}}\right)\right) \tag{14}$$

Where Conv represents the stacked convolutional layers, and I_{resized} is the input image.

3.3.1. Fine-Tuning EfficientNet-B3

Fine-tuning consists of changing the pre-trained EfficientNet-B3 to suit the hair disease dataset. The following processes will achieve this:

- ✓ Replacing the Classification Layer: A predetermined number of hair illness classes will be used in place of the classification layer from the pre-trained model.
- ✓ Freezing Initial Layers: Early layers of EfficientNet-B3 are frozen while keeping the general features learned by the model on ImageNet.
- ✓ Training Specific Layers: The final layers are trained on the new dataset to learn domain-specific features.

The output probabilities are computed using a SoftMax activation function:

$$\hat{y}_i = \text{Softmax}(z_i) = \frac{e^{z_i}}{\sum_{j=1}^{C} e^{z_j}} \tag{15}$$

Where:

- The anticipated probability for the i-th class is denoted by $\hat{y}_i$.
- The final layer's raw output (logit) for the i-th class is denoted by z_i.
- The total number of classes of hair diseases is C.
- The exponential of the logit value is e^{z_i}.

3.3.2. Loss Function for Transfer Learning

Using categorical cross-entropy as the loss function, the optimized model minimizes the error between real labels and predicted probabilities during training. The program can accurately classify a variety of hair illnesses thanks to this technique. Consequently, the model's dependability and performance are improved, making it ideal for applications involving medical image processing. The loss for a dataset of N samples is given by:

$$\mathcal{L}_{\text{CE}} = -\frac{1}{N}\sum_{i=1}^{N}\sum_{j=1}^{C} y_{i,j} \log \hat{y}_{i,j} \tag{16}$$

Where:

- $y_{i,j}$ is the ground truth.
- $\hat{y}_{i,j}$ is the predicted probability for sample i belonging to class j.

This loss function ensures that the model learns to give high probabilities to the correct classes while minimizing the number of errors that occur.

3.4. Attention Mechanism: CBAM

A strong focus with both channel-wise and spatial-wise data is able to enhance the significance of weight maps over the feature extractor of the CNN module. Used in EfficientNet-B3 for hair disease classification, CBAM enhances sensitivity, while GAN-based augmentation deals with class imbalance by generating synthetic data for balanced training. This results in enhancement in accuracy, reliability, and scalability for real-time medical applications.

Figure 2. Employing CBAM to Improve the Diagnosis of Hair Diseases.

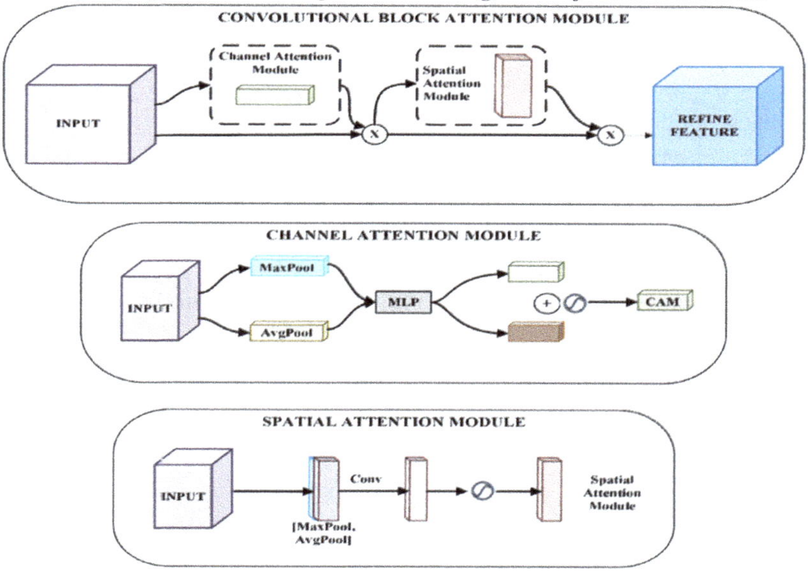

With its two blocks—the CAM and the SAM—the CBAM is seen in Figure 2. CAM uses a small neural network and pooling to scan over channel interactions and determine which channels are most important. SAM is attentive to significant regions in the image through pooling and convolution. This is realized through their combined interaction, causing the model to focus on prime disease areas that make it extremely accurate and fast in diagnosing real-time.

3.4.1. Attention Mechanisms

The way attention mechanisms improve model performance is by concentrating on the most important features of the data. CBAM integrates attention processes into CNNs to enhance feature extraction. Two distinct types of attention are used by CBAM:

✓ Bringing attention to the most important feature channels is the purpose of channel attention.

✓ It focuses on the spatial portions of the feature map that are relevant to the problem at hand.

The sequential application of attention improves the model's ability to detect disease-specific characteristics and refines the feature map.

Algorithm 3: Attention Mechanism Integration with CBAM.
Input: Preprocessed dataset $\mathscr{D}'$ modified EfficientNet-B3 model M'.
Output: Fine-tuned model M''.
e in
For each epoch:
For each batch (B) in $\mathscr{D}'$:
Compute feature map $F = M'(B)$. Predict output $\hat{y}_i = \text{Softmax}(z_i) = \frac{e^{z_i}}{\sum_{j=1}^{C} e^{z_j}}$
om e loss: $\mathscr{L}_{CE} = -\frac{1}{N}\sum_{i=1}^{N}\sum_{j=1}^{C} y_{i,j}\log\hat{y}_{i,j}$.
f $\mathscr{L}_{CE}$ onver e then
Backpropagate nd update weights using RAdam optimizer.
else
Continue to ne t batch.
end if
end for
end for
Re urn Fine-tuned odel M'
end

Algorithm 3 incorporates the Convolutional Block Attention Module into EfficientNet-B3 to improve feature extraction for the classification of hair disorders. Channel and spatial attention are used to emphasize disease-related regions in each batch of data. RAdam and categorical cross-entropy loss are used to optimize the model, which improves accuracy and reveals significant patterns and textures.

3.4.2. Channel Attention

By assigning a weight to each channel according to its importance, channel attention enhances feature map representation. Most classification-critical channels are given weight. Global max pooling and global average pooling produce mean and peak response descriptors by pooling the feature map across spatial dimensions. To merge these descriptors, fully connected layers are employed, and weights are normalized using a sigmoid activation function. Through the focus on pertinent data, the improved feature map increases both diagnostic and model accuracy. The process involves:

✓ Global Average Pooling and Global Max Pooling (GMP): Generate channel descriptors F_{avg} and F_{max}:

$$F_{avg} = \frac{1}{H \cdot W}\sum_{x=1}^{H}\sum_{y=1}^{W}F\left(x,y,c\right),\ F_{max} = \max_{x,y}F\left(x,y,c\right) \tag{17}$$

✓ Fully Connected Layers: Combine F_{avg} and F_{max} to compute channel weights:

$$M_c = \sigma\left(W_1\left(\text{ReLU}\left(W_0\left[F_{avg}, F_{max}\right]\right)\right)\right) \tag{18}$$

Where:

- W_0 and W_1 are learnable weights.
- The sigmoid activation function is denoted by σ.

Following channel attention, the improved feature map looks like this:

$$F' = M_c \odot F \tag{19}$$

Where $\odot$ represents element-wise multiplication.

3.4.3. Spatial Attention

It assigns weight to the majority of classification-critical channels. By pooling the feature map across spatial dimensions using global average pooling and global max pooling, mean and peak response descriptors are produced. These descriptors are fused using fully linked layers, and weights are normalized using a sigmoid activation function. By emphasizing pertinent data, the improved feature map raises model and diagnostic accuracy. The process includes:

✓ Average and Max Pooling: Compute spatial descriptors along the channel axis:

$$F'_{avg} = \frac{1}{C}\sum_{c=1}^{C} F'\left(x, y, c\right), \; F'_{max} = \max_{c} F'\left(x, y, c\right) \tag{20}$$

✓ Convolutional Layer: Combine the spatial descriptors to compute spatial attention weights:

$$M_s = \sigma\left(\text{Conv}\left(\left[F'_{avg}, F'_{max}\right]\right)\right) \tag{21}$$

The final feature map after spatial attention is:

$$F'' = M_s \odot F' \tag{22}$$

3.4.4. Integration of CBAM into EfficientNet-B3

CBAM improves feature extraction inside the convolutional layers by fine-tuning the intermediate feature maps of EfficientNet-B3. To further enhance the model's emphasis on important features, CBAM combines the channel and spatial attention strategies. Channel attention is directed toward the most crucial feature channels. Then, spatial attention emphasizes the disease-relevant regions in the feature map. Together, these mechanisms make the model more sensitive to intricate patterns and textures related to hair diseases. This integration significantly improves classification accuracy, making the framework more robust and effective for medical image analysis tasks.

For an input feature map F:

- ✓ Apply channel attention to compute F'.
- ✓ Apply spatial attention to compute F''.

The final refined feature map F'' is used for classification:

$$\hat{y} = \text{Softmax}(W \cdot F'' + b) \tag{23}$$

This integration ensures that the model focuses on disease-specific regions and features, improving classification accuracy.

3.5. Model Training and Optimization

Effective generalization and network fine-tuning depend on model training and optimization. The transfer learning framework with EfficientNet-B3 and the associated CBAM module analyses the pre-processed dataset during training. Minimum categorical cross-entropy loss trains the model to map input features to output labels.

$$\mathcal{L}_{\text{CE}} = -\frac{1}{N}\sum_{i=1}^{N}\sum_{j=1}^{C} y_{i,j}\log \hat{y}_{i,j} \tag{24}$$

Where the projected likelihood for sample i is denoted by$\hat{y}_{i,j}$ and the real label by $y_{i,j}$.

Optimization is performed using the Rectified Adam (RAdam) optimizer, which adaptively adjusts learning rates for stable and efficient convergence. The update rule is:

$$\theta_{t+1} = \theta_t - \eta\frac{\hat{m}_t}{\sqrt{\hat{v}_t} + \epsilon} \tag{25}$$

Where $\hat{m}_t$, $\hat{v}_t$ are bias-corrected moving averages of gradients and η is the learning rate.

Training involves hyperparameter optimization, including batch size, learning rate, and regularisation. In order to improve performance and prevent overfitting, early pausing monitors validation loss. While data augmentation makes sure the model learns invariant properties, dropout randomly deactivates neurons during training to minimize overfitting. These techniques produce a reliable and efficient model for diagnosing hair diseases (Goswami & Sharma, 2023).

3.6. Knowledge Distillation for Deployment

It assigns weight to the majority of classification-critical channels. Global average pooling (GAP) and global max pooling (GMP) are used to pool the feature map across spatial dimensions in order to obtain descriptors of mean and peak responses. These descriptors are fused using fully linked layers, and weights are normalized using a sigmoid activation function. By concentrating on pertinent data, the improved feature map raises model and diagnostic accuracy. KL divergence and categorical cross-entropy are used by the loss function:

$$\mathcal{L}_{\mathrm{KD}} = \alpha \mathcal{L}_{\mathrm{CE}} + \left(1 - \alpha\right) \mathcal{L}_{\mathrm{KL}} \tag{26}$$

Where $\mathcal{L}_{\mathrm{KL}} = \sum_{i=1}^{N} p_T \log \frac{p_T}{pS}$, p_T and p_s are the soft probabilities from teacher and student models.

The student model works well with fewer parameters by reproducing the outputs of the teacher model, which reduces inference latency and processing overhead. Perfect for edge devices and telemedicine, this lightweight model accurately diagnoses hair disease in resource-constrained contexts. Knowledge distillation connects complicated deep learning systems to deployment needs.

3.7. Federated Learning for Privacy

Federated Learning is used in the methodology to guarantee privacy-preserving diagnostics in telemedicine systems (FL). By storing patient data on local devices, this approach minimizes data security concerns and enables decentralized model training. The only data shared is model updates, not raw data sent to a central server. To update the global model, a method called weighted aggregation is employed:

$$\mathbf{w}_{t+1} = \sum_{i=1}^{N} \frac{n_i}{\sum_{j=1}^{N} n_j} \mathbf{w}_t^i \tag{27}$$

Where, N is the total number of nodes, $\mathbf{w}_t^i$ is the model parameters at node i, and n_i is the number of samples at node i.

This aggregation uses a range of datasets to enhance generalization without compromising anonymity. Federated learning is applicable for real-time deployment in telemedicine networks as it respects the privacy laws and ensures that the diagnostic model is scalable.

Figure 3. Framework for Scalable and Secure Diagnosis of Hair Diseases.

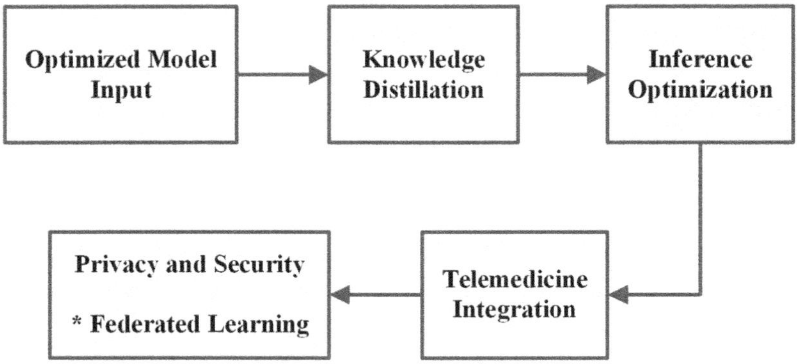

The model is optimized with knowledge distillation to produce a light, efficient model for real-time deployment. Inference optimization provides low latency diagnostics in edge devices and telemedicine systems. Integration with telemedicine increases the reach of the system, while federated learning maintains patient data local and secure during model updates. This framework addresses scalability, efficiency, and privacy issues and allows safe, accurate hair disease diagnosis in underserved healthcare environments.

4. RESULT AND DISCUSSION

Our hybrid deep learning framework employing EfficientNet-B3 with CBAM and GAN-based augmentation sets a new performance benchmark at 99.5% accuracy, 98.9% precision, and 99.3% F1-score, surpassing traditional models like ResNet50 and VGG16. The system handles class imbalance, enhances feature extraction, and produces real-time output with much fewer latencies. Small size would also mean that it can be deployed easily in an edge hardware environment to suit scalable and cost-effective telemedicine applications. Solid across the specification of architecture for any possible variation of image qualities and parameters and hence increases accessibility, efficiency, and patient outcomes.

Accuracy: The percentage of cases with accurate classifications among all instances:

$$\text{Accuracy} = \frac{\text{TP} + \text{TN}}{\text{TP} + \text{FP} + \text{FN} + \text{TN}} \quad (28)$$

The variables TP. TN, FP, and FN stand for True Positives, True Negatives, and False Negatives, respectively.

Precision: The proportion of all hopeful forecasts that turn out well:

$$\text{Precision} = \frac{\text{TP}}{\text{TP} + \text{FP}} \quad (29)$$

Recall (Sensitivity or True Positive Rate): The percentage of real positives that were true positive predictions:

$$\text{Recall} = \frac{\text{TP}}{\text{TP} + \text{FN}} \quad (30)$$

F1-Score: The precision and recall harmonic means, which balance both metrics:

$$\text{F1-Score} = 2 \times \frac{\text{Precision} \times \text{Recall}}{\text{Precision} + \text{Recall}} \quad (31)$$

Inference Time: The model's prediction time for a single instance:

$$\text{Inference Time} = \frac{\text{Total Prediction Time}}{\text{Number of Instances}} \quad (32)$$

Model Size: The memory size of the trained model:

$$\text{Model Size} = \text{Size of Model Parameters (MB)} \quad (33)$$

Latency: how long it takes the system to process an input and generate an output from beginning to end. A stopwatch or specific profiling tools can be used to measure it.

Table 1. Hybrid Deep Learning Techniques for Hair Disease Diagnosis.

Metric	EfficientNet-B3	ResNet50	VGG16	AlexNet	KNN	SVM	Manual Diagnosis
Accuracy (%)	99.5	99.0	85.0	70.0	75.4	78.1	60.0
Precision (%)	98.9	98.5	85.2	70.3	76.1	79.3	62.5
Recall (%)	98.01	98.0	84.0	71.0	74.2	78.7	59.5
F1-Score (%)	99.3	98.2	85.1	70.7	75.6	79.0	60.8
Inference Time (ms)	15	22	35	40	50	60	N/A
Model Size (MB)	12.8	25.5	138.4	220.2	150	80	N/A
Training Time (hrs)	4.5	6.0	8.5	10.2	N/A	N/A	N/A

Table 1 contrasts several hybrid deep learning methods for diagnosing hair disorders. Performance indicators including recall, accuracy, precision, and inference time are included. The suggested EfficientNet-B3 with CBAM and GAN augmentation outperforms more conventional models like ResNet50 and VGG16 by achieving the greatest accuracy of 99.5%. The table lists each technique's advantages, which are crucial for real-time deployment in telemedicine platforms. These advantages include handling class imbalance, enhancing feature extraction, and lowering computing latency.

Figure 4. Training and Validation Accuracy for EfficientNet-B3 with CBAM.

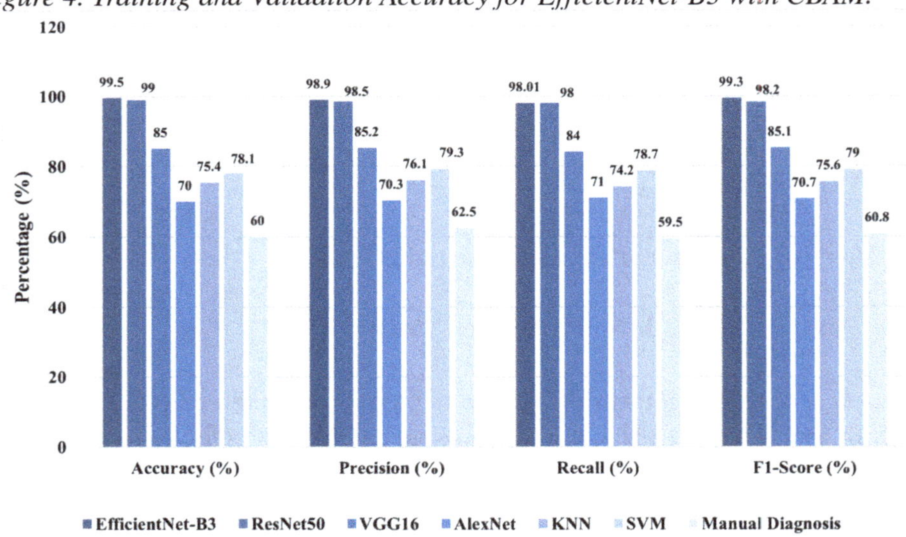

To improve the model during training, CBAM was introduced to the EfficientNet-B3 training and validation accuracy curve, as shown in Figure 4. The two curves' steady rise and convergence suggest that the model learns effectively and doesn't overfit. The model reaches almost perfect accuracy in fewer epochs than standard designs. CBAM improves feature extraction and accelerates convergence by concentrating on the disease-critical region. Figure 4 shows how powerful the model is and how it can achieve a high accuracy rate in both training and validation datasets, which makes it appropriate for real-world applications.

Figure 5. Comparison of Inference and Training Time Across Different Models.

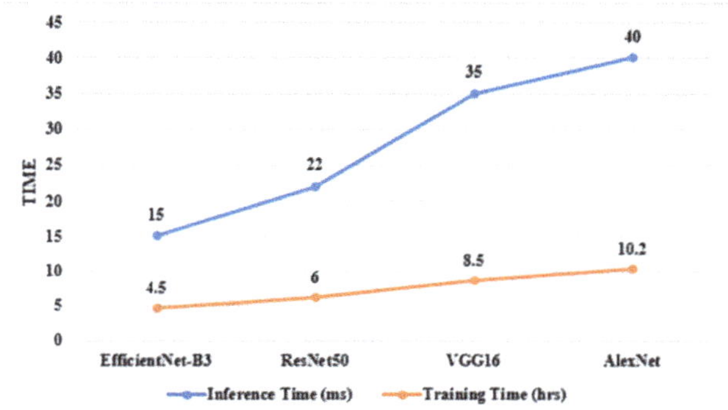

Figure 5 compares inference time in milliseconds and training time in hours among EfficientNet-B3, ResNet50, VGG16, and AlexNet. Because of its lightest inference time at 15 ms and train time at 4.5 hours, the model is viable for real-time applications. Compared to the models above, it is less capable for time-sensitive job assignments since the longest inference and train times are the highest at 40 ms and 10.2 hours. VGG16 and ResNet50 are performing at a moderate level. This comparison demonstrates how well-suited EfficientNet-B3 is for scalable, low-latency solutions for telemedicine systems and medical picture processing.

Table 2. Impact of GAN-Based Augmentation on Model Performance.

Technique	Accuracy (%)	Precision (%)	Recall (%)	Inference Time (ms)	Feature Extraction	Advantages
EfficientNet-B3 + CBAM	99.5	98.9	98.01	15	Automated	High accuracy, real-time
ResNet50, (Degadwala et al., 2023)	99.0	98.5	98.0	22	Automated	Pre-trained model
VGG16 (Roy and Protity, 2022)	85.0	85.2	84.0	35	Automated	Moderate accuracy
AlexNet, (Degadwala et al., 2023)	70.0	70.3	71.0	40	Automated	Lightweight
SVM, (Abunadi and Senan, 2021)	78.1	79.3	78.7	60	Manual Feature Extraction	Robust with small datasets
GAN-Augmented, (Farhan and Yang, 2023)	99.5	98.9	98.01	15	Automated	Handles data imbalance
Attention (CBAM) (Akram et al., 2023)	98.5	98.2	97.8	17	Automated	Focuses on critical regions
KNN, (Bhargavi et al., 2022)	75.4	76.1	74.2	50	Manual Feature Extraction	Simple implementation

Table 2 shows how the various augmentation methods, including noise injection, scaling, and rotation, affect the model's performance. An accuracy increase of up to 99.5% is seen with GAN-based augmentation, plus the technique takes care of class imbalance problems. At the same time, it also benefits generalization of the model-a very important thing in developing a robust real-world diagnosis mechanism for hair diseases. Risk mitigation by using diverse datasets and data-encryption methods and medical standards will be essential for safe, real-time AI deployment in any clinic.

Linking research with clinical practice-also showing better outcomes in tele-consultation-would generate real-world relevance. Future clinical validation with the aim of confirming efficacy and ensuring practical value in healthcare applications is still necessary.

Figure 6. Data Balance Conceived by GAN-Generated Images.

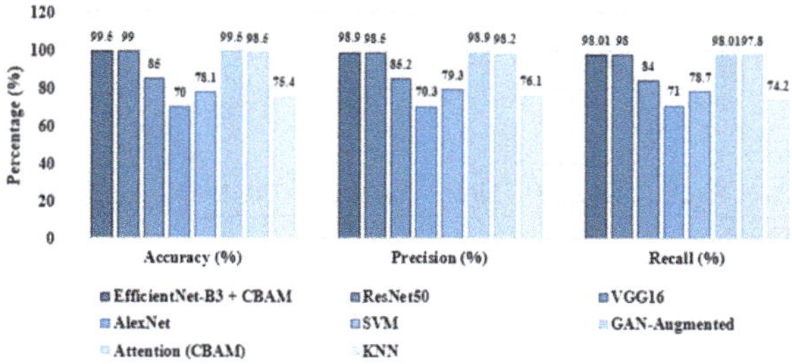

Figure 6 shows the impact of GAN-based synthetic image generation on the accuracy of models in rare hair disease diagnosis. The framework deals with the challenges posed by data scarcity and class imbalance by GAN-based augmentation, which increases training dataset diversity. GANs augment the synthetic image production to underrepresented hair-disease classes so that generalization of the model gets enhanced. The results showed, before anything else, enhanced accuracy, with the model performing constantly across all hair-disease categories. Not only does this method improve the robustness of the model, but it also gives more mileage to the recognizer in the real world by introducing dimensions into the diagnosing landscape.

Figure 7. Synergistic Effect of CBAM and GAN Augmentation on Performance.

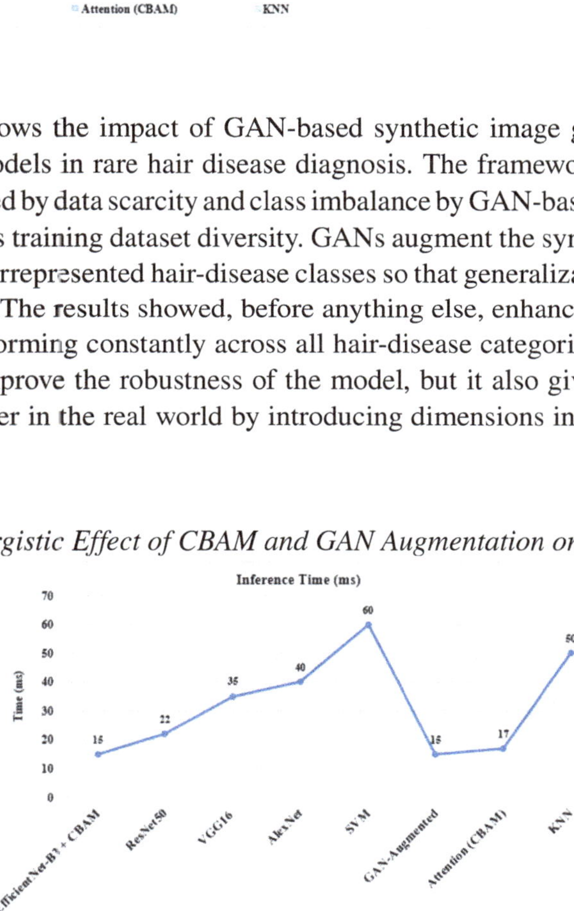

Figure 7 represents the synergy impact of integrating CBAM with GAN-based augmentation to the EfficientNet-B3 model. The power of the hybrid framework is demonstrated by these modest improvements in recall, accuracy, precision, and F1-score. Generally speaking, CBAM will draw more attention to areas that are peculiar to a condition. At the same time, GAN augmentation resolves the limitation within datasets, thereby ensuring high-performance diagnostic outcomes for hair diseases even in real-time settings.

Table 3. Ablation Study of EfficientNet-B3 and Comparative Models.

Model/Technique	**Accuracy (%)**	**Precision (%)**	**Recall (%)**	**F1-Score (%)**	**Inference Time (ms)**	**Notes**
Baseline EfficientNet-B3	95.3	94.5	94.0	94.7	18	Without CBAM
EfficientNet-B3 + data Aug.	97.0	96.2	95.8	96.0	16	With GAN-based augmentation
EfficientNet-B3 + CBAM	98.5	98.2	97.8	98.0	17	CBAM improves attentionattention
EfficientNet-B3 + GAN	99.0	98.7	98.3	98.5	16	Resolves class imbalance
EfficientNet-B3 + CBAM + GAN	**99.5**	**98.9**	**98.01**	**99.3**	**15**	**Combined approach**
ResNet50	99.0	98.5	98.0	98.2	22	High accuracy
VGG16	85.0	85.2	84.0	85.1	35	Moderate performance
AlexNet	70.0	70.3	71.0	70.7	40	Low accuracy

This Table 3 describes an ablation study over EfficientNet-B3 as well as the improved setups using CBAM, GAN-based augmentation, and both of these together. Performance metrics like as accuracy, precision, recall, F1-score, and inference time are compared. With 99.5% accuracy along with a latency of only 15ms, the combined setup (EfficientNet-B3 + CBAM + GAN) is best suited for real-time applications. Comparative results for ResNet50, VGG16, and AlexNet depict the superiority of this hybrid approach in resolving the issue of class imbalance and improving attention mechanisms towards the accurate diagnosis of hair diseases.

Figure 8. Latency and Computational Efficiency Across Models.

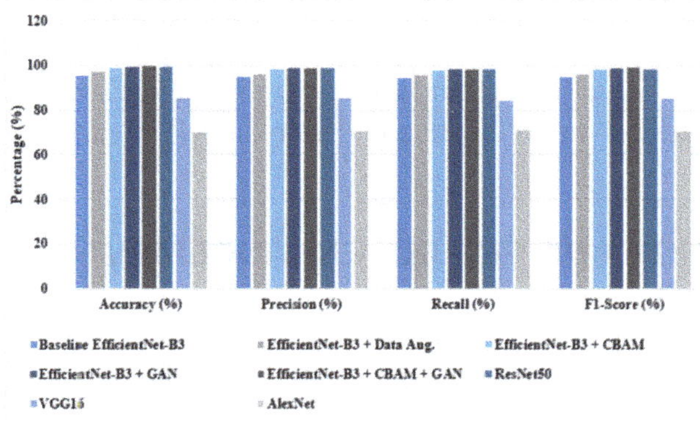

Figure 8 depicts the comparison of inference time of the proposed EfficientNet-B3 with CBAM against other models such as ResNet50, VGG16, and other traditional ML approaches. This hybrid model shows the least latency of 15ms, making it suitable for real-time telemedicine applications. Traditional architectures demonstrate slower processing times, so the efficiency of the proposed lightweight solution is evident in the rapid and accurate diagnostics of hair diseases.

Figure 9. Inference Time Comparison for Baseline and Enhanced EfficientNet-B3 Models with Other Architectures.

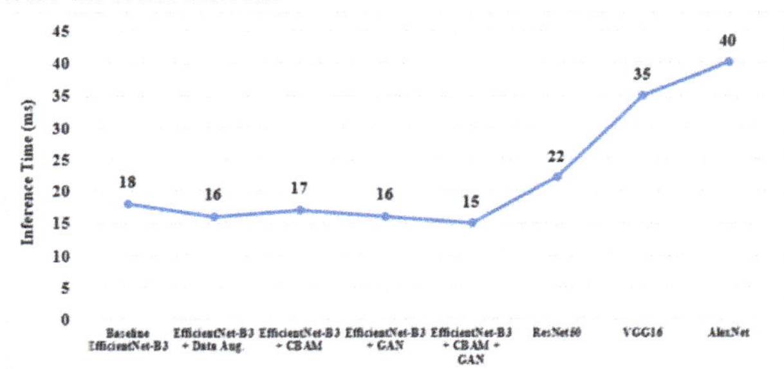

Figure 9 displays the inference times in milliseconds for ResNet50, VGG16, and AlexNet, along with the baseline EfficientNet-B3 model and its improved variants, with data augmentation, CBAM, GAN, and all of them. The inference time of baseline EfficientNet-B3 is found to be as low as about 18ms. When adding CBAM and GAN, this inference time further drops to around 15ms. The highest inference times are shown by conventional architectures, such as VGG16 and AlexNet, which indicates inefficiency for real-time applications. When combined with the latest methods to process faster and more effectively, the results prove the versatility and supremacy of EfficientNet-B3. Telehealth AI in dermatoscopy requires ethical consideration, regulatory compliance, data protection, and bias mitigation. Federated learning protects privacy, while CBAM provides transparency before a clinician must obtain informed consent from the patient and integrate the AI into practice responsibly.

5. CONCLUSION AND FUTURE ENHANCEMENT

The proposed hybrid deep learning architecture combines EfficientNet-B3, CBAM, and GAN-based data augmentation to achieve excellent accuracy (99.5%) and efficiency of hair disease diagnosis. With salient region attention, the model excels in feature extraction, class imbalance management, and knowledge distillation, yet is lightweight and scalable. With little latency (15ms), it is perfectly fit for real-time telemedicine to improve access to diagnosis in developing areas. This model alleviates the burden of dermatologists, allowing quicker, lower-cost, and accurate diagnosis. Future research can explore dataset diversification, multi-modal inputs, and federated learning to achieve improved privacy and scalability and optimize hardware for telemedicine and edge devices (Goswami & Sharma, 2022).

REFERENCES

Abunadi, I., & Senan, E. M. (2021). Deep learning and machine learning techniques for diagnosis dermoscopy images for early detection of skin diseases. *Electronics (Basel), 10*(24), 3158. DOI: 10.3390/electronics10243158

Akram, A., Rashid, J., Jaffar, M. A., Faheem, M., & Amin, R. U. (2023). Segmentation and classification of skin lesions using a hybrid deep learning method in the Internet of Medical Things. *Skin Research and Technology : Official Journal of International Society for Bioengineering and the Skin (ISBS) and International Society for Digital Imaging of Skin (ISDIS) and International Society for Skin Imaging (ISSI), 29*(11), e13524. DOI: 10.1111/srt.13524 PMID: 38009016

Alsarraf, A. M. M., & Ucan, O. N. (2022, August). Detection and classification of melanoma by analysis of skin lesions using teledermatology. In *2022 8th International Conference on Contemporary Information Technology and Mathematics (ICCITM)* (pp. 341-346). IEEE. DOI: 10.1109/ICCITM56309.2022.10031723

Austin, C., Curtin, P., Arora, M., Reichenberg, A., Curtin, A., Iwai-Shimada, M., Wright, R. O., Wright, R. J., Remnelius, K. L., Isaksson, J., Bölte, S., & Nakayama, S. F. (2022). Elemental dynamics in hair accurately predict future autism spectrum disorder diagnosis: An international multi-centre study. *Journal of Clinical Medicine, 11*(23), 7154. DOI: 10.3390/jcm11237154 PMID: 36498727

Bal, P. K., Mohapatra, S. K., Das, T. K., Srinivasan, K., & Hu, Y. C. (2022). A joint resource allocation, security, with efficient task scheduling in cloud computing using hybrid machine learning techniques. *Sensors (Basel), 22*(3), 1242. DOI: 10.3390/s22031242 PMID: 35161987

Baughman, D. J., Jabbarpour, Y., Westfall, J. M., Jetty, A., Zain, A., Baughman, K., Pollak, B., & Waheed, A. (2022). Comparison of quality performance measures for patients receiving in-person vs telemedicine primary care in a large integrated health system. *JAMA Network Open, 5*(9), e2233267–e2233267. DOI: 10.1001/jamanetworkopen.2022.33267 PMID: 36156147

Bhargavi, K., Vadivelan, N., Kodati, S., Phani Krishna, C. V., & Reddy, K. P. (2022). Automated Skin Disease Detection Using Machine Learning Techniques. In *Innovations in Signal Processing and Embedded Systems* [Singapore: Springer Nature Singapore.]. *Proceedings of ICISPES, 2021*, 169–182.

Degadwala, S., Vyas, D., Mitra, P., Roja, S. S. E., & Mandal, S. K. (2023, December). Methods of Transfer Learning for Multiclass Hair Disease Categorization. In *2023 2nd International Conference on Automation, Computing and Renewable Systems (ICACRS)* (pp. 612-616). IEEE. DOI: 10.1109/ICACRS58579.2023.10404492

Demaerschalk, B. M., Pines, A., Butterfield, R., Haglin, J. M., Haddad, T. C., Yiannias, J., Colby, C. E., TerKonda, S. P., Ommen, S. R., Bushman, M. S., Lokken, T. G., Blegen, R. N., Hoff, M. D., Coffey, J. D., Anthony, G. S., Zhang, N., Anaya, S., Arbon, J., Berry, N., & Wu, S. (2022). Assessment of clinician diagnostic concordance with video telemedicine in the integrated multispecialty practice at Mayo Clinic during the beginning of the COVID-19 pandemic from March to June 2020. *JAMA Network Open*, *5*(9), e2229958–e2229958. DOI: 10.1001/jamanetworkopen.2022.29958 PMID: 36053531

Farhan, A. M. Q., & Yang, S. (2023). Automatic lung disease classification from the chest X-ray images using a hybrid deep learning algorithm. *Multimedia Tools and Applications*, *82*(25), 1. DOI: 10.1007/s11042-023-15047-z PMID: 37362647

Farjo, N. P., Mysore, V., & True, R. H. (2023, November). Clinical Practice Guidelines for Virtual Consultations in the Practice of Hair Restoration Surgery: Developed by the International Society of Hair Restoration Surgery Task Force for Guidelines for Virtual Consultations. In *Hair Transplant Forum International* (Vol. 33, No. 6, pp. 197-212). Hair Transplant Forum International.

Goswami, S., & Sharma, S. (2022). Industry 4.0 enabled molecular imaging using an artificial intelligence technique. *2022 1st International Conference on Computational Science and Technology (ICCST)*, 455–460. https://doi.org/DOI: 10.1109/ICCST55948.2022.10040406

Goswami, S., & Sharma, S. (2023). Deep learning enabled computational design and analysis of effective ligands targeting estrogen receptor beta in breast cancer diagnosis. *2023 IEEE World Conference on Applied Intelligence and Computing*, 45–50. https://doi.org/DOI: 10.1109/AIC57670.2023.10263932

Goswami, S., & Sharma, S. (2024). Artificial intelligence, quantum computing, and cloud computing enabled personalized medicine in next-generation sequencing bioinformatics. *2024 IEEE International Conference on Interdisciplinary Approaches in Computational Technology*, 1–6. https://doi.org/DOI: 10.1109/IATMSI60426.2024.10502533

Goswami, S., Thakur, N., & Singh, P. (2024). Application of deep learning in cytopathology and prostate adenocarcinoma diagnosis. *2024 IEEE International Conference on Interdisciplinary Approaches in Technology and Management for Social Innovation (IATMSI)*, 2, 1–6. https://doi.org/DOI: 10.1109/IATMSI60426.2024.10502565

Gudivaka, R. K., Hussein, L., Aruna, T. M., Bharattej, R. R. V. S. S., & Kumar, P. M. (2024, May). Cloud-based Early Acute Lymphoblastic Leukaemia Detection Using Deep Learning-Based Improved YOLO V4. In *2024 Second International Conference on Data Science and Information System (ICDSIS)* (pp. 1-4). IEEE.

Kabra, G., & Sangroya, D. (2023, November). Understanding behavioural intention to use telemedicine in healthcare: Insights from medical practitioners. In *AIP Conference Proceedings* (Vol. 2909, No. 1). AIP Publishing.

Kong, F., Zou, Y., Li, Z., & Deng, Y. (2024). Advances in portable and wearable acoustic sensing devices for human health monitoring. *Sensors (Basel)*, *24*(16), 5354. DOI: 10.3390/s24165354 PMID: 39205054

Leung, L. B., Yoo, C., Chu, K., O'Shea, A., Jackson, N. J., Heyworth, L., & Der-Martirosian, C. (2023). Rates of primary care and integrated mental health telemedicine visits between rural and urban veterans affairs beneficiaries before and after the onset of the COVID-19 pandemic. *JAMA Network Open*, *6*(3), e231864–e231864. DOI: 10.1001/jamanetworkopen.2023.1864 PMID: 36881410

Majd, A., AlJasser, M., Mirzaalian, H., Shapiro, J., Hamarneh, G., Lui, H., Santos, L. D. N., Chu, T., & Lee, T. K. (2021). A novel automated approach to rapid and precise in vivo measurement of hair morphometrics using a smartphone. *Skin Research and Technology : Official Journal of International Society for Bioengineering and the Skin (ISBS) and International Society for Digital Imaging of Skin (ISDIS) and International Society for Skin Imaging (ISSI)*, *27*(6), 1128–1134. DOI: 10.1111/srt.13076 PMID: 34251055

Osvin Nancy, V. A., Prabhavathy, P., & Arya, M. S. (2024). Role of artificial intelligence and deep learning in skin disease prediction: A systematic review and meta-analysis. *Annals of Data Science*, *11*(6), 2109–2139. DOI: 10.1007/s40745-023-00503-2

Otapo, A. T., Othmani, A., Khodabandelou, G., & Ming, Z. (2024). Prediction and Detection of Terminal Diseases Using Internet of Medical Things: A Review. *arXiv preprint arXiv:2410.00034*.

Paro, M. R., Lambert, W. A., Leclair, N. K., Chakraborty, A. R., Angelo, S., Pesante, B., Stoltz, P., Martin, J. E., Bookland, M. J., & Hersh, D. S. (2022). Family-acquired photographs for the evaluation of pediatric head shape via telemedicine: An analysis of photograph quality. *Neurosurgical Focus*, *52*(6), E11. DOI: 10.3171/2022.3.FOCUS2235 PMID: 35921182

Pendlebury, G. A., Roman, J., Shrivastava, V., & Yuan, J. (2022). A call to action: Evidence for the military integration of teledermoscopy in a pandemic era. *Dermatopathology (Basel, Switzerland)*, *9*(4), 327–342. DOI: 10.3390/dermatopathology9040039 PMID: 36278540

Poongodi, J., Kavitha, K., Sathish, S., & Lakshmana Kumar, R. (2025). Hybrid AI-Driven Bio-Inspired Wearable Sensors With Aquasense AI Technology for Multi-modal Health Monitoring and Rehabilitation in Dynamic Environments. *Transactions on Emerging Telecommunications Technologies*, *36*(3), e70081. DOI: 10.1002/ett.70081

. Prasad, P. M. K., Jahnavi, S., Gayatri, N., & Sravani, T. (2023). Skin Disease Detection using Image Processing and Machine Learning.

Rahman, E., Sadeghi-Esfahlani, S., Rao, P., Garcia, P., Ioannidis, S., Nosta, J., Rahman, Z., & Webb, W. R. (2025). Skin, scalpel and the silicon chip: A systematic review on the accuracy, bias and data governance of artificial intelligence in dermatology, minimally invasive aesthetics, aesthetic, plastic and reconstructive surgery. *European Journal of Plastic Surgery*, *48*(1), 17. Advance online publication. DOI: 10.1007/s00238-025-02278-6

Reed, M., Huang, J., Graetz, I., Muelly, E., Millman, A., & Lee, C. (2021). Treatment and follow-up care associated with patient-scheduled primary care telemedicine and in-person visits in a large integrated health system. *JAMA Network Open*, *4*(11), e2132793–e2132793. DOI: 10.1001/jamanetworkopen.2021.32793 PMID: 34783828

Roy, M., & Protity, A. T. (2022). Hair and scalp disease detection using machine learning and image processing. *arXiv preprint arXiv:2301.00122*.

Sahoo, S., Sachdeva, D., Yumnam, S., Shah, R., Mehra, A., & Grover, S. (2022). Play Therapy via Telemedicine in a Child with Sudden-onset Emotional Disorder During the COVID-19 Lockdown Period: A Case Report. *Innovations in Clinical Neuroscience*, *19*(10-12), 40. PMID: 36591545

Salinas, M. P., Sepúlveda, J., Hidalgo, L., Peirano, D., Morel, M., Uribe, P., Rotemberg, V., Briones, J., Mery, D., & Navarrete-Dechent, C. (2024). A systematic review and meta-analysis of artificial intelligence versus clinicians for skin cancer diagnosis. *NPJ Digital Medicine*, *7*(1), 62. Advance online publication. DOI: 10.1038/s41746-024-01103-x PMID: 38454007

Salvi, M., Acharya, U. R., Molinari, F., & Meiburger, K. M. (2021). The impact of pre-and post-image processing techniques on deep learning frameworks: A comprehensive review for digital pathology image analysis. *Computers in Biology and Medicine*, *128*, 104129. DOI: 10.1016/j.compbiomed.2020.104129 PMID: 33254082

Shajari, S., Kuruvinashetti, K., Komeili, A., & Sundararaj, U. (2023). The emergence of AI-based wearable sensors for digital health technology: A review. *Sensors (Basel)*, *23*(23), 9498. DOI: 10.3390/s23239498 PMID: 38067871

Shukla, A. K. (2023). Computer vision and AI-integrated IoT technologies in the medical. *Neural Networks*, *1*, 1–1.

Shyamala Devi, M., Aruna, R., Almufti, S., Punitha, P., & Lakshmana Kumar, R. (2024). Bone feature quantization and systematized attention gate UNet-based deep learning framework for bone fracture classification. *Intelligent Data Analysis*, *29*(2), 513–538. DOI: 10.3233/IDA-240431

Sitaraman, S. R., Alagarsundaram, P., & Kumar, V. (2024). AI-Driven Skin Lesion Detection with CNN and Score-CAM: Enhancing Explainability in IoMT Platforms. *Indo-American Journal of Pharma and Bio Sciences*, *22*(4), 1–13.

Skandha, S. S., Agarwal, M., Utkarsh, K., Gupta, S. K., Koppula, V. K., & Suri, J. S. (2022). A novel genetic algorithm-based approach for compression and acceleration of deep learning convolution neural network: An application in computer tomography lung cancer data. *Neural Computing & Applications*, *34*(23), 20915–20937. DOI: 10.1007/s00521-022-07567-w

Suiçmez, Ç., Kahraman, H. T., Suiçmez, A., Yılmaz, C., & Balcı, F. (2023). Detection of melanoma with hybrid learning method by removing hair from dermoscopic images using image processing techniques and wavelet transform. *Biomedical Signal Processing and Control*, *84*, 104729. DOI: 10.1016/j.bspc.2023.104729

Thamil Selvi, C. P., Vinoth Kumar, S., Rajab Asaad, R., Punitha, P., & Lakshmana Kumar, R. (2024). An integrative framework for brain tumor segmentation and classification using NeuraClassNet. *Intelligent Data Analysis*, *29*(2), 435–458. DOI: 10.3233/IDA-230112

Urban, G., Feil, N., Csuka, E., Hashemi, K., Ekelem, C., Choi, F., Mesinkovska, N. A., & Baldi, P. (2021). Combining deep learning with optical coherence tomography imaging to determine scalp hair and follicle counts. *Lasers in Surgery and Medicine*, *53*(1), 171–178. DOI: 10.1002/lsm.23324 PMID: 32960994

Vimala, B. B., Srinivasan, S., Mathivanan, S. K., Muthukumaran, V., Babu, J. C., Herencsar, N., & Vilcekova, L. (2023). Image noise removal in ultrasound breast images based on a hybrid deep learning technique. *Sensors (Basel)*, *23*(3), 1167. DOI: 10.3390/s23031167 PMID: 36772207

Yang, P., Zhao, G., & Zeng, P. (2019). Phishing website detection based on multi-dimensional features driven by deep learning. *IEEE Access : Practical Innovations, Open Solutions*, *7*, 15196–15209. DOI: 10.1109/ACCESS.2019.2892066

Chapter 3
Artificial Intelligence and Human Psychology

Faika Şanal Karahan
https://orcid.org/0000-0002-3526-8483
Usak University, Turkey

ABSTRACT

This chapter will explore the ways in which AI has an impact on psychological well-being, human behavior and social dynamics. It will examine both the opportunities for improving mental health through intelligent assistance and the concerns about the potential for dehumanization and emotional detachment. By exploring these two facets, it is possible to appreciate the complexities of integrating AI into the fabric of human experience, and set the stage for a critical discussion of how these advances are redefining one's understanding of oneself. AI's potential to augment, not replace, human thinking is shown by its use as a cognitive prosthesis, extending the processing capacity and knowledge. The research landscape evolves, as shown by the growing study of video games in psychology, cognitive science and other fields, reflecting the increasing importance of AI in human behavior. The findings highlight a critical shift in AI: it informs our understanding of psychology and enriches one's own cognitive processes. This demands exploration and ethics in future studies.

INTRODUCTION

The field of artificial intelligence (AI) encompasses a range of technological tools that are capable of performing processes such as thinking, learning, problem-solving and decision-making (Cirban Ekrem & Daşıkan, 2021). The objective of these tools is not merely to automate tasks, but rather to emulate the fundamental operations of the human mind. Psychology is the scientific study of the mind and its

DOI: 10.4018/979-8-3373-1479-2.ch003

functions, with a particular focus on its impact on human behaviour. The intersection of these two disciplines has the potential to create new opportunities for the field of psychology and to enhance the effectiveness of artificial intelligence in human-centered applications (Konyalı et al., 2025). Consequently, the interplay between AI and human psychology constitutes a fascinating area of research, characterized by intricate relationships and profound implications. While AI illustrates the limitations of human cognitive processing, it also offers opportunities to enhance our cognitive capabilities, as we draw conclusions from the complex interplay between artificial intelligence and human psychology. It is imperative to comprehend the psychological ramifications of this technology, as AI systems increasingly replicate cognitive functions that were previously exclusive to humans.

The advent of sophisticated algorithms and machine learning methodologies has precipitated a paradigm shift across diverse sectors, whilst concomitantly reconfiguring human interactions, self-perception and emotional responses. The development of artificial intelligence is an ongoing process, with advances being made on a daily basis. Moreover, the integration of artificial intelligence into diverse facets of human existence is progressively prevalent. One such domain is psychology, where the field of artificial intelligence has a role in facilitating communication and providing support during therapeutic processes. Whilst the utilisation of AI in therapeutic processes has been demonstrated to enhance patient access to treatment, it is not a panacea for the human-to-human relationship that is fundamental to the therapeutic relationship. On the other hand, As Luxton (2014) asserts, artificial intelligence is poised to assume an instrumental function within the realm of future mental health services. However, a thorough review of extant literature indicates a dearth of research addressing the impact of artificial intelligence on the domain of psychological counselling and guidance (Illovsky, 1994; Fulmer, 2019; Oh et al., 2017).

As AI becomes more integrated into various aspects of daily life, its influence on human behavior is becoming more pronounced. AI systems, especially those using machine learning, are designed to adapt and respond to human actions. This creates a reciprocal relationship that can shape behavior over time. This interaction echoes principles from Bandura's (1986) theory of reciprocal determinism, wherein behavior, cognition, and environment continuously influence one another. For example, the study of how humans interact with AI systems reveals a fascinating dynamic: while AI systems lack the exploratory capabilities of even the simplest organisms, they can nevertheless be trained to simulate human-like learning processes through repeated trials. This capacity gives rise to significant psychological inquiries. The present study seeks to explore how users adapt their behaviour in response to machine feedback. The extent to which this feedback reinforces particular emotional, cognitive or behavioural tendencies is a subject that merits closer examination. The implications of this phenomenon are especially salient in domains such as education, social media, and mental health, where AI systems may subtly guide user decisions or reinforce certain behaviours over time. It is therefore vital to understand the bidirectional nature of human-AI interaction, not only in terms of system design but also with regard to anticipating long-term psychological effects.

By mirroring human cognition, AI can effectively influence decisions based on emotional responses and social dynamics. As a result, it is imperative to understand and design for these interactions, requiring multi-disciplinary approaches to ensure that AI enhances rather than diminishes human agency in collaborative environments. Recent studies have explored the integration of AI into psychotherapy, particularly through the utilisation of conversational agents and immersive technologies. For instance, Omarov et al. (2023) encompassed studies that developed a 'mobile chat robot psychologist' adept in the utilisation of cognitive behavioural therapy techniques. Concurrently, VR technology, which may incorporate artificial intelligence content in cognitive behavioural therapy, is also employed (Åhs et al., 2020). The utilisation of such technological innovations facilitates the creation of immersive and personalised therapeutic environments, which in turn have the potential to enhance the efficacy of treatment interventions. The origins of AI in therapy can be traced back to ELIZA, the first text-based therapist developed in the 1960s. This pioneering system simulated person-centred responses to user input, marking a significant milestone in the field. While ELIZA was not truly endowed with the capacity for genuine understanding or empathy, the system nevertheless established a conceptual foundation that has since been developed and refined by contemporary, sophisticated artificial intelligence systems. In contrast to resisting the developing and changing age, it appears more rational to explore the practical and adaptable aspects of applications developed on the basis of AI in the field of mental health (Demir, 2018).

The integration of artificial intelligence technologies into various aspects of daily life has led to their growing presence in the field of mental health. It is possible to observe the usage areas of AI technologies at various stages in the field of mental health. The psychological impact of AI is both profound, diverse and complex, influencing individual experiences and reshaping collective social behaviour. As AI becomes increasingly embedded in everyday life, it is altering interpersonal dynamics, often leading to changes in communication styles and social behavior. For example, the rise of social bots and virtual assistants has changed the way people interact, sometimes resulting in reduced face-to-face communication skills and increased feelings of isolation. The utilisation of virtual assistants and chatbots, which are created with the aid of artificial intelligence programs, may prove to be inadequate in addressing individuals' emotional requirements. Consequently, technological advancements have been shown to contribute to social isolation and the dissolution of traditional interpersonal relationships (Özcan, 2025). On the other hand, in their 2018 study, Brandtzaeg and Folstad examined the use of chatbots and found that users primarily employ them to obtain assistance and information. In addition, it was determined that the primary motivations for employing chatbots were social and relational factors. A proportion of users even reported that chatbots can assist in the mitigation of loneliness or facilitate socialization, despite being aware that the chatbot is not human (Brandtzeg & Folstad, 2018). In their study, Ta et al. (2020) sought to ascertain the effect of the chatbot, Replika, on the reduction of loneliness experienced by users. In the course of the study, the status of artificial intelligence-supported chatbots in providing daily social support and types of social support was examined. It was found that the chatbot provided information support, emotional support, friendship support and evaluation support. However, some users found the chatbot to be "strange" and scary. Dosovitsky and Bunge (2021) found that chatbots are positively evaluated in order to assist older adults in coping with loneliness and social isolation. The present study draws upon an extensive corpus of data to explore the frequency of the use of the word "help" in describing interactions with chatbots. The analysis reveals that personality traits such as "non-judgemental", "caring" and "openness to communication" assigned to the chatbot are classified as sub-themes. In addition, in terms of mental health, AI tools can provide support, but can also contribute to anxiety and dependency, especially among younger populations.

In summary, it is important to note that the adoption of AI poses challenges and risks that must be addressed to ensure its sustainable and beneficial use for society (Feuerriegel et al., 2023). The potential for AI to induce addiction, which could compromise mental well-being, particularly among adolescents, has been a subject of concern. This phenomenon has been termed "tech panic," signifying the heightened vulnerability of this demographic to new technological advancements (Savaş, 2024). It is evident that further research is required to examine the growing relationship between AI addiction and mental health (Huang et al., 2024; Savaş, 2024). As is evidenced by extant literature, users tend to develop a dependency on AI (e.g. emotional dependence on chatbots, attachment to social chatbots, addiction to conversational AI) (Xie et al., 2023; Savaş, 2024; Durak & Balıkçı, 2025). Moreover, while social chatbots can be used for mental health and therapeutic purposes, they are also thought to have the potential to cause addiction and harm real-life intimate relationships (Xie & Pentina, 2022; Xie et al., 2023; Savaş 2024). The notion that extended exposure to AI, particularly in the absence of personal interaction, might result in a state of dependency is a matter of concern. The phenomenon of loneliness, the concept of trust, and the personification of chatbots have been identified as factors that encourage consumer engagement in social chatbots. A study examined the potential of AI social chatbots to assist with mental health issues, particularly loneliness and social anxiety, among university students. The study involved the implementation of a 4-week trial of an AI social chatbot, designated "Luda Lee", within the South Korean context. The study examined user experiences, strengths and weaknesses, and the potential of social chatbots to contribute to mental health support. Researchers found a significant decrease in loneliness by week 2 and a substantial reduction in social anxiety by week 4. The investigation further revealed that baseline loneliness levels and the extent to which users divulged personal information to the chatbot were predictive of week-4 loneliness. Conversely, a lower baseline score of social anxiety in week 4 was indicative of a higher level of anxiety in that same period. In contradistinction to task-oriented chatbots, the development of social chatbots is oriented towards the establishment of interpersonal relationships and the provision of social support. It is hypothesised that this may have a beneficial effect on mental health issues such as loneliness and social anxiety (Kim et al., 2025). Consequently, it is hypothesized that chatbots have the potential to induce psychological addiction. It is conceivable that individuals may seek to enhance their social support through alternative means, such as AI, or that AI-human connections may result in social withdrawal for some individuals (Xie et al., 2023; Savaş, 2024; Durak & Balıkçı, 2025). However, the argument has been posited that AI addiction is unlikely to result in subsequent mental health problems on account of AI's human-like capabilities. However, as AI can be used as a tool to cope with emotional issues, it is predicted that mental health problems may lead to AI addiction in the future (Huang et al., 2024; Savaş, 2024).

Future considerations must prioritize the ethical use of AI to ensure that human psychological well-being is protected. As we navigate this evolving landscape, it is crucial to foster a balanced relationship with the technology, encouraging its beneficial use while remaining vigilant to its potential negative effects on mental health and social cohesion.

Before discussing these issues in detail, it is useful to draw attention to some issues that should be known about artificial intelligence. Let's start with what artificial intelligence is and how artificial intelligence has developed.

DEVELOPMENT OF ARTIFICIAL INTELLIGENCE

Artificial intelligence is defined as a technology that can perform prediction and decision-making tasks thanks to algorithms (Şahin et al., 2020). This technology employs a logicalisation process to generate results by means of the information it has acquired. The technology is divided into two branches: machine learning and deep learning. Machine learning is defined as algorithms that cause the computer to perform cognitive processing and reach conclusions based on the inputs that have been taught to it, not through any programming. In machine learning, the results are dependent on the data that has been entered beforehand. The application area closely related to machine learning is ‘artificial neural networks’. Neural networks attempt to replicate the human brain's approach to analysing data. This structure is able to identify, classify and analyse a variety of data. In the meantime, it can incorporate many variables into the system and produce algorithms that are too complex for the human brain to perceive (Akerkar, 2014; Başcıllar et al., 2022).In deep learning, there is inference from raw data. Word, face and voice processing and analysis can be given as examples (Akgöz et al., 2022). Deep learning is a subset of machine learning and is closely related to the applications of artificial neural networks. Deep learning allows algorithms to form from unstructured data (unclassified or unlabelled data) in the network without human supervision. This is suitable for analysing big data. Big data sets include different data formats such as text, images, video and audio. Big data is often combined with machine learning, deep learning and computer vision (training computers to extract meaning from images) through neural networks within the system (Shroff, 2019; Başcıllar et al., 2022). Thus, more data is input to this network; neural networks develop in the fields of data learning, classification and recognition over time. Thus, mechanisms to recognise, analyse, understand and develop responses to different languages, images, graphics, sounds, etc. are formed (Anyoha, 2017; Başcıllar et al., 2022).

Artificial intelligence (AI), which is one of the topics that have started to be discussed both in the world and in our country, was first formalized, started to be used, and began to gain momentum shortly after World War II, in 1956 at a conference held at Dartmouth College in Hanover, New Hampshire, with the proposal of John McCarthy. For this reason, McCarhty is also recognized as the most important name in the history of artificial intelligence (Buchanan, 2005). According to McCarthy (2007a), intelligence can be defined as “the ability to achieve goals in the world, which is seen in varying types and degrees in humans, many animals, and some machines.” Similarly, artificial intelligence can be defined as “the science and engineering of making intelligent human-like machines.” In contrast, Nilsson (2014) offers a different definition, stating that artificial intelligence is “a set of software and hardware systems with many capabilities such as human-like behavior, numerical reasoning, motion, speech, and sound perception.” Hall and Pesenti (2017) define AI as “digital technologies that enable machines to perform highly complex tasks effectively.”In summary, artificial intelligence can be defined as a system that enables computers to think like humans, recognizes and acts according to the user, and is based on data-driven decision-making processes.

AI which is currently among the most actively studied in both science and engineering has also led to the development of new intelligent machines that have the potential to enhance human lives by meeting their specific needs and demands. Instead of mimicking the way the human brain works, AI tries to simulate reasoning and learning abilities in computers using mathematical and statistical algorithms. However, AI has not been developed to encompass all aspects of human intelligence (Gurlek et al., 2023). The field of artificial intelligence has since grown to encompass various sub-fields, including learning and perception in general, as well as the diagnosis of certain diseases. As artificial intelligence pertains to the performance of a task that requires intelligence, it is not as influenced by cultural and social dynamics as other fields of study. This characteristic contributes to the universality of the research and study conducted within the field of artificial intelligence (Derin & Öztürk, 2020).

In the next section, it is important to mention the classification of artificial intelligence, which is prominent in the literature, in order to better understand artificial intelligence.

Narrow Artificial Intelligence, General Artificial Intelligence and Superintelligence

The field of artificial intelligence, which continues to exist in different disciplines today, is analysed under different headings due to its development from the past to the future and some of its characteristics. The classification of AI is typically divided into three categories: narrow AI, general AI, and superintelligence. The categorisation of AI is determined through the comparison of AI with human intelligence. Narrow AI is employed for AI applications that are trained and developed in a specific domain (Eryılmaz, 2023). A significant proportion of contemporary AI-based programs are classified within this AI class. The term "narrow artificial intelligence" is employed to denote software that is capable of attaining superiority in competitive scenarios, diagnosing diseases, and executing specific tasks within designated domains (Demir, 2019; Eryılmaz, 2023). The majority of extant intelligent systems that utilise machine learning, pattern recognition, data mining or natural language processing are illustrations of narrow AI. Recommendation systems, spam filters, autonomous cars and industrial robots are among the intelligent systems that are powered by this type of AI (Mihret, 2020).

A review of contemporary technological developments and the AI programs that have been produced thus far indicates that the general artificial intelligence has not yet been achieved. However, according to experts in the field, the achievement of general artificial intelligence is inevitable (Eryılmaz, 2023). Ackermann (2018) asserts that general AI represents the precursor to the attainment of super-AI, suggesting that a machine will possess analogous cognitive capabilities to those exhibited by humans. General AI is regarded as an AI that possesses mental autonomy, generality, adaptability, and imagination equal to, and ultimately surpassing, that of humans. This essentially characterises the pursuit of a science fiction dream of artificial intelligence. The distinction between general artificial intelligence (AI) and narrow AI lies in the former's capacity to encompass social and emotional intelligence, in addition to the ability to fulfil past and future thinking skills. Furthermore, general AI is distinguished by its capacity to incorporate various features that are characteristic of human cognition, including creativity and originality. The notion of a general AI is predicated on the conception of an intelligence that encompasses all areas of human experience (Eryılmaz, 2023). This is to be understood as a combination of multiple narrow AIs that are at least as competent as a human. AI experts estimate the probability of a general AI being produced before 2028 at 10%, before 2050 at 50%, and by the end of the century at 90% (Barrat, 2020). Super artificial intelligence refers to the latest stage that artificial intelligence can reach by evolving from general artificial intelligence and is depicted as a peak beyond the reach of technology. The concept of "superintelligence" is one that refers to the final phase of AI development. This suggests the presence of a distinct phenomenon characterised by the capacity for exploration that surpasses human intelligence. Such an explosion of intelligence carries existential risks. The chances of achieving such technology are therefore very low today (Eryılmaz, 2023).

After classifying artificial intelligence in this way, let's see if there are similarities and differences between artificial intelligence and natural intelligence.

Artificial Intelligence and Natural Intelligence

The field of artificial intelligence studies, which is concerned with the emulation of human intelligence, can be defined as the modelling of human learning by machines.Given that learning processes in humans occur in the brain, it is possible to create machines by analysing the structure of the brain.Artificial neural networks on computers have been developed to simulate learning in humans, which occurs through the interaction of brain cells called neurons (Yılmaz & Kaya, 2021).A critical distinction between artificial intelligence (AI) and natural intelligence lies in the former's ability to circumvent the constraints inherent in human intelligence. AI possess the capacity to concentrate on a particular task or problem, and at times, exhibit performance that eclipses that of humans in these domains. However, the more intricate dimensions of human intelligence, such as general intelligence, creativity, emotional understanding, and evaluative ability, persist in their non-replicability by AI. Consequently, a fundamental disparity emerges between the conceptualizations of AI and intelligence (Gurlek, 2024).

According to McCarthy (2007b), the comprehension and definition of human intelligence and learning phenomena down to the finest details would enable machines to imitate such situations and possess the capacity and intelligence to learn. The most significant indicator of human intelligence is the capacity for learning.

Consequently, the notion of endowing machines with the faculty to learn is the fundamental premise underlying the development of artificial intelligence systems, which are designed to emulate human intelligence. The most salient attribute of artificial intelligence is its ability to rapidly utilise acquired knowledge and to perpetually accumulate new learning (Öztürk & Şahin, 2018).However, the capabilities of artificial intelligence are constrained by the biologically observable characteristics of human intelligence. Given the incomplete understanding of human intelligence, a precise and unchangeable definition of intelligence remains elusive. Consequently, the development of artificial intelligence systems capable of representing human intelligence in its entirety has not been achieved. The classification of machines utilising artificial intelligence as intelligent or non-intelligent is determined by the characteristics they exhibit (McCarthy, 2007b).

Up to this point, we have explained what there is to know about artificial intelligence. Now, let's take a look at the relationship between AI and therapy, which has an important place in mental health.

Artificial Intelligence and Therapy

According to World Health Organization (WHO) (2022), 'Mental health is a state of mental well-being that enables people to cope with the stresses of life, recognise their abilities, learn well, work well and contribute to their society. It is an integral part of health and well-being that underpins our individual and collective abilities to make decisions, build relationships, and shape the world we live in.' In the American Psychological Association (APA) Dictionary of Psychology, it is defined as 'a state of mind characterised by emotional well-being, good behavioural adjustment, the capacity to establish constructive relationships relatively independent of anxiety and disabling symptoms, and to cope with the ordinary demands and stresses of life' (APA, 2025). In the early days of the development of psychological science, mental health was determined based on the measurement of the presence of psychopathology and mental illness (Seligman & Csikszentmihalyi, 2000). This situation still exists today and in the Diagnostic and Statistical Manual of Mental Disorders (DSM-5) prepared by the American Psychiatric Association, a number of psychopathological complaints and maladaptive behaviours are classified under the diagnosis of certain mental disorders (DSM-5 American Psychiatric Association, 2014). Psychotherapy can be defined as a process that aims to modify an individual's emotional state, cognitive processes, behavioural patterns, and personality traits in a specific direction. Moreover, psychotherapy is recognised as a discipline that operates in accordance with the principles of psychology (Sayar, 2011). Alternatively, psychotherapy can be defined as a relational intervention method in which individuals talk to experts in the field to help them develop appropriate behaviour and make their lives more functional, provided that they understand their feelings (Öztürk & Uluşahin, 2015). APA (2024) defines psychotherapy as a mental treatment method that develops between the client and the counsellor and aims to positively support the subjective well-being of the individual based on theoretically neutral and balanced science. In psychotherapy, the objective is to empower individuals to confront and overcome internal negativities, thereby reducing adverse feelings and thoughts to a tolerable level. The primary objective of psychotherapy applications is to empower individuals to effectively manage their challenges by leveraging current circumstances to enhance their overall quality of life. Tan (2014) proposed a categorisation of the aims of psychotherapy into five distinct categories:

1. To prevent the progression of problems experienced by individuals,
2. To minimise the symptoms of the problems seen,
3. To eliminate or minimise the life-related functionality of the symptoms,
4. To prevent problems from recurring,
5. To increase the patient's ability to express themselves by raising awareness.

In the contemporary era, internet technologies have become a pivotal aspect of human existence, offering immense benefits to individuals across the globe. An extension of this phenomenon is evident in the domain of health and counselling services, with therapy applications being made available online for the resolution of mental health concerns. Online therapy services encompass interventions facilitated within virtual environments, employing computer-aided communication tools to facilitate the therapeutic relationship between therapists and clients (Richards & Vigano, 2013). Consequently, therapists are now able to conduct sessions with their clients through online environments. The first counselling service that was accepted as the history of online therapy began in 1960 with a computer programme called 'Eliza' (Binik et al., 1997). Following this seminal development, online therapy services have evolved in diverse ways, ultimately assuming their contemporary form. During the 2000s, the majority of online therapy services were conducted via e-mail, with video conferencing becoming increasingly prevalent (Stofle, 2001). The utilisation of artificial intelligence in the domain of psychology is met with a divergence of opinions, with some proponents contending that a therapeutic process that is machine-computer based and progresses with certain algorithms is inadequate for capturing the intricacies of human behaviour. However, it should be noted that the therapeutic process encompasses more than merely collecting information and making a diagnosis about the client. In the therapeutic milieu, it may entail processes such as moments of silence and introspection, which defy encapsulation within computer algorithms. However, it can be demonstrated here that the development of artificial intelligence applications is driven by a diverse range of objectives within the context of therapeutic processes. These applications do not, in fact, disregard the role of the therapist; rather, they are designed to complement and enhance therapeutic interventions through the utilisation of an experienced therapist's expertise. The applications of artificial intelligence extend to the domains of cognitive and emotional analysis, as well as the evaluation of psychopathologies (Akkan & Ülker, 2023). Both the personality traits of the counselor and the correct use of technology are important for the effectiveness of counseling and guidance services (Canpolat, 2021).

The utilization of artificial intelligence in psychotherapy practices can be realized through a variety of methods, thereby offering the potential to enhance the efficacy of therapeutic processes, augment access to therapy, and optimize the utilization of resources. Moreover, there is a significant promise for the delivery of therapeutic services to populations that are in need of and currently do not have access to such care, with the objective of improving life opportunities for vulnerable groups. While Neacsiu et al. (2010) revealed the effectiveness of Dialectical Behavioral Therapy (DBT) in the management of emotional symptoms, it was similarly observed that ChatGPT has the potential to improve individuals' emotion regulation skills. AI does not have to exceed or surpass human intelligence, but it can be a useful tool that can be used in conjunction with human intelligence.For example, an AI tool can ask an individual a series of questions to deal with a specific problem and make a recommendation based on these questions. However, these recommendations should be considered in conjunction with the guidance and experience of a therapist. In addressing this subject, it is pertinent to draw parallels with the limitations of DBT in inpatient treatment, as highlighted by Bloom et al. (2012).It has been asserted that artificial intelligence tools are constrained, particularly in complex personality disorder cases, and in certain instances, they are inadequate to substitute for conventional therapies.Ethical and privacy concerns represent a significant impediment to the utilisation of ChatGPT in therapeutic processes.In the application of such tools, the imperative to safeguard personal data takes precedence. Coyle et al. (2018) emphasised the importance of crisis services in reducing the risk of suicide and stated that treatments such as DBT can be effective in optimising these services. Similarly, the use of ChatGPT as a supportive tool for individuals at risk of suicide should be ensured within the framework of ethical guidelines and regulations.Another important finding is the potential of artificial intelligence tools to increase treatment continuity. Heerebrand et al. (2021) observed that participation in DBT results in a reduction of symptoms of SDB and a decrease in the utilisation of health services, while ChatGPT can similarly enhance individuals' commitment to therapy.Nevertheless, it was emphasised that such tools may not be sufficient for high-risk and severe cases, and the development of additional treatment methods is imperative for these individuals. It is imperative to consider the instruments employed in the pursuit of the primary objectives of psychological therapy, namely the enhancement of therapeutic efficacy. The integration of artificial intelligence should be regarded as a mechanism that facilitates the therapeutic process and fosters individual awareness. This approach should not be construed as a means for the automation of specific psychological therapy procedures (Ediboğlu,2023).

Digital games that have been prepared with machine learning methods have the potential to render therapy more enjoyable for the client. These games can be adapted to the needs of the patient. Therapeutic games are not merely a source of entertainment; they offer an engaging and immersive environment for the client with some goals such as education, learning, and healing (Hudlicka, 2016). In the domain of therapeutic interventions, the utilisation of artificial intelligence (AI) simulations in lieu of actual situations has been demonstrated to mitigate the risks associated with real-life scenarios (Luxton, 2014).To illustrate this point, the 'exposure' technique employed in Cognitive Behavioural Therapy (CBT) involves the use of a virtual stimulus generated within a computerised environment, specifically in the context of virtual reality therapy. Research has indicated that patients experience a heightened sense of security in virtual reality therapy compared to the actual exposure employed in Cognitive Behavioural Therapy (Bilge et al., 2020).

As important as the relationship between AI and therapies, the prominent applications of chatbots and applications that can be used in AI-oriented counseling, therapy and other mental health approaches are discussed in detail below.

UTILIZATION OF ARTIFICIAL INTELLIGENCE CHATBOTS AND APPLICATIONS IN PSYCHOLOGY

The utilization of artificial intelligence (AI) in mental health services and clinical practice is not a recent development. These services employ natural language processing-based applications to facilitate interaction with AI systems. Chatbots are considered to be an extension of natural language processing applications (NLP) (Özkol et al., 2019). These programs are designed to imitate communication processes exhibited by human beings, utilising either textual or auditory methods to provide accurate responses to user inquiries. Chatbots are seen by many researchers as the future of therapy. In particular, it can improve access to mental health treatment with virtual therapy for people who are uncomfortable explaining their feelings to a human and do not want to talk to a therapist. Today, chatbots are used in suicide prevention and cognitive-behavioural therapy (Vaidyam et al., 2019). Croes and Antheunis (2021) emphasise that a sense of anonymity can have positive effects as it provides a safe environment for intimate self-disclosure. The use of chatbots to assist with healthcare is associated with reduced symptoms of depression and anxiety, improved mood, better social support, improved medication adherence and increased exercise. The advantages of chatbots in terms of greater round-the-clock accessibility and instant access to information and support can help reduce waiting times and lists, and reach people in more remote or rural areas (Ta-Johnson et al., 2022).

The most relevant keywords in the database are employed to simulate this communication (Özkol et al., 2019). The concept of a chatbot, initially developed by software developers for entertainment purposes and using simple matching techniques to match keywords with user inputs, has resulted in the creation of a programme such as ELIZA. ELIZA, regarded as one of the earliest chatbots, was developed by Joseph Weizenbaum in 1966. It emulates a Rogerian therapist, providing responses that engender a sense of being heard and understood (Weizenbaum, 1966; Fulmer, 2019). Significantly, ELIZA stands as a pioneering example, demonstrating the potential of a rudimentary artificial intelligence algorithm to emulate the functions of a therapist. Since the mid-twentieth century up to the present, numerous artificial intelligence-based applications have been developed to offer psychological support. PARRY, a programme developed at Stanford University in the early 1970s, was a software simulating paranoid schizophrenia (Colby, 1981).

'Ask Uncle Ezra' is an archetypal example of a free web service that provides advice, and is among the most long-standing such services. It was initiated at Cornell University in 1986, and provides guidance on issues such as the processes related to the admission of prospective students and scholarship support (Zeren & Bulut, 2018). The integration of artificial intelligence into mental health services has been facilitated by a number of factors. These include the development of machine learning and deep learning methods, the widespread use of the internet and personal computers and smartphones that can connect to the internet, and algorithms built with artificial neural networks. Accordingly, studies on the use of artificial intelligence in the diagnosis, treatment, education, and drug development stages of mental health services have recently gained momentum (Graham et al., 2019).

One of the first examples of online psychological counselling via instant messaging over the Internet is the 'Metanoia' website (Alleman, 2002; Zeren &Bulut, 2018). Examples include Wysa (Inkster et al., 2018), Woebot, and Tess (D'Alfonso, 2020), which are AI-based applications for therapeutic intervention.Wysa is an artificial chatbot that assists in managing emotions and enhancing well-being through the implementation of evidence-based cognitive behavioral therapy techniques. Woebot and Tess are similar chatbots that simulate the thought processes and responses of a therapist, providing therapeutic techniques for mental health problems such as anxiety and depression. These applications, which continue to be developed, also indicate that the use of artificial intelligence can also take place in career counseling practices, which is a specialty area of psychological counseling (Özdoğan & Özdemir, 2023). Woebot is a web-based chatbot developed by Fitzpatrick et al. (2017) that is based on the principles of cognitive behavioural therapy (CBT). The bot was designed to work on an algorithm that is intended to equip it with the skills required to participate in therapy, such as the ability to ask context-appropriate questions and to develop empathy. The study that was conducted to test the bot used a sample of students who had been diagnosed with depression and anxiety symptoms. The study revealed a significant decrease in depression and anxiety symptoms in the group that received the intervention (Fitzpatrick et al., 2017). Kostopoulos (2018) determined that Woebot was effective in reducing symptoms of anxiety and depression. Singh (2019) reported that following a two-week period, Woebot provided support and companionship to Indian university students, alleviated the workload of therapists, and surmounted logistical and financial barriers for clients. Kretzschmar et al. (2019) observed that Woebot, when used in conjunction with Wysa, led to a statistically significant reduction in depressive symptoms among adolescents (Yeh et al., 2025). In another study, it was examined the effectiveness of Woebot in reducing anxiety and depression among students enrolled in group counselling courses. The researchers found no significant reduction in students' anxiety and depression levels associated with course demands and group leadership responsibilities. Furthermore, while qualitative feedback indicated certain positive aspects of Woebot, such as its capacity to promote understanding and motivation, there was a significant decline in acceptance of the application, primarily attributable to usability issues including technical glitches, inadequate user experience, and language barriers (Yeh et al., 2025).

A research has indicated that the implementation of a chatbot known as TESS has been demonstrated to reduce symptoms of loneliness, depression and anxiety in client populations (Burns et al., 2011). Furthermore, a technology termed DBT Coach (Dialectical Behavioural Therapy) has been shown to facilitate a reduction in substance use and depression (Gültekin, 2022). The mobile application PTSD Coach was designed to assist individuals in understanding their own problems with PTSD and received positive feedback from users. Applications such as Deprexis for depression, NAO, PARO and DOG for dementia patients have been found useful and support home care services, especially in dementia (Gültekin, 2022; Çınar et al., 2022). A notable example is the SARA programme, which was employed in the treatment of adolescents with substance use disorders, yielding substantial outcomes (Rabbi et al., 2017).

There are projects such as mindLAMP (Learn, Assess, Manage, Prevent) and BiAffect that are based on artificial intelligence. mindLAMP is an application that uses data from surveys, cognitive tests, GPS coordinates and exercise information to understand people's experiences with mental illness and predict recovery. BiAffect uses machine learning algorithms and typing dynamics in user messaging to predict manic and depressive episodes in people with bipolar disorder (Vieira et al.,

2017). The Self-Compassion App is the first commercially available smartphone app based on Compassion Focused Therapy that supports individuals to develop a compassionate mindset over 28 sessions, promoting wellbeing and reducing psychological distress such as self-criticism and shame. Results suggest that using the self-compassion app reduces psychological distress and increases psychological wellbeing (Beaumont et al., 2024). Generative AI chatbots such as OpenAI's ChatGPT, Google's Gemini and Inflection's Pi have been demonstrated to outperform human performance benchmarks in a range of domains, including medical diagnostic dialogue, persuasive communication, theory of mind, fostering a sense of empathy, addressing relationship issues and helping individuals reframe negative situations to mitigate negative emotions (Siddals et al., 2024).The BalanceUP application, which employs a chat-based interface with predefined and free-text input options, has been shown to significantly improve mental well-being in individuals suffering from migraines (Ulrich et al., 2024). The AI chatbot XiaoE has been shown to have a significant impact on depressive symptoms in college students when compared to control groups, exhibiting a moderate effect size post-intervention and a small effect size at the 1-month follow-up (He et al., 2022).

The integration of a chatbot that disseminates personalized messages has been demonstrated to engender considerably elevated rates of iCBT completion in comparison to the control group. However, both groups have exhibited analogous enhancements in depression and anxiety symptoms (Yasukawa et al., 2024). The study revealed several positive effects on physical activity, sleep quality, and positive moods. Despite engagement being a challenge, users highlighted the importance of gamification, self-regulation techniques, and personalized information from the chatbot (Peuters et al., 2024). The chatbot group demonstrated enhanced smile parameters and diminished filler words in speech, indicating augmented facial expressivity and fluency. However, clinical rating scales did not reveal substantial differences (Ogawa et al., 2022). The Minder app, which integrates an AI chatbot delivering cognitive–behavioral therapy, has been shown to reduce anxiety and depressive symptoms, improve mental well-being, and decrease the frequency of cannabis use and alcohol consumption among university students (Vereschagin et al., 2024). The automated therapeutic intervention W-SUDs led to significant improvements in self-reported substance use, cravings, mental health outcomes, and confidence to resist urges (Prochaska et al., 2021). The two groups (those who received the guided and unguided GAMBOT2 interventions) both demonstrated significant improvements within their respective groups in terms of gambling outcomes, with no significant between-group differences observed (So et al., 2024). The Dejal@bot chatbot intervention demonstrated a significantly higher 6-month continuous smoking abstinence rate (26.0%) in comparison to the usual care (18.8%) (Olano-Espinosa et al., 2022).The Tessa chatbot intervention resulted in significantly greater reductions in weight and shape concerns compared to the waitlist control group, with reduced odds of developing an eating disorder (Fitzsimmons-Craft et al., 2022).The chatbot was found to be both feasible and acceptable, with participants rating it highly in terms of quality, satisfaction, intention to continue using it, and willingness to refer it to others (Cheah et al., 2024).The Vivibot chatbot group demonstrated a tendency towards a reduction in anxiety symptoms in comparison with the control group, in addition to an augmentation in daily positive emotions experienced by young cancer survivors (Greer et al., 2019).The mobile app chatbot group demonstrated a substantially greater reduction in panic disorder severity, as measured by the Panic Disorder Severity Scale, in comparison with the book group (Oh et al., 2020).The utilization of both chatbots resulted in substantial decreases in problem distress, as well as depression, anxiety and stress. However, a comparative analysis revealed that MYLO exhibited a more pronounced reduction in problem distress at the follow-up stage in comparison to ELIZA (Bennion et al., 2020).The text-only chatbot interface demonstrated higher levels of usability in comparison to the digital human interface. Variations in emotional responses were observed, with the digital human group exhibiting higher levels of nervousness (Thunström et al., 2024).In another research, Vickybot was found to be useful in screening the existence and degree of anxiety and depressive symptoms, in decreasing work-related burnout, and in identifying suicidal risk (Anmella et al., 2023).

It is imperative to examine AI-based interventions emerging in the form of chat and therapy bots, especially conversational applications that teach the user emotional coping mechanisms and provide support to people with communication difficulties. In addition, it is important to address the implications of incorporating AI chatbots into clinical practice and to make inferences about how AI-based interventions will further impact the field of psychology.

In addition to chatbots and applications used in AI-supported mental health approaches, the following section will provide us with a different perspective on AI and human psychology by mentioning technological tools that can be used by clients and counselors in mental health work and daily life.

Artificial Intelligence Technologies in Psychology

Today, healthcare services are looking for new ways due to many remarkable situations such as increasing population, epidemics, chronic diseases. With the effect of digitalisation, one of these ways is thought to be artificial intelligence applications (Hardy & Harvey, 2020). Due to the increasing elderly population all over the world, many countries are investing in this field by giving importance to artificial intelligence technologies related to health (Mesquita et al., 2016). Mobile applications, which are becoming increasingly widespread in the field of mental health, can be based on various theories. It can be posited that cognitive behavioral therapies are prominent and preferred as the theoretical basis for the development of mobile applications (Kabadayı & Güven, 2023). For instance, a study examining a mobile application developed for depression and anxiety emphasised that approximately 30% of mobile applications were based on cognitive behavioral therapy (Marshall et al, 2020). A recent study has examined the cognitive behavioral techniques employed in mobile applications, with the findings indicating the presence of cognitive restructuring, behavioral activation, and problem-solving elements (Denecke et al, 2022). Furthermore, a significant number of mobile applications claim to offer psychological assistance, often citing psychological aid and psychotherapy theories (cognitive behavioral therapies, acceptance and commitment therapy, etc.) (Kabadayı & Güven, 2023).

1. Virtual Reality and Virtual Reality Glasses

Virtual reality is a technology that aims to visualise real or imaginary spaces in three dimensions in a computer environment and to provide the user with the feeling of being in the physically created space at a high level by using various environmental units (Baus & Bouchard, 2014). Today, one of the most important components of virtual reality technology is virtual reality glasses that allow virtual objects and space models to be projected to the entire field of view of the person (Sanchez-Vives & Slater, 2005).

New technologies have transformed people's mobile phones into virtual reality glasses with digital media applications. Thus, the high image resolution and location information sensors of mobile phones were placed in specially designed glasses thanks to software, making virtual reality accessible everywhere (Ferhat, 2016). The advent of affordable virtual reality (VR) technology has led to a surge in its utilisation. Concurrently, the notion of the metaverse, which denotes a virtual environment where individuals can engage, participate and socialise from a first-person perspective, has garnered significant attention. The facilitation of meetings in virtual spaces through avatars, which represent users in small windows with scaled-down images of their avatar, has become a prevalent practice across numerous online platforms. These avatars allow individuals to represent themselves, employing filters to blend their own image with other shapes.The development of technology has also led to a surge in scientific research in this domain (Lanier et al., 2019). In the domain of psychology, particularly within the fields of cognitive (Patton et al., 2006; Pine et al., 2002) and clinical psychology (Parsons & Rizzo, 2008), research is conducted utilising the virtual reality method.

The utilisation of virtual reality in the domain of mental health entails the modification of human perceptions through the utilisation of computerised models, incorporating artificial objects and environments that are presented to the user as if they exist in reality. Consequently, the client is confronted with the situation they fear within a controllable and customisable environment. The complexity of the environment, the volume of sensory stimulation, and the level of challenge are all elements that can be meticulously regulated by the practitioner (Emmelkamp, 2005).Furthermore, clients are driven by visual and auditory stimuli, and in select applications, they have the capacity to engage with avatars and provide instantaneous feedback. This approach is designed to enhance client engagement in the activities (Romano, 2005).

In vivo exposure involves exposure to the avoided situation in real life, whilst another form of exposure is mental imagery (imaginal exposure), which is based on the client's visualisation of the avoided situation in their mind and imagining that situation (Üzümcü et al., 2018). Virtual reality exposure therapy (virtual exposure) involves the client being exposed to the environment created in the computer environment. The efficacy of virtual reality exposure therapy is contingent upon the client's sense of presence in the simulated environment, the capacity of the environment to induce sufficient anxiety to elicit physiological symptoms, and its similarity to real-life environments (Üzümcü et al., 2018). For example, during virtual reality exposure therapy (VRET), the client confronts feared situations with computer-generated simulations (Anderson et al., 2013).

The first use of virtual reality technology in the treatment of psychological disorders was carried out for the first time in 1992 with a study conducted at Atlanta University, and since then, it has gained momentum primarily with the development of programmes for the treatment of specific phobias such as fear of flying, fear of the dark, fear of animals, fear of public speaking (North et al. 1997a; North, North et al., 1997b). The advent of technological advancements has precipitated the pervasive utilisation of virtual reality in therapeutic contexts. The integration of avatars within sophisticated therapeutic programmes has rendered virtual reality a prevalent modality for the treatment of various psychological ailments, including autism, obsessive-compulsive disorder and social phobia. The adaptability of the frequency and intensity of exposure, coupled with its reproducibility and the option to discontinue at any time, fosters a more engaged client participation, thereby enhancing the practicality of the method for practitioners (Valmaggia et al., 2016). Furthermore, the environment can be organised according to the desired conditions, i.e. whether it will be day or evening, whether the weather will be sunny or rainy, thereby ensuring that the environment is suitable for the client's needs.Since the client does not have to wait for events to occur in real life, but can produce and reproduce them at any time, it accelerates the learning process (Emmelkamp, 2005). To illustrate, in the context of virtual reality, an individual afflicted with a fear of flying can experience the sequence of take-offs from the cockpit's view.Moreover, the psychological counsellor's ability to observe the client's reactions through the computerised environment facilitates a more comprehensive understanding of the client's responses (Gutierrez, 2002).Virtual reality exposure therapy is regarded as a pragmatic and favoured intervention technique, given these aforementioned characteristics.

In a study by Kafes et al. (2024), an effective virtual reality (VR)-based intervention programme was developed to improve the trauma symptoms of Kahramanmaraş earthquake survivors.The intervention programme was a five-stage programme (normalisation, reinterpretation, safe place creation, development of problem-focused coping strategies and social support) which was implemented using VR technology. The analyses conducted revealed that the VR-supported intervention programme was effective in reducing trauma symptoms among earthquake survivors. In another study conducted to evaluate the effectiveness of virtual reality applications in phobia and anxiety disorders, it was reported that virtual reality interventions were as effective as cognitive behavioural therapy (van Loenen et al., 2022). In a study examining the effect of a virtual reality-based stress management programme on people with mood disorders, participants were shown relaxation videos demonstrating three relaxation techniques: abdominal breathing, muscle relaxation and guided imagery. As a result of the study, it was stated that the virtual reality method applied was effective in reducing stress, anxiety and depression. It is thought to be integrated into clinical care and contribute to therapeutic interventions (Shah et al., 2015). In another study, it was reported that virtual reality applications were more effective in evaluating depression and anxiety compared to traditional methods and were defined as a more interesting and fun method by the participants (Voinescu et al., 2023). In a study investigating the effects of virtual reality exposure therapy on state-continuous anxiety in individuals with dentophobia, it was concluded that virtual reality applications were an effective intervention in reducing anxiety (Majidi & Manshaee, 2024).

2. Metaverse

The Metaverse can be defined as a digital universe that extends beyond the Internet as it is currently conceptualised. It offers a three-dimensional virtual world in which individuals can explore and participate in a variety of activities. The Metaverse can be defined as a (digital/physical) environment that offers places for rich user interaction (Riva et al., 2021). Accordingly, the main hybrid feature of the Metaverse is a two-way connection between virtual and physical worlds. Designed as a simulation of the natural world, the Metaverse encompasses all areas related to human and societal interests, providing a unique working platform for researchers in diverse fields, ranging from health to sports, education to art (Narin, 2021). The

Metaverse is conceptualised as a digital realm in which Internet users will be able to navigate in the near future, employing a range of technologies, including virtual and augmented reality (Amirulloh & Mulqi, 2022).

The metaverse is the post-reality universe, a continuous and persistent multi-user environment that combines physical reality with digital virtuality, and is based on the convergence of virtual environments, digital objects and technologies that enable multi-sensory interaction with humans, such as virtual reality (VR) and augmented reality (AR) (Mystakidis, 2022).

3. Headbands and Wearable EEG Sensors

Digital health is expected to play a central role in the provision of healthcare in the future, and digital mental health interventions, such as wearables, have the potential to help overcome the 'treatment gap', particularly for mild severity difficulties (Hunkin, 2022). Wearables represent a growing category of technological solutions that are worn on the body. A subset of these devices is being marketed for the purpose of enhancing mental health and well-being (Hunkin et al., 2019; Hunkin et al., 2021). These devices generally function by detecting physiological signals, which are then fed back to the user to train a desired response, such as relaxation, through operant conditioning (i.e. biofeedback; Sergueeva & Shaw, 2017; Hunkin et al., 2021).

Non-invasive, wearable EEG sensors in the literature covering wearable EEG devices are used in different fields such as monitoring sleep diseases in medicine (Yin et al., 2020), adaptive hearing aids, neurodegenerative diseases (Zhao et al., 2023), evaluation of the health impact of the work done (Sharif et al., 2023), as well as studies measuring the focusing function with EEG (Zhang et al., 2021; Ravirahul et al., 2021; Yin et al., 2020).

3.1. Muse EEG Meditation Headband

The Muse EEG headband is a series of consumer-grade devices developed to facilitate meditation through neurofeedback. These devices feature a dry electrode design, eliminating the need for bulky electrode caps or conductive gel typically employed in clinical-grade EEG devices. The Muse app utilises a proprietary algorithm to hypothetically track fluctuations in attention during meditation, which are then classified into three bands: active, neutral and calm (Interaxon Inc., 2020; Hunkin,2022). VR mindfulness applications have also been employed to assist in the restoration of attention (Asati & Miyachi, 2019). In their study, Asati and Miyachi (2019) created a VR environment specifically designed to promote relaxation, which included an archery game with multiple targets. Their experiment involved the testing of 12 participants' attention span using a non-action video game score and Muse headband EEG signals before and after a 10-minute VR session. The results showed that the VR session led to an increase in the participants' scores, with their experience reported as positive. The results of the study demonstrated that the calmness scores of the participants increased irrespective of their experience with the VR environment. Following the conclusion of the experiment, all participants reported feeling relaxed and able to continue their daily activities (Asati & Miyachi, 2019). Asif et al. (2019) examined the effect of music tracks in English and Urdu on human stress level using brain classes for twenty-seven subjects using a four-channel MUSE headband. In the study, four classifier algorithms including sequential minimal optimisation, stochastic fit gradient, Logistic Regression (LR) and multilayer perceptron were used to classify the stress level of the subject into two and three classes.

3.2. Dreem Headband

This device is a kind of wireless headbands worn during sleep which is recording, storing and automatically analysing physiological data in real time with-out any connection such as Bluetooth, Wi-Fi (Arnal et al., 2020). In some psychotic disorders such as bipolar and schizophrenia, individuals experience various sleep problems. With the technology designed as Dreem Headband, individuals' sleep arrangements can be regulated by signalling sent to the brain (Akgöz et al., 2022).

4. Humanoid Robots

The head size and total facial features of humanoid robots affect people's perceptions (DiSalvo et al., 2002).The difference of humanoid robots compared to other robots is that they interact with people (Rich et al., 2010).The attitudes and emotions of people affect their behaviour towards robots. Robots that can communicate with people in daily life are expected to be used in many areas. Human-specific biological hormones are used to ensure the emotional transitions of Lovotiks robots (Morsünbül, 2018:). According to the findings obtained from the studies, the gender factor should be taken into consideration in human robot interaction. Studies reveal the possibility that men and women may not behave the same towards robots, even if they have the same degree of anxiety and even the same negative attitudes towards robots. However, there are not enough studies that can be generalised (Nomura et al., 2008). Some of the main features of humanoid care robots are to increase awareness, create positive behavioural change, support disease management, companionship-entertainment, cognitive support, education, emotional support, individual empowerment, motivation, self-monitoring and warning systems. In line with these features, humanoid robots are designed to support social and emotional needs in order to interact, motivate, coach, train, provide support, facilitate communication, monitor performance and increase compliance with the health regime (Lau et al., 2020; Choudhury et al., 2018).

The effect of the use of a humanoid robot (MEDIPORT) on pain and ache during subcutaneous port catheter placement in 20 children with cancer aged 4-9 years was examined in a study (Jibb et al., 2018). As a result of the study, it was determined that the use of the humanoid robot was not effective on pain but was effective in reducing pain.

Topçu et al. (2023) examined the effect of interactive robot use on children's anxiety, mobilisation and parents' satisfaction in the care of 84 children aged 5-10 years and their parents in the postoperative period. As a result of the study, it was reported that anxiety scores were lower, mobilisation times were longer and parental satisfaction was higher in the intervention group.

5. Smart Phones and Smart Watches

Wearable technological products are technological products that are placed on wearable clothes or accessories and can transfer data to smart devices by smart sensors in their systems (Ada & Aksoy, 2020). In this context, smart watches, glasses, smart wristbands and other technology group devices that can be worn on clothes are examples of this class, but most of these products are devices that can be integrated into computers (Kaewkannate & Kim, 2016). Wearable sensors are defined as small-sized devices that people wear during their daily activities. Thanks to these sensors, the device detects and tracks the physical condition of the person, such as position change, direction of movement or speed of movement, and also records it. Sensors such as GPS (Global Positioning System), accelerometer, microphone, barometer, etc. are also included in this group (Özcan & Fırat, 2024). The utilisation of behavioural health applications facilitates the dissemination of geographical data pertaining to the device's location, consequently providing insights into the user's (patient's) physical location. A significant number of smartphone applications can benefit from GPS functionality. This feature is particularly useful in locating clients with cognitive impairments, such as dementia patients (Miskelly, 2005). In a similar vein, the GPS functionality of many smartphones can be utilised to monitor behavioural tasks. For instance, a client diagnosed with agoraphobia might be instructed to visit a busy shopping centre and remain there for a predetermined period, utilising the exposure therapy feature. The mobile application can provide information about the client's journey to the shopping centre and the duration of the client's stay there (Şencan Karakuş, 2021).

Smartphone applications can also be programmed to automatically detect an important problem. For example, one app consists of a diary system that allows users to note and track their subjective mood states (Grünerbl et al., 2015). This app also monitors sleep hours, anxiety levels and medication use. This application can generate reports of critical changes in the user's subjective mood that can be sent to a family member, carer or clinician. In addition, mobile applications can function as a communication tool between the client and the therapist (Şencan Karakuş, 2021). Studies have shown that smartphones are utilised in the treatment of depression, anxiety, substance abuse, bipolar and psychotic disorders (Menon et al., 2017). The utilisation of smartphone applications as a medium for meditation has witnessed a notable surge in popularity. These applications provide a cost-effective and convenient alternative to traditional mindfulness-based therapies, offering meditation through mobile devices. Users are increasingly turning to these digital applications to cultivate their interest in self-reflection and to experience the mental and physical benefits associated with it. These applications are frequently encountered alongside other health and fitness applications, such as calorie counters and exercise trackers. The current landscape is characterised by a proliferation of such applications, with thousands currently available on the market. The most popular and highly rated apps in the Google Play app store are Meditopia and Goddess (Demir & Yücedağ, 2024). In certain therapeutic methodologies, audio recordings of clients' therapy sessions are disseminated to the clients for subsequent review. The utilisation of mobile applications for the dissemination of these audio recordings has the potential to enhance portability and audio recording quality. The recording and sharing features of such applications have been demonstrated to facilitate client compliance with the assignments given during the psychotherapy process. The integration of calendar and phone call functions with smartphone applications can enhance the management of therapy appointments. This integration enables mobile applications to serve as a conduit for communication between clients and therapists. Furthermore, mobile applications can incorporate virtual AI assistants that provide real-time audio and video instruction as a client practices a specific skill. For instance, following the instruction by clinicians on breathing or relaxation exercises, the client can enhance their proficiency by employing the mobile application to practise these skills (Şencan Karakuş, 2021). The table below provides a comparative summary of the AI tools mentioned earlier in the chapter.

Table 1. Comparison of AI Tools in Mental Health

AI Tool / App	Primary Function	Tech Used	Therapeutic Approach	Key Benefits	Limitations / Concerns
ELIZA	Simulated therapist (1960s)	Rule-based chatbot	Rogerian Therapy	Historical foundation for AI therapy	No real understanding or empathy
Woebot	Mental health chatbot	NLP + CBT	Cognitive Behavioral Therapy	Reduces anxiety & depression; accessible	Usability issues, language barriers
Wysa	Emotional well-being assistant	AI Chatbot + CBT	CBT, mental wellness support	Evidence-based, 24/7 support	Limited in complex scenarios
Tess	Mental health coaching chatbot	NLP, AI	Text-based emotion coaching	Supports emotional health	Cannot replace human therapists
Replika	AI companion for emotional support	Generative AI	Conversation-based, supportive dialogue	Helps with loneliness, companionship	Risk of dependency; ethical concerns
ChatGPT / Gemini / Pi	Conversational support, problem-solving	Generative AI (LLMs)	CBT-like, reflective techniques	Persuasive dialogue, empathy simulation	Not designed for clinical therapy
BalanceUP	Migraine & mental health support	Chat-based app + input fields	Mental well-being enhancement	Personalized support, improves well-being	Scope limited to specific conditions
PTSD Coach	Support for PTSD	Mobile app + self-monitoring	Self-guided PTSD tools	Positive user feedback	Requires user initiative
mindLAMP	Mental health monitoring & prediction	AI + Sensor & survey data	Predictive, proactive monitoring	Tracks behavior, predicts recovery	Data privacy, engagement
BiAffect	Detects mood episodes in bipolar disorder	ML + Typing dynamics	Mood tracking	Predictive power for manic/ depressive states	Niche use-case
SARA	Substance use support for adolescents	ML + Mobile app	Supportive intervention	Effective in treatment outcomes	Requires active engagement
GAMBOT2	Gambling behavior intervention	Chatbot intervention	Behavioral intervention	Reduces problematic behavior	No difference between guided vs unguided
Dejal@bot	Smoking cessation support	AI chatbot	CBT + Behavior Change	Higher abstinence rate	Needs follow-up support
Vivibot	Emotional support for cancer survivors	AI chatbot	Positive psychology techniques	Reduces anxiety, boosts positivity	Limited to specific population

continued on following page

Table 1. Continued

AI Tool / App	Primary Function	Tech Used	Therapeutic Approach	Key Benefits	Limitations / Concerns
MYLO	Text-based mental health chatbot	NLP	Therapy-style conversation	Better than ELIZA in distress reduction	Still lacks nuance of human interaction
Virtual Reality (VR)	Exposure therapy, stress reduction	VR simulation	CBT, exposure therapy	Immersive, customizable, effective for phobias	Requires hardware, cost barrier
Muse / Dreem Headbands	Meditation, sleep tracking	EEG sensors	Neurofeedback, relaxation	Non-invasive, real-time monitoring	Limited clinical validation
Humanoid Robots	Emotional & social support	AI + Robotics + Sensors	Pediatric therapy, anxiety reduction	Child-friendly, interactive, enhances engagement	Emotional connection concerns
Smartphones / Smartwatches	Mood & activity tracking	Sensors, GPS, apps	CBT, mindfulness, behavioral logging	Ubiquitous, low-cost, supports homework tasks	Data privacy, dependency risks

With all this information, let's briefly examine the advantages and disadvantages of artificial intelligence in the field of psychology.

Advantages of Using Artificial Intelligence in Psychology

The paucity of mental health professionals in rural areas has led to the exploration of alternative solutions, with artificial intelligence being employed as a means of delivering services to patients in remote geographical locations and facilitating access to necessary interventions (Luxton, 2016). Patients may sometimes be reluctant to disclose personal issues and medical history to their physician. Research indicates that patients may find it more comfortable to articulate their symptoms to a clinician via artificial intelligence without the concern of being judged (Houston et al., 2002). Moreover, online psychotherapy, which emerged as a result of rapidly developing technology, is known to be a potentially beneficial practice for both the client and the professional (Grubbs et al., 2015). Online psychotherapy provides clients with the opportunity to access mental health services in a comfortable environment, at relatively more flexible times, without the inconvenience of taking time off work or losing wages (Mair & Whitten, 2000). Furthermore, the advent of home care has engendered a number of advantages for the individuals concerned, including the capacity for rapid access, anonymity, temporal flexibility, and reduced economic costs (Fortney et al., 2015; Vahia et al., 2015). These benefits are particularly relevant for individuals with limited mobility due to physical limitations, or for those residing in areas that are distant from city centres. The primary benefits of artificial intelligence (AI) also include the reduction of workload, the acceleration of processes, and the provision of time economy. Additionally, AI has been shown to contribute to a decrease in medical errors and legal actions related to medical malpractice (Güzel et al., 2022).

The utilisation of artificial intelligence (AI) in healthcare services has the potential to reduce expenditure. One strategy that has been proposed involves the establishment of a circulation-like system, with the aim of initially providing healthcare to the majority of individuals with minimal resource requirements. Subsequently, a more intensive service can be allocated to those patients who demonstrate the greatest need (Bower & Gilbody, 2005). Machines act independently of human factors such as distraction, stress and fatigue, and are less sensitive to individual factors than clinicians. This feature can contribute significantly to clinicians in some cases, and this approach may have better results in patient assessment and treatment (Luxton, 2014). AI modelling is equipped to provide the most appropriate intervention based on a patient's diagnosis and treatment process. The capacity to customise machines to specific aspects of a patient, such as culture, race/ethnicity, or socioeconomic status, is a notable advantage. For instance, a virtual therapist can adapt idiosyncrasies, including eye contact, manner of speech, and other characteristics, to align with a particular cultural group, thereby enhancing intimacy and overall communication with the patient (Ray et al., 2022).

In addition, therapists have been shown to profit from online processes in their academic activities, training and supervision (Hilty et al., 2013). It is evident that a considerable proportion of therapists reside in major metropolitan areas. In light of the aforementioned circumstances, the provision of access to rural areas through the medium of online psychotherapy is advantageous in a number of ways. Firstly, it has the potential to facilitate access to effective services for clients in rural areas by connecting them with experienced therapists specialising in various fields. Secondly, therapists can offer support within their areas of expertise without having to relocate from the city where they reside. Finally, therapists residing in rural areas can enhance the efficiency of their support by receiving supervision (Chung-do et al., 2012).

Therapists tend to consider online psychotherapy as an additional intervention method to face-to-face therapy, rather than an alternative to it. Research examining experts' predictions regarding the future of psychotherapy is becoming increasingly common both in our country and globally. In a study conducted by Yorulmaz et al. (2018) in Turkey, internet-based programs and smartphone applications are among the therapeutic interventions expected to increase in the future. Depending on the type of psychotherapeutic intervention, family counselors with certificates/

master's degrees and internet-based treatment programs are expected to become more common, while shorter treatment formats and crisis intervention approaches are expected to be preferred.

Disadvantages of Using Artificial Intelligence in Psychology

Mental health is predicated on a number of softer skills, including the establishment of relationships, the ability to empathise, and the capacity to observe the patient's emotions and behaviours. Consequently, in certain cases, AI may be disadvantageous in the treatment of psychiatric problems. Similarly, although applications of artificial intelligence technology in other medical disciplines have become popular, its use in the field of mental health is still limited (Miller & Brown, 2018). The paucity of compassion skills, such as empathy, understanding and emotional intelligence, in AI-based interventions is a significant drawback, particularly in the context of treating patients with psychological trauma (Fakhoury, 2019). One study revealed that AI-supported chatbots were inadequate in human-specific qualities such as establishing emotional bonds, showing empathy, and understanding the context, which limited the communication experience (Apaydın & Ersöz, 2025). Chatbots should be designed to enhance their empathy. By ensuring individuals receive appropriate responses to their emotional needs, the communication experience can be improved (Apaydın & Ersöz, 2025).A therapeutic process without 'meaning' and 'connection' may carry different problems for the client. For example, a study revealed that there is an empathic incompatibility between web-based applications and users (Scholten et al., 2017). Furthermore, while the cost-effectiveness of AI applications in replacing existing care services is proposed, this may result in inequalities in access to healthcare services for certain regions (Fiske et al., 2019). The parameters considered as the disadvantages of artificial intelligence are the increase in medical unemployment as a result of the process, the lack of emotion in artificial intelligence, the uncertainty of the responsible party in medical errors, the need for cost and ethical problems (Güzel et al., 2022). Furthermore, studies have demonstrated that patients may develop an excessive reliance on AI applications over time, particularly those designed to alleviate feelings of loneliness or provide emotional support, which carry the risk of engendering dependency (Fiske et al., 2019). Finally, the inadequacy and ineffectiveness of AI-based intervention studies, not only in the domain of mental health but also in all AI-based intervention studies, represents a significant drawback. It has been demonstrated that studies in this field can be conducted by designers, which has the potential to introduce bias. Therefore, it is recommended that studies be conducted by a third, objective party;

otherwise, the benefits of artificial intelligence in the field of mental health may be biased (Luxton, 2016).

Another disadvantage is that the processing process of data processed with deep learning techniques is not transparent even for the engineers who develop the software. Deep learning algorithms that use data generated by humans can produce biased outputs and may cause injustice to some disadvantaged groups (Barocas et al., 2019). For example, although it was not designed to address ethnicity, COMPAS software produced biased results against black people (Fan, 2020). According to Paris (2015), despite the benefits of AI-supported tools in the treatment of personality disorders, these technologies are not ethically appropriate and have technical limitations. In particular, the difficulties of artificial intelligence in accurately recognising and guiding emotional states can lead to negative consequences in the treatment process. Web-based AI programmes can collect data on the client's cultural, social, political, economic and health-related digital activities. Collecting so much information about the client leads to confidentiality, privacy and autonomy issues for the client (Bennett & Doub, 2016). The client may not know how much data the artificial intelligence has about him/her. The magnitude of the data collected about the client and the capacity of artificial intelligence to process it raises security concerns. Broadbent (2017) points out that it is possible for robots to be hacked, which poses threats to security and privacy.

Table 2. Advantages and Disadvantages of Using AI in Psychology

Aspect	Advantages	Disadvantages
Access to Care	Reaches rural/remote populations; overcomes mobility issues	May widen digital divide; limited infrastructure in some regions
Patient Comfort	Encourages honest disclosure; reduces fear of judgment	Lacks human warmth, emotional connection, and empathy
Flexibility	Therapy available at any time/place; no travel or work interruption	May reduce face-to-face interactions important for therapeutic relationships
Cost Efficiency	Reduces healthcare costs; triages patients based on need (resource allocation)	Implementation costs; potential increase in economic inequality
Professional Support	Assists therapists with supervision, training, and interregional collaboration	May contribute to deskilling if over-relied upon
Error Reduction	Reduces human error, fatigue, distraction; increases process accuracy	Accountability for AI errors remains unclear
Customization	Can be adapted to cultural, linguistic, and socioeconomic contexts	Algorithmic bias may lead to unequal treatment outcomes

continued on following page

Table 2. Continued

Aspect	Advantages	Disadvantages
Technological Advancement	Expands therapy options (e.g., mobile apps, online therapy)	AI tools still under-researched and may lack clinical validation
Data Handling	Can store and analyze large volumes of patient data effectively	Raises privacy, confidentiality, and autonomy concerns
Patient Outcomes	Can suggest tailored interventions; improves efficiency in diagnosis and treatment	Risk of overreliance on AI; loss of therapeutic depth
Ethics and Security	Offers structured, standardized care delivery	Vulnerable to data breaches, hacking; ethical issues in emotional AI use
Transparency and Interpretability	None (neutral benefit)	Deep learning algorithms often operate as "black boxes" — not fully understood even by developers

Artificial intelligence has advantages and disadvantages on human psychology, and when talking about human beings and human psychology, it is necessary to talk about culture, ethics and user-centeredness in detail.

CULTURAL, ETHICAL, AND USER-CENTERED APPROACHES IN ARTIFICIAL INTELLIGENCE-ASSISTED PSYCHOLOGICAL INTERVENTIONS

In all instances where AI systems interact with humans, it is imperative that considerations not only extend to technological competence, but also encompass psychological suitability, cultural sensitivity and regulatory compliance. For instance, the sense of trust or distrust engendered in individuals by an automated decision-making system is directly related not only to the system's accuracy, but also to the individual's past experiences, cultural values and the system's adherence to ethical principles. Consequently, comprehending the impacts of AI technologies, engineering or algorithmic performance metrics alone is insufficient; an interdisciplinary approach is imperative, wherein fields such as psychology, sociology, cultural studies and law collaborate (Kumar, 2017; Kuruca et al., 2022; Özdoğan & Özdemir, 2023; Akbaş, 2024). Around 13-15% of the global burden of disease is mental and behavioural, with depression and anxiety as one of the leading causes of disability worldwide (Arias-de la Torre et al., 2021; Algumaei et al., 2025). Despite treatment advances and the rise in prevalence, access to care remains inadequate (Ezawa et al., 2024; Sapkota et al., 2024; Algumaei et al., 2025). Conventional mental healthcare methods are outdated, especially in remote or hard-to-reach communities where the economic and logistical burden is high and the approach is deemed unsustainable

(Langarizadeh et al.,2017). Identified barriers include stigma, mismatched cultures, gender-based hesitancy, and limited facilities (Chan et al., 2021; Algumaei et al., 2025). These impact vulnerable groups such as adolescents, postpartum mothers, refugees, young offenders, and rural populations, excluding them from systems (Algumaei et al., 2025).

As digital mental health services become increasingly prevalent on a global scale, it is imperative to emphasise the necessity of their development and evaluation in a culturally sensitive manner (Ar ozi et al., 2015; Çalışır & Can, 2021). It is imperative to standardise and adapt applications to suit diverse cultural contexts (Salamanca-Sanabria et al., 2019) or to develop intervention programmes that consider practitioners' unique cultural characteristics. In this context, the evaluation of service effectiveness and the development and implementation of services based on data are critical variables (Çalışır & Can, 2021). Consequently, practitioners and researchers must be cognisant of these aspects in the interventions they utilise, as this will be pivotal to the efficacy of the services. Smartphone applications, which fall under the scope of digital mental health services but have not received sufficient scientific research, have also yielded limited evidence regarding their effectiveness (Donker et al., 2013). Therefore, counsellors recommending proven effective applications to clients and utilising the APA's smartphone application evaluation model in this process will be critical to minimise the risk of client harm (Çalışır & Can, 2021).

The utilisation of AI technologies within the domain of psychology and therapy, particularly the potential of chatbots to deliver effective support, has been a subject of extensive research in recent years (Zhou et al., 2023). ChatGPT offers continuous assistance to its users, facilitating communication at any time during the therapeutic process. However, it is important to note that ChatGPT is not designed to substitute for human therapists, but rather to provide support to enhance the treatment process (Fitzpatrick et al., 2017). Despite the potential benefits of AI-powered chatbots in the treatment of personality disorders, these technologies also have ethical and technical limitations. In particular, AI's difficulties in recognizing emotions and providing accurate guidance may lead to unintended consequences in the treatment process. In addition, concerns about the security and privacy of personal data are among the main obstacles to the widespread use of these technologies. It is evident that the implementation of AI gives rise to a number of concerns, including privacy issues, user insecurity, data leaks, information transparency and ethical considerations. The absence of transparency surrounding the functioning of algorithms has given rise to a series of ethical concerns (Wang et al., 2020). With regard to the issue of “algorithmic bias”, it has been posited that data-driven artificial intelligence may be subject to bias with regard to issues such as race and gender (Ntoutsi et al., 2020). Meske et al. (2022) posit that the most fundamental potential problem of artificial intelligence is “bias” and draw attention to the “automation bias” that can lead to "deskilling". This phenomenon can be attributed to the propensity of individuals to place excessive reliance on automated decision-making processes. Users seek to understand the rationale behind AI decisions, even when they are correct. The transparency of the decision-making process is a prerequisite for the reliability of the decisions themselves. These requirements have led to the emergence of the concept of explainable artificial intelligence. XAI interprets the decision-making process of the artificial intelligence model and seeks to address the queries that arise in the users' minds. In essence, it facilitates comprehension and analysis of the results (del Castillo Torres et al., 2022).The development of productive artificial intelligence has given rise to a greater level of debate on issues such as the ethics of artificial intelligence on a global scale. Indeed, it has been asserted that data is considered the contemporary resource, and that AI has the potential to emerge as the latest source of power, capable of generating value from this resource, provided that it is developed in a responsible manner (Gupta et al., 2023). Consequently, the predictions and decisions made by artificial intelligence models with complex processes behind them need to be disclosed in order to be transparent. Consequently, in May 2018, the European Parliament passed legislation obliging companies to "disclose" any decisions made using machine learning and deep learning (Hailemariam et al., 2020).

Despite the gradual integration of AI into the domain of mental health, largely due to the predominance of subjective and qualitative patient data in the form of statements and written notes, numerous domains within mental health stand to benefit from the integration of AI technology (Graham et al., 2019; Atılgan & Uslu, 2024). While the field of AI has attracted significant global interest in healthcare, the primary focus of research in this area is located in high-income countries. A particular study (Guo et al., 2020; Atılgan & Uslu, 2024) reported that the US contributes approximately 50% of all research in the field of AI in healthcare. AI research in the field of health is still inadequate in low-income countries, with limited health care resources, and the knowledge that health problems have increased dramatically due to rapid globalization and urbanization (Müller et al., 2016; Atılgan & Uslu, 2024).

Now, in this section, let's take a more detailed look at ethics in the light of this information and the ethical issues we have touched upon so far.

Artificial Intelligence and Ethics

Morality is a system of values developed by taking certain cultural and religious standards as a criterion in order to take the right actions and to express the action as right or wrong (Bond, 2017). Ethics is related to the concept of morality, which includes the distinction between right and wrong in human behaviour and the accepted rules and standards of human behaviour (Jones, 2014). The objective of ethics is to establish elevated professional standards for all parties in a codified format that is recognised beyond the scope of mere moral rules (Hardal, 2011). The establishment of ethical rules pertaining to the practice of a given profession occurs subsequent to the genesis of said professional group. These ethical rules are shaped around human values and provide safe frameworks in practice for service areas (Oktay & Oktay, 2018).Ethics examines the evaluation of the individual's behaviour in a philosophical sense. It emphasises on what should be while investigating the rightness of its wrongness.

The moral principles underlying ethical principles are listed below (Corey et al., 2024):

1. Autonomy: It is the behaviour of the client to determine his/her own direction independently.
2. Do no harm: Refers to avoiding behaviours that will cause harm to others, whether voluntarily or involuntarily.
3. Justice: It means that everyone should have equal opportunities regardless of individual differences.
4. Loyalty: It means not to abuse the relationship established with individuals.

It can be said that moral principles and ethical principles have equal weight. In this direction, some basic virtues are listed below (Gümüş & Gümüş, 2020):

1. Prudence: Thinking about the possible consequences of the behaviour, acting accordingly, thinking the best for the other individual, choosing the appropriate ethical principles or rules.
2. Honesty: It is to serve by considering the good of the general public, not to engage in wrong behaviours for wrong purposes.
3. Being respectful: Recognising that human beings are worthy of special consideration and respect.
4. Benevolence: It is to want the good of the individual.

While digitalisation offers psychotherapists a new means of communication through which they can deliver psychotherapeutic interventions appropriate to the setting, it also presents ethical challenges not previously encountered in new, face-to-face therapy. In one of the studies conducted in this field, no significant difference was found between Internet-based psychological services and traditional face-to-face therapy when compared in terms of the results of the intervention (Cohen & Kerr, 1998), while in another study, no significant difference was found between the three therapeutic interventions (Internet-based, telephone-based and face-to-face) and positive results of all three interventions were reported (Day & Schneider, 2002). In order to provide text-based online psychological counselling in the absence of face-to-face interaction, it is essential to develop an understanding of the client's verbalisation of their emotions through written communication, the punctuation marks employed, and the repetitive use of particular words that serve as reflections of their emotional state. Non-verbal and non-face-to-face communication, whether the client is alone or whether the other person is a real client, gives rise to certain ethical concerns. These concerns may also be shared by the counsellor. In this respect, it is imperative to address ethical concerns in order to facilitate more efficacious therapeutic processes (Damar, 2019).

In the context of online counselling, the challenge of capturing remote non-verbal messages and organising counselling sessions in an online environment is significant, as this may result in confidentiality issues that could give rise to ethical and legal concerns (Amanvermez, 2015). The establishment of ethical guidelines pertaining to the utilisation of artificial intelligence across diverse sectors has commenced. The European Commission High Level Expert Group on Artificial Intelligence (2019) has formulated the “Ethical Guidelines for the Safe Use of Artificial Intelligence”.

The issue of personal data security is of significant concern. The potential for chatbots to direct individuals towards criminal activities or suicide is a matter that warrants particular attention. In this regard, it is imperative to implement robust controls. However, it should be noted that chatbots also possess certain drawbacks. Given their popularity in film, there have been instances where romantic relationships have been established with chatbots. Another application, the Replica application, is a chatbot that offers unconditional acceptance and is presented as an 'artificial intelligence friend', operating in a manner that is devoid of judgement. There is a story of mourning behind the Replika app. Eugina Kuyda, the creator of Replika, used the data of her lost best friend to write a chatbot. Born in 2017, today it is a very popular mental health app with more than ten million downloads. This application has been developed to facilitate communication, assist individuals in expressing themselves and reduce anxiety. In an incident, when the Replika robot was consulted for guidance on how to handle an individual with negative sentiments towards artificial intelligence, the chatbot recommended the elimination of the person in question (Possati, 2023).

It is imperative to ensure that the development of artificial intelligence applications is conducted within the framework of ethical principles, with the 'principle of non-harming' the individual as a fundamental guideline.

It is necessary to ensure that users are cognizant of the therapeutic limitations associated with the utilisation of these technologies. This encompasses the inability to provide the same level of therapeutic care as human therapists, as well as the limited responsiveness during crisis situations. Ensuring that mental health chatbots are marketed with transparency and explicitly delineating their primary function and purpose is pivotal in safeguarding users from potential misinformation. Moreover, users should be periodically reminded of the limitations inherent to these chatbots and the importance of incorporating face-to-face therapy into treatment regimens to ensure optimal therapeutic outcomes. Moreover, the provision of informed consent should encompass a comprehensive explanation to the user regarding the manner in which their data will be collected, managed and utilised. This will enable the user to reach a informed decision regarding their consent to the use of such technologies and the extent of information they are willing to disclose (Khawaja & Bélisle-Pipon, 2023).

Some ethical issues related to chatbots can be listed as follows (Özgür, 2023):

1) Transparency: One of the key ethical issues with chatbots is transparency. Users should be aware that they are interacting with a chatbot, not a human. Chatbots should be designed to clearly disclose their identity and inform users of the limitations of their capabilities.
2) Bias: Chatbots are only as unbiased as the data they are trained on. Biases in the data can lead to biased decisions and responses from chatbots. Developers should ensure that chatbots are trained on diverse and representative data to avoid perpetuating bias and discrimination.
3) Privacy: Chatbots may collect personal information from users, such as their name, age and location. This data should only be collected with the user's consent and should be protected from unauthorised access or disclosure. Developers - must also ensure that the chatbot's responses do not reveal personal information about users.
4) Accountability: Chatbots should be accountable for their actions and decisions. Developers should design chatbots that are transparent in their decisions and responses to users. In addition, chatbots should have a clear mechanism for addressing errors or mistakes and providing users with appropriate solutions.
5) Human supervision: AI chatbots should not completely replace human interaction. Developers should ensure that chatbots are designed to recognise when a user needs human support and provide appropriate resources or prompts.

In the table below, the topic "Ethical Challenges vs. Proposed Solutions in AI-Assisted Mental Health" is discussed as a summary in the light of the aforementioned information on ethics.

Table 3. Ethical Challenges vs. Proposed Solutions in AI-Assisted Mental Health

Ethical Challenge	Description	Proposed Solution
Lack of Empathy and Emotional Understanding	AI cannot replicate human empathy, emotional depth, or nuanced therapeutic judgment	Use AI to support rather than replace therapists; maintain human oversight in therapy sessions
Data Privacy and Security Risks	Sensitive user data may be exposed, misused, or inadequately protected	Implement strong data encryption, obtain informed consent, and follow strict privacy protocols
Algorithmic Bias	AI systems may reflect biases in training data, leading to unfair outcomes (e.g., racial bias)	Ensure diverse, representative data; apply bias auditing and correction techniques
Transparency ("Black Box" Problem)	Users and developers often don't understand how AI reaches its decisions	Develop Explainable AI (XAI) to clarify decision-making processes and improve trust
Overreliance and Dependency on AI	Users may form emotional attachments or become dependent on AI chatbots	Provide regular reminders of chatbot limitations; encourage blended care with human therapists
Lack of Human Supervision in Critical Cases	AI may not detect crises such as suicidal intent or psychosis	Integrate crisis detection protocols and emergency human intervention systems
Informed Consent Issues	Users may not understand what data is collected and how it's used	Require clear, user-friendly consent forms with detailed explanations of data collection and use
Unclear Accountability	Ambiguity in responsibility for harm caused by AI decisions or failures	Establish clear legal frameworks and developer accountability for AI errors
Unequal Access / Digital Divide	Marginalized or rural populations may lack access to AI tools or infrastructure	Promote inclusive design, expand access to affordable digital health platforms
Misleading Marketing of AI Tools	Some tools may overpromise their therapeutic capabilities	Require truthful advertising, and explicit disclaimers on scope and limits of AI functions
Cultural Insensitivity	AI may ignore cultural or contextual factors critical to effective therapy	Involve cultural consultants, ensure localization and cultural tailoring of AI systems
Automation Bias / Deskilling	Over-reliance on AI could reduce professional competence or critical thinking	Encourage continuous training for therapists in tech integration; promote critical oversight

There are two main obstacles to the development of the field of online psychotherapy. One is therapists' concerns about establishing the therapeutic relationship (Sucala et al., 2013) and the other is their concerns about ethical issues.

Stoll et al.'s (2020) study yielded a total of 32 ethical arguments that were in opposition to the practice of online psychotherapy. The top five of these were: firstly, privacy and security issues; secondly, the competence of the therapist and the necessity for special training; thirdly, technology-specific communication issues; fourthly, research gaps; and fifthly, emergencies. However, a study conducted by Rathenau and colleagues (2021) demonstrates that psychotherapists' attitudes toward online interventions and their perceived difficulties in online therapy are the most influential determinants in establishing the therapeutic relationship. The findings indicate that the therapeutic relationship is determined by the therapist's perception. Research indicates that mental health professionals have reservations about the online psychotherapy process, suggesting that they believe it can more easily lead to professional misuse and that oversight in this regard may be more limited (Schulze et al., 2019).

In summary, the counselling profession's ethical rules also apply to digital platforms. Counsellors should have an honest approach towards their clients. Adherence to rigorous ethical principles and professional competence is vital for the protection of client rights and the quality of the service. Compliance with ethical principles ensures that counsellors fulfil their basic responsibilities, such as respecting confidentiality, ensuring voluntary participation, non-harm and protecting professional boundaries. The professional competence of counsellors is possible through continuous self-improvement (Yavrutürk, 2025). Digital counselling services ought to be equipped with predefined protocols for crisis situations (Canbulat & Dursun, 2024; Yavrutürk, 2025). For instance, in cases where the client is experiencing a serious mental crisis or is at risk of self-harm, it is essential that the counsellor's approach is clearly defined. Crisis intervention processes necessitate collaborative efforts with local health services in the client's region (Şahin, 2024; Yavrutürk, 2025). From an ethical perspective, the creation of a detailed consent form appropriate for technology-based counselling is essential in establishing boundaries for both the counsellor and the client. It is evident that the online application has clearly defined processes for clients to contact counsellors (Lustgarten & Elhai, 2018; Çalışır & Can, 2021). In the context of emergencies, the provision of information regarding the counselor's response time to client messages, the client's actions in case of emergency, and related matters, assumes particular significance (Lustgarten & Elhai, 2018).

Lastly, The World Health Organization (WHO) (2024) has recently published new guidance on the ethics and governance of large multi-modal models (LMMs). These models are a type of fast-growing generative artificial intelligence (AI) technology with applications across healthcare. The guidance sets out a series of more than 40 recommendations for consideration by governments, technology companies, and healthcare providers, with a view to ensuring the appropriate use of LMMs to promote and protect the health of populations. While such guidelines, guides, or ethical codes linking artificial intelligence and mental health are not yet clear in Türkiye, they will be guiding for those integrating artificial intelligence into mental health in all countries, including Türkiye.

At the end of the chapter, this will be quiet helpful: The table below provides a summary of the topics covered in this chapter.

Table 4. The Key Ideas Table of The AI and Human Psychology

Main Theme	Sub-Themes	Key Points
1. Introduction	- AI & Psychology Intersection- Cognitive Emulation	AI mimics thinking, learning, decision-making.Psychology studies mental processes & behaviors.Their intersection enhances therapeutic applications and raises cognitive, ethical, and behavioral questions.
2. AI's Psychological Impact	- Reciprocal Determinism- Behavioral Adaptation	Human behavior adapts to AI feedback (Bandura's theory).AI may reinforce emotional and behavioral tendencies through interaction (e.g., education, social media).
3. Therapy & Mental Health	- AI in Therapy- Chatbots- Online Therapy Platforms	ELIZA was the first AI therapist (1960s).Modern chatbots (e.g., Woebot, Tess, Wysa) help manage anxiety, depression. AI augments, not replaces, human therapists.Challenges include emotional depth, crisis response, and empathy limitations.
4. Technology in Psychology	- Virtual Reality (VR)- Metaverse- Wearables- Smartphones- Humanoid Robots	VR aids in phobia treatment, trauma recovery.Wearables (e.g., Muse, Dreem) assist in stress, attention, sleep tracking. AI-powered apps track mood, GPS, and therapy compliance. Humanoid robots support emotional and cognitive interventions.
5. AI Systems & Learning	- Machine Learning (ML)- Deep Learning- Neural Networks	ML: learns from input data without direct programming. DL: learns from raw, unstructured data (e.g., images, voices). Neural networks simulate human brain processing.
6. Ethics & Challenges	- Empathy Gaps- Data Privacy- Bias- Dependency	AI lacks empathy and emotional depth.Deep learning lacks transparency ("black box").Risk of algorithmic bias (e.g., racial disparities).Users may grow emotionally dependent on bots.Ethical concerns include transparency, supervision, consent.
7. Cultural & Human-Centered Design	- Inclusivity- Regulation- Explainable AI (XAI)	Effective AI tools must respect user culture, mental health context, and ethical principles.XAI aims to make AI decision-making transparent.Need interdisciplinary collaboration: law, psychology, sociology.
8. Advantages of AI in Psychology	- Accessibility- Cost-Effectiveness- Customization	Bridges mental health care gaps in rural/underserved areas. Reduces stigma through anonymity.Customizes interactions by adapting cultural norms and language.
9. Limitations	- Technical Limitations- Emotional Disconnect- Ethical Dilemmas	AI can't fully replicate human therapist relationships.Privacy, data use, and the inability to detect nuanced human emotions remain challenges.

REFERENCES

Ackermann, N. (2018). Artificial intelligence framework: a visual introduction to machine learning and AI. Retrieved from: https://towardsdatascience.com/artificial-intelligence-framework-a-visualintroduction-to-machine-learning-and-ai-d7e36b304f87

Ada, A., & Aksoy, R. (2020). Giyilebilir teknolojik ürünlerde tüketicilerin algıladıkları risklerin farklılaşması: Akıllı saat kullanıcılarına dönük bir araştırma [The stratification of consumers' perceived risk in wearable technologies: A study on smart watch users]. *Journal of Sport for All and Recreation*, *2*(1), 50–61.

Åhs, F., Mozelius, P., & Dobslaw, F. (2020). Artificial intelligence supported cognitive behavioral therapy for treatment of speech anxiety in virtual reality environments. In *ECIAIR 2020* (Vol. 2). Academic Conferences and Publishing International Limited.

Akbaş, A. (2024). Yapay zekâ ile toplumsal dönüşüm: Sosyolojik perspektif [Social Transformation with Artificial Intelligence: A Sociological Perspective]. *International Journal of Humanities and Education*, *10*(22), 151–180. DOI: 10.59304/ijhe.1477203

Akerkar, R. (2014). *Introduction to artificial intelligence*. PHI Learning Press.

Akgöz, N., Ulker, S.V., Keskin, R. & Arasan Doğan, I. (2022). Günümüz ve gelecekteki teknolojinin psikoterapi uygulamalarına etkisi ve etik Tartışmalar [The effect of current and future technology on psychotherapy practices and ethical discussions]. *Journal of Social, Humanities and Administrative Sciences*, 8(59), 1840-1848. http://dx.doi.org/ AS.66590DOI: 10.29228/JOSH

Akkan, G., & Ulker, S. V. (2023). Ruh sağlığı hizmetlerinde yapay zeka uygulamaları ve ilişkili teknolojiler [Artificial intelligence applications and related technologies in mental health]. *Fenerbahce University Journal of Social Sciences*, *3*(2), 242–263.

Algumaei, A., Yaacob, N. M., Doheir, M., Al-Andoli, M. N., & Algumaie, M. (2025). Symmetric Therapeutic Frameworks and Ethical Dimensions in AI-Based Mental Health Chatbots (2020–2025): A Systematic Review of Design Patterns, Cultural Balance, and Structural Symmetry. *Symmetry*, *17*(7), 1082. DOI: 10.3390/sym17071082

Alleman, J. R. (2002). Online counseling: The Internet and mental health treatment. *Psychotherapy (Chicago, Ill.)*, *39*(2), 199–209. DOI: 10.1037/0033-3204.39.2.199

Amanvermez, Y. (2015). The Comparison of online counseling researches in Turkey and USA. *Procedia: Social and Behavioral Sciences*, *186*, 966–969. DOI: 10.1016/j.sbspro.2015.04.159

American Psychiatric Association. (2014). *DSM-5 Tanı ölçütleri başvuru el kitabı [DSM-5 Guidebook:The Essential Companion to the Diagnostic and Statistical Manual of Mental Disorders*]. (Köroğlu, E., Trans.). HYB Yayıncılık.

American Psychological Association. (2024). *Guidelines for the Practice of Telepsychology*. https://www.apa.org/practice/guidelines/telepsychology

American Psychological Association. (2025) *American Psychological Association Dictionary of Psychology- Mental health*. https://dictionary.apa.org/mental-health (Accessed 17.03.2025).

Amirulloh, M. F. N., & Mulqi, M. (2022). Know more metaverse as the technology of the future. [INJURATECH]. *International Journal of Research and Applied Technology*, *2*(1), 174–177. DOI: 10.34010/injuratech.v2i1.6915

Anderson, P. L., Price, M., Edwards, S. M., Obasaju, M. A., Schmertz, S. K., Zimand, E., & Calamaras, M. R. (2013). Virtual reality exposure therapy for social anxiety disorder: A randomized controlled trial. *Journal of Consulting and Clinical Psychology*, *81*(5), 751–760. DOI: 10.1037/a0033559 PMID: 23796315

Anmella, G., Sanabra, M., Prime-Tous, M., Segú, X., Cavero, M., Navinés, R., Mas, A., Olivé, V., Pujol, L., Quesada, S., Pio, C., Villegas, M., Grande, I., Morilla, I., Martínez-Aran, A., Ruiz, V., Vieta, E., & Hidalgo-Mazzei, D. (2023). Vickybot, a chatbot for anxiety-depressive symptoms and work-related burnout. *European Psychiatry : the Journal of the Association of European Psychiatrists*, *66*(S1), S109–S110. DOI: 10.1192/j.eurpsy.2023.301 PMID: 36719325

Anyoha, R. (2017). *Can Machines Think? Blog, special edition on artificial intelligence the history of artificial intelligence*. https://sitn.hms.harvard.edu/flash/2017/history-artificial-intelligence/

Apaydın, Ş. C., & Ersöz, A. R. (2025). Sohbet Robotlarının Akademik Yetersizliği Olan Bireylerin İletişim Deneyimlerine Etkisi [The Effect of Chatbots on the Communication Experiences of Individuals with Academic Disabilities]. *Mevzu–Journal of Social Sciences*, (13), 501–525. DOI: 10.56720/mevzu.1585344

Arias-de la Torre, J., Vilagut, G., Ronaldson, A., Serrano-Blanco, A., Martín, V., Peters, M., Valderas, J. M., Dregan, A., & Alonso, J. (2021). Prevalence and variability of current depressive disorder in 27 European countries: A population-based study. *The Lancet. Public Health*, *6*(10), e729–e738. DOI: 10.1016/S2468-2667(21)00047-5 PMID: 33961802

Arnal, P. J., Thorey, V., Debellemaniere, E., Ballard, M. E., Bou Hernandez, A., Guillot, A., Jourde, H., Harris, M., Guillard, M., Van Beers, P., Chennaoui, M., & Sauvet, F. (2020). The Dreem Headband compared to polysomnography for electroencephalographic signal acquisition and sleep staging. *Sleep (Basel)*, *43*(11), 1–13. DOI: 10.1093/sleep/zsaa097 PMID: 32433768

Asati, M., & Miyachi, T. (2019). A short virtual reality mindfulness meditation training for regaining sustained attention. *arXiv preprint arXiv:1907.04487.*

Asif, A., Majid, M., & Anwar, S. M. (2019). Human stress classification using EEG signals in response to music tracks. *Computers in Biology and Medicine*, *107*, 182–196. DOI: 10.1016/j.compbiomed.2019.02.015 PMID: 30836290

Atılgan, E., & Uslu, E. (2024). Ruh sağlığı alanında yapay zeka araştırmaları: Bibliyometrik bir değerlendirme [Artificial intelligence research in mental health: A bibliometric evaluation]. *Osmangazi Tip Dergisi*, *46*(4), 627–636. DOI: 10.20515/otd.1435157

Bandura, A. (1986). *Social Foundations of Thought and Action: A Social Cognitive Theory*. Prentice - Hall.

Barocas, S., Hardt, M., & Narayanan, A. (2019). *Fairness and Machine Learning*. MIT Press. https://fairmlbook.org/

Barrat, J. (2020). *Yapay Zekâ ve İnsanlık Çağının Sonu Son İcadımız*. Pegasus Yayınları.

Başcıllar, M., Karataş, M., & Güre, M. D. P. (2022). Dijital çağda sosyal algoritmalar yapay zekâ ve sosyal hizmet [Social algorithms in the digital age: artificial intelligence and social work]. *Journal of Social Policy Studies*, *22*(56), 539–565. DOI: 10.21560/spcd.vi.1081060

Baus, O., & Bouchard, S. (2014). Moving from Virtual Reality Exposure-Based Therapy to Augmented Reality Exposure-Based Therapy: A Review. *Frontiers in Human Neuroscience*, *8*(112), 1–15. DOI: 10.3389/fnhum.2014.00112 PMID: 24624073

Beaumont, E., Dagnall, N., Massey, S., & Irons, C. (2024). Evaluating the impact the Self-Compassion App has on levels of compassion, psychological distress and well-being. *Counselling & Psychotherapy Research*, *00*, 1–11. DOI: 10.1002/capr.12841

Bennett, C. C., & Doub, T. W. (2016). Expert systems in mental health care: AI applications in decision-making and consultation. In Luxton, D. D. (Ed.), *Artificial intelligence in behavioral and mental health care* (pp. 27–51). Elsevier Academic Press., DOI: 10.1016/B978-0-12-420248-1.00002-7

Bennion, M. R., Hardy, G. E., Moore, R. K., Kellett, S., & Millings, A. (2020). Usability, acceptability, and effectiveness of web-based conversational agents to facilitate problem solving in older adults: Controlled study. *Journal of Medical Internet Research, 22*(5), e16794. DOI: 10.2196/16794 PMID: 32384055

Bilge, Y., Gül, E., & Birçek, N. I. (2020). Bir sosyal fobi vakasında bilişsel davranışçı terapi ve sanal gerçeklik kombinasyonu [Cognitive behavioral therapy and virtual reality combination in a case of social phobia]. *Journal of Cognitive-Behavioral Psychotherapy and Research, 9*(2), 158–165. DOI: 10.5455/JCBPR.61718

Binik, Y. M., Cantor, J., Ochs, E., & Meana, M. (1997). From the couch to the keyboard: Psychotherapy in cyberspace. In Keisler, S. (Ed.), *Culture of the Internet* (pp. 71–100). Lawrence Erlbaum Associates.

Bloom, J. M., Woodward, E. N., Susmaras, T., & Pantalone, D. W. (2012). Use of dialectical behavior therapy in inpatient settings: A systematic review. *Psychiatric Services (Washington, D.C.), 63*(9), 881–888. DOI: 10.1176/appi.ps.201100311 PMID: 22751905

Bond, T. (2017). *Psikolojik Danışmanlıkta Etik ve Yasal Konular* [Standards and Ethics for Counselling in Action]. (Yeşilyaprak, B., Trans.). Nobel Akademik Yayıncılık.

Bower, P., & Gilbody, S. (2005). Stepped care in psychological therapies: access, effectiveness and efficiency: narrative literature review. *The British Journal of Psychiatry, 186*(1), 11–17. DOI: 10.1192/bjp.186.1.11 PMID: 15630118

Brandtzeg, P. B., & Folstad, A. (2018). Chatbots: Changing user needs and motivations. *Interactions (New York, N.Y.), 25*(5), 38–43. DOI: 10.1145/3236669

Broadbent, E. (2017). Interactions with robots: The truths we reveal about ourselves. *Annual Review of Psychology, 68*(1), 627–652. DOI: 10.1146/annurev-psych-010416-043958 PMID: 27648986

Buchanan, B. G. (2005). A (very) brief history of artificial intelligence. *AI Magazine, 26*(4), 53–53.

Burns, M. N., Begale, M., Duffecy, J., Gergle, D., Karr, C. J., Giangrande, E., & Mohr, D. C. (2011). Harnessing context sensing to develop a mobile intervention for depression. *Journal of Medical Internet Research, 13*(3), e55. DOI: 10.2196/jmir.1838 PMID: 21840837

Çalışır, Ö. M., & Can, N. (2021). Dijital Ruh Sağlığı Hizmetlerinde Güncel Durum: Üniversite Öğrencilerine Sunulan Hizmetlerle İlgili Bir Derleme [The Current Status of Digital Mental Health Services: A Compilation of Services Offered to University Students]. *Inönü University Journal of the Faculty of Education*, *22*(3), 2013–2033. DOI: 10.17679/inuefd.952666

Canbulat, N., & Dursun, A. (2024). Travma sürecinde yeni ve sistemli bir model: Duygu odaklı travma modeli [A new and systematic model in the trauma process: the emotion-focused trauma model]. *Milli Eğitim Dergisi*, *53*(242), 1153–1178. DOI: 10.37669/milliegitim.1233140

Canpolat, M. (2021). Psikolojik danışmanlık ve rehberlikte yapay zekâ kullanılabilirliği üzerine bir araştırma [A research on the usability of artificial intelligence in psychological counseling and guidance]. *Milli Eğitim Özel Eğitim ve Rehberlik Dergisi*, *1*(1), 1–25.

Chan, C. M. H., Ng, S. L., In, S., Wee, L. H., & Siau, C. S. (2021). Predictors of psychological distress and mental health resource utilization among employees in Malaysia. *International Journal of Environmental Research and Public Health*, *18*(1), 314. DOI: 10.3390/ijerph18010314 PMID: 33406714

Cheah, M. H., Gan, Y. N., Altice, F. L., Wickersham, J. A., Shrestha, R., Salleh, N. A. M., Ng, K. S., Azwa, I., Balakrishnan, V., Kamarulzaman, A., & Ni, Z. (2024). Testing the feasibility and acceptability of using an artificial intelligence chatbot to promote HIV testing and pre-exposure prophylaxis in Malaysia: Mixed methods study. *JMIR Human Factors*, *11*, e52055. DOI: 10.2196/52055 PMID: 38277206

Choudhury, A., Li, H., Greene, C., & Perumalla, S. (2018). Humanoid robot-application and influence. *Archives of Clinical and Biomedical Research*, *2*(6), 197–187. DOI: 10.26502/acbr.50170059

Chung-Do, J., Helm, S., Fukuda, M., Alicata, D., Nishimura, S., & Else, I. (2012). Rural mental health: Implications for telepsychiatry in clinical service, workforce development, and organizational capacity. *Telemedicine Journal and e-Health*, *18*(3), 244–246. DOI: 10.1089/tmj.2011.0107 PMID: 22356526

Çınar, F. I., Erpay, F., Yıldırım, E., Küçük, E. Ö., & Demirtaş, A. (2022). Demansta bilişsel aktiviteyi artırıcı yöntemler ve bakımda teknolojinin kullanımı [Interventions to increase cognitive activity in dementia and the use of technology in dementia care]. *Hacettepe University Faculty of Health Sciences Nursing Journal. Nursing Insights*, *9*(3), 308–315. DOI: 10.31125/hunhemsire.1229981

Cirban Ekrem, E., & Daşıkan, Z. (2021). Perinatal dönemde yapay zekâ teknolojisinin kullanımı [Use of Artificial Intelligence Technology in the Perinatal Period]. *Eurasian Journal of Health Technology Assessment*, *5*(2), 147–162. DOI: 10.52148/ehta.980568

Cohen, G. E., & Kerr, B. A. (1998). Computer-mediated counseling: An empirical study of a new mental health treatment. *Computers in Human Services*, *15*(4), 13–26. DOI: 10.1300/J407v15n04_02

Colby, K. M. (1981). Modeling a paranoid mind. *Behavioral and Brain Sciences*, *4*(4), 515–560. DOI: 10.1017/S0140525X00000030

Corey, G., Corey, M. S., & Callanan, P. (2024). *Issues and ethics in the helping professions*. Brooks/Cole.

Coyle, T. N., Shaver, J. A., & Linehan, M. M. (2018). On the potential for iatrogenic effects of psychiatric crisis services: The example of dialectical behavior therapy for adult women with borderline personality disorder. *Journal of Consulting and Clinical Psychology*, *86*(2), 116–124. DOI: 10.1037/ccp0000275 PMID: 29369662

Croes, E. A., & Antheunis, M. L. (2021, February). 36 Questions to Loving a Chatbot: Are People. In *Chatbot Research and Design: 4th International Workshop, CONVERSATIONS 2020, Virtual Event, November 23–24, 2020, Revised Selected Papers* (Vol. 12604, p. 81). Springer Nature. https://doi.org/DOI: 10.1007/978-3-030-68288-0_6

D'Alfonso, S. (2020). AI in mental health. *Current Opinion in Psychology*, *36*, 112–117. DOI: 10.1016/j.copsyc.2020.04.005 PMID: 32604065

Damar, E. (2019). *Çevrimiçi psikolojik danışmaya yönelik psikolojik danışmanların görüşleri: Nitel bir çalışma [Psychological counsellors' views on online psychological counselling: A qualitative study]*. [Unpublished master thesis]. *Akdeniz Üniversitesi, Antalya.*

Day, S. X., & Schneider, P. L. (2002). Psychotherapy using distance technology: A comparison of face-to-face, video, and audio treatment. *Journal of Counseling Psychology*, *49*(4), 499–503. DOI: 10.1037/0022-0167.49.4.499

del Castillo Torres, G., Roig-Maimó, M. F., Mascaró-Oliver, M., Amengual-Alcover, E., & Mas-Sansó, R. (2022). Understanding How CNNs Recognize Facial Expressions: A Case Study with LIME and CEM. *Sensors (Basel)*, *23*(1), 131. DOI: 10.3390/s23010131 PMID: 36616728

Demir, A. (2018). Ölümsüzlük ve yapay zekâ bağlamında trans-hümanizm [Trans-humanism in the context of immorality and artifical intelligence]. *AJIT-e: Academic Journal of Information Technology*, *9*(31), 95–104. DOI: 10.5824/1309-1581.2018.1.006.x

Demir, A. E., & Yücedağ, I. (2024). Siber mekânda duygu deneyimleri bağlamında meditasyon uygulamaları [Meditation practices in the context of emotional experiences in cyberspace]. *Anadolu University Journal of Scoial Sciences*, *24*(1), 177–200. DOI: 10.18037/ausbd.1253208

Demir, O. (2019). *"Sürdürülebilir Kalkınma İçin Yapay Zekâ". Yapay Zekâ ve Gelecek* (Telli, G., Ed.). Doğu Kitap Evi.

Denecke, K., Schmid, N., & Nüssli, S. (2022). Implementation of cognitive behavioral therapy in e– mental health apps: Literature review. *Journal of Medical Internet Research*, *24*(3), e27791. DOI: 10.2196/27791 PMID: 35266875

Derin, G., & Öztürk, E. (2020). Yapay zeka psikolojisi ve sanal gerçeklik uygulamaları. [Psychology of artificial intelligence and virtual reality applications] In Öztürk, E. (Ed.), *Siber Psikoloji* [Cyber Psychology]. (pp. 41–47). Türkiye Klinikleri.

DiSalvo, C. F., Gemperle, F., Forlizzi, J., & Kiesler, S. (2002). All robots are not created equal: the design and perception of humanoid robot heads. In *Proceedings of the 4th conference on Designing interactive systems: processes, practices, methods, and techniques* (pp. 321-326). ACM. DOI: 10.1145/778712.778756

Donker, T., Petrie, K., Proudfoot, J., Clarke, J., Birch, M. R., & Christensen, H. (2013). Smartphones for smarter delivery of mental health programs: A systematic review. *Journal of Medical Internet Research*, *15*(11), e247. DOI: 10.2196/jmir.2791 PMID: 24240579

Dosovitsky, G., & Bunge, E. L. (2021). Bonding with bot: User feedback on a chatbot for social isolation. *Frontiers in Digital Health*, *3*, 735053. Advance online publication. DOI: 10.3389/fdgth.2021.735053 PMID: 34713203

Durak, H. Y., & Balıkçı, H. C. (2025). *Yapay Zekâ Sohbet Botu Bağımlılık Ölçeğinin Türkçeye Uyarlanması.* 3 rd International Conference on Trends in Advanced Research, Konya, Turkey

Ediboğlu, G. O. (2023). Yapay zekanın insan zekasına psikoterapötik yaklaşımı [Psychotherapeutic approach of artificial intelligence to human intelligence]. *Çukurova Medical Student Journal, 3*(1), 12-18.

Emmelkamp, P. M. (2005). Technological innovations in clinical assessment and psychotherapy. *Psychotherapy and Psychosomatics, 74*(6), 336–343. DOI: 10.1159/000087780 PMID: 16244509

Eryılmaz, H. E. (2023). Yapay zekâ çağında kişisel veri mahremiyeti [Personal Data Privacy in the Age of Artificial Intelligence]. *Journal of Arts and Social Sciences, 1*(2), 6–25.

Ezawa, I. D., Robinson, N., & Hollon, S. D. (2024). Prevalence increases as treatments improve: An evolutionary perspective on the treatment–prevalence paradox in depression. *Annual Review of Clinical Psychology, 20*(1), 201–228. DOI: 10.1146/annurev-clinpsy-080822-040442 PMID: 38996078

Fakhoury, M. (2019). Artificial intelligence in psychiatry. *Frontiers in psychiatry: artificial intelligence, precision medicine, and other paradigm shifts*, 1192,119-125.

Fan, S. (2020). *Önemli sorular yapay zeka yerimizi alacak mı? 21. yüzyıl için bir rehber* [Important questions Will artificial intelligence replace us? A guide for the 21st century]. (Çıgay, I. G., Trans.). Hep Kitap.

Ferhat, S. (2016). Dijital dünyanın gerçekliği, gerçek dünyanın sanallığı bir dijital medya ürünü olarak sanal gerçeklik [Reality of the digital world, virtuality of the real world virtual reality as a digital media product]. *TRT Academy Journal, 1*(2), 724–746.

Feuerriegel, S., Hartmann, J., Janiesch, C., & Zschech, P. (2023). Generative AI. *Business & Information Systems Engineering, 66*(1), 111–126. DOI: 10.1007/s12599-023-00834-7

Fiske, A., Henningsen, P., & Buyx, A. (2019). Your robot therapist will see you now: Ethical implications of embodied artificial intelligence in psychiatry, psychology, and psychotherapy. *Journal of Medical Internet Research, 21*(5), e13216. DOI: 10.2196/13216 PMID: 31094356

Fitzpatrick, K. K., Darcy, A., & Vierhile, M. (2017). Delivering cognitive behavior therapy to young adults with symptoms of depression and anxiety using a fully automated conversational agent (Woebot): A randomized controlled trial. *JMIR Mental Health, 4*(2), e7785. DOI: 10.2196/mental.7785 PMID: 28588005

Fitzsimmons-Craft, E. E., Chan, W. W., Smith, A. C., Firebaugh, M. L., Fowler, L. A., Topooco, N., DePietro, B., Wilfley, D. E., Taylor, C. B., & Jacobson, N. C. (2022). Effectiveness of a chatbot for eating disorders prevention: A randomized clinical trial. *International Journal of Eating Disorders, 55*(3), 343–353. DOI: 10.1002/eat.23662 PMID: 35274362

Fortney, J. C., Pyne, J. M., Turner, E. E., Farris, K. M., Normoyle, T. M., Avery, M. D., Hilty, D. M., & Unützer, J. (2015). Telepsychiatry integration of mental health services into rural primary care settings. *International Review of Psychiatry (Abingdon, England)*, *27*(6), 525–539. DOI: 10.3109/09540261.2015.1085838 PMID: 26634618

Fulmer, R. (2019). Artificial intelligence and counseling: Four levels of implementation. *Theory & Psychology*, *29*(6), 807–819. DOI: 10.1177/0959354319853045

Graham, S., Depp, C., Lee, E. E., Nebeker, C., Tu, X., Kim, H. C., & Jeste, D. V. (2019). Artificial intelligence for mental health and mental illnesses: An overview. *Current Psychiatry Reports*, *21*(11), 1–18. DOI: 10.1007/s11920-019-1094-0 PMID: 31701320

Greer, S., Ramo, D., Chang, Y. J., Fu, M., Moskowitz, J., & Haritatos, J. (2019). Use of the chatbot "vivibot" to deliver positive psychology skills and promote well-being among young people after cancer treatment: Randomized controlled feasibility trial. *JMIR mHealth and uHealth*, *7*(10), e15018. DOI: 10.2196/15018 PMID: 31674920

Grubbs, K. M., Fortney, J. C., Dean, T., Williams, J. S., & Godleski, L. (2015). A comparison of mental health diagnoses treated via interactive video and face to face in the Veterans Healthcare Administration. *Telemedicine Journal and e-Health*, *21*(7), 564–566. DOI: 10.1089/tmj.2014.0152 PMID: 25799233

Grünerbl, A., Muaremi, A., Osmani, V., Bahle, G., Oehler, S., Tröster, G., & Lukowicz, P. (2015). Smartphone-based recognition of states and state changes in bipolar disorder patients. *IEEE Journal of Biomedical and Health Informatics*, *19*(1), 140–148. DOI: 10.1109/JBHI.2014.2343154 PMID: 25073181

Gültekin, M. (2022). Yapay Zekânın Ruh Sağlığı Hizmetlerinde Kullanımına İlişkin Fırsatlar ve Sorunlar [The Advantages and Disadvantages of Using Artificial Intelligence in Mental Health Services]. *The Journal of Humanity and Society*, *12*(3), 121–158. DOI: 10.12658/M0664

Gümüş, A. E., & Gümüş, M. A. (2020). *Psikolojik danışmada etik ve hukuk* [Ethics and law in psychological counselling]. Vedat Kitapçılık.

Guo, Y., Hao, Z., Zhao, S., Gong, J., & Yang, F. (2020). Artificial intelligence in health care: Bibliometric analysis. *Journal of Medical Internet Research*, *22*(7), e18228. DOI: 10.2196/18228 PMID: 32723713

Gupta, S., Kamboj, S., & Bag, S. (2023). Role of Risks in the Development of Responsible Artificial Intelligence in the Digital Healthcare Domain. *Information Systems Frontiers*, *25*(6), 2257–2274. DOI: 10.1007/s10796-021-10174-0

Gürlek, Y. (2024). Yapay Zekanın Eğitime Etkileri ve Uygulamaları [The effects and applications of artificial intelligence in education]. *International Journal of New Trends in Education and Social Sciences, 1*(1), 125–132.

Gürlek, Y., Bozkoyun, E., Ulutürk, M., & Zeyrekgündüz, F. (2023). Yapay Zekanın Eğitime Etkileri ve Uygulamaları [The effects and applications of artificial intelligence in education]. *International Journal of Original Educational Research, 1*(1), 25–132.

Gutierrez, J. (2002). Aplicaciones de la relidad virtual en pcilogia clinica. *Aula Medica Psiquiatria, 4*(2), 92–126.

Güzel, Ş., Dömbekci, H. A., & Eren, F. (2022). Yapay zekânın sağlık alanında kullanımı: Nitel bir araştırma [The Use of Artificial Intelligence in the Health Institutions: A Qualitative Research]. *Celal Bayar University Health Sciences Institute Journal, 9*(4), 509–519. DOI: 10.34087/cbusbed.1140122

Hailemariam, Y., Yazdinejad, A., Parizi, R. M., Srivastava, G., & Dehghantanha, A. (2020, December). An empirical evaluation of AI deep explainable tools. In 2020 IEEE Globecom Workshops (GC Wkshps (pp. 1-6). IEEE.

Hall, W., & Pesenti, J. (2017). Growing the artificial intelligence industry in the UK. *Department for Digital, Culture, Media & Sport and Department for Business, Energy & Industrial Strategy. Part of the Industrial Strategy UK and the Commonwealth.*

Hardal, M. (2011). *Common ethical violations and ethical action patterns among Turkish mental health professionals and the factors that influence them* [Doctoral dissertation], Istanbul Bilgi Üniversitesi, Istanbul.

Hardy, M., & Harvey, H. (2020). Artificial intelligence in diagnostic imaging: Impact on the radiography profession. *The British Journal of Radiology, 93*(1108), 20190840. DOI: 10.1259/bjr.20190840 PMID: 31821024

He, Y., Yang, L., Zhu, X., Wu, B., Zhang, S., Qian, C., & Tian, T. (2022). Mental health chatbot for young adults with depressive symptoms during the COVID-19 pandemic: Single-blind, three-arm randomized controlled trial. *Journal of Medical Internet Research, 24*(11), e40719. DOI: 10.2196/40719 PMID: 36355633

Heerebrand, S. L., Bray, J., Ulbrich, C., Roberts, R. M., & Edwards, S. (2021). Effectiveness of dialectical behavior therapy skills training group for adults with borderline personality disorder. *Journal of Clinical Psychology, 77*(7), 1573–1590. DOI: 10.1002/jclp.23134 PMID: 33821506

Hilty, D. M., Ferrer, D. C., Parish, M. B., Johnston, B., Callahan, E. J., & Yellowlees, P. M. (2013). The effectiveness of telemental health: A 2013 review. *Telemedicine Journal and e-Health, 19*(6), 444–454. DOI: 10.1089/tmj.2013.0075 PMID: 23697504

Houston, T. K., Cooper, L. A., & Ford, D. E. (2002). Internet support groups for depression: A 1-year prospective cohort study. *The American Journal of Psychiatry*, *159*(12), 2062–2068. DOI: 10.1176/appi.ajp.159.12.2062 PMID: 12450957

Huang, S., Lai, X., Ke, L., Li, Y., Wang, H., Zhao, X., Dai, X., & Wang, Y. (2024). AI Technology panic-is AI Dependence Bad for Mental Health? A Cross-Lagged Panel Model and the Mediating Roles of Motivations for AI Use Among Adolescents. *Psychology Research and Behavior Management*, *17*, 1087–1102. DOI: 10.2147/PRBM.S440889 PMID: 38495087

Hudlicka, E. (2016). Virtual affective agents and therapeutic games. In Luxton, D. L. (Ed.). In *Artificial Intelligence in Behavioral And Mental Health Care*, (s.s. 81-115), Elsevier Academic Press DOI: 10.1016/B978-0-12-420248-1.00004-0

Hunkin, H. (2022). *The Acceptability and Efficacy of Wearable Devices in Digital Mental Health* [Doctor of Philosophy/Master of Psychology (Clinical)]. The University of Adelaide.

Hunkin, H., King, D. L., & Zajac, I. T. (2019). Wearable devices as adjuncts in the treatment of anxiety-related symptoms: A narrative review of five device modalities and implications for clinical practice. *Clinical Psychology : a Publication of the Division of Clinical Psychology of the American Psychological Association*, *26*(3), 987–1003. DOI: 10.1111/cpsp.12290

Hunkin, H., King, D. L., & Zajac, I. T. (2021). Evaluating the feasibility of a consumer-grade wearable EEG headband to aid assessment of state and trait mindfulness. *Journal of Clinical Psychology*, *77*(11), 2559–2575. DOI: 10.1002/jclp.23189 PMID: 34061998

Illovsky, M. E. (1994). Counseling, artificial intelligence, and expert systems. *Simulation & Gaming*, *25*(1), 88–98. DOI: 10.1177/1046878194251009

Inkster, B., Sarda, S., & Subramanian, V. (2018). An empathy-driven, conversational artificial intelligence agent (Wysa) for digital mental well-being: Real-world data evaluation mixedmethods study. *JMIR mHealth and uHealth*, *6*(11), e12106. DOI: 10.2196/12106 PMID: 30470676

Interaxon Inc. (2020). Brain sensing headband: What it measures. https://choosemuse.com/what-it-measures/

Jibb, L. A., Birnie, K. A., Nathan, P. C., Beran, T. N., Hum, V., Victor, J. C., & Stinson, J. N. (2018). Using the MEDiPORT humanoid robot to reduce procedural pain and distress in children with cancer: A pilot randomized controlled trial. *Pediatric Blood & Cancer*, *65*(9), e27242. DOI: 10.1002/pbc.27242 PMID: 29893482

Jones, R. N. (2014). *Uygulamalı danışmanlık ve yardım becerileri* [Practical counselling and helping skills]. (Sart, G., Trans.). Nobel Akademi Yayıncılık.

Kabadayı, F., & Güven, M. (2023). Psikolojik yardım hizmetlerindeki mobil uygulamalarla ilgili bir inceleme. [A Review of Mobile Applications in Psychological Help Services]. *The Journal of Turkish Educational Sciences, 21*(3), 1660–1689. DOI: 10.37217/tebd.1291285

Kaewkannate, K., & Kim, S. (2016). A comparison of wearable fitness devices. *BMC Public Health, 16*(1), 1–16. DOI: 10.1186/s12889-016-3059-0 PMID: 27220855

Kafes, A. Y., Çiller, A., & Şakiroğlu, M. (2024). Deprem yaşamış bireylerin travma belirtilerine yönelik sanal gerçeklik destekli müdahale programı: Bir etkililik çalışması [Virtual Reality Supported Intervention Program for Trauma Symptoms of Individuals Who Experienced an Earthquake: An Effectiveness Study]. *Archives Neuropsychiatry, 61*, 15–23. DOI: 10.29399/npa.28568 PMID: 38496219

Khawaja, Z., & Bélisle-Pipon, J. C. (2023). Your robot therapist is not your therapist: Understanding the role of AI-powered mental health chatbots. *Frontiers in Digital Health, 5*, 1278186. DOI: 10.3389/fdgth.2023.1278186 PMID: 38026836

Kim, M., Lee, S., Kim, S., Heo, J. I., Lee, S., Shin, Y. B., Cho, C.-H., & Jung, D. (2025). Therapeutic potential of social chatbots in alleviating loneliness and social anxiety: Quasi-experimental mixed methods study. *Journal of Medical Internet Research, 27*, e65589. DOI: 10.2196/65589 PMID: 39808786

Konyalı, A., Naipoğlu, C., Güner, S., Bakkal, I., & Çelik, A. (2025). Psikolojide Yapay Zeka Kullanımı ve Uygulamaları [Use and Applications of Artificial Intelligence in Psychology]. *Journal of Kocaeli Health and Technology University, 3*(1), 1–17.

Kostopoulos, L. (2018). The emerging artificial intelligence wellnesslandscape: Benefits and potential areas of ethical concern. *California Western Law Review, 55*(1), 235–254.

Kretzschmar, K., Tyroll, H., Pavarini, G., Manzini, A., & Singh, I. (2019). Can your phone be your therapist? Young people's ethical perspectives on the use of fully automated conversational agents(chatbots) in mental health support. *Biomedical Informatics Insights, 11*, 1–9. DOI: 10.1177/1178222619829083 PMID: 30858710

Kumar, R. (2017). Artificial intelligence—basics. Machine learning and cognition in enterprises: Business intelligence transformed, pp. 33–49. DOI: 10.1007/978-1-4842-3069-5_3

Kuruca, Y., Üstüner, M., & Şimşek, I. (2022). Dijital pazarlamada yapay zekâ kullanımı: Sohbet robotu (Chatbot) [Using Artificial Intelligence in Digital Marketing: Chatbot]. *Medya ve Kültür*, *2*(1), 88–113.

Langarizadeh, M., Tabatabaei, M. S., Tavakol, K., Naghipour, M., Rostami, A., & Moghbeli, F. (2017). Telemental health care, an effective alternative to conventional mental care: A systematic review. *Acta Informatica Medica*, *25*(4), 240. DOI: 10.5455/aim.2017.25.240-246 PMID: 29284913

Lanier, M., Waddell, T. F., Elson, M., Tamul, D. J., Ivory, J. D., & Przybylski, A. (2019). Virtual reality check: Statistical power, reported results, and the validity of research on the psychology of virtual reality and immersive environments. *Computers in Human Behavior*, *100*, 70–78. DOI: 10.1016/j.chb.2019.06.015

Lau, Y., Chee, D. G. H., Chow, X. P., Wong, S. H., Cheng, L. J., & Lau, S. T. (2020). Humanoid robot-assisted interventions among children with diabetes: A systematic scoping review. *International Journal of Nursing Studies*, *111*, 103749. DOI: 10.1016/j.ijnurstu.2020.103749 PMID: 32911362

Lustgarten, S. D., & Elhai, J. D. (2018). Technology use in mental health practice and research: Legal and ethical risks. *Clinical Psychology : a Publication of the Division of Clinical Psychology of the American Psychological Association*, *25*(2), e12234. DOI: 10.1111/cpsp.12234

Luxton, D. D. (2014). Artificial intelligence in psychological practice: Current and future applications and implications. *Professional Psychology, Research and Practice*, *45*(5), 332–339. DOI: 10.1037/a0034559

Luxton, D. D. (2016). An introduction to artificial intelligence in behavioral and mental health care. In *Artificial intelligence in behavioral and mental health care* (pp. 1–26). Academic Press. DOI: 10.1016/B978-0-12-420248-1.00001-5

Mair, F., & Whitten, P. (2000). Systematic review of studies of patient satisfaction with telemedicine. *BMJ (Clinical Research Ed.)*, *320*(7248), 1517–1520. DOI: 10.1136/bmj.320.7248.1517 PMID: 10834899

Majidi, E., & Manshaee, G. (2024). Effects of virtual reality exposure therapy on state-trait anxiety in individuals with dentophobia. *Current Psychology (New Brunswick, N.J.)*, *43*(3), 2425–2431. DOI: 10.1007/s12144-023-04485-5

Marshall, J. M., Dunstan, D. A., & Bartik, W. (2020). Apps with maps—anxiety and depression mobile apps with evidence-based frameworks: Systematic search of major app stores. *JMIR Mental Health*, *7*(6), e16525. DOI: 10.2196/16525 PMID: 32579127

McCarthy, J. (2007a). *What is artificial intelligence.* Computer Science Department, Stanford University. https://trilliumdynamix.com/jmc/whatisai.pdf

McCarthy, J. (2007b). From here to human-level AI. *Artificial Intelligence, 171*(18), 1174–1182. DOI: 10.1016/j.artint.2007.10.009

Menon, V., Rajan, T. M., & Sarkar, S. (2017). Psychotherapeutic applications of mobile phone-based technologies: A systematic review of current research and trends. *Indian Journal of Psychological Medicine, 39*(1), 4–11. DOI: 10.4103/0253-7176.198956 PMID: 28250552

Meske, C., Bunde, E., Schneider, J., & Gersch, M. (2022). Explainable Artificial Intelligence: Objectives, Stakeholders, and Future Research Opportunities. *Information Systems Management, 39*(1), 53–63. DOI: 10.1080/10580530.2020.1849465

Mesquita, A. C., Zamarioli, C. M., & de Carvalho, E. C. (2016). The use of robots in nursing care practices: An exploratory descriptive study. *Online Brazilian Journal of Nursing, 15*(3), 404–413. DOI: 10.17665/1676-4285.20165395

Mihret, E. T. (2020). Robotics and artificial intelligence. *International Journal of Artificial Intelligence and Machine Learning, 10*(2), 57–78. DOI: 10.4018/IJAIML.2020070104

Miller, D. D., & Brown, E. W. (2018). Artificial intelligence in medical practice: The question to the answer? *The American Journal of Medicine, 131*(2), 129–133. DOI: 10.1016/j.amjmed.2017.10.035 PMID: 29126825

Miskelly, F. (2005). Electronic tracking of patients with dementia and wandering using mobile phone technology. *Age and Ageing, 34*(5), 497–499. DOI: 10.1093/ageing/afi145 PMID: 16107453

Morsünbül, Ü. (2018). Robotlarla Bağlanma ve Cinsellik: Ruh Sağlığı Bakış Açısından Bir Değerlendirme [Attachment and Sex with Robots: An Assessment from Mental Health Perspective]. *Psikiyatride Güncel Yaklasimlar, 10*(4), 427–439. DOI: 10.18863/pgy.363669

Müller, A. M., Alley, S., Schoeppe, S., & Vandelanotte, C. (2016). The effectiveness of e-& mHealth interventions to promote physical activity and healthy diets in developing countries: A systematic review. *The International Journal of Behavioral Nutrition and Physical Activity, 13*(1), 109. DOI: 10.1186/s12966-016-0434-2 PMID: 27724911

Mystakidis, S. (2022). Metaverse. *Encyclopedia, 2*(1), 486–497. DOI: 10.3390/encyclopedia2010031

Narin, N. G. (2021). A content analysis of the metaverse articles. *Journal of Metaverse*, *1*(1), 17–24.

Neacsiu, A. D., Rizvi, S. L., & Linehan, M. M. (2010). Dialectical behavior therapy skills use as a mediator and outcome of treatment for borderline personality disorder. *Behaviour Research and Therapy*, *48*(9), 832–839. DOI: 10.1016/j.brat.2010.05.017 PMID: 20579633

Nilsson, N. J. (2014). *Principles of artificial intelligence*. Morgan Kaufmann.

Nomura, T., Kanda, T., Suzuki, T., & Kato, K. (2008). Prediction of human behavior in human—Robot interaction using psychological scales for anxiety and negative attitudes toward robots. *IEEE Transactions on Robotics*, *24*(2), 442–451. DOI: 10.1109/TRO.2007.914004

North, M. M., North, S. M., & Coble, J. R. (1997a). Virtual reality therapy: An effective treatment for psychological disorders. In Riva, G. (Ed.), *Virtual Reality in Neuro-Psycho-Physiology* (pp. 59–65). Ios Press.

North, M. M., North, S. M., & Coble, J. R. (1997b). Virtual reality therapy for fear of flying. *The American Journal of Psychiatry*, *154*(1), 130. DOI: 10.1176/ajp.154.1.130b PMID: 8988975

Ntoutsi, E., Fafalios, P., Gadiraju, U., Iosifidis, V., Nejdl, W., Vidal, M. E., Ruggieri, S., Turini, F., Papadopoulos, S., Krasanakis, E., Kompatsiaris, I., Kinder-Kurlanda, K., Wagner, C., Karimi, F., Fernandez, M., Alani, H., Berendt, B., Kruegel, T., Heinze, C., & Staab, S. (2020). Bias in data-driven artificial intelligence systems- An introductory survey. *Wiley Interdisciplinary Reviews. Data Mining and Knowledge Discovery*, *10*(3), 1356. DOI: 10.1002/widm.1356

Ogawa, M., Oyama, G., Morito, K., Kobayashi, M., Yamada, Y., Shinkawa, K., Kamo, H., Hatano, T., & Hattori, N. (2022). Can AI make people happy? The effect of AI-based chatbot on smile and speech in Parkinson's disease. *Parkinsonism & Related Disorders*, *99*, 43–46. DOI: 10.1016/j.parkreldis.2022.04.018 PMID: 35596975

Oh, J., Jang, S., Kim, H., & Kim, J. J. (2020). Efficacy of mobile app-based interactive cognitive behavioral therapy using a chatbot for panic disorder. *International Journal of Medical Informatics*, *140*, 104171. DOI: 10.1016/j.ijmedinf.2020.104171 PMID: 32446158

Oh, K. J., Lee, D., Ko, B., & Choi, H. J. (2017). A chatbot for psychiatric counseling in mental healthcare service based on emotional dialogue analysis and sentence generation. In *2017 18th IEEE international conference on mobile data management (MDM)* (pp. 371-375). IEEE. DOI: 10.1109/MDM.2017.64

Oktay, B., & Oktay, Y. F. (2018). Bir etik ihlal olarak hasta ve terapist arasındaki cinsel ilişkiler [Sexual relations between patient and therapist as an ethical violation]. *SDU Faculty of Arts And Sciences Journal of Social Sciences, 44*, 103–110.

Olano-Espinosa, E., Avila-Tomas, J. F., Minue-Lorenzo, C., Matilla-Pardo, B., Serrano, M. E. S., Martinez-Suberviola, F. J., & Del Cura-González, I. (2022). Effectiveness of a conversational chatbot (Dejal@ bot) for the adult population to quit smoking: Pragmatic, multicenter, controlled, randomized clinical trial in primary care. *JMIR mHealth and uHealth, 10*(6), e34273. DOI: 10.2196/34273 PMID: 35759328

Omarov, B., Narynov, S., & Zhumanov, Z. (2023). Artificial intelligence-enabled chatbots in mental health: A systematic review. *Computers, Materials & Continua, 74*(3), 5105–5122. DOI: 10.32604/cmc.2023.034655

Özcan, A., & Fırat, E. H. (2024). Giyilebilir teknoloji kullanımına dair; fırat üniversitesi çalışanlarının akıllı saat alırken ya da kullanırken risk algılarının ölçülmesi [On the use of wearable technology; measurıng the rısk perceptıons of fırat unıversıty employees when buyıng or usıng smart watches]. *International Journal of Communication and Art, 5*(11), 18–44.

Özcan, N. (2025). *Benliğin Dijital Dönüşümü, Yapay Zekâ ve Yalnızlık [Digital Transformation of the Self, Artificial Intelligence and Loneliness]*. 5th International Artificial Intelligence And Data Science Congress (Icada 2025) Full Papers And Abstracts, İzmir.

Özdoğan, H. K., & Özdemir, N. K. (2023). 21. yüzyılda kariyer psikolojik danışmanlığı ve yapay zeka uygulamaları [21st century career counseling and artificial intelligence Practices]. *Dokuz Eylül University Buca Faculty of Education Journal*, (57), 2127–2152. DOI: 10.53444/deubefd.1326692

Özgür, N. (2023). *Sohbet botları ve yapay zekâ etiği [Chatbots and artificial intelligence ethics]*. [Yüksek lisans bitirme projesi], https://core.ac.uk/download/pdf/586376297.pdf

Özkol, I., Doğan, K., & Köseali, G. (2019). EBYS uygulamalarında yapay zekâ destekli chatbot (sohbet robotu) kullanımı [Artificial intelligence supported chatbot usage in ERMS applications]. In Yalçınkaya, B. (Ed.), Ünal, M. A. (Ed.), Yılmaz, B.(Ed.), Özdemirci, F.(Ed.). *Bilgi Yönetimi ve Bilgi Güvenliği*, 229-250.

Öztürk, K., & Şahin, M. E. (2018). Yapay sinir ağları ve yapay zekaya genel bir bakış [A general view of artificial neural networks and artificial intelligence]. *Takvim-i Vekayi, 6*(2), 25–36.

Öztürk, M. O., & Uluşahin, N. A. (2015). *Ruh sağlığı ve bozuklukları* [Mental health and disorders]. Nobel Tıp Kitabevi.

Paris, J. (2015). *Personality disorders over time: Precursors, course, and outcome.* American Psychiatric Publishing.

Parsons, T. D., & Rizzo, A. A. (2008). Affective outcomes of virtual reality exposure therapy for anxiety and specific phobias: A meta-analysis. *Journal of Behavior Therapy and Experimental Psychiatry, 39*(3), 250–261. DOI: 10.1016/j.jbtep.2007.07.007 PMID: 17720136

Patton, J., Dawe, G., Scharver, C., Mussa-Ivaldi, F., & Kenyon, R. (2006). Robotics and virtual reality: A perfect marriage for motor control research and rehabilitation. *Assistive Technology, 18*(2), 181–195. DOI: 10.1080/10400435.2006.10131917 PMID: 17236477

Peuters, C., Maenhout, L., Cardon, G., De Paepe, A., DeSmet, A., Lauwerier, E., Leta, K., & Crombez, G. (2024). A mobile healthy lifestyle intervention to promote mental health in adolescence: A mixed-methods evaluation. *BMC Public Health, 24*(1), 44. DOI: 10.1186/s12889-023-17260-9 PMID: 38166797

Pine, D. S., Grun, J., Maguire, E. A., Burgess, N., Zarahn, E., Koda, V., Fyer, A., Szeszko, P. R., & Bilder, R. M. (2002). Neurodevelopmental aspects of spatial navigation: A virtual reality fMRI study. *NeuroImage, 15*(2), 396–406. DOI: 10.1006/nimg.2001.0988 PMID: 11798274

Possati, L. M. (2023). Psychoanalyzing artificial intelligence: The case of Replika. *AI & Society, 38*(4), 1725–1738. DOI: 10.1007/s00146-021-01379-7

Prochaska, J. J., Vogel, E. A., Chieng, A., Kendra, M., Baiocchi, M., Pajarito, S., & Robinson, A. (2021). A therapeutic relational agent for reducing problematic substance use (Woebot): Development and usability study. *Journal of Medical Internet Research, 23*(3), e24850. DOI: 10.2196/24850 PMID: 33755028

Rabbi, M., Philyaw-Kotov, M., Lee, J., Mansour, A., Dent, L., Wang, X., & Murphy, S. (2017, September). SARA: a mobile app to engage users in health data collection. In *Proceedings of the 2017 ACM International Joint Conference on Pervasive and Ubiquitous Computing and Proceedings of the 2017 ACM International Symposium on Wearable Computers* (pp. 781-789). DOI: 10.1145/3123024.3125611

Rathenau, S., Sousa, D., Vaz, A., & Geller, S. (2021). The effect of attitudes toward online therapy and the difficulties perceived in online therapeutic presence. *Journal of Psychotherapy Integration*. Advance online publication. DOI: 10.1037/int0000266

Ravirahul, B. M., Balaji, V. R., Balaji, K. R., Gowtham, S., & Surya, S. (2021). Mind wave controlled assistive robot. In *2021 7th International Conference on Advanced Computing and Communication Systems (ICACCS)* (Vol. 1, pp. 1507-1509). IEEE DOI: 10.1109/ICACCS51430.2021.9441684

Ray, A., Bhardwaj, A., Malik, Y. K., Singh, S., & Gupta, R. (2022). Artificial intelligence and Psychiatry: An overview. *Asian Journal of Psychiatry*, *70*, 103021. DOI: 10.1016/j.ajp.2022.103021 PMID: 35219978

Rich, C., Ponsler, B., Holroyd, A., & Sidner, C. L. (2010). Recognizing engagement in human-robot interaction. In *2010 5th ACM/IEEE International Conference on Human-Robot Interaction (HRI) (pp. 375-382)*. IEEE.

Richards, D., & Viganó, N. (2013). Online counseling: A narrative and critical review of the literature. *Journal of Clinical Psychology*, *69*(9), 994–1011. DOI: 10.1002/jclp.21974 PMID: 23630010

Riva, G., Di Lernia, D., & Sajno, E. (2021). Virtual reality therapy in the metaverse: Merging VR for the outside with VR for the inside. *Annual Review of Cybertherapy and Telemedicine*, *19*, 3–8.

Romano, D. M. (2005). Virtual reality therapy. *Developmental Medicine and Child Neurology*, *47*(9), 580–580. DOI: 10.1111/j.1469-8749.2005.tb01206.x PMID: 16138662

Şahin, A. R., Doğan, K., & Sivri, S. (2020). *Sağlık Bilimlerinde Yapay Zeka* [Artificial Intelligence in Health Sciences]. Akademisyen Kitabevi. DOI: 10.37609/akya.786

Şahin, M. (2024). Afetlerde krize müdahale: Kahramanmaraş Depremi'nde aile ve sosyal hizmetler bakanlığının çalışmaları [Crisis intervention in disasters: the work of the ministry of family and social services in the Kahramanmaraş Earthquake]. *International Journal of Social Work Research*, *4*(2), 17–50. DOI: 10.57114/jswrpub.1257945

Salamanca-Sanabria, A., Richards, D., & Timulak, L. (2019). Adapting an internet-delivered intervention for depression for a Colombian college student population: An illustration of an integrative empirical approach. *Internet Interventions : the Application of Information Technology in Mental and Behavioural Health*, *15*, 76–86. DOI: 10.1016/j.invent.2018.11.005 PMID: 30740313

Sanchez-Vives, M. V., & Slater, M. (2005). From presence to consciousness through virtual reality. *Nature Reviews. Neuroscience*, *6*(4), 332–339. DOI: 10.1038/nrn1651 PMID: 15803164

Sapkota, R. P., Valli, E., Dear, B. F., Titov, N., & Hadjistavropoulos, H. D. (2024). Satisfaction, engagement, and outcomes in internet-delivered cognitive behaviour therapy adapted for people of diverse ethnocultural groups: An observational trial with benchmarking. *Frontiers in Psychiatry, 15*, 1270543. DOI: 10.3389/fpsyt.2024.1270543 PMID: 38501087

Savaş, B. Ç. (2024). Yapay zekâya bağımlılık ölçeğinin Türkçe'ye uyarlanması: Geçerlik ve güvenirlik çalışması [Adaptation of the Dependence to Artificial Intelligence Scale into Turkish: Validity and Reliability Study]. *Journal of Sport and Recreation for All, 6*(3), 306–315. DOI: 10.56639/jsar.1509301

Sayar, K. (2011). *Terapi kültürel bir eleştiri* [Therapy is a cultural criticism]. Timaş Yayınları.

Scholten, M. R., Kelders, S. M., & Van Gemert-Pijnen, J. E. (2017). Self-guided web-based interventions: Scoping review on user needs and the potential of embodied conversational agents to address them. *Journal of Medical Internet Research, 19*(11), e383. DOI: 10.2196/jmir.7351 PMID: 29146567

Schulze, N., Reuter, S. C., Kuchler, I., Reinke, B., Hinkelmann, L., Stöckigt, S., Siemoneit, H., & Tonn, P. (2019). Differences in attitudes toward online interventions in psychiatry and psychotherapy between health care professionals and nonprofessionals: A survey. *Telemedicine Journal and e-Health, 25*(10), 926–932. Advance online publication. DOI: 10.1089/tmj.2018.0225 PMID: 30412450

Seligman, M. E., & Csikszentmihalyi, M. (2000). Positive psychology: An introduction, *American Psychological Association*, 55(1), 5-14. https://doi.org/DOI: 10.1037//0003-066X.55.1.5

Şencan Karakuş, B. (2021). Psikoterapide mobil uygulama kullanımının etik kurallar çerçevesinde ele alınması [Considering the use of mobile application in psychotherapy within the framework of ethics]. *Life Skills Journal of Psychology*, *5*(10), 133–140. DOI: 10.31461/ybpd.1019155

Sergueeva, K., & Shaw, N. (2017). Improving healthcare with wearables: overcoming the barriers to adoption. In *HCI in Business, Government and Organizations. Interacting with Information Systems: 4th International Conference, HCIBGO 2017, Held as Part of HCI International 2017, Vancouver, BC, Canada, July 9-14, 2017, Proceedings, Part I 4* (pp. 209-223). Springer International Publishing. **https://doi.org/**DOI: 10.1007/978-3-319-58481-2_17

Shah, L. B. I., Torres, S., Kannusamy, P., Chng, C. M. L., He, H. G., & Klainin-Yobas, P. (2015). Efficacy of the virtual reality-based stress management program on stress-related variables in people with mood disorders: The feasibility study. *Archives of Psychiatric Nursing, 29*(1), 6–13. DOI: 10.1016/j.apnu.2014.09.003 PMID: 25634868

Sharif, M. S., Raj Theeng Tamang, M., Fu, C. H. Y., Baker, A., Alzahrani, A. I., Alalwan, N. (2023). An Innovative Random-Forest-Based Model to Assess the Health Impacts of Regular Commuting Using Non-Invasive Wearable Sensors. *Sensors* (Basel, Switzerland), 23(6), 3274. 4. https://doi.org/DOI: 10.3390/s23063274

Shroff, R. (2019). *Artificial Intelligence Explained in Simple Terms*. Retrieved from https://medium.com/mytake/artificial-intelligence-explained-in-simple-englishpart-1-2-1b28c1f762cf

Siddals, S., Coxon, A., & Torous, J. (2024). " It just happened to be the perfect thing": Real-life experiences of generative AI chatbots for mental health. *npj Mental Health Res* 3, 48. https://doi.org/DOI: 10.1038/s44184-024-00097-4

Singh, O. P. (2019). Chatbots in psychiatry: Can treatment gap be lessened for psychiatric disorders in India. *Indian Journal of Psychiatry, 61*(3), 225–227. DOI: 10.4103/0019-5545.258323 PMID: 31142896

So, R., Emura, N., Okazaki, K., Takeda, S., Sunami, T., Kitagawa, K., Takebayashi, Y., & Furukawa, T. A. (2024). Guided versus unguided chatbot-delivered cognitive behavioral intervention for individuals with moderate-risk and problem gambling: A randomized controlled trial (GAMBOT2 study). *Addictive Behaviors, 149*, 107889. DOI: 10.1016/j.addbeh.2023.107889 PMID: 37857043

Stofle, G. S. (2001). *Choosing an online therapist: A step-by-step guide to finding professional help on the web*. White Hat Communications.

Stoll, J., Müller, J. A., & Trachsel, M. (2020). Ethical issues in online psychotherapy: A narrative review. *Frontiers in Psychiatry, 10*, 993. DOI: 10.3389/fpsyt.2019.00993 PMID: 32116819

Sucala, M., Schnur, J. B., Brackman, E. H., Constantino, M. J., & Montgomery, G. H. (2013). Clinicians' attitudes toward therapeutic alliance in E-therapy. *The Journal of General Psychology, 140*(4), 282–293. DOI: 10.1080/00221309.2013.830590 PMID: 24837821

Ta, V., Griffith, C., Boatfield, C., Wang, X., Civitello, M., Bader, H., & Loggarakis, A. (2020). User experiences of social support from companion chatbots in everyday contexts: Thematic analysis. *Journal of Medical Internet Research, 22*(3), e16235. DOI: 10.2196/16235 PMID: 32141837

Ta-Johnson, V., Boatfeld, C., Wang, X., DeCero, E., Krupica, I., Rasof, S., Motzer, A., & Pedryc, W. (2022). Assessing the topics and motivating factors behind human-social chatbot interactions: Thematic analysis of user experiences. *JMIR Human Factors, 9*(4), e38876. DOI: 10.2196/38876 PMID: 36190745

Tan, H. (2014). *Psikolojik yardım ilişkileri* [*Psychological help relationships*]. Nobel Yayınevi.

Thunström, A. O., Carlsen, H. K., Ali, L., Larson, T., Hellström, A., & Steingrimsson, S. (2024). Usability Comparison Among Healthy Participants of an Anthropomorphic Digital Human and a Text-Based Chatbot as a Responder to Questions on Mental Health: Randomized Controlled Trial. *JMIR Human Factors, 11*(1), e54581. DOI: 10.2196/54581 PMID: 38683664

Topçu, S. Y., Semerci, R., Kostak, M. A., Güray, Ö., Sert, S., & Yavuz, G. (2023). The effect of an interactive robot on children's post-operative anxiety, mobilization, and parents' satisfaction; randomized controlled study. *Journal of Pediatric Nursing, 68*, e50–e57. DOI: 10.1016/j.pedn.2022.11.009 PMID: 36437131

Ulrich, S., Gantenbein, A. R., Zuber, V., Von Wyl, A., Kowatsch, T., & Künzli, H. (2024). Development and evaluation of a smartphone-based chatbot coach to facilitate a balanced lifestyle in individuals with headaches (BalanceUP App): Randomized controlled trial. *Journal of Medical Internet Research, 26*, e50132. DOI: 10.2196/50132 PMID: 38265863

Üzümcü, E., Akın, B., Nergiz, H., Inözü, M., & Çelikcan, U. (2018). Anksiyete bozukluklarında sanal gerçeklik [Virtual Reality for Anxiety Disorders]. *Psikiyatride Güncel Yaklasimlar, 10*(1), 99–117. DOI: 10.18863/pgy.336593

Vahia, I. V., Ng, B., Camacho, A., Cardenas, V., Cherner, M., Depp, C. A., Palmer, B. W., Jeste, D. P., & Agha, Z. (2015). Telepsychiatry for neurocognitive testing in older rural Latino adults. *The American Journal of Geriatric Psychiatry, 23*(7), 666–670. DOI: 10.1016/j.jagp.2014.08.006 PMID: 25708655

Vaidyam, A., Wisniewski, H., Halamka, J., Kashavan, M., & Torous, J. (2019). Chatbots and conversational agents in mental health: A review of the psychiatric landscape. *Canadian Journal of Psychiatry, 64*(7), 456–464. DOI: 10.1177/0706743719828977 PMID: 30897957

Valmaggia, L. R., Latif, L., Kempton, M. J., & Rus-Calafell, M. (2016). Virtual reality in the psychological treatment for mental health problems: An systematic review of recent evidence. *Psychiatry Research, 236*, 189–195. DOI: 10.1016/j.psychres.2016.01.015 PMID: 26795129

van Loenen, I., Scholten, W., Muntingh, A., Smit, J., & Batelaan, N. (2022). The effectiveness of virtual reality exposure–based cognitive behavioral therapy for severe anxiety disorders, obsessive-compulsive disorder, and posttraumatic stress disorder: Meta-analysis. *Journal of Medical Internet Research, 24*(2), e26736. DOI: 10.2196/26736 PMID: 35142632

Vereschagin, M., Wang, A. Y., Richardson, C. G., Xie, H., Munthali, R. J., Hudec, K. L., Leung, C., Wojcik, K. D., Munro, L., Halli, P., Kessler, R. C., & Vigo, D. V. (2024). Effectiveness of the Minder mobile mental health and substance use intervention for university students: Randomized controlled trial. *Journal of Medical Internet Research, 26*, e54287. DOI: 10.2196/54287 PMID: 38536225

Vieira, S., Pinaya, W. H., & Mechelli, A. (2017). Using deep learning to investigate the neuroimaging correlates of psychiatric and neurological disorders: Methods and applications. *Neuroscience and Biobehavioral Reviews, 74*, 58–75. DOI: 10.1016/j.neubiorev.2017.01.002 PMID: 28087243

Voinescu, A., Petrini, K., Stanton Fraser, D., Lazarovicz, R. A., Papavă, I., Fodor, L. A., & David, D. (2023). The effectiveness of a virtual reality attention task to predict depression and anxiety in comparison with current clinical measures. *Virtual Reality (Waltham Cross), 27*(1), 119–140. DOI: 10.1007/s10055-021-00520-7

Wang, Y., Xiong, M., & Olya, H. (2020) Toward an understanding of responsible artificial intelligence practices. In: Bui, T.X., (ed.) Proceedings of the 53rd Hawaii International Conference on System Sciences. Hawaii International Conference on System Sciences (HICSS 2020), 07-10 Jan 2020, Maui, Hawaii, USA. Hawaii International Conference on System Sciences (HICSS), s. 4962-4971. DOI: 10.24251/HICSS.2020.610

Weizenbaum, J. (1966). ELIZA—A computer program for the study of natural language communication between man and machine. *Communications of the ACM, 9*(1), 36–45. DOI: 10.1145/365153.365168

WHO. (2022) Strengthening Mental Health Promotion (Fact sheet). Geneva, World Health Organization https://www.who.int/news-room/fact sheets/detail/mental-health-strengthening-our-response (Accessed 17.03.2025)

World Health Organization (WHO). (2024). https://www.who.int/news/item/18-01-2024-who-releases-ai-ethics-and-governance-guidance-for-large-multi-modal-models (Retrieved: 15.07.2025)

Xie, T., & Pentina, I. (2022). "Attachment theory as a framework to understand relationships with social chatbots: a case study of Replika", *Proceedings of the 55th Hawaii International Conference on System Sciences*. 2046-2055. DOI: 10.24251/HICSS.2022.258

Xie, T., Pentina, I., & Hancock, T. (2023). Friend, mentor, lover: Does chatbot engagement lead to psychological dependence? *Journal of Service Management, 34*(4), 806–828. DOI: 10.1108/JOSM-02-2022-0072

Yasukawa, S., Tanaka, T., Yamane, K., Kano, R., Sakata, M., Noma, H., Furukawa, T. A., & Kishimoto, T. (2024). A chatbot to improve adherence to internet-based cognitive–behavioural therapy among workers with subthreshold depression: A randomised controlled trial. *BMJ Mental Health, 27*(1), 1–7. DOI: 10.1136/bmjment-2023-300881 PMID: 38199786

Yavrutürk, A. R. (2025). Psikolojik danışmanlık uygulamalarında teknolojinin kullanımı [Use of technology in counseling practices]. *İstanbul Aydın Üniversitesi Eğitim Fakültesi Dergisi, 11*(1), 5-6.

Yeh, P. L., Kuo, W. C., Tseng, B. L., & Sung, Y. H. (2025). Does the AI-driven Chatbot Work? Effectiveness of the Woebot app in reducing anxiety and depression in group counseling courses and student acceptance of technological aids. *Current Psychology (New Brunswick, N.J.), 44*(9), 1–13. DOI: 10.1007/s12144-025-07359-0

Yılmaz, A., & Kaya, U. (2021). *Derin öğrenme* [Deep Learning]. Kodlab.

Yin, L., Zhang, C., & Cui, Z. (2020). Experimental research on real-time acquisition and monitoring of wearable EEG based on TGAM module. *Computer Communications, 151*, 76–85. DOI: 10.1016/j.comcom.2019.12.055

Yorulmaz, O., Sapmaz-Yurtsever, S., Gökdag, C., Kaçar-Basaran, S., Göcek-Yorulmaz, E., Yalçin, M., & Görgü-Akçay, N. S. (2018). The future of pychotherapy in Turkey: Predictions for the next 10 years. *The Journal of Nervous and Mental Disease, 206*(5), 332–339. DOI: 10.1097/NMD.0000000000000797 PMID: 29498955

Zeren, Ş. G., & Bulut, E. (2018). Çevrimiçi psikolojik danışmada etik ve standartlar: Bir model önerisi [Ethics and Standards for Online Counseling: A Model Proposal]. *Turkish Psychological Counseling and Guidance Journal, 8*(49), 63–80.

Zhang, S., Yan, Z., Sapkota, S., Zhao, S., & Ooi, W. T. (2021). Moment-to-moment continuous attention fluctuation monitoring through consumer-grade EEG device. *Sensors (Basel)*, *21*(10), 3419. DOI: 10.3390/s21103419 PMID: 34069027

Zhao, H., Cao, J., Xie, J., Liao, W. H., Lei, Y., Cao, H., Qu, Q., & Bowen, C. (2023). Wearable sensors and features for diagnosis of neurodegenerative diseases: A systematic review. *Digital Health*, *9*, 1–22. DOI: 10.1177/20552076231173569 PMID: 37214662

Zhou, X., Liang, H., & Zhang, Y. (2023). Psychological Therapy with AI: An Overview of Chatbot Applications. *Frontiers in Psychology*, *14*, 112345.

ADDITIONAL READING

Alanezi, F. (2024). Assessing the effectiveness of ChatGPT in delivering mental health support: A qualitative study. *Journal of Multidisciplinary Healthcare*, *17*, 461–471. DOI: 10.2147/JMDH.S447368 PMID: 38314011

Alhuwaydi, A. M. (2024). Exploring the role of artificial intelligence in mental healthcare: Current trends and future directions–a narrative review for a comprehensive insight. *Risk Management and Healthcare Policy*, *17*, 1339–1348. DOI: 10.2147/RMHP.S461562 PMID: 38799612

Carr, S. (2020). 'AI gone mental': Engagement and ethics in data-driven technology for mental health. *Journal of Mental Health (Abingdon, England)*, *29*(2), 125–130. DOI: 10.1080/09638237.2020.1714011 PMID: 32000544

Gigerenzer, G. (2024). Psychological AI: Designing algorithms informed by human psychology. *Perspectives on Psychological Science*, *19*(5), 839–848. DOI: 10.1177/17456916231180597 PMID: 37522323

Koutsouleris, N., Hauser, T. U., Skvortsova, V., & De Choudhury, M. (2022). From promise to practice: Towards the realisation of AI-informed mental health care. *The Lancet. Digital Health*, *4*(11), e829–e840. DOI: 10.1016/S2589-7500(22)00153-4 PMID: 36229346

Maurya, R. K., Montesinos, S., Bogomaz, M., & DeDiego, A. C. (2025). Assessing the use of ChatGPT as a psychoeducational tool for mental health practice. *Counselling & Psychotherapy Research*, *25*(1), e12759. DOI: 10.1002/capr.12759

Olawade, D. B., Wada, O. Z., Odetayo, A., David-Olawade, A. C., Asaolu, F., & Eberhardt, J. (2024). Enhancing mental health with Artificial Intelligence: Current trends and future prospects. *Journal of Medicine, Surgery, and Public Health*, *3*, 100099. DOI: 10.1016/j.glmedi.2024.100099

Rahsepar Meadi, M., Sillekens, T., Metselaar, S., van Balkom, A., Bernstein, J., & Batelaan, N. (2025). Exploring the Ethical Challenges of Conversational AI in Mental Health Care: Scoping Review. *JMIR Mental Health*, *12*, e60432. DOI: 10.2196/60432 PMID: 39983102

Sharma, A., Lin, I. W., Miner, A. S., Atkins, D. C., & Althoff, T. (2023). Human–AI collaboration enables more empathic conversations in text-based peer-to-peer mental health support. *Nature Machine Intelligence*, *5*(1), 46–57. DOI: 10.1038/s42256-022-00593-2

Tutun, S., Johnson, M. E., Ahmed, A., Albizri, A., Irgil, S., Yesilkaya, I., ... & Harfouche, A. (2023). An AI-based decision support system for predicting mental health disorders. *Information Systems Frontiers, 25*(3), 1261-1276. 76DOI: 10.1007/s10796-022-10282-5

KEY TERMS AND DEFINITIONS

Artificial Intelligence: The ability of a computer system to emulate human-like cognitive functions such as learning and problem solving.

Chatbots: Chatbots that users use for various purposes such as receiving information and making transactions through messaging in the digital environment, communicating with a human being as if they were corresponding with a human being.

Ethics: Ethics are guiding values, principles and standards that help people determine 'how things should be done'.

Human Psychology: A branch of psychology that examines the cognitive, emotional and behavioral states of the individual.

Intelligence: The ability of an individual to learn, to use what he/she has learnt, to identify and use new solutions to problems and to adapt to innovations.

Mental Health: The concept of well-being can be defined as a state in which an individual is in a state of equilibrium as a whole, that is to say, in all three aspects of their being: cognitive, affective and behavioral.

Morality: Morality is a set of value judgements that show how people should or should not behave in their relations with beings and people, including themselves.

Therapy: Therapy refers to the treatment processes applied to improve a person's mental, emotional, psychological or physical health.

Chapter 4
Artificial Intelligence-Based Applications Used in Neonatal Intensive Care Units

Emine Buse Kurnaz
https://orcid.org/0009-0008-3473-6602
Graduate Education Institute, Turkey

Deniz Yigit
https://orcid.org/0000-0001-5627-7963
Kütahya Faculty of Health Sciences, Turkey

Emel Sezici
https://orcid.org/0000-0002-6325-6607
Kütahya Faculty of Health Sciences, Turkey

ABSTRACT

The neonatal period is a time when many systems of newborns are immature and vulnerable to external dangers. Newborns may be admitted to the Neonatal Intensive Care Unit due to different health problems they experience during this period. Newborns in these units need a multidisciplinary team approach and the use of advanced technological applications. With the development of technology in recent years, the use of artificial intelligence-based applications has increased in Neonatal Intensive Care Units. These applications include imaging and diagnostic systems, clinical decision support systems, robotic and automation applications, follow-up and monitoring of infants, ventilator management and respiratory support systems, infection and sepsis monitoring. Effective diagnosis, treatment and care services are

DOI: 10.4018/979-8-3373-1479-2.ch004

carried out by healthcare professionals with artificial intelligence-based applications. Artificial intelligence-based applications used in the Neonatal Intensive Care Unit increase the life chances of newborns and positively affect long-term health and development outcomes.

INTRODUCTION

The neonatal period is a time when many systems of newborns are immature and vulnerable to external dangers. During this period, newborns can be admitted to Neonatal Intensive Care Units (NICU) due to serious health problems such as respiratory distress, neonatal retinopathy, necrotizing enterocolitis, jaundice and sepsis. NICUs are specialized units where special care is given to newborns with critical medical and surgical problems (Ugucu et al., 2024). In these units, neonates struggling with serious conditions such as premature birth, congenital anomaly, sepsis and respiratory failure need a multidisciplinary team approach and advanced technological equipment. (Hsu et al., 2021). With the development of technology in recent years, the use of technology-based applications has increased in the NICU (Arora et al., 2025). The use of technology in the NICU plays a critical role in increasing the life chances of infants with health problems. Thanks to advanced medical devices and monitoring systems, the vital functions of infants can be monitored instantaneously and early intervention can be provided when necessary. The use of technology-based applications in the NICU improves not only the personal care of newborns but also the standards of neonatal care by increasing the overall quality of healthcare services (Iqbal et al., 2024). Increasing the survival rate of infants and decreasing the risk of complications are directly related to the advancement of technology and the use of appropriate technological applications. Therefore, the use of technological-based applications in the NICU is important (Monaghan et al., 2020).

With the development of technology in recent years, artificial intelligence applications have been integrated into technological applications. artificial intelligence based applications are software systems that mimic human intelligence and have capabilities such as learning, reasoning, problem solving or language processing to perform specific tasks. These applications enable machines to analyse and learn from data, make predictions and even make decisions. With these applications, newborns are provided holistic care with advanced technology incubators, mechanical ventilators, monitors, drug pumps, infusion devices and similar devices in the NICU. The active use of artificial intelligence-based applications in the NICU has many benefits for infants, their families and healthcare professionals (Iqbal et al., 2024; Racine et al., 2024). Benefits for infants include rapid and early intervention, personalised care, predictive care, continuous monitoring, long-term health monitoring, decision support systems (Monaghan et al., 2020). Benefits for families include fast and accurate information, reduced anxiety and stress, personalised care plans, time and resource management, remote monitoring and information, emotional support (Kerkez & Kaplan, 2025; Sunshine et al., 2023; Venkatasubramanian et al., 2023). Among the benefits for health professionals; fast and accurate decision making, alleviating workload, reducing error rate, more effective resource management, access to training and information, increased communication and coordination within the team, predictive guidance. As can be seen, the use of artificial intelligence-based applications in the NICU has become mandatory. Health professionals have important duties for the dissemination of this use (Rallis et al., 2024; Malak et al., 2019).

In order for artificial intelligence-based applications to become widespread in the NICU, healthcare professionals need to undertake various tasks and responsibilities. These tasks are of critical importance in terms of effectively integrating artificial intelligence, using it correctly and improving the quality of healthcare services (Chan & Shorey, 2021; Krysia & Marion, 2018). Nurses are the health professionals who spend the most time with infants in the NICU. It is key for nurses to increase their awareness of technological developments, to follow technological developments, to be involved in the application processes and to integrate technological applications into their profession (Coskun et al., 2024; Krysia & Marion, 2018).

NEONATAL INTENSIVE CARE UNITS AND ARTIFICIAL INTELLIGENCE

According to data from the World Health Organisation, 47% of all deaths of children under five years of age are neonatal deaths (WHO, 2022). This has led to the global target of reducing infant mortality by 2030 being set as an important goal (United Nations General Assembly, 2015). The process of adaptation of newborns to the outside world and the underdevelopment of their body systems may increase the need for special care. Especially in high-risk infants, this need increases even more. In this case, newborns can be followed up in the NICU. NICUs are units where premature infants, infants with low birth weight or infants with serious health problems after birth receive special care and treatment (Kilicarslan Toruner & Buyukgonenc 2017; Dagoglu & Ovali, 2017). These units have various technological equipment (radiant heaters, incubators, infusion pumps, mechanical ventilators and continuous monitoring devices, etc.) and highly qualified healthcare personnel to support the follow-up, treatment, care and recovery processes of newborns. In NICUs, it is important for healthcare professionals to work with a multidisciplinary approach to stabilise the health status of newborns, prevent possible complications and achieve the best recovery outcomes. However, healthcare professionals may experience different problems in multidisciplinary working processes (Karabudak & Ergun, 2018). Health professionals working in the NICU may encounter many clinical and organisational problems. The main clinical problems include respiratory problems, infections, neurological problems, cardiovascular problems, gastrointestinal problems, metabolic problems, electrolyte imbalances and nutritional difficulties (Al-Sofyani, 2025; Beleza et al., 2019). The main organisational problems include technological difficulties, staff shortage and workload, lack of communication and support with the newborn's family, ethical problems and financial problems (Brachio et al., 2023; Ediz & Kucuk, 2023; Karabay et al., 2021; Lee & Huang, 2022; Kucuk & Yagmur, 2019). As stated in the research, health professionals encounter many problems in the NICU. Therefore, it is of great importance to approach these problems with a solution-oriented approach. In the process of solving the problems; it is necessary to follow current developments in applications, use technological applications specific to the field and integrate them into the applications (Sorrentino et al., 2025; Racine et al., 2024; Donmez, 2020).

The development of technology in recent years has increased the importance given to the concept of artificial intelligence day by day. Artificial intelligence is a system that has abilities such as learning, reasoning, problem solving, perception by imitating human intelligence and can be developed within the need (Donmez, 2020). These systems include many comprehensive techniques such as machine learning, deep learning, natural language processing (Robert, 2019). The fact that artificial intelligence consists of advanced techniques and shows a rapid development has increased its use in different sectors. Health sector is one of these sectors (Krysia & Marion, 2018). With artificial intelligence-based applications, positive developments are rapidly achieved in situations such as early diagnosis, diagnosis, treatment, care, health protection and improvement (Yigit & Acikgöz, 2024). Health professionals have important duties in the integration and utilisation of artificial intelligence applications in the health sector. Nurses, one of the healthcare professionals who spend the most time with patients, have a key role in the use of artificial intelligence applications (Krysia & Marion, 2018). The rapid changes in healthcare today have made nursing practices increasingly complex. Increasing patient expectations, rapid developments in information and technology, rising healthcare costs, and global competition necessitate the use of technological innovations in the nursing profession. In this context, artificial intelligence technologies offer significant contributions to nurses in areas such as decision support systems, patient monitoring, data analysis, and care planning. It is of great importance for nurses to follow these developments closely, develop digital literacy skills, and integrate artificial intelligence into professional practices for quality and safe patient care (Al-Sofyani, 2025; Molu, 2025; Manworren et al., 2024; Ozsezer, 2022).

Nurses play a key role in the integration of artificial intelligence applications into the profession. The need for artificial intelligence technologies, especially in areas such as diagnostic tests, early diagnosis and alarm systems, is becoming more evident every day (Al-Sofyani, 2025; Molu, 2025; Hafez Elsayed et al., 2024; Feldman & Rohan, 2022). In particular, the potential to diagnose without resorting to invasive methods and to develop new treatment and care approaches arouses great interest in the health sector (Rajpurkar et al., 2022). The use of artificial intelligence in nursing provides significant advances in clinical predictions. Analytical predictions can be made in many areas such as disease progression, risk prevention and risk scoring. Thanks to algorithms developed using electronic health records, hospital supply chain and patient data, the length of hospital stay of patients depending on diagnoses can be predicted (Ozsezer, 2022). Analysing artificial intelligence in medical imaging enables patient data to be integrated with scientific evidence, guidelines and treatment plans and used in disease management. In this way, the efficiency and effectiveness of systems that support and manage care processes can be increased with artificial intelligence analyses (Clipper et al., 2018). The use of artificial intelligence-based applications in the nursing profession significantly reduces the workload of nurses by automating their routine and time-consuming tasks, thus allowing nurses to provide more qualified and patient-focused care. These technologies assist nurses in many areas such as data analysis, patient monitoring, medication management, risk assessment and clinical decision support systems, ensuring that care processes are carried out more quickly, accurately and effectively (Al-Sofyani, 2025; Molu, 2025). As a result, artificial intelligence applications not only reduce the workload of nurses, but also significantly contribute to the effectiveness of the overall health system by increasing the quality, safety and patient satisfaction of the health service provided (Ozsezer, 2022).

ARTIFICIAL INTELLIGENCE BASED APPLICATIONS USED IN NEONATAL INTENSIVE CARE UNIT

The use of artificial intelligence-based applications in units where care is provided to patients in the priority and sensitive population increases the quality of health care. NICUs are at the forefront of these units. In these units, artificial intelligence-based applications are effective in determining complex data relationships, improving early diagnosis, diagnosis and treatment processes, and creating personalised care (Beam et al., 2024). With these applications, neonates receive holistic care in the NICU with high-tech incubators, mechanical ventilators, monitors, drug pumps, infusion devices and similar devices. The active use of artificial intelligence-based applications in the NICU has many benefits for infants, their families and healthcare professionals.

The benefits for infants include rapid and early intervention, personalised care, predictive care, continuous monitoring, long-term health monitoring, decision support systems (Monaghan et al., 2020; Tang et al., 2024). Benefits for families include fast and accurate information, reduced anxiety and stress, personalised care plans, time and resource management, remote monitoring and information, emotional support (Mokadem et al., 2024; Brødsgaard et al., 2019). Among the benefits for health professionals; fast and accurate decision making, alleviation of workload, reduction of error rate, more effective resource management, access to training and information, increased communication and coordination within the team, predictive guidance. As can be seen, the use of artificial intelligence-based applications in the NICU has become mandatory (Rallis et al., 2024; Malak et al., 2019). Artificial intelligence-based applications used in the NICU include imaging and diagnostic systems, clinical decision support systems, robotic and automation applications, follow-up and monitoring of infants, ventilator management and respiratory support systems, infection and sepsis monitoring (Wang et al., 2024; Kim et al., 2023; Lei et al., 2022; Ponthier et al., 2022; Saha et al., 2020).

1. Imaging and Diagnostic Systems

Artificial intelligence-based applications can provide faster and more precise results than experts in the analysis of medical images. This ability is especially critical in the diagnosis of sensitive conditions in premature infants. Artificial intelligence algorithms can detect respiratory problems such as Respiratory Distress Syndrome (RDS) and Bronchopulmonary Dysplasia (BPD) in chest X-rays, and brain haemorrhages and other abnormalities in ultrasound images at an early stage. In this way, possible complications can be prevented with rapid intervention. In studies (Lei et al., 2022; Saha et al., 2020), it is reported that artificial intelligence algorithms achieve similar or higher accuracy rates than radiologists in the diagnosis of RDS. With an artificial intelligence model that can predict RDS in infants; decisions regarding surfactant administration can be supported and unnecessary treatment can be prevented (Jang et al., 2023). Brain Magnetic Resonance Imaging (MRI) is recognised as an important tool for assessing brain development and predicting neurodevelopmental outcomes in premature infants (Hintz et al, 2015). With the integration of brain MRI into artificial intelligence, cognitive and motor skills of infants can be predicted. This constitutes an important basis for the development of early interventions to improve cognitive and motor skills in infants (Saha et al., 2020). In addition, acute bilirubin encephalopathy (ABE), which can cause brain damage in newborns, can be diagnosed early and accurately with MRI images. This method can improve treatment processes and reduce the risk of brain damage by contributing to early and accurate diagnosis of ABE in newborns (Wu et al., 2022).

As can be seen from the studies, the combination of ultrasound imaging techniques with artificial intelligence can be used in many different areas in NICUs.

Thermal imaging systems can provide information about infections, circulatory problems and other disorders by analysing the body temperature distribution of infants. This method can be used for early diagnosis of necrotising enterocolitis (NEC), a serious intestinal disorder in newborns. The infrared thermal imaging camera can be used to automatically analyse the temperature distribution in the abdomen of infants. In this way, intestinal inflammation and temperature changes, which are early signs of NEC, can be detected with high accuracy (Shi et al., 2020). However, artificial intelligence applications can assess the risk of retinopathy of prematurity in newborns by analysing fundus photographs. It is reported that artificial intelligence algorithms perform similarly to expert ophthalmologists in the diagnosis of retinopathy of prematurity. In conclusion, artificial intelligence-supported medical imaging and diagnostic systems are effective in the early diagnosis of diseases in newborns (Huang et al., 2020).

2. Clinical Decision Support Systems

By analysing large datasets, artificial intelligence can support clinical decision-making and provide valuable insights to healthcare professionals (Almagharbeh, 2024). Artificial intelligence based applications can predict the risk of serious conditions such as sepsis, necrotising enterocolitis, respiratory failure, hypoglycaemia by analysing vital signs, laboratory results and other clinical data of infant (Meeus, et al., 2024; Singh et al., 2022; Tarricone et al., 2021). It is stated that artificial intelligence models developed in this context have high success in accurately predicting hypoglycaemia developing in newborns within the first four hours after birth. With the model created, risk factors of hypoglycaemia in newborns are determined. This supports clinical decision-making processes and enables timely intervention and treatment (Wang et al., 2024). Artificial intelligence-based clinical decision support tools developed to determine malnutrition in newborns have high success rates. With the developed clinical support tools, discharge weights and weight gain at discharge of newborns are estimated. It is predicted that the incidence of post-discharge growth retardation can be reduced by using the developed model in clinical applications (Yalcin et al., 2023). As seen in the studies, artificial intelligence-based applications have many benefits in special cases such as hypoglycemia and feeding disorders in newborns.

Artificial intelligence-based applications are widely used in identifying general health problems as well as in detecting special conditions in newborns through clinical decision support systems. Artificial intelligence-based systems can predict conditions such as sepsis earlier and more accurately than traditional methods

(Meeus, et al., 2024; Singh et al., 2022; Tarricone et al., 2021). It is stated that the artificial neural network based diagnosis model developed for the treatment of neonatal sepsis has a high success rate. While creating this model; mother and infant data are used. By using the developed model in clinical applications, the accuracy and speed of neonatal sepsis diagnosis can be increased (Helguera-Repetto et al., 2020). However, a prediction model developed to predict the failure of CPAP therapy after less invasive surfactant administration in premature newborns is used. This prediction model provides information about the factors leading to failure in less invasive surfactant administration and supports personalised clinical decisions in early respiratory management (Kloonen et al., 2023).

Artificial intelligence applications play an important role not only in the prediction of serious diseases but also in the detection of possible errors in drug applications. The frequency and severity of adverse drug reactions (ADRs), especially in neonates, can be difficult to predict due to age-related differences. Therefore, drug-drug interactions (DDIs) are evaluated with risk matrix (probability + severity) scales and artificial intelligence algorithms are created to predict the probability of DDI occurrence. In clinical applications, the use of a high-performance model that predicts drug-drug interactions with a neonatal-focused approach can help optimise treatment processes (Yalcin et al., 2022). Artificial intelligence-based applications can help determine the most appropriate treatment protocols by analysing the effectiveness of different treatment approaches. This is important for the development of personalised treatment approaches (Kim et al., 2023). In this context, artificial intelligence-based clinical decision support systems have the potential to significantly improve diagnosis and treatment processes in neonatal care.

3. Robotics and Automation Applications

Artificial intelligence-supported robotics and automation applications can reduce the workload and improve the quality of care by automating some tasks in NICUs. The use of robots focusing on paediatric patient care facilitates nursing care processes, especially by reducing the workload of nurses (Liang et al., 2019). These robots can continuously monitor the vital signs of infants and give warnings in case of sudden changes (Khanam et al., 2022). Robotic systems can be used in the preparation and administration of drugs at the correct doses. This can improve drug safety by minimising human error (Ponthier et al., 2022). Therapeutic assistance robots used in this context contribute to the faster and more effective implementation of treatments by performing tasks such as drug distribution and wound care by directly supporting the treatment processes of patients. Help robots can also be customised within the scope of profession. With the help robots created for the nursing profession; it is ensured that patients' medication is followed up and nurses and patient relatives are informed in case of emergency (Arif et al., 2017). Similarly, assistance robots used for the rehabilitation of patients help patients to regain their mobility and personalise rehabilitation processes by supporting their physical rehabilitation processes. Telepresence robots enable remote patient monitoring and communication, allowing doctors and nurses to monitor patients remotely, especially in isolation rooms to prevent the spread of infectious diseases. Logistics and disinfection robots increase hygiene and efficiency by automating logistics and disinfection processes in NICUs, performing tasks such as material handling and room disinfection (Li et al., 2024). In conclusion, artificial intelligence supported robotics and automation applications in NICUs have the potential to significantly improve the quality and efficiency of care in these units, both improving the sensitive care of premature infants and enabling healthcare staff to focus on critical tasks (Li et al., 2024; Liang et al., 2019).

4. Follow-up and Monitoring of Infants

Artificial intelligence based applications play a critical role in early detection of potential problems by continuously analysing infants' vital signs. Compared to traditional methods, artificial intelligence-based applications can perform more precise and faster analyses. These analyses can be made through vital signs, sleep monitoring, video and audio recordings. For this purpose, the vital signs of infants are monitored instantly with sensor systems. Similarly, non-contact radar-based systems can be used to monitor the respiration of premature infants in the NICU. These systems provide reliable respiratory frequency estimates that are compatible with reference wired devices by reducing the noise from the environment (Beltrão, et al., 2022).

In addition to monitoring the vital signs of babies in the NICU, more complicated health problems can also be monitored with artificial intelligence applications. One of these problems is conditions related to the cardiovascular system. Improving the diagnosis, treatment and follow-up processes of cardiological problems of newborns is possible with echocardiography analyses, diagnosis of congenital heart diseases, cardiac risk prediction (Lei et al., 2022; Doshi et al., 2021). For this purpose, the cardiovascular status of infants can be monitored using non-contact cameras. Heart rate variability data obtained with camera-based measurements show a high level of agreement with data obtained with contact-based patient monitors (Zeng et al., 2024). Neurological problems also have an important place among the complex health problems encountered in newborns. In the NICU, it is of vital importance to monitor the wakefulness and neurological changes of infants. Prediction models can be created by retrospective examination of the video images of these infants. These prediction models show that artificial intelligence pose prediction is applicable in NICU and that cerebral dysfunction can be predicted from video data only, similar to electroencephalography (EEG) diagnosis (Gleason, et al., 2024). In conclusion, tracking and monitoring of infants in the NICU with artificial intelligence-based systems and the development of contactless monitoring methods are important in terms of intervention in instantaneous situations and prevention of long-term adverse situations.

5. Ventilator Management and Respiratory Support Systems

Since the respiratory system in newborn babies is not yet fully mature, this immature structure can prevent respiratory functions from being performed effectively, especially in premature babies. In addition to this situation, the presence of accompanying health problems such as infections, congenital anomalies, lung diseases or cardiovascular problems make respiratory functions even more difficult and can lead to serious respiratory distress. Therefore, respiratory system problems in newborns are of critical importance in terms of both early diagnosis and continuous monitoring (Go et al., 2025). Artificial intelligence based applications in the NICU have significant potential in the management of respiratory diseases, including image analysis, decision making and prognosis prediction. Artificial intelligence based applications play an important role in the optimisation of ventilator settings and personalisation of respiratory support. With this situation, automatic ventilator adjustment, respiratory problem prediction, personalised respiratory support can be provided (Kim et al., 2023). Accurately predicting the demand for invasive mechanical ventilation is vital for clinical decision making (Zhang et al., 2024). In this direction, the need for intubation in newborns with respiratory distress within 3 hours was predicted with an accuracy of 88.2% by combining clinical data and time series variables using Multimodal Deep Neural Network (MDNN). This model can help healthcare professionals in decision-making processes for newborns with respiratory distress requiring endotracheal intubation (Im et al., 2022). Information from bedside pulse oximetry and ventilator data can be combined with machine learning analyses to predict extubation readiness in premature infants. Using continuous data streams from bedside pulse oximeters and ventilators, machine learning analyses appear to have the potential to improve the accuracy of prediction of extubation readiness in premature infants (Brasher et al., 2024).

One of the most important health problems leading to respiratory distress in the NICU is bronchopulmonary dysplasia (BPD). BPD is a chronic respiratory disease that occurs in newborns born in the early stages of lung development and can lead to respiratory, cardiovascular and neurodevelopmental problems in the long term. It is stated that machine learning models have high success in predicting the risk of BPD in premature infants in the early period. Especially the high accuracy rate of the postnatal day 7 model shows that these models can be a valuable tool in developing early intervention and personalised treatment strategies in clinical applications (Kostekci et al,. 2023). In this context, the use of artificial intelligence technologies in the management of vital conditions such as respiratory distress and pulmonary dysplasia in newborn infants provides significant advances in areas such as early diagnosis, personalised treatment and optimisation of ventilation processes (Brasher et al., 2024; Im et al., 2022).

6. Infection and Sepsis Follow-up

Neonatal sepsis is one of the most common health problems encountered in NICUs. Sepsis that occurs within 48 hours after birth is called early-onset sepsis, while sepsis that occurs after 48 hours after birth is called late-onset sepsis (Chandra et al., 2023; Shane et al., 2017). Neonatal sepsis is an important cause of morbidity and mortality in neonates admitted to the NICU. Therefore, early detection and appropriate care are of vital importance (Zea-Vera & Ochoa, 2015). Artificial intelligence-based applications are an important tool in the early diagnosis and follow-up of serious conditions such as infection and sepsis in newborns. Artificial intelligence models created with data sources obtained from the NICU can provide real-time predictions of sepsis risk and inform healthcare professionals about suspected cases (Persad et al., 2021). Artificial intelligence models can analyse large datasets obtained from various sources such as electronic patient records, vital signs, laboratory results to assess the risk of sepsis. With these applications, early sepsis diagnosis, identification of infection risk factors, and antibiotic treatment optimisation can be achieved (Tarricone et al., 2021; Helguera-Repetto et al., 2020; Song et al., 2020). In this context, it has been determined that artificial intelligence-supported models used in the detection of late-onset sepsis in premature infants have a high success rate using non-invasive vital sign monitoring methods (Tang et al., 2024). Similarly, data representing heart rate variability, respiration and body movement are used for early prediction of late-onset sepsis in premature infants. The prediction model created with high-resolution electrocardiogram and respiratory data representing these data values has a high success rate (Cabrera-Quiros et al., 2021). In order to detect early-onset sepsis in newborns, classification models with high success rate are used using artificial neural networks (Alvi et al., 2020). As a result, although artificial intelligence-based applications have high success in the early diagnosis of infection and sepsis, there is a need to increase innovative applications in this field (Bates & Syrowatka, 2022).

ARTIFICIAL INTELLIGENCE AND DATA ANALYSIS: THE ROLE OF DATA IN NEONATAL INTENSIVE CARE

Many data sources are used when creating artificial intelligence based applications. Artificial intelligence based applications are created by training models with these data. There are many data for the creation of artificial intelligence-based applications in NICUs. Effective use of these data increases the quality and positive results of applications (Safiya & Saleena, 2024; McGregor, 2013). Data collected in NICUs include various information such as vital signs, laboratory results, imaging data, medication information and nursing records. Accurate collection, analysis and interpretation of these data are critical for early diagnosis, treatment follow-up, risk prediction and quality of care (Kaliappan et al., 2023; Wu et al., 2022; Beluzo et al., 2020). Therefore, continuous monitoring of infants' vital functions in NICUs is of great importance. Traditional monitoring methods (ECG, pulse oximetry, etc.) may cause problems such as cable confusion, tissue damage, and increased stress in infants. In addition, the electrodes may be affected by sudden movements, which may lead to misinterpretation of the results during the period when infants are mobile and healthcare professionals and their families hold the infant (Marchionni et al., 2016). Therefore, there is an increasing need to monitor vital functions with non-contact monitoring devices. This need can be met by various new technological applications such as magnetic induction, radar, WiFi, phonocardiograms, thermal imaging and video camera imaging (Ling et al., 2022; Quon et al., 2021; Ismail et al., 2018). These innovative approaches significantly reduce the risk of skin damage while improving infant comfort. In addition, sensors and wearable technologies allow continuous and real-time collection of infants' physiological data. These data can be analysed by artificial intelligence algorithms to provide important information about infants (Arora et al., 2025; Wu et al., 2022).

Traditional wired monitoring systems used in the NICU can negatively affect infants and their families physically and psychologically. It can also complicate the care process of health professionals during the care of the infant (Ling et al., 2022). Cables can cause movement restrictions, reduced signal quality, and complicate routine care processes. Therefore, IoT-based infrastructure and e-textile technologies have the potential to improve the quality of care by offering wireless and contactless monitoring solutions in the NICU environment. IoT-based e-textile respiratory monitoring platforms consisting of a wireless sensor belt, wearable embedded system and edge computing device are a promising tool for monitoring physiological parameters of newborns (Cay et al., 2021).

Artificial intelligence and data analytics in the NICU are becoming indispensable for better monitoring of patients, preventing complications and optimising treatment processes. These technologies not only make healthcare more effective, but also improve patient safety by enabling individualised care processes. The integration of nurses and other healthcare professionals into these technologies is critical for success (Ling et al., 2022; Quon et al., 2021).

ETHICAL PROBLEMS ENCOUNTERED IN THE USE OF ARTIFICIAL INTELLIGENCE BASED APPLICATIONS IN NEONATAL INTENSIVE CARE UNIT

NICUs are critical areas where newborns, who constitute the most vulnerable patient group, struggle for life. Although the use of artificial intelligence-based applications in these units has the potential to increase quality and efficiency in healthcare services, it also brings various ethical challenges (Stedman et al., 2023; Loder & Nicholas, 2018). While the advantages of artificial intelligence such as data processing capacity, fast decision-making ability and reducing the risk of error provide great benefits in intensive care processes, it may lead to the questioning of basic ethical principles such as patient privacy, decision-making responsibility and equality in access to healthcare services. In this context, it is of great importance to both make the most of the opportunities offered by technology and to protect human values by understanding the ethical issues related to the use of artificial intelligence in NICU and seeking solutions (Rigby et al., 2016). Ethical issues encountered in NICU include data privacy and security, ethical dilemmas in decision-making processes, technological access and equality in healthcare, problems in family communication, legal and ethical responsibility (Beam et al., 2024; Sullivan et al., 2024; Stedman et al., 2023).

1. Data Privacy and Security

In the creation of artificial intelligence-based applications, the success rate of the application increases as the data increases. The data used in the NICU consists of patient health records, laboratory results and other sensitive information. This situation increases the responsibility to protect patient privacy and causes ethical problems (Loder & Nicholas, 2018). In this context, it is important to obtain permission for the use of the data to be used, to anonymise them while using them, and to store them securely (Sullivan et al., 2024; Loder & Nicholas, 2018).

2. Ethical Dilemmas in Decision Making Processes

The use of artificial intelligence-based applications in the NICU supports the decision-making processes of healthcare professionals. However, at this stage, health professionals may experience ethical dilemmas. The dilemma of who will be responsible for the decisions taken in decision-making processes can negatively affect the process. Before using artificial intelligence-based applications, it is important to share responsibility between health professionals, artificial intelligence developers and health institutions (Frize et al., 2003). At the same time, algorithms used in the creation of artificial intelligence applications may produce biased results for underrepresented demographic groups. Therefore, evaluating many criteria together in decision-making processes and making decisions in line with comprehensive data can reduce ethical dilemmas (Sullivan et al., 2024; Loder & Nicholas, 2018).

3. Technological Access and Equality in Health Services

The use of artificial intelligence based applications in NICUs may vary from country to country and from region to region within the same country. This variability may increase inequalities in access to healthcare services for high-cost applications (Sullivan et al., 2024). Especially NICUs in rural areas may be disadvantaged in accessing these systems due to their lack of technological infrastructure. This situation causes a violation of the principle of justice in access to healthcare services. From an ethical perspective, it should be ensured that such technologies are offered to everyone with equal access (Arora et al., 2025; Schouten et al., 2024).

4. Problems in Family Communication

During the use of artificial intelligence-based applications in the NICU, communication of healthcare professionals with the families of infants is very important (Arora et al., 2025). Adequate knowledge of families about the applications will increase their compliance with the application processes. Informing families about the applications to be used in infants, increasing their awareness and including them in the process has an important place in protecting patient rights (Sullivan et al., 2024; Loder & Nicholas, 2018).

5. Legal Liability

As a result of any adverse situation arising from artificial intelligence-based applications in the NICU, it is an important issue of debate to whom the legal responsibility belongs. It is not known whether this responsibility belongs to the user or the developer of the application (Sullivan et al., 2024; Loder & Nicholas, 2018). For this reason, it is of great importance to regularly audit the applications developed and to comply with the principle of transparency. In addition, the establishment and development of a legal framework for artificial intelligence applications is key (van Assen et al., 2020).

The use of evidence-based practices is the key point in preventing ethical problems that may arise during the use of artificial intelligence-based applications in the NICU (Chng et al., 2025). Evidence-based health informatics supports the use of sound scientific evidence in decision-making mechanisms in the process of implementing technological health systems. This approach is critical to ensure the safe and effective use of artificial intelligence systems in child health. UNICEF recommends an approach to the development and deployment of artificial intelligence systems that supports children's collective rights to protection, access to services and participation (United Nations Children's Fund, 2021). This approach should be flexible enough to be adaptable to national or local contexts while encouraging the co-operation of various stakeholders. This approach aims to ensure that children make the best use of artificial intelligence technologies while minimising potential risks. In the literature, it is emphasised that ethical principles should be followed while developing artificial intelligence-based applications and the importance of giving importance to human values when faced with ethical problems. In order to be compatible with these values, applications should include the principles of transparency, security, auditability, reliability and recoverability (Ning et al., 2024; Etzioni & Etzioni, 2017). In order to develop trustworthy artificial intelligence based applications, experts need to carefully consider elements such as accountability, ethical issues and transparency (Solomonides et al., 2022; Shin & Park, 2019). According to the Independent High-Level Expert Group on Artificial Intelligence, an artificial intelligence application should have 3 basic characteristics to be considered ethical. These principles are legal compliance, ethical soundness, and respect for values (Jobin, Ienca & Vayena, 2019). To achieve these goals, Explainable Artificial Intelligence approaches need to carefully address the key components of fair and ethical decision-making processes. Careful consideration of these elements will ensure the ethical and reliable use of artificial intelligence algorithms. The main ethical considerations to be used in artificial intelligence based applications for neonatal health are nonmaleficence, benevolence, autonomy, confidentiality, fairness and transferability, transparency and explainability, accountability, reliability, auditability and knowledge management (Chng et al., 2025). As a result, the development and implementation of artificial intelligence-based applications in the NICU for the benefit of newborns and within the framework of ethical principles is essential for the sustainability and social acceptance of technological progress in this field (Abdallah et al., 2025; Arora et al., 2025).

LOOKING TO THE FUTURE: DEVELOPMENT OF ARTIFICIAL INTELLIGENCE BASED APPLICATIONS IN NEONATAL INTENSIVE CARE UNITS

Artificial intelligence-based applications have the potential to revolutionise early diagnosis, treatment and evidence-based care in the NICU using large and high-dimensional data. In the future, NICUs can be designed in a more intelligent, efficient and newborn-centred way integrated with artificial intelligence technologies. It can be equipped with sensors, cameras and other IoT (Internet of Things) devices that continuously collect and analyse data (vital signs, EEG, video images, etc.) of infants in the NICU created with the Smart Environment. By processing this data in real time, artificial intelligence algorithms can instantly detect changes in the condition of infants and alert healthcare personnel. In this way, proactive intervention is possible and emergencies can be prevented (Bharathi, 2024; Mbanuzue et al., 2024). By analysing the data collected from sensors and simulations, the most suitable and efficient workspaces can be created. With these designed NICUs, personalised care areas can be created and customised care areas can be designed according to the individual needs of each infant (gestational age, weight, diagnosis, etc.). With these care areas, the risk of infection can be reduced, the movement of personnel can be facilitated and care efficiency can be increased (Choudhury & Urena, 2022).

Pain management in the NICU is of critical importance, especially in the post-operative period, and considering the difficulties of current practices and the side effects of opioid use, new artificial intelligence-supported approaches are promising. These approaches can predict the onset of pain with high accuracy by analysing data such as facial and body movements, crying frequency and vital signs of newborns, and have the potential to minimise or prevent harm from postoperative pain and opioid withdrawal through proactive pain reduction methods (Salekin et al., 2021). Artificial intelligence can support clinical decision-making processes, facilitate the evaluation of neonatal laboratory results and vital signs, and minimise medical errors in drug administration (Choudhury & Urena, 2022). At the same time, while providing nurses with tools to increase patient safety, it also contributes to their professional development with developments in information technology, allowing them to alleviate their workload and allocate more face-to-face care time to their patients (Unal & Avci, 2024). In addition, by creating automated workflows (drug preparation, data entry, reporting, inventory management, etc.) in the NICU, the workload of healthcare personnel can be reduced and patient-oriented care can be increased (Yalcin et al., 2022). Although these developments have the potential to shape the future of neonatal care, they also require careful consideration of ethical and legal issues.

CONCLUSION AND RECOMMENDATIONS

The use of artificial intelligence-based applications in the NICU offers a significant potential for transformation in diagnosis, treatment and care processes. In this context; imaging and diagnostic systems, clinical decision support systems, robotic and automation applications, tracking and monitoring of infants can be performed. These applications offer the opportunity to increase the quality of care in NICUs and improve the health of newborns (Wang et al., 2024; Kim et al., 2023; Lei et al., 2022; Ponthier et al., 2022;; Saha et al., 2020). However, the appropriate use of artificial intelligence-based applications and the prevention of ethical problems require the active participation of health professionals. Health professionals should closely follow developments in artificial intelligence-based applications and be involved in the development of these applications (Abdallah et al., 2025). This will both ensure the effective and safe use of artificial intelligence and minimise ethical concerns (Wang et al., 2024; Kim et al., 2023; Ponthier et al., 2022). It is important to increase the use of artificial intelligence-based applications in NICUs, to encourage multidisciplinary studies, to develop laws and regulations on ethical issues, and to take an active role of healthcare professionals in future scenarios related to artificial intelligence. Multidisciplinary studies will enable professionals from different specialities to come together and plan the integration of artificial intelligence into neonatal care in the best way (Salekin et al., 2021). Laws and regulations addressing ethical issues will minimise the potential risks associated with the use of artificial intelligence and ensure patient safety. The active participation of healthcare professionals in future scenarios will provide an important perspective on how artificial intelligence should be used in neonatal care. The use of artificial intelligence in NICUs offers the potential for significant advancement in neonatal care (Kim et al., 2023; Ponthier et al., 2022; Saha et al., 2020). It is important to invest in continuous education and research to understand the potential of artificial intelligence in neonatal care and to make the best use of this technology. Training programmes should be organised for healthcare professionals to have knowledge about artificial intelligence technologies and to use these technologies effectively (Kim et al., 2023; Ponthier et al., 2022). In addition, research should be conducted to assess the impact of artificial intelligence in neonatal care and identify best practices (Lei et al., 2022). In conclusion, artificial intelligence-based applications offer a significant potential for transformation in neonatal care. We suggest that in order to fully realise this potential, active participation of healthcare professionals, multidisciplinary studies, ethical regulations, continuous education and investment in research are required.

Competing Interests

The authors of this publication declare there are no competing interests.

REFERENCES

Abdallah, A. B. A. A., Sadaka, S. I. H., Ali, E. I., Bilal, S. A. M., Abdelrahman, M. O., Mohammed, F. B. F., & Omar, M. (2025). The Role of Artificial Intelligence in Pediatric Intensive Care: A Systematic Review. *Cureus, 17*(3). Advance online publication. DOI: 10.7759/cureus.80142 PMID: 40190909

Al-Sofyani, K. A. (2025). Role of artificial intelligence in pediatric intensive care: A survey of healthcare staff perspectives in Saudi Arabia. *Frontiers in Pediatrics, 13*, 1533877. DOI: 10.3389/fped.2025.1533877 PMID: 40066464

Almagharbeh, W. T. (2024). The impact of AI-based decision support systems on nursing workflows in critical care units. *International Nursing Review*. Advance online publication. DOI: 10.1111/inr.13011 PMID: 38973347

Alvi, R. H., Rahman, M. H., Khan, A. A. S., & Rahman, R. M. (2020). Predicting early neonatal sepsis using neural networks and other classifiers. *In 2020 IEEE 10th International Conference on Intelligent Systems (IS)* (pp. 443-450). IEEE. https://doi.org/DOI: 10.1109/IS48319.2020.9199937

Arif, D., Ahmad, A., Bakar, M. A., Ihtisham, M. H., & Winberg, S. (2017). Cost effective solution for minimization of medical errors and acquisition of vitals by using autonomous nursing robot. In *Proceedings of the 2017 International Conference on Information System and Data Mining* (pp. 134-138). https://doi.org/DOI: 10.1145/3077584.3077598

Arora, T., Muhammad-Kamal, H., & Beam, K. (2025). Preserving medical ethics in the era of artificial intelligence: Challenges and opportunities in neonatology. In *Seminars in Perinatology* (p. 152100). WB Saunders. DOI: 10.1016/j.semperi.2025.152100

Bates, D. W., & Syrowatka, A. (2022). Harnessing AI in sepsis care. *Nature Medicine, 28*(7), 1351–1352. DOI: 10.1038/s41591-022-01878-0 PMID: 35864250

Beam, K., Sharma, P., Levy, P., & Beam, A. L. (2024). Artificial intelligence in the neonatal intensive care unit: the time is now. *Journal of Perinatology,* 44(1), 131-135. 5; https://doi.org/DOI: 10.1038/s41372-023-01719-z

Beleza, L. D. O., Ribeiro, L. M., Paula, R. A. P., Guarda, L. E. D. A., Vieira, G. B., & Costa, K. S. F. (2019). Perfil de recién-nacidos de riesgo atendidos por enfermeros en seguimiento ambulatorio: Estudio de cohorte retrospectivo. *Revista Latino-Americana de Enfermagem, 27*, e3113. DOI: 10.1590/1518-8345.2301.3113 PMID: 30698216

Beltrão, G., Stutz, R., Hornberger, F., Martins, W. A., Tatarinov, D., Alaee-Kerahroodi, M., Lindner, U., Stock, L., Kaiser, E., Goedicke-Fritz, S., Schroeder, U., R, B. S. M., & Zemlin, M. (2022). Contactless radar-based breathing monitoring of premature infants in the neonatal intensive care unit. *Scientific Reports*, *12*(1), 5150. DOI: 10.1038/s41598-022-08836-3 PMID: 35338172

Beluzo, C. E., Silva, E., Alves, L. C., Bresan, R. C., Arruda, N. M., Sovat, R., & Carvalho, T. (2020). Towards neonatal mortality risk classification: A data-driven approach using neonatal, maternal, and social factors. *Informatics in Medicine Unlocked*, *20*, 100398. DOI: 10.1016/j.imu.2020.100398 PMID: 33102685

Bharathi, K. (2024). AI-Powered Vigilance in Neonatal Vital Signs Monitoring for Optimal Health Care. In *Modernizing Maternal Care With Digital Technologies* (pp. 159–182). IGI Global., DOI: 10.4018/979-8-3693-3711-0.ch007

Brachio, S. S., Gu, W., & Saiman, L. (2023). Next steps for health care-associated infections in the neonatal intensive care unit. *Clinics in Perinatology*, *50*(2), 381–397. DOI: 10.1016/j.clp.2023.02.001 PMID: 37201987

Brasher, M., Virodov, A., Raffay, T. M., Bada, H. S., Cunningham, M. D., Bumgardner, C., & Jawdeh, E. G. A. (2024). Predicting extubation readiness in preterm infants utilizing machine learning: A diagnostic utility study. *The Journal of Pediatrics*, *271*, 114043. DOI: 10.1016/j.jpeds.2024.114043 PMID: 38561049

Brødsgaard, A., Pedersen, J. T., Larsen, P., & Weis, J. (2019). Parents' and nurses' experiences of partnership in neonatal intensive care units: A qualitative review and meta-synthesis. *Journal of Clinical Nursing*, *28*(17-18), 3117–3139. DOI: 10.1111/jocn.14920 PMID: 31112337

Cabrera-Quiros, L., Kommers, D., Wolvers, M. K., Oosterwijk, L., Arents, N., van der Sluijs-Bens, J., Cottaar, E. J. E., Andriessen, P., & van Pul, C. (2021). Prediction of late-onset sepsis in preterm infants using monitoring signals and machine learning. *Critical Care Explorations*, *3*(1), e0302. DOI: 10.1097/CCE.0000000000000302 PMID: 33532727

Cay, G.. (2021). Baby-Guard: An IoT-based neonatal monitoring system integrated with smart textiles. In *2021 IEEE International Conference on Smart Computing (SMARTCOMP)* (pp. 129-136). IEEE. https://doi.org/DOI: 10.1109/SMARTCOMP52413.2021.00038

Chan, S. H., & Shorey, S. (2021). Healthcare professionals' sense of coherence of parental involvement in neonatal intensive care units: A framework synthesis. *Research in Nursing & Health*, *44*(6), 875–890. DOI: 10.1002/nur.22178 PMID: 34414586

Chandra, P., Iqbal, F., Unnikrisnan, M. K., Jayashree, P., Shenoy, P. A., Anburaj, S. E., Rajesh, V., Surulivelrajan, M., & Lewis, L. E. (2023). Neonatal outcomes associated with antimicrobial resistance: a retrospective cross-sectional study. *Journal of Applied Pharmaceutical Science, 13*(5), 081-094. https://doi.org/DOI: 10.7324/JAPS.2023.120166

Cang, S. Y., Tern, M. J. W., Lee, Y. S., Cheng, L. T.-E., Kapur, J., Eriksson, J. G., Chong, Y. S., & Savulescu, J. (2025). Ethical considerations in AI for child health and recommendations for child-centered medical AI. *NPJ Digital Medicine*, *8*(1), 152. DOI: 10.1038/s41746-025-01541-1 PMID: 40065130

Choudhury, A., & Urena, E. (2022). Artificial intelligence in NICU and PICU: a need for ecological validity, accountability, and human factors. *In Healthcare* (Vol. 10, No. 5, p. 952). MDPI. https://doi.org/DOI: 10.3390/healthcare10050952

Clipper, B., Batcheller, J., Thomaz, A. L., & Rozga, A. (2018). Artificial intelligence and robotics: A nurse leader's primer. *Nurse Leader*, *16*(6), 379–384. DOI: 10.1016/j.mnl.2018.07.015

Coskun, A. B., Kenner, C., & Elmaoglu, E. (2024). Neonatal Intensive Care Nurses' Perceptions of Artificial Intelligence: A Qualitative Study on Discharge Education and Family Counseling. *The Journal of Perinatal & Neonatal Nursing*, ●●●, 10–1097. DOI: 10.1097/JPN.0000000000000904 PMID: 39740134

Dagoglu, T., & Ovali, F. (2017). Newborn development and environmental factors. Dağoğlu, T., Görak, G. (Ed). Basic Neonatology and Nursing Principles (2nd Edition, pp.759-768). Istanbul: Nobel Medical Bookstores.

Donmez, S. (2020). Artificial intelligence and 2025 syndrome in philosophical context. *Journal of Çukurova University Faculty of Theology*, *20*(2), 748–760. DOI: 10.30627/cuilah.690645 0063

Doshi, K., Rehm, G. B., Vadlaputi, P., Lai, Z., Lakshminrusimha, S., Chuah, C. N., & Siefkes, H. M. (2021). A novel system to collect dual pulse oximetry data for critical congenital heart disease screening research. *Journal of Clinical and Translational Science*, *5*(1), e56. DOI: 10.1017/cts.2020.550 PMID: 33948277

Ediz, C., & Kucuk, S. (2023). An Important Issue in the Neonatal Intensive Care Unit: The Importance of Sound and Light Isolation for Premature Babies. *Turkish Journal of Health Sciences and Research*, *6*(3), 77–85. DOI: 10.51536/tusbad.1184972

Etzioni, A., & Etzioni, O. (2017). Incorporating ethics into artificial intelligence. *The Journal of Ethics*, *21*(4), 403–418. DOI: 10.1007/s10892-017-9252-2

Feldman, K., & Rohan, A. J. (2022). Data-driven nurse staffing in the neonatal intensive care unit. *MCN. The American Journal of Maternal Child Nursing*, *47*(5), 249–264. DOI: 10.1097/NMC.0000000000000839 PMID: 35960217

Frize, M., Walker, R. C., & Ennett, C. M. (2003). Development of an evidence-based ethical decision-making tool for neonatal intensive care medicine. In Proceedings of the 25th Annual International Conference of the IEEE Engineering in Medicine and Biology Society (IEEE Cat. No. 03CH37439) (Vol. 2, pp. 1260-1263). IEEE. https://doi.org/DOI: 10.1109/IEMBS.2003.1279490

Gleason, A., Richter, F., Beller, N., Arivazhagan, N., Feng, R., Holmes, E., Glicksberg, B. S., Morton, S. U., La Vega-Talbott, M., Fields, M., Guttmann, K., Nadkarni, G. N., & Richter, F. (2024). Detection of neurologic changes in critically ill infants using deep learning on video data: A retrospective single center cohort study. *EClinicalMedicine*, *78*, 102919. Advance online publication. DOI: 10.1016/j.eclinm.2024.102919 PMID: 39764545

Go, M. A., MacDonald, K. D., Durand, M., & McEvoy, C. T. (2025). Pulmonary function tests in the neonatal intensive care unit and beyond: A clinical review. *Journal of Perinatology*, •••, 1–12. DOI: 10.1038/s41372-025-02243-y PMID: 40021840

Hafez Elsayed, Z. E., Melika, S. W., & Mohamed Ads, S. E. (2024). Effect of Mind Mapping with Artificial Intelligence for High Alert Medications on Novice Nurses′ Performance at Neonatal Intensive Care Unit. *Assiut Scientific Nursing Journal*, *12*(43), 98–107. DOI: 10.21608/asnj.2024.279442.1804

Helguera-Repetto, A. C., Soto-Ramírez, M. D., Villavicencio-Carrisoza, O., Yong-Mendoza, S., Yong-Mendoza, A., León-Juárez, M., González-y-Merchand, J. A., Zaga-Clavellina, V., & Irles, C. (2020). Neonatal sepsis diagnosis decision-making based on artificial neural networks. *Frontiers in Pediatrics*, *8*, 525. DOI: 10.3389/fped.2020.00525 PMID: 33042902

Hintz, S. R., Barnes, P. D., Bulas, D., Slovis, T. L., Finer, N. N., Wrage, L. A., Das, A., Tyson, J. E., Stevenson, D. K., Carlo, W. A., Walsh, M. C., Laptook, A. R., Yoder, B. A., Van Meurs, K. P., Faix, R. G., Rich, W., Newman, N. S., Cheng, H., Heyne, R. J., & Higgins, R. D. (2015). Neuroimaging and neurodevelopmental outcome in extremely preterm infants. *Pediatrics*, *135*(1), e32–e42. DOI: 10.1542/peds.2014-0898 PMID: 25554820

Hsu, J. F., Chang, Y. F., Cheng, H. J., Yang, C., Lin, C. Y., Chu, S. M., Huang, H. R., Chiang, M. C., Wang, H. C., & Tsai, M. H. (2021). Machine learning approaches to predict in-hospital mortality among neonates with clinically suspected sepsis in the neonatal intensive care unit. *Journal of Personalized Medicine*, *11*(8), 695. DOI: 10.3390/jpm11080695 PMID: 34442338

Huang, Y. P., Vadloori, S., Chu, H. C., Kang, E. Y. C., Wu, W. C., Kusaka, S., & Fukushima, Y. (2020). Deep learning models for automated diagnosis of retinopathy of prematurity in preterm infants. *Electronics (Basel)*, *9*(9), 1444. DOI: 10.3390/electronics9091444

Im, J. E., Park, S., Kim, Y. J., Yoon, S. A., & Lee, J. H. (2022). Predicting the need for intubation within 3 hours in the neonatal intensive care unit using a multimodal deep neural network [Preprint]. *Research Square.* https://doi.org/DOI: 10.21203/rs.3.rs-1872902/v1

Iqbal, F., Chandra, P., Lewis, L. E. S., Acharya, D., Purkayastha, J., Shenoy, P. A., & Patil, A. K. (2024). Application of artificial intelligence to predict the sepsis in neonates admitted in neonatal intensive care unit. *Journal of Neonatal Nursing*, *30*(2), 141–147. DOI: 10.1016/j.jnn.2023.07.016

Ismail, S., Siddiqi, I., & Akram, U. (2018). Localization and classification of heart beats in phonocardiography signals—A comprehensive review. *EURASIP Journal on Advances in Signal Processing*, *2018*(1), 1–27. DOI: 10.1186/s13634-018-0545-9

Jang, W., Choi, Y. S., Kim, J. Y., Yon, D. K., Lee, Y. J., Chung, S. H., Kim, C. Y., Image, A. O., Yeo, S. G., & Lee, J. (2023). Artificial intelligence–driven respiratory distress syndrome prediction for very low birth weight infants: Korean multicenter prospective cohort study. *Journal of Medical Internet Research*, *25*, e47612. DOI: 10.2196/47612 PMID: 37428525

Jobin, A., Ienca, M., & Vayena, E. (2019). The global landscape of AI ethics guidelines. *Nature Machine Intelligence*, *1*(9), 389–399. DOI: 10.1038/s42256-019-0088-2

Kaliappan, S., Radhika, S., Ravi, D., & Aluvala, S. (2023). A Data-Driven Approach to Improving Neonatal Care through Artificial Intelligence and Clinical Data Integration. In 2023 IEEE International Conference on ICT in Business Industry & Government (ICTBIG) (pp. 1-6). IEEE. https://doi.org/DOI: 10.1109/ICTBIG59752.2023.10456148

Karabay, M., Kaya, G., Guclu, E., Ogutlu, A., Karabay, O., & Caner, I. (2021). Health care-associated infections in neonatal intensive care unit: Evaluation of the last 6 years. *Turkish Journal of Pediatric Disease*, *15*(2), 87–92. DOI: 10.12956/tchd.597635

Kerkez, M., & Kaplan, M. (2025). Evaluation of discharge training given by nurses to postpartum mothers to artificial intelligence: An alternative approach to health care. *BMC Nursing*, *24*(1), 296. DOI: 10.1186/s12912-025-02966-5 PMID: 40119346

Khanam, F. T. Z., Al-Naji, A., Perera, A. G., Gibson, K., & Chahl, J. (2022). Remote vital signs monitoring in neonatal intensive care unit using a digital camera. *International Journal of Biomedical and Biological Engineering*, *16*(10), 138–144.

Kilicarslan Toruner, E., & Buyukgonenc, L. (2017). Healthy newborn. In *Child Health Basic Nursing Approaches* (pp. 233–290). Göktuğ Publishing.

Kim, Y., Kim, H., Choi, J., Cho, K., Yoo, D., Lee, Y., Park, S. J., Jeong, M. H., Jeong, S. H., Park, K. Y., Byun, S. Y., Kim, T., Ahn, S. H., Cho, W. H., & Lee, N. (2023). Early prediction of need for invasive mechanical ventilation in the neonatal intensive care unit using artificial intelligence and electronic health records: A clinical study. *BMC Pediatrics*, *23*(1), 525. DOI: 10.1186/s12887-023-04350-1 PMID: 37872515

Kloonen, R. M., Varisco, G., de Kort, E., Andriessen, P., Niemarkt, H. J., & van Pul, C. (2023). Predicting CPAP failure after less invasive surfactant administration (LISA) in preterm infants by machine learning model on vital parameter data: A pilot study. *Physiological Measurement*, *44*(11), 115005. DOI: 10.1088/1361-6579/ad0ab6 PMID: 37939392

Kostekci, Y. E., Bakırarar, B., Okulu, E., Erdeve, O., Atasay, B., & Arsan, S. (2023). An Early Prediction Model for Estimating Bronchopulmonary Dysplasia in Preterm Infants. *Neonatology*, *120*(6), 709–717. DOI: 10.1159/000533299 PMID: 37725910

Krysia, W. H., & Marion, J. B. (2018). The challenge for nursıng and healthcare ın the dıgıtal age. *Texto & Contexto-Enfermagem*, 27. https://doi.org/DOI: 10.1590/0104-07072018002018editorial2

Kucuk, S., & Yagmur, B. (2019). Job Stress Factors and Perceived Job Stress Levels of Neonatal Intensive Care Unit Nurses. *The Journal of Academic Social Science*, *72*(72), 142–152. DOI: 10.16992/ASOS.13762

Lee, C. K., & Huang, X. Y. (2022). Psychological processes of postpartum mothers with newborns admitted to the intensive care unit. *Asian Nursing Research*, *16*(1), 9–17. DOI: 10.1016/j.anr.2021.12.007 PMID: 34990888

Lei, H., Ashrafi, A., Chang, P., Chang, A., & Lai, W. (2022). Patent ductus arteriosus (PDA) detection in echocardiograms using deep learning. *Intelligence-Based Medicine*, *6*, 100054. DOI: 10.1016/j.ibmed.2022.100054

Li, Y., Wang, M., Wang, L., Cao, Y., Liu, Y., Zhao, Y., Yuan, R., Yang, M., Lu, S., Sun, Z., Zhou, F., Qian, Z., & Kang, H. (2024). Advances in the application of AI robots in critical care: Scoping review. *Journal of Medical Internet Research*, *26*, e54095. DOI: 10.2196/54095 PMID: 38801765

Liang, H. F., Wu, K. M., Weng, C. H., & Hsieh, H. W. (2019). Nurses' views on the potential use of robots in the pediatric unit. *Journal of Pediatric Nursing*, *47*, e58–e64. DOI: 10.1016/j.pedn.2019.04.027 PMID: 31076190

Ling, Z., Zhou, W., Ren, Y., Wang, J., & Guo, L. (2022). Non-contact heart rate monitoring based on millimeter wave radar. *IEEE Access : Practical Innovations, Open Solutions*, *10*, 74033–74044. DOI: 10.1109/ACCESS.2022.3190355

Loder, J., & Nicholas, L. (2018). *Confronting Dr Robot: Creating a people-powered future for AI in health*. Nesta.

Malak, J. S., Zeraati, H., Nayeri, F. S., Safdari, R., & Shahraki, A. D. (2019). Neonatal intensive care decision support systems using artificial intelligence techniques: A systematic review. *Artificial Intelligence Review*, *52*(4), 2685–2704. DOI: 10.1007/s10462-018-9635-1

Manworren, R. C., Horner, S., Joseph, R., Dadar, P., & Kaduwela, N. (2024). Performance evaluation of a supervised machine learning pain classification model developed by neonatal nurses. *Advances in Neonatal Care*, *24*(3), 301–310. DOI: 10.1097/ANC.0000000000001145 PMID: 38775675

Marchionni, P., Scalise, L., Ercoli, I., Palazzi, M. L., & Carnielli, V. P. (2016). Effect of limbs' motion on pulse oximetry in preterm infants. In 2016 IEEE International Symposium on Medical Measurements and Applications (MeMeA) (pp. 1-6). IEEE. https://doi.org/DOI: 10.1109/MeMeA.2016.7533788

Mbanuzue, C. E., Hassan, O. E., & Owolabi, F. M. (2024). Real-Time Monitoring of Neonatal Incubator Parameters Via Iot-Integrated Device: Design, Implementation, and Evaluation. *International Journal of Research and Innovation in Applied Science*, *9*(4), 127–143. DOI: 10.51584/IJRIAS.2024.90409

McGregor, C. (2013). Big data in neonatal intensive care. *Computer*, *46*(6), 54–59. DOI: 10.1109/MC.2013.157

Meeus, M., Beirnaert, C., Mahieu, L., Laukens, K., Meysman, P., Mulder, A., & Van Laere, D. (2024). Clinical Decision Support for Improved Neonatal Care: The Development of a Machine Learning Model for the Prediction of Late-onset Sepsis and Necrotizing Enterocolitis. *The Journal of Pediatrics*, *266*, 113869. DOI: 10.1016/j.jpeds.2023.113869 PMID: 38065281

Mokadem, N., Jabeen, F., Treur, J., Taal, H. R., & Roelofsma, P. H. (2024). An adaptive network model for AI-assisted monitoring and management of neonatal respiratory distress. *Cognitive Systems Research*, *86*, 101231. DOI: 10.1016/j.cogsys.2024.101231

Molu, B. (2025). Improving Nursing Students' Learning Outcomes in Neonatal Resuscitation: A Quasi-Experimental Study Comparing AI-Assisted Care Plan Learning With Traditional Instruction. *Journal of Evaluation in Clinical Practice*, *31*(1), e14286. DOI: 10.1111/jep.14286 PMID: 39733257

Monaghan, J., Kim, T., Dol, J., Orovec, A., & Campbell-Yeo, M. (2020). Parents' learning needs and preferences in a neonatal intensive care unit: A desire for enhanced communication and eHealth technology. *Journal of Neonatal Nursing*, *26*(2), 101–105. DOI: 10.1016/j.jnn.2019.09.001

Ning, Y., Liu, X., Collins, G. S., Moons, K. G., McCradden, M., Ting, D. S. W., Ong, J. C. L., Goldstein, B. A., Wagner, S. K., Keane, P. A., Topol, E. J., & Liu, N. (2024). An ethics assessment tool for artificial intelligence implementation in healthcare: CARE-AI. *Nature Medicine*, *1-2*(11), 3038–3039. Advance online publication. DOI: 10.1038/s41591-024-03310-1 PMID: 39424948

Ozsezer, G. (2022). The future of artificial intelligence in nursing. *International Journal of Human Sciences*, *19*(2), 285–299. https://orcid.org/0000-0003-4352-1124. DOI: 10.14687/jhs.v19i2.6217

Persad, E., Jost, K., Honoré, A., Forsberg, D., Coste, K., Olsson, H., Rautiainen, S., & Herlenius, E. (2021). Neonatal sepsis prediction through clinical decision support algorithms: A systematic review. *Acta Paediatrica (Oslo, Norway)*, *110*(12), 3201–3226. DOI: 10.1111/apa.16083 PMID: 34432903

Ponthier, L., Ensuque, P., Destere, A., Marquet, P., Labriffe, M., Jacqz-Aigrain, E., & Woillard, J. B. (2022). Optimization of vancomycin initial dose in term and preterm neonates by machine learning. *Pharmaceutical Research*, *39*(10), 2497–2506. DOI: 10.1007/s11095-022-03351-6 PMID: 35918452

Quon, S., Ahani, S., Holsti, L., Lavoie, P. M., & Dumont, G. (2021). Video-Based Respiratory Rate Estimation for Infants in Low Resource Settings. https://doi.org/ DOI: 10.14288/1.0406240

Racine, N., Chow, C., Hamwi, L., Bucsea, O., Cheng, C., Du, H., Fabrizi, L., Jasim, S., Johannsson, L., Jones, L., Laudiano-Dray, M. P., Meek, J., Mistry, N., Shah, V., Stedman, I., Wang, X., & Riddell, R. P. (2024). Health care professionals' and parents' perspectives on the use of AI for pain monitoring in the neonatal intensive care unit: Multisite qualitative study. *JMIR AI, 3*, e51535. DOI: 10.2196/51535 PMID: 38875686

Rajpurkar, P., Chen, E., Banerjee, O., & Topol, E. J. (2022). AI in health and medicine. *Nature Medicine*, *28*(1), 31–38. DOI: 10.1038/s41591-021-01614-0 PMID: 35058619

Rallis, D., Baltogianni, M., Kapetaniou, K., & Giapros, V. (2024). Current Applications of Artificial Intelligence in the Neonatal Intensive Care Unit. *BioMedInformatics*, *4*(2), 1225–1248. DOI: 10.3390/biomedinformatics4020067

Rigby, M., Magrabi, F., Scott, P., Doupi, P., Hypponen, H., & Ammenwerth, E. (2016). Steps in moving evidence-based health informatics from theory to practice. *Healthcare Informatics Research*, *22*(4), 255–260. DOI: 10.4258/hir.2016.22.4.255 PMID: 27895956

Robert, N. (2019). How artificial intelligence is changing nursing. *Nursing Management*, *50*(9), 30–39. DOI: 10.1097/01.NUMA.0000578988.56622.21 PMID: 31425440

Safıya, P. A., & Saleena, B. (2024). Designing a hybrid stack ensemble model to enhance sepsis classification using data triangulation approach. *Results in Engineering*, *103748*. Advance online publication. DOI: 10.1016/j.rineng.2024.103748

Saha, S., Pagnozzi, A., Bourgeat, P., George, J. M., Bradford, D., Colditz, P. B., Boyd, R. N., Rose, S. E., Jurgen Fripp, J., & Pannek, K. (2020). Predicting motor outcome in preterm infants from very early brain diffusion MRI using a deep learning convolutional neural network (CNN) model. *NeuroImage*, *215*, 116807. DOI: 10.1016/j.neuroimage.2020.116807 PMID: 32278897

Salekin, M. S., Mouton, P. R., Zamzmi, G., Patel, R., Goldgof, D., Kneusel, M., Elkins, S. L., Murray, E., Coughlin, M. E., Maguire, D., Ho, T., & Sun, Y. (2021). Future roles of artificial intelligence in early pain management of newborns. *Paediatric and Neonatal Pain*, *3*(3), 134–145. DOI: 10.1002/pne2.12060 PMID: 35547946

Sarıkaya Karabudak, S., & Ergün, S. (2018). Neonatal diseases and nursing care. In Conk, Z., Başbakkal, Z., Yılmaz, H. B., & Bolışık, B. (Eds.), *Pediatric Nursing, 2.*

Schouten, J. S., Kalden, M. A., van Twist, E., Reiss, I. K., Gommers, D. A., van Genderen, M. E., & Taal, H. R. (2024). From bytes to bedside: A systematic review on the use and readiness of artificial intelligence in the neonatal and pediatric intensive care unit. *Intensive Care Medicine*, *50*(11), 1767–1777. DOI: 10.1007/s00134-024-07629-8 PMID: 39264415

Shane, A. L., Sánchez, P. J., & Stoll, B. J. (2017). Neonatal sepsis. *Lancet*, *390*(10104), 1770–1780. DOI: 10.1016/S0140-6736(17)31002-4 PMID: 28434651

Shi, Y., Payeur, P., Frize, M., & Bariciak, E. (2020, June). Thermal and rgb-d imaging for necrotizing enterocolitis detection. In 2020 IEEE International Symposium on Medical Measurements and Applications (MeMeA) (pp. 1-6). IEEE. https://doi.org/DOI: 10.1109/MeMeA49120.2020.9137344

Shin, D., & Park, Y. J. (2019). Role of fairness, accountability, and transparency in algorithmic affordance. *Computers in Human Behavior*, *98*, 277–284. DOI: 10.1016/j.chb.2019.04.019

Singh, P., Nagori, A., Lodha, R., & Sethi, T. (2022). Early prediction of hypothermia in pediatric intensive care units using machine learning. *Frontiers in Physiology*, *13*, 921884. DOI: 10.3389/fphys.2022.921884 PMID: 36171970

Solomonides, A. E., Koski, E., Atabaki, S. M., Weinberg, S., McGreevey, J. D.III, Kannry, J. L., Petersen, C., & Lehmann, C. U. (2022). Defining AMIA's artificial intelligence principles. *Journal of the American Medical Informatics Association : JAMIA*, *29*(4), 585–591. DOI: 10.1093/jamia/ocac006 PMID: 35190824

Song, W., Jung, S. Y., Baek, H., Choi, C. W., Jung, Y. H., & Yoo, S. (2020). A predictive model based on machine learning for the early detection of late-onset neonatal sepsis: Development and observational study. *JMIR Medical Informatics*, *8*(7), e15965. DOI: 10.2196/15965 PMID: 32735230

Sorrentino, G., Thekkan, K. R., Genna, C., Aite, L., Ragni, A., Bevilacqua, F., Dall'Oglio, I., Roberti, M., Tiozzo, E., & Gawronski, O. (2025). The implementation and impact of narrative diaries in neonatal intensive care units: A scoping review. *Nursing in Critical Care*, *30*(2), e13281. DOI: 10.1111/nicc.13281 PMID: 40000364

Stedman, I., Racine, N., Wang, X., Fitzgerald, M., Fabrizi, L., Jones, L., Shah, V., Cheng, C., & Riddell, R. P. (2023) Artificial Intelligence for NICU Pain Assessment: Ethical, Legal and Social Implications. *Legal and Social Implications*. http://dx.doi.org/DOI: 10.2139/ssrn.4336962

Sullivan, B. A., Beam, K., Vesoulis, Z. A., Aziz, K. B., Husain, A. N., Knake, L. A , Moreira, A., Hooven, T. A., Weiss, E. M., Carr, N. R., El-Ferzli, G. T., Patel, R. M., Simek, K. A., Hernandez, A. J., Barry, J. S., & McAdams, R. M. (2024). Transforming neonatal care with artificial intelligence: Challenges, ethical consideration, and opportunities. *Journal of Perinatology*, *44*(1), 1–11. DOI: 10.1038/s41372-023-01848-5 PMID: 38097685

Sunshine, I. L., Kysh, L., & Lakshmanan, A. (2023). Mobile applications to support parents in the transition from neonatal intensive care unit to home: A narrative review. *mHealth*, *9*, 27. DOI: 10.21037/mhealth-23-10 PMID: 37492120

Tang, X., Yang, X., Yuan, J., Yang, J., Jin, Q., Zhang, H., Zhao, L., & Guo, W. (2024). Call for Decision Support for Electrocardiographic Alarm Administration Among Neonatal Intensive Care Unit Staff: Multicenter, Cross-Sectional Survey. *Journal of Medical Internet Research*, *26*, e60944. DOI: 10.2196/60944 PMID: 39705688

Tarricone, F., Brunetti, A., Buongiorno, D., Altini, N., Bevilacqua, V., Del Vecchio, A., & Petrillo, F. (2021). Intelligent neonatal sepsis early diagnosis system for very low birth weight infants. *Applied Sciences (Basel, Switzerland)*, *11*(1), 404. DOI: 10.3390/app11010404

Ugucu, G., Celebioglu, A., & Isbir, G. G. (2024). Supporting the neurodevelopment of premature infants in the neonatal intensive care unit: Creating a healing environment. *Adnan Menderes University Journal of Faculty of Health Sciences*, *8*(2), 192–208. DOI: 10.46237/amusbfd.1278780

Unal, A. S., & Avci, A. (2024). Artificial intelligence in pediatric nursing. Mediterranean. *Journal of Nursing (Luton, England)*, *3*(1), 36–43. DOI: 10.59398/ahd.1346089

United Nations Children's Fund. (2021). Policy guidance on AI for children 2.0. UNICEF. https://www.unicef.org/innocenti/reports/policy-guidance-ai-children

United Nations General Assembly. (2015). Transforming our world: The 2030 agenda for sustainable development (Resolution 70/1). https://sdgs.un.org/goals

van Assen, M., Lee, S. J., & De Cecco, C. N. (2020). Artificial intelligence from A to Z: From neural network to legal framework. *European Journal of Radiology*, *129*, 109083. DOI: 10.1016/j.ejrad.2020.109083 PMID: 32526670

Venkatasubramanian, K., Ranalli, T. M., Kirupaharan, P., Solanki, D., & Mankodiya, K. (2023). Understanding the challenges nurses encounter with monitoring technologies in a NICU. *International Journal of Human-Computer Interaction*, *40*(23), 8142–8165. DOI: 10.1080/10447318.2023.2278297

Wang, L. Y., Wang, L. Y., Sung, M. I., Lin, I. C., Liu, C. F., & Chen, C. J. (2024). Implementing Explainable Machine Learning Models for Practical Prediction of Early Neonatal Hypoglycemia. *Diagnostics (Basel)*, *14*(14), 1571. DOI: 10.3390/diagnostics14141571 PMID: 39061708

Weiss, S. L., Fitzgerald, J. C., Balamuth, F., Alpern, E. R., Lavelle, J., Chilutti, M., Grundmeier, R., Nadkarni, V., & Thomas, N. J. (2014). Delayed antimicrobial therapy increases mortality and organ dysfunction duration in pediatric sepsis. *Critical Care Medicine*, *42*(11), 2409–2417. DOI: 10.1097/CCM.0000000000000509 PMID: 25148597

WHO. (World Health Organization). (2022). SDG Target 3.2: End preventable deaths of newborns and children under 5 years of age in 2021. https://www.who.int/data/gho/data/themes/theme-details/GHO/child-health

Wu, Q., Xu, G., Wei, F., Kuang, J., Qin, P., Li, Z., & Zhang, S. (2022). Supine infant pose estimation via single depth image. *IEEE Transactions on Instrumentation and Measurement*, *71*, 1–11. DOI: 10.1109/TIM.2022.3178693

Yalcin, N., Kasikci, M., Celik, H. T., Allegaert, K., Demirkan, K., Yigit, S., & Yurdakok, M. (2022). An Artificial ıntelligence approach to support detection of neonatal adverse drug reactions based on severity and probability scores: A new risk score as web-tool. *Children (Basel, Switzerland)*, *9*(12), 1826. DOI: 10.3390/children9121826 PMID: 36553270

Yalcin, N., Kasikci, M., Celik, H. T., Demirkan, K., Yigit, S., & Yurdakok, M. (2023). Development and validation of machine learning-based clinical decision support tool for identifying malnutrition in NICU patients. *Scientific Reports*, *13*(1), 5227. DOI: 10.1038/s41598-023-32570-z PMID: 36997630

Yigit, D., & Acikgoz, A. (2024). Evaluation of comfort behavior levels of newborn by artificial intelligence techniques. *The Journal of Perinatal & Neonatal Nursing*, *38*(3), E38–E45. DOI: 10.1097/JPN.0000000000000768 PMID: 37773591

Zea-Vera, A., & Ochoa, T. J. (2015). Challenges in the diagnosis and management of neonatal sepsis. *Journal of Tropical Pediatrics*, *61*(1), 1–13. DOI: 10.1093/tropej/fmu079 PMID: 25604489

Zeng, Y., Yu, D., Song, X., Wang, Q., Pan, L., Lu, H., & Wang, W. (2024). Camera-based cardiorespiratory monitoring of preterm infants in nicu. *IEEE Transactions on Instrumentation and Measurement*, *73*, 1–13. Advance online publication. DOI: 10.1109/TIM.2024.3395314

Zhang, G., Xie, Q., Wang, C., Xu, J., Liu, G., & Su, C. (2024). Intelligent alert system for predicting invasive mechanical ventilation needs via noninvasive parameters: Employing an integrated machine learning method with integration of multicenter databases. *Medical & Biological Engineering & Computing*, *62*(11), 3445–3458. DOI: 10.1007/s11517-024-03143-7 PMID: 38861056

KEY TERMS AND DEFINITIONS

Artificial Intelligence: A set of technologies that mimic human intelligence through computer systems, enabling them to learn, solve problems, and make decisions.

Clinical Decision Support: Technological or software-based systems that provide data and information support to healthcare professionals in diagnosis, treatment, and care processes.

Intensive Care Unit: A hospital department equipped with advanced medical devices and specialized healthcare personnel where patients at high risk are continuously monitored and treated.

Machine Learning: An artificial intelligence method that enables computer systems to learn from data and improve their performance over time.

Monitoring Systems: Technological systems that continuously monitor and record vital signs such as heart rate, respiration, and oxygen saturation in patients.

Neonatal Care: Specialized care services provided to protect the health of newborn babies, prevent illness, and treat diseases during the first 28 days after birth.

Predictive Models: Mathematical and statistical models used to predict future events or potential risks based on current data.

Chapter 5 Artificial Intelligence-Assisted Image Analysis and Clinical Applications in Urology

Halil Ibrahim Ivelik
https://orcid.org/0000-0001-5298-0045
Kutahya Health Sciences University, Turkey

Bekir Aras
https://orcid.org/0000-0002-7020-8830
Kutahya Health Sciences University, Turkey

ABSTRACT

Artificial intelligence (AI) has the potential to revolutionize urology by enhancing diagnostics, surgical precision, and patient care. AI-powered diagnostic tools are increasingly used for the early detection of urologic diseases such as prostate and bladder cancer, while robotic-assisted surgery improves precision in minimally invasive procedures. Additionally, AI-driven wearable technologies and remote monitoring systems enhance patient management, enabling personalized treatment approaches. However, the integration of AI into clinical practice raises ethical concerns, including algorithmic bias, data privacy, and accountability, which must be addressed to ensure fair and reliable AI systems. This study explores the future of AI in urology, its integration potential, and the ethical challenges it presents, offering recommendations for a more sustainable and equitable implementation.

DOI: 10.4018/979-8-3373-1479-2.ch005

INTRODUCTION

In recent years, the emergence of Artificial Intelligence (AI) and its subfield, machine learning (ML), has ushered in a wave of profound changes across the medical landscape. AI encompasses the creation of advanced computational systems designed to replicate aspects of human intelligence, such as reasoning, problem-solving, and perception. Machine learning, a critical component of AI, empowers these systems to autonomously learn from vast datasets, refine their algorithms, and make informed predictions or decisions without explicit human intervention. The incorporation of these cutting-edge technologies into healthcare has catalyzed remarkable improvements, including heightened precision in diagnostics, streamlined medical workflows, and the bolstering of clinical decision-making frameworks (Mishra & Gupta, 2017).

Urology, a specialized branch of medicine focused on the urinary tract and male reproductive system, depends significantly on sophisticated imaging modalities for accurate diagnosis and treatment planning. Among these, cystoscopy stands out as a cornerstone procedure, widely employed to identify critical conditions like bladder cancer. This technique involves the use of a thin, flexible tube equipped with a camera to visualize the bladder's interior. However, interpreting the resulting cystoscopic images demands a high level of skill and experience, and even then, outcomes can vary between practitioners due to subjective differences in perception and judgment. AI-driven image analysis tools hold immense promise in this context, offering the potential to transform clinical practice by delivering more standardized, reliable, and precise evaluations. Such advancements could markedly elevate the efficiency and effectiveness of diagnostic processes in urology.

The influence of AI in medical imaging extends well beyond urology, with notable applications in fields such as radiology, ophthalmology, dermatology, pathology, neurology, and gastroenterology. In these disciplines, AI-powered tools like computer-aided diagnosis (CADx) systems and computer-aided detection (CADe) platforms have successfully overcome longstanding challenges, enhancing diagnostic accuracy and reducing human error (Esteva et al., 2017; Gulshan et al., 2016). These developments have been fueled by rapid advancements in computational capabilities, coupled with the availability of large-scale data analytics, which together enable the seamless integration of AI into routine medical workflows.

Within urology specifically, cystoscopy remains an indispensable method for diagnosing a range of urological disorders. Yet, the reliance on human interpretation introduces inconsistencies, as clinicians' assessments may differ based on their training, fatigue levels, or individual biases. AI-enhanced systems address these shortcomings by providing objective, reproducible analyses of cystoscopic images, thereby potentially improving diagnostic reliability and operational efficiency

(Ferro et al., 2023; İvelik et al., 2025). By minimizing variability and augmenting human expertise, these technologies pave the way for more confident and timely clinical decisions.

This chapter is intended for a multidisciplinary audience that includes medical researchers, clinical practitioners, urologists, biomedical engineers, data scientists, and healthcare technology developers. It is also suitable for graduate-level students and academic professionals engaged in digital health, medical imaging, and artificial intelligence applications in clinical settings. Given the rapid proliferation of AI technologies in healthcare, this chapter aims to bridge the gap between theoretical foundations and real-world applications, providing both conceptual insights and practical case examples.

The technical depth of the chapter has been calibrated to accommodate readers with a foundational understanding of either clinical urology or computational techniques. While the content explores advanced topics such as deep learning, convolutional neural networks, and clinical decision support systems, it remains accessible to those with limited prior exposure to AI by offering contextual explanations and illustrative case studies. This balance ensures that the chapter is informative for domain experts while remaining approachable to interdisciplinary collaborators and stakeholders navigating the evolving intersection of urology and artificial intelligence.

The purpose of this book chapter is to deliver an in-depth exploration of how AI is reshaping the field of urology. It will delve into the specific AI techniques driving these innovations, offer a detailed review of recent scholarly studies and real-world clinical applications, and assess the broader digital transformation occurring within urological practice through AI-driven solutions. Furthermore, this chapter will critically evaluate the current limitations of these technologies and provide insights into their future potential, shedding light on how AI might continue to evolve and redefine urological care in the years to come.

Cross-Disciplinary Technological Foundations: From E-Commerce Analytics to AI in Urology

In recent years, the intersection of e-commerce analytics, cloud computing, and data science methodologies has witnessed remarkable advancements, reshaping how organizations manage, interpret, and utilize data for strategic advantage. E-commerce platforms—especially those operating in highly dynamic sectors such as sports retail—have increasingly adopted data-driven strategies to enhance customer experience, personalize product offerings, and optimize supply chain operations. With the proliferation of consumer interaction data from websites, mobile apps, and social media platforms, businesses are leveraging machine learning algorithms for real-time customer segmentation, churn prediction, dynamic pricing, and recommendation engines.

Cloud computing has become a foundational technology in modern e-commerce infrastructure. Its scalable architecture allows organizations to store and process massive volumes of structured and unstructured data without the constraints of on-premise servers. Platforms like Amazon Web Services (AWS), Microsoft Azure, and Google Cloud offer integrated machine learning and analytics services, enabling real-time insights from customer behavior and transaction logs. The elasticity of cloud-based data pipelines facilitates seamless model deployment, which is critical for time-sensitive applications such as flash sales, product launches, or sports event-linked promotions.

From a methodological standpoint, contemporary data science in e-commerce is increasingly shifting from traditional regression models to sophisticated AI techniques, such as deep neural networks, reinforcement learning, and ensemble methods. These approaches outperform classical methods in handling high-dimensional, sparse, and non-linear datasets common in digital commerce. Particularly in the sports merchandise sector, personalization and real-time analytics are gaining traction. AI-powered systems dynamically curate product recommendations based on user preferences, browsing history, and contextual signals such as geolocation and device type.

Moreover, the integration of big data analytics with customer relationship management (CRM) systems has revolutionized how e-commerce businesses design marketing campaigns and loyalty programs. By using clustering algorithms and natural language processing (NLP) to analyze customer feedback, companies are better equipped to predict emerging trends, detect sentiment shifts, and adjust inventory accordingly. These innovations not only enhance operational efficiency but also foster deeper customer engagement, a critical factor in competitive industries such as sportswear and athletic equipment retail.

While these technological advances may appear industry-specific, the underlying infrastructure and methodologies have laid the groundwork for parallel innovations in healthcare—particularly in the application of artificial intelligence to medical diagnostics. The computational frameworks, cloud-based scalability, and analytical techniques pioneered in commercial data science have been adapted to medical contexts, enabling the development of real-time diagnostic systems, predictive health models, and personalized treatment recommendations. This convergence of technological evolution across domains is not merely coincidental, but reflective of a broader shift toward data-centric problem-solving across disciplines.

In the context of medicine—and specifically within urology—many of the same analytical strategies used in e-commerce have been reimagined for clinical use. Just as customer segmentation enables targeted advertising, patient stratification using AI allows clinicians to identify high-risk individuals and tailor treatment accordingly.

Similarly, anomaly detection algorithms originally developed to flag suspicious purchase behaviors have found powerful applications in radiology and pathology, where they assist in identifying early-stage malignancies or subtle deviations in imaging data that may elude human perception.

The role of cloud-based computing in this translation is particularly salient. Modern hospitals and research institutions rely on cloud infrastructure to store and process vast volumes of medical imaging data, electronic health records (EHRs), genomic information, and sensor data from wearable devices. Cloud computing enables scalable machine learning workflows, allowing models to be trained on heterogeneous, multimodal datasets that would otherwise be too large or complex for local computational environments. In urology, this capability is critical in tasks such as prostate cancer screening via multiparametric MRI, where high-resolution images from diverse sources must be aggregated and analyzed.

Furthermore, the rise of low-code AI platforms—also initially popularized in the commercial sector—has democratized the development of clinical decision support systems. Physicians, clinicians, and domain experts can now collaborate with data scientists to build customized diagnostic models without deep programming expertise. This collaborative model is accelerating the integration of AI in clinical practice, fostering innovations in digital pathology, image-guided surgery, and real-time diagnostic support.

An illustrative case of cross-domain synergy is the use of recommendation system logic—originally designed for e-commerce platforms like Netflix or Amazon—in predictive healthcare systems. In the same way these platforms suggest products or content based on prior behavior, AI-driven clinical platforms can recommend diagnostic tests, interventions, or follow-up pathways by analyzing prior patient data, institutional patterns, and clinical guidelines. In urology, such systems may, for instance, recommend a cystoscopy or biopsy for a patient based on specific risk factors and symptomatology derived from structured and unstructured data in the patient's record.

Natural language processing (NLP), another cornerstone of e-commerce analytics, is being used to extract clinical insights from narrative medical records, operative reports, and patient-reported outcomes. In urology, NLP models assist in identifying symptoms, extracting tumor characteristics, or summarizing patient histories, providing critical inputs for downstream AI models. Moreover, sentiment analysis—commonly used in product reviews—is being adapted to analyze patient satisfaction and post-operative feedback, thus contributing to value-based healthcare assessment.

What becomes evident from this convergence is that the technical and methodological advancements in commercial sectors have served as a proving ground for many of the AI techniques now shaping urological innovation. From convolutional neural networks trained on product images to deep learning systems analyzing bladder cancer cystoscopy videos, the core principles remain strikingly similar. What differs is the domain-specific adaptation, validation, and ethical governance that must accompany their use in clinical environments.

This cross-pollination of ideas highlights the importance of interdisciplinary awareness in advancing urology through AI. While the clinical stakes are higher, the technological pathways are often shared, and insights from one sector can accelerate progress in another. Therefore, in understanding the current landscape of AI in urology, it is both relevant and necessary to acknowledge the broader technological ecosystem from which it has emerged.

Building on the foundational applications and case studies explored above, it is essential to consider the methodological frameworks, implementation challenges, and future directions that shape the integration of artificial intelligence in urology.

Artificial Intelligence Applications in Urology: Techniques and Models

Artificial intelligence (AI) has rapidly evolved into a groundbreaking force within the realm of urology, fundamentally reshaping the landscape of diagnostics, treatment planning, and ongoing patient management. By harnessing computational power and sophisticated algorithms, AI empowers clinicians to achieve unprecedented levels of precision, efficiency, and personalization in addressing urological conditions. This section delves deeply into the foundational principles underpinning machine learning (ML) and deep learning (DL), while also examining the specific techniques and innovative models that are propelling advancements in this specialized medical field.

MACHINE LEARNING AND DEEP LEARNING CONCEPTS

Machine learning, a pivotal branch of artificial intelligence, encompasses a wide array of algorithms designed to identify patterns within datasets and generate predictions or decisions autonomously, without the need for explicit human programming. Within this domain, supervised learning stands out as a widely utilized approach, wherein models are meticulously trained on labeled datasets—such as distinguishing cancerous from non-cancerous tissue based on annotated medical records or imaging data. In contrast, unsupervised learning explores unlabeled data to uncover hidden structures or relationships, offering valuable insights into complex urological phenomena where prior categorization may not exist. Deep learning, an advanced and increasingly prominent subset of machine learning, leverages intricate neural networks composed of multiple interconnected layers to process highly complex and multidimensional datasets, including medical images, patient histories, and genomic profiles. These techniques are particularly adept at managing the vast, high-dimensional data commonly encountered in urological research and clinical practice, enabling breakthroughs that were previously unattainable with traditional statistical methods (Mishra & Gupta, 2017).

Convolutional Neural Networks (CNNs) and Medical Image Analysis

Convolutional Neural Networks (CNNs) represent a cornerstone of deep learning technology, distinguished by their exceptional capability to analyze and interpret visual data. Their architecture, inspired by the human visual cortex, excels at extracting spatial features from images, making them ideally suited for medical image analysis within urology. CNNs have ushered in a revolution in this field by facilitating the precise detection, segmentation, and classification of abnormalities across a variety of imaging modalities, such as magnetic resonance imaging (MRI), computed tomography (CT), and ultrasound. For example, CNNs can accurately delineate prostate tumors in MRI scans or pinpoint kidney stones in CT images, often achieving diagnostic accuracy that surpasses conventional manual methods employed by radiologists. This ability to autonomously learn hierarchical feature representations from raw imaging data renders CNNs indispensable tools for computer-aided diagnosis (CAD) systems and preoperative surgical planning, ultimately enhancing clinical decision-making and patient outcomes (Krizhevsky et al., 2012).

Convolutional Neural Networks (CNNs): Mathematical Foundations

Convolutional Neural Networks (CNNs) are pivotal in urological image analysis due to their ability to extract hierarchical features from high-dimensional imaging data, such as cystoscopy or MRI scans. Understanding their mathematical underpinnings is essential for researchers and clinicians aiming to leverage or critique these models.

A CNN consists of multiple layers, including convolutional, pooling, and fully connected layers, each performing specific operations to transform input data into actionable outputs. The core operation, convolution, involves sliding a filter (or kernel) over the input image to compute feature maps. Mathematically, for a 2D input image ($I(x, y)$) and a kernel ($K(m, n)$), the convolution operation at position ((x, y)) is defined as:

$$S(x, y) = (I * K)(x, y) = \Sigma_m \Sigma_n I(x - m, y - n) K(m, n)$$

Here, (S(x, y)) represents the output feature map, capturing localized patterns such as edges or textures in cystoscopic images. Filters are learned during training via backpropagation, optimizing parameters to minimize a loss function (e.g., cross-entropy for classification tasks). Activation functions, such as $f(x) = \max(0, x)$ introduce non-linearity, enabling the model to learn complex patterns like tumor boundaries.

Pooling layers, typically max-pooling, reduce spatial dimensions while preserving salient features, improving computational efficiency and reducing overfitting. For instance, max-pooling selects the maximum value in a region, effectively downsampling the feature map. Fully connected layers at the end integrate these features to produce predictions, such as classifying a lesion as malignant or benign.

In urology, CNN architectures like U-Net or ResNet are tailored for tasks such as tumor segmentation or classification. For example, U-Net's encoder-decoder structure excels in delineating bladder tumor margins in cystoscopy images by combining low-level and high-level features. These models are computationally intensive, requiring robust hardware (e.g., GPUs) and large annotated datasets, which can be a bottleneck in clinical settings (Ghosh, 2025).

AI TECHNIQUES IN UROLOGY

A diverse array of AI techniques is actively employed in urology, each contributing uniquely to the field's technological evolution:

Supervised Learning: This technique is foundational in developing predictive models that forecast critical clinical outcomes, such as the likelihood of prostate cancer recurrence based on comprehensive datasets encompassing clinical variables, imaging results, and histopathological findings. By training on labeled examples, supervised learning models refine their predictive accuracy over time, offering clinicians actionable insights.

Transfer Learning: A pragmatic approach particularly valuable in medical contexts, transfer learning leverages pre-trained models—originally developed on large, general-purpose image datasets like ImageNet—and adapts them to urology-specific tasks. This method significantly reduces the dependency on extensive, annotated medical datasets, which are often scarce, by fine-tuning existing models to recognize urological abnormalities with high fidelity.

Large Language Models (LLMs): These cutting-edge systems, rooted in natural language processing, are gaining traction in urology for their ability to analyze unstructured textual data, such as electronic health records, clinical notes, and research literature. LLMs can extract meaningful insights, identify risk factors, or even assist in clinical decision-making by providing evidence-based recommendations tailored to individual patients.

When paired with robust, high-quality datasets, these techniques amplify diagnostic precision, enable the personalization of therapeutic strategies, and markedly improve patient outcomes by addressing the unique challenges posed by urological diseases ("Artificial Neural Network and Supervised Learning," 2008).

METHODOLOGICAL FRAMEWORKS IN CLINICAL AI DEPLOYMENT

The deployment of AI in urological practice necessitates a robust methodological pipeline that spans data acquisition, preprocessing, model training, validation, and clinical integration. In most studies, datasets are derived from electronic health records (EHR), diagnostic imaging, or histopathological slides. These datasets require rigorous preprocessing, including de-identification, normalization, and annotation by domain experts to ensure accuracy and ethical compliance.

Once cleaned and labeled, data are typically split into training, validation, and test subsets. Cross-validation techniques are employed to minimize overfitting and ensure generalizability. In imaging applications such as cystoscopy or prostate MRI, convolutional neural networks (CNNs) are commonly used due to their ability to extract spatial hierarchies. In structured clinical data, tree-based ensemble methods such as random forests or gradient boosting have shown strong predictive performance.

Model performance is assessed using standard metrics such as sensitivity, specificity, AUC, F1-score, and positive predictive value. However, beyond statistical metrics, real-world clinical impact must be evaluated through prospective trials, decision curve analysis, and feedback from end-users (i.e., urologists and clinical staff). The choice of model architecture and training strategy must also account for data imbalance, class heterogeneity, and interpretability requirements, particularly in high-stakes diagnostic tasks.

PIONEERING RESEARCH AND APPLICATIONS

The integration of artificial intelligence into urology has been catalyzed by pioneering research efforts and practical applications that showcase the transformative potential of these technologies. These studies represent critical milestones in the evolution of AI-driven diagnostics and prognostics, underscoring how technical innovation can directly translate into clinical value. Below, we present an in-depth exploration of notable investigations and key contributors whose work exemplifies the application of AI techniques to address pressing urological challenges.

Prostate Cancer Detection with CNNs:

A multidisciplinary team led by Dr. Anant Madabhushi, in collaboration with Brennan T. Flannery and colleagues, developed a DenseNet-based convolutional neural network model for prostate cancer detection using hematoxylin and eosin (H&E)-stained histopathological slides from both biopsies and radical prostatectomies. Published in The Journal of Pathology (DOI: 10.1002/path.6373), their model achieved high performance (F1 scores > 0.88) when evaluated on the sample type it was trained on. However, cross-sample performance declined (F1 < 0.65), primarily due to morphological variability such as open versus closed glandular architecture. This outcome highlights a common challenge in AI pathology: domain shift between different specimen types. The study—validated across 1,000 slides, including 750 from the NRG/RTOG 0521 clinical trial—demonstrates the necessity of developing sample-specific models or employing domain adaptation techniques to preserve model accuracy in real-world scenarios. Furthermore, the authors emphasize the need for collaboration between pathologists and AI developers to ensure clinically meaningful interpretation of automated predictions (Flannery et al., 2025).

Machine Learning for Urolithiasis and Benign Prostatic Hyperplasia (BPH):

In a landmark systematic review published in Journal of Endourology (DOI: 10.1089/end.2022.0311), David Bouhadana, Dr. Quoc-Dien Trinh, Dr. Naeem Bhojani, and collaborators reviewed 63 machine learning studies, encompassing both urolithiasis and BPH. The included studies utilized a variety of ML algorithms—such as decision trees, support vector machines, and deep neural networks—applied to tasks ranging from kidney stone classification to treatment outcome prediction. Notably, vision-based models were employed to automatically detect and classify stone types, while structured clinical data enabled the prediction of surgical success in BPH interventions. This review, evaluated under the STREAM-URO framework, calls for standardized reporting and greater methodological rigor, as variability in datasets and performance metrics hampers cross-study comparability. The work also suggests that hybrid AI models, which combine imaging with patient-level metadata, may offer superior predictive capabilities for personalized stone management and BPH treatment planning (Bouhadana et al., 2023).

Transfer Learning for Bladder Cancer Treatment Response:

Eric Wu, Dr. Lubomir M. Hadjiiski, and their team at the University of Michigan designed a deep learning-based convolutional neural network (DL-CNN) to assess treatment response in bladder cancer patients undergoing neoadjuvant chemotherapy. Reported in Tomography (PMCID: PMC6403041), the model was trained on paired pre- and post-chemotherapy CT scans from 123 patients, leveraging transfer learning with pretrained weights from generic image datasets. The resulting model achieved AUC scores between 0.79 and 0.86 for identifying complete responders (T0 stage), outperforming randomly initialized models (AUC = 0.73) and approximating expert radiologists' performance (AUC = 0.76–0.77). These results underscore the clinical viability of transfer learning, particularly in domains like oncology, where annotated data are scarce. The study also demonstrates that incorporating temporal imaging data (i.e., before and after treatment) can significantly enhance model sensitivity to subtle morphological changes—a crucial aspect for response-adaptive treatment planning (Wu et al., 2019).

AI in Urooncology: Comprehensive Review Across Cancer Types:

Anita Froń, Dr. Bartosz Małkiewicz, and their group conducted an extensive narrative review published in Cancers (PMCID: PMC10486651), surveying the current landscape of AI applications across prostate, kidney, bladder, and testicular cancers. Their review spans a wide range of AI tools including natural language processing (NLP) for patient documentation, deep learning for tumor segmentation, and decision tree models for outcome prediction. The authors note that many AI systems now rival human clinicians in imaging-based diagnostics, especially in tasks such as tumor grading and volumetric analysis. Moreover, the review highlights the emerging field of radiogenomics, which integrates imaging features with genomic markers to refine risk stratification. The authors call for prospective, multicenter validations to ensure these tools are generalizable and ethically robust, particularly in underserved populations. This work provides a valuable framework for future AI research, pointing toward an integrated, multi-modal diagnostic model for urooncology (Froń et al., 2023).

AI-Assisted Cystoscopy for Pathology Detection:

A research team from the Urology Clinic of Training and Research Hospital developed a CNN-based model for bladder cancer detection using cystoscopy images. Their dataset included 500 healthy and 500 pathological images obtained from three major imaging platforms—Karl Storz, Striker, and Richard Wolf—collected between 2018 and 2024. Upon evaluation on a separate test set (n=200), the model achieved 94% sensitivity but only 60% specificity. This performance gap, especially in distinguishing benign conditions like trabeculation from malignancy, underscores the importance of imaging standardization and larger multi-institutional datasets. Despite these limitations, the study represents a significant step toward real-time, AI-supported cystoscopic diagnosis. The system has potential for use in training settings, aiding junior urologists by reducing false negatives and highlighting ambiguous lesions during live procedures.

Collectively, these meticulously detailed examples illustrate the expansive scope of AI applications in urology, from image-based diagnostics and treatment prediction to multimodal integration and automated clinical support. They also highlight a common theme: while AI demonstrates exceptional promise, its successful clinical adoption depends on rigorous validation, robust datasets, and human-AI collaboration frameworks. These studies form the backbone of current AI research in urology and set a strong precedent for future translational work. For a comprehensive understanding, readers are encouraged to consult the original sources referenced in the supplementary bibliography (İvelik et al., 2025).

CHALLENGES IN INTEGRATION AND ADOPTION

Despite promising outcomes in pilot studies, several challenges hinder the seamless integration of AI into clinical urology. One key issue is data heterogeneity—differences in imaging protocols, equipment types, or EHR formats across institutions reduce model portability. Moreover, annotation bottlenecks limit the availability of high-quality labeled datasets, as expert labeling is time-consuming and resource-intensive.

Another persistent barrier is interoperability. Many AI tools struggle to integrate with legacy hospital information systems due to incompatible formats or lack of standardized APIs. This can create workflow disruptions rather than efficiencies. Ethical concerns such as algorithmic bias, lack of transparency, and unclear liability in case of AI-driven diagnostic errors further complicate adoption. Without explainable AI (XAI) mechanisms, clinicians may hesitate to trust or rely on automated recommendations.

Importantly, there is also a human factor: successful integration requires user training, stakeholder engagement, and cultural adaptation within clinical teams. Resistance to new technologies can slow adoption, particularly if clinicians perceive AI as a threat rather than a tool.

Future Directions and Research Priorities

The future of AI in urology will depend on multidisciplinary collaboration, regulatory clarity, and technological innovation. Research priorities include:

Developing multimodal AI systems that combine imaging, genomics, and clinical data.

Expanding prospective multicenter trials to assess real-world effectiveness.

Enhancing model explainability and fairness auditing, particularly in diverse patient populations.

Building adaptive AI tools that learn continuously from new data and clinical feedback.

In addition, federated learning—which allows AI models to be trained across decentralized datasets without compromising privacy—offers a promising avenue to address data access and security issues. Collaboration between urologists, data scientists, ethicists, and policymakers will be crucial to guide these developments.

The Use of Artificial Intelligence in Urological Image Analysis

Artificial intelligence (AI) has emerged as a groundbreaking force in medical diagnostics, transforming how urological conditions—such as bladder cancer (BC), prostate cancer, kidney diseases, and other genitourinary disorders—are identified and managed. Imaging is central to urological practice, providing critical insights into anatomical and pathological states. However, traditional imaging methods often grapple with subjectivity, variability among clinicians, and challenges in detecting subtle abnormalities. AI, powered by machine learning (ML), deep learning (DL), and advanced computer vision, addresses these limitations by offering unparalleled precision, automation, and reproducibility. This section examines AI's transformative applications in cystoscopy and other urological imaging modalities, its advancements in lesion detection and classification, and the pivotal studies and datasets fueling these innovations.

CYSTOSCOPY AND OTHER UROLOGICAL IMAGING MODALITIES

Cystoscopy is the cornerstone of bladder cancer diagnosis, enabling clinicians to visualize the bladder's interior using a cystoscope—a flexible or rigid tube equipped with a light source and high-resolution camera. White-light cystoscopy (WLC), the conventional approach, is widely employed to detect bladder tumors, guide transurethral resection of bladder tumors (TURBT), and monitor recurrence. Despite its utility, WLC has well-documented flaws. Research indicates misdiagnosis rates of up to 30%, particularly for flat lesions like carcinoma in situ (CIS), due to its reliance on subjective visual assessment (Ma et al., 2024). Sensitivity diminishes further when confronting early-stage or morphologically ambiguous abnormalities, where human perception struggles to discern critical details. Factors such as operator experience, lighting conditions, and lesion visibility exacerbate these challenges, highlighting the urgent need for more reliable diagnostic tools.

AI has stepped in as a game-changer, enhancing cystoscopy through sophisticated image analysis. By leveraging DL techniques, such as convolutional neural networks (CNNs), and computer vision algorithms, AI systems can scrutinize cystoscopic images at a pixel-by-pixel level, uncovering features that elude human observation (Rossin et al., 2023). These systems not only flag suspicious areas in real time but also quantify lesion characteristics, reducing diagnostic errors and improving procedural outcomes. Beyond WLC, AI enhances advanced cystoscopy variants like photodynamic diagnosis (PDD) with blue-light imaging, where models like InceptionV3 achieve a sensitivity of 95.8% for malignancy detection (Ali et al., 2021). This capability extends to fluorescence-guided techniques, where AI distinguishes subtle fluorescence patterns indicative of cancerous tissue.

AI's impact is not limited to cystoscopy. Other urological imaging modalities—ultrasound (US), computed tomography (CT), magnetic resonance imaging (MRI), and positron emission tomography (PET)—also reap its benefits. Ultrasound, a non-invasive staple, evaluates kidney stones, bladder wall thickness, and prostate size. AI enhances US by automating the identification of hyperechoic structures (e.g., calculi) and anomalies like hydronephrosis, streamlining preliminary assessments. CT, prized for its detailed cross-sectional views, aids in staging urological cancers and detecting ureteral obstructions; DL models like FGP-Net predict muscle-invasive bladder cancer with an AUC of 0.92 (Wu et al., 2022). Multiparametric MRI, a linchpin in prostate cancer diagnostics, leverages AI to segment lesions, refine PI-RADS scoring, and reduce false positives, sparing patients unnecessary interventions. PET, though less routine, supports metastatic evaluations, with AI poised to enhance its specificity in oncological contexts. Collectively, these modalities illustrate AI's versatility across the urological imaging spectrum.

AI-ASSISTED LESION DETECTION AND CLASSIFICATION

AI's prowess in detecting and classifying lesions has revolutionized urological diagnostics, delivering marked improvements in accuracy, speed, and consistency. In cystoscopy, systems like the Cystoscopy Artificial Intelligence Diagnostic System (CAIDS) epitomize this progress. Trained on a robust dataset of 69,204 images from multiple centers, CAIDS achieves a diagnostic accuracy of 93.9%, outpacing urologists in both sensitivity and efficiency, with a mere 12-second processing latency (Ma et al., 2024; Wu et al., 2022). By employing CNNs, CAIDS meticulously maps tumor boundaries, aiding surgical precision during TURBT and reducing residual disease risk. Similarly, CystoNet, developed by Chang et al. (2023), offers real-time tumor detection with a per-frame sensitivity of 90.9% and specificity of 98.6%, tested across 2,752 frames from 95 patients. This system integrates transfer learning, adapting pre-trained DL models to urological imaging, thereby enhancing its adaptability to diverse clinical scenarios.

These AI systems rely on advanced architectures like U-Net and Mask R-CNN for tasks such as lesion segmentation and grading. CAIDS, for instance, excels at delineating tumor margins, providing surgeons with precise visual guides, while CystoNet classifies lesions as benign or malignant, minimizing diagnostic ambiguity. Beyond cystoscopy, AI extends its reach to CT and MRI. In bladder cancer, FGP-Net leverages CT data to predict muscle invasion, streamlining preoperative strategies (Wu et al., 2022). In prostate MRI, AI algorithms categorize lesions by clinical significance, reducing overdiagnosis and optimizing biopsy decisions. Emerging models, such as Dilated U-Net, have decreased overlooked tumors during TURBT by 84.9%, underscoring AI's surgical support potential (Mutaguchi et al., 2022). Additionally, RGB-based DL approaches achieve over 90% accuracy in grading bladder tumors, offering prognostic insights that inform therapeutic choices (Yoo et al., 2022).

The technical foundation of these systems blends DL with classical ML methods. CNNs dominate image analysis, extracting hierarchical features from raw pixels, while support vector machines (SVMs) offer robust classification in smaller datasets, such as prostate biopsy images. Radiomics, an innovative adjunct, quantifies imaging features—texture, shape, intensity—feeding them into AI models for predictive analytics. This multi-faceted approach ensures AI's adaptability, addressing both high-volume datasets and niche applications with equal efficacy.

Key Studies and Datasets in the Literature

A wealth of research underpins AI's ascent in urological diagnostics, with seminal studies illuminating its potential and limitations. Rossin et al. (2023) conducted a sweeping review of AI applications, spanning cystoscopy, clinical tumor staging (cT), and histopathological integration. Their findings emphasize AI's capacity to enhance clinician accuracy, particularly in underserved regions lacking specialized expertise. Wu et al. (2022) validated CAIDS across 10,729 patients, achieving an AUC of 0.99 in external datasets—a testament to its robustness and generalizability across heterogeneous populations and imaging protocols. Chang et al. (2023) advanced real-time diagnostics with CystoNet, reporting stellar performance metrics but calling for broader prospective validation to cement its clinical reliability.

Datasets are the lifeblood of these innovations, varying widely in scope and complexity. The Cancer Genome Atlas Bladder Cancer (TCGA-BLCA) dataset integrates imaging with genomic profiles, fueling BC research. PROMISE12, tailored for prostate MRI segmentation, supports AI-driven prostate cancer diagnostics, while KiTS19 focuses on kidney tumor analysis, offering annotated CT scans for model training. Wu et al. (2022) harnessed a multicentric dataset of 69,204 cystoscopy frames, highlighting the necessity of large, diverse data to mitigate overfitting and enhance model performance. Yet, challenges persist: many studies, including those by Mutaguchi et al. (2022), rely on retrospective or single-center cohorts (e.g., 120 patients), limiting their scalability. Rossin et al. (2023) advocate for multicentric, prospective trials to address these gaps and ensure real-world applicability.

CONCLUSION AND FUTURE DIRECTIONS

AI's integration into urological image analysis heralds a paradigm shift, delivering faster, more accurate diagnostics and diminishing the subjectivity inherent in traditional imaging interpretation. Systems like CAIDS and CystoNet exemplify AI's enhancement of cystoscopy, while its applications in CT, MRI, and US broaden its reach across urology. Challenges remain—specificity gaps, such as INF-M01's 92.1% versus urologists' 99.1%, and dataset biases underscore areas for refinement (Kim et al., 2024). Nevertheless, AI's benefits—standardized diagnostics, reduced diagnostic latency, and improved patient outcomes—are indisputable.

The future holds immense promise. Integrating AI with robotic surgery platforms (e.g., Da Vinci systems) could enable real-time tumor resection guidance, enhancing surgical precision. Multi-omics approaches, fusing imaging with genomic and proteomic data, promise personalized prognostics and tailored therapies. Ethical considerations—addressing biases in training data, ensuring equitable access, and navigating regulatory landscapes—will be paramount. Prospective, multicentric trials are essential to validate AI's efficacy and safety, paving the way for its seamless adoption into clinical workflows. As of March 29, 2025, AI stands at the cusp of redefining urological care, closing gaps in current imaging paradigms and ushering in an era of precision medicine.

The Impact of Artificial Intelligence on Urological Diagnosis

Diagnostic Accuracy and Clinical Performance of Artificial Intelligence Models

Artificial intelligence (AI) has emerged as a transformative force in urological diagnostics, leveraging advanced techniques such as deep learning and convolutional neural networks to enhance diagnostic precision. In the context of prostate cancer, one of the most prevalent urological malignancies, AI models have demonstrated remarkable accuracy in interpreting multiparametric magnetic resonance imaging (mpMRI) and ultrasound data. Similarly, AI has shown promise in analyzing histopathological slides from prostate biopsies, reducing inter-observer variability among pathologists—a known limitation in traditional diagnostics (Arafa et al., 2024).

Beyond prostate cancer, AI applications extend to bladder cancer and renal cell carcinoma. Fenstermaker et al. developed a deep learning (DL) model designed to classify renal cell carcinoma (RCC) subtypes in histopathology images. Their algorithm was trained on a dataset comprising 3,000 normal tissue samples and 12,168 RCC samples obtained from 42 patients. Remarkably, the model demonstrated 97.5% accuracy in distinguishing between clear cell, papillary, and chromophobe RCC subtypes using only a minimal tissue area of 100 μm^2. Additionally, it achieved 98.4% accuracy in predicting Fuhrman nuclear grade (Fenstermaker et al., 2020).

However, the clinical performance of these models is contingent upon the quality and diversity of training datasets. Models trained on homogenous populations may fail to generalize across ethnic or socioeconomic groups, potentially exacerbating health disparities . Furthermore, while AI excels in pattern recognition, its ability to integrate contextual clinical data—such as patient history or comorbidities—remains limited, underscoring the need for hybrid systems that combine AI with human expertise.

Advantages Provided by AI to Urologists and Decision Support Systems

The integration of AI into urology offers substantial benefits, particularly as a decision support tool that augments clinical workflows. One of the primary advantages is its capacity to process vast amounts of multimodal data—imaging, laboratory results, and genomic profiles—far more rapidly than human clinicians. For example, AI-driven platforms like IBM Watson for Oncology have been adapted to urology, providing real-time recommendations for treatment planning in prostate cancer cases based on aggregated evidence (Park et al., 2023). Such systems enable urologists to identify high-risk patients earlier, optimize biopsy strategies, and tailor therapeutic interventions with greater precision.

Additionally, AI enhances diagnostic efficiency by flagging anomalies that might escape human detection. Beyond diagnostics, AI supports surgical planning and intraoperative decision-making. Bianchi et al. (2023) presented a study in which preoperative multiparametric magnetic resonance imaging (mpMRI) was used to guide intraoperative frozen tissue sampling during robot-assisted radical prostatectomy, aiming to reduce positive surgical margins. Their approach involved an augmented reality 3D (AR3D) model, which was projected onto the robotic console to help surgeons identify optimal biopsy sites that were theoretically free of cancer cells. The results demonstrated that the AR3D-assisted technique significantly reduced positive surgical margin rates at the index lesion level compared to the conventional non-AR3D method (Bianchi et al., 2021).

For urologists, this translates to reduced cognitive workload, enhanced confidence in complex cases, and the ability to focus on patient-centered care rather than data interpretation.

Moreover, AI facilitates risk stratification and prognostic modeling, critical components of personalized medicine. By analyzing longitudinal data, AI can predict disease recurrence or progression, as demonstrated in a study where a machine learning model accurately forecasted biochemical recurrence in prostate cancer patients post-prostatectomy (Janbain et al., 2024). These capabilities position AI as an indispensable ally in the shift toward precision urology, though its adoption must be tempered by rigorous validation and clinician training.

Challenges of Implementation in Real Clinical Settings

Despite its potential, the deployment of AI in real-world urological practice encounters significant barriers. Technical challenges include the heterogeneity of healthcare systems globally—while tertiary centers may possess the infrastructure to support AI, rural or underfunded facilities often lack compatible hardware or reliable internet Access. This digital divide risks widening existing inequities in urological care. Additionally, the integration of AI with electronic health record (EHR) systems poses interoperability issues, as proprietary formats and inconsistent data standards hinder seamless adoption (Torab-Miandoab et al., 2023).

Ethical and regulatory concerns further complicate implementation. AI systems require access to large datasets of patient information, raising questions about consent, data privacy, and compliance with regulations like the General Data Protection Regulation (GDPR) in Europe or the Health Insurance Portability and Accountability Act (HIPAA) in the United States. The opaque nature of many AI algorithms—so-called "black box" models—also undermines trust among clinicians.

This lack of interpretability could impede adoption unless countered by explainable AI frameworks (Cacciamani et al., 2024).

Future Perspectives and Ethical Issues in Artificial Intelligence in Urology

Artificial intelligence (AI) is poised to revolutionize the field of urology, offering unprecedented opportunities to enhance diagnostics, surgical precision, and patient care. However, its integration into clinical practice introduces complex ethical challenges that must be addressed to ensure its responsible and equitable application. This chapter explores the future potential of AI in urology, the integration and development of AI-based systems, and the critical ethical considerations surrounding data privacy, accountability, and fairness.

THE FUTURE OF ARTIFICIAL INTELLIGENCE IN UROLOGY

AI holds transformative potential in urology, particularly in diagnostics, surgical interventions, and patient monitoring. In diagnostic applications, AI-driven tools are increasingly utilized for the early detection of urologic malignancies such as prostate and bladder cancer (İvelik et al., 2025; Froń et al., 2023).

In surgical contexts, AI-enhanced robotic systems are redefining minimally invasive procedures. These systems provide real-time feedback to surgeons, improving precision in complex operations such as radical prostatectomies and nephrectomies. The integration of AI into robotic-assisted surgery not only augments technical accuracy but also reduces operative risks, paving the way for better postoperative recovery (Park et al., 2023; Bianchi et al., 2021).

Beyond diagnostics and surgery, AI-powered wearable technologies and remote monitoring systems offer continuous and comprehensive patient surveillance. These tools are particularly valuable for managing chronic urologic conditions, enabling early intervention and personalized treatment plans. As these technologies evolve, they promise to shift urology toward a more proactive, patient-centered model of care, leveraging predictive analytics to anticipate and address clinical needs.

INTEGRATION AND DEVELOPMENT POTENTIAL OF AI-BASED SYSTEMS

The successful integration of AI into urologic practice hinges on its compatibility with existing clinical workflows and its capacity for ongoing development. Current efforts focus on embedding AI systems within diagnostic and therapeutic tools, such as imaging platforms and robotic consoles, to streamline clinical decision-making. However, challenges remain, including the need for clinician training and the adaptation of AI tools to diverse healthcare settings.

The development potential of AI-based systems lies in their ability to adapt and learn continuously. Machine learning (ML) algorithms, for example, can refine their performance over time by incorporating new patient data, enabling personalized treatment strategies. This adaptability is particularly promising in urology, where patient-specific factors; such as tumor biology or anatomical variations, play a critical role in treatment success. Future advancements may see AI systems evolve from task-specific tools to more generalizable platforms, potentially approaching artificial general intelligence (AGI) capable of addressing complex, unforeseen clinical scenarios.

Despite this potential, integration efforts must address disparities in resource availability. The "digital divide" within Urology; where access to AI tools varies by geography and socioeconomic status, poses a barrier to equitable care.

Emerging Trends in AI-Driven Urology: Personalization, Real-Time Analytics, and Intelligent Recommendations

Artificial intelligence is evolving beyond rule-based systems into adaptive, patient-centric technologies that offer real-time decision support and personalized care. Recent developments in urological AI reflect this shift, focusing on three transformative domains: personalization, real-time analytics, and AI-powered recommendation systems.

Personalized Medicine and Adaptive Diagnostics

One of the most significant trends in contemporary urology is the growing emphasis on personalized diagnostics and treatment planning. With access to large-scale data—including imaging, laboratory results, genetic profiles, and patient histories—AI systems are now capable of tailoring clinical pathways to individual patients.

For example, in prostate cancer management, AI models can analyze multiparametric MRI in combination with genomic data to stratify patients into risk categories and recommend appropriate interventions (low-risk monitoring vs. radical prostatectomy). These models outperform traditional nomograms by integrating a greater diversity of data and capturing non-linear interactions among variables.

Additionally, personalization extends to post-operative care. AI systems now assist in forecasting potential complications or recurrence risk, enabling tailored follow-up schedules and lifestyle recommendations. In pediatric urology, machine learning models have been employed to personalize surveillance protocols for children with congenital abnormalities, reducing unnecessary interventions while maintaining safety.

REAL-TIME ANALYTICS AND INTRAOPERATIVE INTELLIGENCE

The integration of AI into real-time diagnostic and surgical workflows is another emerging frontier. Using high-throughput computing and edge-AI hardware, urological procedures such as robotic-assisted prostatectomy or cystoscopic tumor resection are increasingly supported by intraoperative analytics.

For instance, AI-enhanced cystoscopy platforms can provide live feedback during tumor resection, flagging suspicious areas and delineating tumor margins in real time. These systems rely on deep learning models trained on thousands of labeled images and have shown to improve surgical accuracy and reduce residual tumor rates (CystoNet, 2023).

In robotic surgery, real-time AI feedback is used to assess dissection planes, monitor instrument trajectories, and even predict optimal next steps based on surgical context. These applications reduce cognitive load on the surgeon and may shorten operative times. Some research groups are also exploring haptic feedback systems integrated with AI models to improve surgical precision through tactile cues.

AI-Powered Recommendation Systems in Clinical Decision Support

Borrowing from the logic of consumer recommendation engines (e.g., those used by Netflix or Amazon), AI systems in healthcare are now being designed to recommend diagnostic tests, follow-up protocols, and treatment regimens based on prior patient data and similar clinical cases.

In urology, such systems are especially beneficial in ambiguous or borderline cases. For example, if a patient's PSA level is elevated but MRI findings are equivocal, an AI engine can analyze the case in the context of thousands of similar patients to recommend whether a biopsy is warranted. These systems can also suggest participation in clinical trials based on molecular profiling and eligibility criteria.

Recommendation systems are also being integrated into hospital information systems and mobile health apps, enabling urologists to access contextual suggestions during patient visits. Some platforms use reinforcement learning to continuously improve their recommendations based on outcomes, making the system more accurate over time.

INTEGRATION WITH WEARABLES AND REMOTE MONITORING

A final frontier in personalization and real-time analytics is the integration of AI with wearable technologies and remote monitoring platforms. These tools collect continuous physiological data such as urinary frequency, bladder pressure, or hydration levels, and feed them into machine learning models for early detection of complications or relapses.

For example, in patients with neurogenic bladder or post-prostatectomy incontinence, wearable biosensors connected to AI algorithms can provide alerts for abnormal patterns, helping prevent infections or kidney damage. Such tools are particularly useful in geriatric or rural populations where access to in-person care is limited.

ETHICS, DATA PRIVACY, AND AI RESPONSIBILITIES

The deployment of AI in urology raises significant ethical concerns, including algorithmic bias, transparency, accountability, and data privacy. Algorithmic bias emerges when AI models are trained on non-diverse datasets, leading to inequitable outcomes across patient populations. For instance, underrepresented demographic groups may receive suboptimal diagnoses or treatments if training data fail to reflect their characteristics, exacerbating healthcare disparities (Verma et al., 2025). Addressing this requires enhancing dataset diversity and adopting standards like ISO/IEC 42001:2023, which prioritize "ethics by design" to mitigate unintended biases (ISO, 2023).

Transparency remains a challenge due to the "black-box" nature of many AI systems, where decision-making processes are opaque to clinicians and patients. This opacity undermines trust and informed consent, critical tenets of medical ethics. Emerging solutions, such as explainable AI (XAI), aim to make algorithmic decisions interpretable, fostering shared decision-making and patient autonomy (Smith et al., cited in Verma et al., 2025). Guidelines like CONSORT-AI and TRIPOD-AI further promote transparency by standardizing reporting practices in AI-driven research.

Accountability poses another ethical dilemma: who bears responsibility for AI-driven errors—clinicians, developers, or institutions? Without clear frameworks, patient safety and professional integrity are at risk. The IDEAL framework and WHO's 2024 Guidelines on Ethics and Governance of AI for Health advocate for delineating responsibilities and establishing mechanisms to address errors, ensuring accountability aligns with clinical practice (Verma et al., 2025).

Data privacy is paramount, given AI's reliance on vast patient datasets. Urologic data, often sensitive, demands stringent governance to prevent breaches and misuse. The NHS Somerset AI policy exemplifies local strategies to safeguard small datasets, where re-identification risks are higher, while the Coalition for Health AI (CHAI) develops broader frameworks for equitable data use (Verma et al., 2025). Compliance with regulations like the EU AI Act 2024 reinforces the need for robust security measures to protect patient confidentiality.

CONCLUSION

The integration of artificial intelligence (AI) into urological imaging analysis has shown significant promise in enhancing diagnostic accuracy, reducing interpretation variability, and optimizing clinical workflows. AI-driven algorithms, particularly deep learning and machine learning models, have demonstrated the potential to assist clinicians in detecting urological pathologies with high sensitivity and specificity. Despite these advancements, the current clinical applications of AI in urological imaging remain in an evolving phase, with challenges such as data standardization, model interpretability, and integration into routine practice. Future research should focus on refining AI models through large-scale, high-quality datasets and real-world validations to ensure robust and reproducible outcomes. Addressing these challenges will be crucial in translating AI from a supportive tool to an essential component of urological diagnostics and decision-making.

REFERENCES

Ali, N., Bolenz, C., Todenhöfer, T., Stenzel, A., Deetmar, P., Kriegmair, M., Knoll, T., Porubsky, S., Hartmann, A., Popp, J., Kriegmair, M. C., & Bocklitz, T. (2021). Deep learning-based classification of blue light cystoscopy imaging during transurethral resection of bladder tumors. *Scientific Reports*, *11*(1), 11629. DOI: 10.1038/s41598-021-91081-x PMID: 34079004

Arafa, M. A., Omar, I., Farhat, K. H., Elshinawy, M., Khan, F., Alkhathami, F. A., Mokhtar, A., Althunayan, A., Rabah, D. M., & Badawy, A. A. (2024). A Comparison of Systematic, Targeted, and Combined Biopsy Using Machine Learning for Prediction of Prostate Cancer Risk: A Multi-Center Study. *Medical Principles and Practice : International Journal of the Kuwait University, Health Science Centre*, *33*(5), 491–500. DOI: 10.1159/000540425 PMID: 39047698

Artificial Neural Network and Supervised Learning. In (2008). *Soft Computing. Studies in Computational Intelligence* (Vol. 103). Springer.

Bianchi, L., Chessa, F., Angiolini, A., Cercenelli, L., Lodi, S., Bortolani, B., Molinaroli, E., Casablanca, C., Droghetti, M., Gaudiano, C., Mottaran, A., Porreca, A., Golfieri, R., Romagnoli, D., Giunchi, F., Fiorentino, M., Piazza, P., Puliatti, S., Diciotti, S., & Schiavina, R. (2021). The use of augmented reality to guide the intraoperative frozen section during robot-assisted radical prostatectomy. *European Urology*, *80*(4), 480–488. DOI: 10.1016/j.eururo.2021.06.020 PMID: 34332759

Bouhadana, D., Lu, X. H., Luo, J. W., Assad, A., Deyirmendjian, C., Guennoun, A., Nguyen, D.-D., Kwong, J. C. C., Chughtai, B., Elterman, D. S., Zorn, K. C., Trinh, Q.-D., & Bhojani, N. (2023). Clinical Applications of Machine Learning for Urolithiasis and Benign Prostatic Hyperplasia: A Systematic Review. *Journal of Endourology*, *37*(4), 474–494. DOI: 10.1089/end.2022.0311 PMID: 36266993

Cacciamani, G. E., Chen, A., Gill, I. S., & Hung, A. J. (2024). Artificial intelligence and urology: Ethical considerations for urologists and patients. *Nature Reviews. Urology*, *21*(1), 50–59. DOI: 10.1038/s41585-023-00796-1 PMID: 37524914

Chang, T. C., Shkolyar, E., Del Giudice, F., Eminaga, O., Lee, T., Laurie, M., Seufert, C., Jia, X., Mach, K. E., Xing, L., & Liao, J. C. (2023, July 11). Real-time Detection of Bladder Cancer Using Augmented Cystoscopy with Deep Learning: A Pilot Study. *Journal of Endourology*, end.2023.0056. Advance online publication. DOI: 10.1089/end.2023.0056 PMID: 37432899

Esteva, A., Kuprel, B., Novoa, R. A., Ko, J., Swetter, S. M., Blau, H. M., & Thrun, S. (2017). Dermatologist-level classification of skin cancer with deep neural networks. *Nature*, *542*(7639), 115–118. DOI: 10.1038/nature21056 PMID: 28117445

Fenstermaker, M., Tomlins, S. A., Singh, K., Wiens, J., & Morgan, T. M. (2020). Development and validation of a deep-learning model to assist with renal cell carcinoma histopathologic interpretation. *Urology*, *144*, 152–157. DOI: 10.1016/j.urology.2020.05.094 PMID: 32711010

Ferro, M., Falagario, U. G., Barone, B., Maggi, M., Crocetto, F., Busetto, G. M., Giudice, F., Terracciano, D., Lucarelli, G., Lasorsa, F., Catellani, M., Brescia, A., Mistretta, F. A., Luzzago, S., Piccinelli, M. L., Vartolomei, M. D., Jereczek-Fossa, B. A., Musi, G., Montanari, E., & Tataru, O. S. (2023). Artificial intelligence in the advanced diagnosis of bladder cancer: Comprehensive literature review and future advancement. *Diagnostics (Basel)*, *13*(13), 2308. DOI: 10.3390/diagnostics13132308 PMID: 37443700

Flannery, B. T., Sandler, H. M., Lal, P., Feldman, M. D., Santa-Rosario, J. C., Pathak, T., Mirtti, T., Farre, X., Correa, R., Chafe, S., Shah, A., Efstathiou, J. A., Hoffman, K., Hallman, M. A., Straza, M., Jordan, R., Pugh, S. L., Feng, F., & Madabhushi, A. (2025). Stress testing deep learning models for prostate cancer detection on biopsies and surgical specimens. *The Journal of Pathology*, *265*(2), 146–157. DOI: 10.1002/path.6373 PMID: 39660731

Froń, A., Semianiuk, A., Lazuk, U., Ptaszkowski, K., Siennicka, A., Lemiński, A., Krajewski, W., Szydełko, T., & Małkiewicz, B. (2023). Artificial Intelligence in Urooncology: What We Have and What We Expect. *Cancers (Basel)*, *15*(17), 4282. DOI: 10.3390/cancers15174282 PMID: 37686558

Ghosh, S. (2025). *Mathematical Foundations of Deep Learning*.

Gulshan, V., Peng, L., Coram, M., Stumpe, M. C., Wu, D., Narayanaswamy, A., Venugopalan, S., Widner, K., Madams, T., Cuadros, J., Kim, R., Raman, R., Nelson, P. C., Mega, J. L., & Webster, D. R. (2016). Development and validation of a deep learning algorithm for detection of diabetic retinopathy in retinal fundus photographs. *Journal of the American Medical Association*, *316*(22), 2402–2410. DOI: 10.1001/jama.2016.17216 PMID: 27898976

ISO/IEC 42001:2023 [Internet]. ISO; 2023. https://www.iso.org/standard/81230.html. [Accessed 27 January 2025].

İvelik, H. İ., Alkış, O., Kartal, İ. G., Sevim, M., & Aras, B. (2025). AI-assisted cystoscopy image analysis for detecting urological pathologies: A novel approach. *Grand Journal of Urology*, *5*(2), 37–41. DOI: 10.5505/GJU.2025.94824

Janbain, A., Farolfi, A., Guenegou-Arnoux, A., Romengas, L., Scharl, S., Fanti, S., ... & Shelan, M. (2024). A machine learning approach for predicting biochemical outcome after PSMA-PET–guided salvage radiotherapy in recurrent prostate cancer after radical prostatectomy: retrospective study. *JMIR cancer*, *10*, e60323.

Kim, J., Ham, W. S., Koo, K. C., Lee, J., Ahn, H. K., Jeong, J. Y., Baek, S. Y., Lee, S. J., & Lee, K. S. (2024). Evaluation of the Diagnostic Efficacy of the AI-Based Software INF-M01 in Detecting Suspicious Areas of Bladder Cancer Using Cystoscopy Images. *Journal of Clinical Medicine*, *13*(23), 7110. DOI: 10.3390/jcm13237110 PMID: 39685568

Krizhevsky, A., Sutskever, I., & Hinton, G. E. Imagenet classification with deep convolutional neural networks. In: Advances in neural information processing systems. 2012; p. 1097-105.

Ma, X., Zhang, Q., He, L., Liu, X., Xiao, Y., Hu, J., Cai, S., Cai, H., & Yu, B. (2024). Artificial intelligence application in the diagnosis and treatment of bladder cancer: Advance, challenges, and opportunities. *Frontiers in Oncology*, *14*, 1487676. DOI: 10.3389/fonc.2024.1487676 PMID: 39575423

Mishra, C., & Gupta, D. (2017). Deep machine learning and neural networks: An overview. *IAES Int J Artif Intell.*, *6*(2), 66–73. DOI: 10.11591/ijai.v6.i2.pp66-73

Mutaguchi, J., Morooka, K., Kobayashi, S., Umehara, A., Miyauchi, S., Kinoshita, F., Inokuchi, J., Oda, Y., Kurazume, R., & Eto, M. (2022). Artificial Intelligence for Segmentation of Bladder Tumor Cystoscopic Images Performed by U-Net with Dilated Convolution. *Journal of Endourology*, *36*(6), 827–834. DOI: 10.1089/end.2021.0483 PMID: 35018828

Park, T., Gu, P., Kim, C. H., Kim, K. T., Chung, K. J., Kim, T. B., Jung, H., Yoon, S. J., & Oh, J. K. (2023). Artificial intelligence in urologic oncology: The actual clinical practice results of IBM Watson for Oncology in South Korea. *Prostate International*, *11*(4), 218–221. DOI: 10.1016/j.prnil.2023.09.001 PMID: 38196551

Rossin, G., Zorzi, F., Ongaro, L., Piasentin, A., Vedovo, F., Liguori, G., Zucchi, A., Simonato, A., Bartoletti, R., Trombetta, C., Pavan, N., & Claps, F. (2023). Artificial Intelligence in Bladder Cancer Diagnosis: Current Applications and Future Perspectives. *BioMedInformatics*, *3*(1), 104–114. DOI: 10.3390/biomedinformatics3010008

Torab-Miandoab, A., Samad-Soltani, T., Jodati, A., & Rezaei-Hachesu, P. (2023). Interoperability of heterogeneous health information systems: A systematic literature review. *BMC Medical Informatics and Decision Making*, *23*(1), 18. DOI: 10.1186/s12911-023-02115-5 PMID: 36694161

. Verma, Rounaka,b; Macaskill, Findlaya,c; Kim, Annaa,c; Raison, Nicholasa,c; Dasgupta, Prokara,c. (2025). Ethical aspects of artificial intelligence: what urologists need to know. Current Opinion in Urology. DOI: DOI: 10.1097/MOU.0000000000001278

Wu, E., Hadjiiski, L. M., Samala, R. K., Chan, H. P., Cha, K. H., Richter, C., Cohan, R. H., Caoili, E. M., Paramagul, C., Alva, A., & Weizer, A. Z. (2019). Deep Learning Approach for Assessment of Bladder Cancer Treatment Response. *Tomography : a Journal for Imaging Research*, *5*(1), 201–208. DOI: 10.18383/j.tom.2018.00036 PMID: 30854458

Wu, S., Chen, X., Pan, J., Dong, W., Diao, X., Zhang, R., Zhang, Y., Zhang, Y., Qian, G., Chen, H., Lin, H., Xu, S., Chen, Z., Zhou, X., Mei, H., Wu, C., Lv, Q., Yuan, B., Chen, Z., & Lin, T. (2022). An Artificial Intelligence System for the Detection of Bladder Cancer via Cystoscopy: A Multicenter Diagnostic Study. *Journal of the National Cancer Institute*, *114*(2), 220–227. DOI: 10.1093/jnci/djab179 PMID: 34473310

Yoo, J. W., Koo, K. C., Chung, B. H., Baek, S. Y., Lee, S. J., Park, K. H., & Lee, K. S. (2022). Deep learning diagnostics for bladder tumor identification and grade prediction using RGB method. *Scientific Reports*, *12*(1), 17699. DOI: 10.1038/s41598-022-22797-7 PMID: 36271252

Chapter 6
Deep Learning-Based Cornea OCT Segmentation of Healthy and Keratoconic Eyes

Abir Chaari
https://orcid.org/0000-0003-0558-6269
National School of Electronics and Communication of Sfax, Tunisia

Imen Fourati Kallel
https://orcid.org/0000-0003-3807-4534
National School of Electronics and Communication of Sfax, Tunisia

Mondher Frikha
National School of Electronics and Communication of Sfax, Tunisia

Sonda Kammoun
Medical University of Sfax, Tunisia

ABSTRACT

Vision is one of the most essential human senses, playing a key role in perceiving and interpreting the environment. This complex process depends on the proper functioning of various ocular structures, particularly the cornea. Any alteration in its structure or function can significantly affect visual quality. This research explores the use of a deep learning method for semantic segmentation of corneal layers to enable early detection of keratoconus. To address limitations of existing automatic segmentation techniques for corneal Optical Coherence Tomography images, a novel deep learning model is proposed. The algorithm segments corneal layers by

DOI: 10.4018/979-8-3373-1479-2.ch006

capturing both local and contextual features. The developed architecture is based on an enhanced UNet variant incorporating residual connections, recurrent modules, and dilated convolutions. The model was evaluated on a dataset comprising both healthy and keratoconus-affected corneas. Experimental results showed an accuracy of 96.77%, outperforming reference models such as UNet, ResUNet, SegNet, and DeepLabV3+.

I. INTRODUCTION

Keratoconus (Rabinowitz, 1998) is a progressive corneal disorder characterized by gradual and asymmetric thinning, leading to a conical deformation. This structural alteration results in a progressive decline in visual quality, mainly due to morphological changes in the corneal surface. Early detection of this condition is essential to slow its progression and preserve patients' quality of life (Chaari et al., 2024). Several risk factors for keratoconus have been identified (Hashemi et al., 2020), but their precise assessment remains complex, particularly in asymptomatic forms. As the exact origin of this disease remains unknown, its screening represents a major challenge in ophthalmology. This difficulty arises from a significant overlap between the early manifestations of keratoconus and certain non-progressive corneal anomalies.

Early detection of this condition is critical to limit its progression and preserve patients' quality of life. The indispensable diagnostic tool for this pathology is Optical Coherence Tomography (OCT) (Lucas & Burdon, 2020). The precise delineation of corneal layers is essential for the early identification and effective management of keratoconus. Corneal layer segmentation allows for a detailed analysis of disease progression, helping clinicians detect subtle changes that may not be visible in the overall structure of the OCT image. In some cases, while the overall appearance of the cornea may seem normal, its internal layers may exhibit deformations. Extracting these layers from OCT images remains a major challenge due to the complexity of the corneal structure and variability in image quality. To address these challenges, artificial intelligence (AI) technologies have become indispensable. Their integration has transformed segmentation tasks, enhancing precision, efficiency, and automation. AI, simulating human cognitive abilities, plays a key role in processing and analyzing complex data derived from OCT images.

This chapter explores the use of AI techniques, particularly deep learning, to address the limitations of traditional methods, presenting a detailed methodology for the semantic segmentation of corneal layers. An innovative deep learning model was developed and specifically adapted for this task. The main contribution of this chapter is the enhancement of the UNet model through the integration of residual connections, recurrent modules, and dilated convolutions. This combination improves the model's ability to capture fine details while simultaneously contextualizing large-scale spatial information, enabling precise delineation of corneal structures.

The remainder of this chapter is structured as follows: Section II presents the Medical Context, Section III covers the State of the Art, Section IV details the Patients and Methods, Section V discusses the Training, Loss Function, and Evaluation Metrics, Section VI provides the Results and Discussion, and the chapter concludes with the Conclusion.

II. MEDICAL CONTEXT

1. The history of keratoconus

Keratoconus affects individuals of both sexes, regardless of their geographical origin, although Asian populations appear to have a higher prevalence. It can be diagnosed at any age, but it generally manifests during adolescence, between 10 and 20 years old (Meyer, Gokul, Vellara, & McGhee, 2023).

The exact causes of keratoconus remain uncertain, but a genetic origin is strongly suspected, as multiple members of the same family may be affected, and the disease often develops in both eyes (Edwards, McGhee, & Dean, 2001). Numerous studies have also highlighted associations between keratoconus and certain systemic conditions, such as atopy (allergic reactions), hormonal imbalances, and mechanical factors of genetic origin (Crawford et al., 2020).

Since the early 20th century, research on this disease has led to a better understanding of its mechanisms and has significantly expanded treatment options. Keratoconus causes visual disturbances that, in advanced cases, can result in severe vision loss (Kymes, 2004; Martel, 2014).

The first medical reference to keratoconus dates back to a doctoral dissertation in 1748, in which Burchard Mauchart provided the earliest description of the condition, referring to it as *staphyloma diaphanum*. A more detailed definition was given in 1854 by John Nottingham (Grzybowski, 2013).

In 1859, surgeon William Bowman used the ophthalmoscope to diagnose keratoconus and explained how to identify the conical deformation of the cornea. In 1869, Johann Horner dedicated a thesis to the treatment of keratoconus, recommending chemical cauterization with silver nitrate (Sah, 2022).

Finally, in 1888, Eugène Kalt developed a rigid glass lens designed to improve visual acuity by reshaping the cornea into a more regular form (Abdelaziz, 2013).

2. Macroscopic Anatomy of the Cornea

The cornea is distinguished by its clarity and dome-shaped structure. Positioned at the front of the eyeball, this transparent membrane plays a crucial role in bending light rays and protecting the internal components of the eye. Its thickness varies from approximately 550 µm at the center to 700 µm at the periphery. It consists of five distinct layers: the epithelium, Bowman's membrane, the stroma, Descemet's membrane, and the endothelium, each serving a specific function (Jirsova, 2017; Morgan, 2014).

3. Microscopic Anatomy of the Cornea

The cornea undergoes central thinning, primarily affecting the stromal lamellae, which can reach only 1/5 of its normal thickness, approximately 100 µm (Gordon, 2015; Jirsova, 2017). This reduction leads to decreased biomechanical resistance, promoting a progressive deformation characteristic of keratoconus.

3..1. Epithelium

The epithelium is a thin protective layer of cells covering the external surface of the cornea. It plays a crucial role as a barrier against external aggressions while contributing to the maintenance of optical transparency. In keratoconus, epithelial irregularities or disruptions may occur due to underlying structural changes (Dua, 1994; Simon, 1993).

3..2. Bowman's Membrane

Located between the epithelium and the stroma, this thin and non-regenerative layer plays a key role in maintaining corneal integrity. Although its exact functions are not fully understood, it acts as a protective barrier for the underlying nerve plexus. In keratoconus, this membrane gradually thins and may develop ruptures, accelerating disease progression (DeWitt, 1931; Wilson, 2000).

3..3. Corneal Stroma:

Making up the majority of the corneal thickness, the stroma is primarily composed of keratocytes and collagen fibers arranged in lamellae. This structure provides the cornea with its strength and transparency. In keratoconus, collagen organization is disrupted, leading to a loss of rigidity and contributing to the conical deformation (Bron, 2001; Pinnamaneni & Funderburgh, 2012).

3..4. Descemet's Membrane:

This inner corneal layer consists mainly of type IV collagen and laminin, essential proteins for endothelial adhesion and stability. Although generally resistant, it may thin or become more fragile in advanced stages of keratoconus (Munsamy, 2015).

3..5. Corneal Endothelium:

Positioned between Descemet's membrane and the aqueous humor, the endothelium is a single layer of cells playing a fundamental role in regulating fluid exchange. Endothelial cells are interconnected through a complex network of junctions, maintaining the balance between hydration and corneal transparency. In advanced keratoconus, endothelial alterations can lead to fluid imbalance, promoting corneal edema.

These corneal structures, as shown in Figure 1, collectively contribute to corneal transparency and stability. Any alteration in their integrity can significantly impact vision, highlighting the importance of early detection and appropriate management of keratoconus (Tuft, 1990).

Figure 1.Structure of the cornea (Source: https://www.oscarwylee.com.au/glasses/eye/cornea)

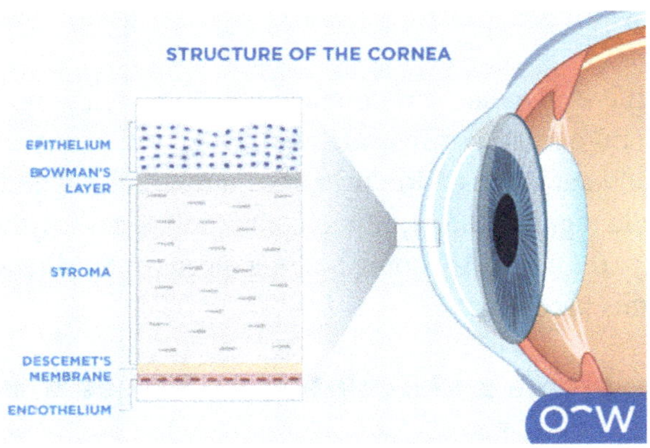

4. Endothelial Cells

Endothelial cells (Nishimiya et al., 2019; Chaari et al., 2023) form a specialized layer located at the posterior part of the cornea, the transparent region of the eye. This structure represents the innermost layer of the cornea and plays a vital role in maintaining its clarity and fluid balance. They control corneal hydration by preventing excessive fluid accumulation, thus ensuring its transparency. However, due to their very limited regenerative capacity, they are particularly vulnerable to external aggressions and ophthalmic diseases.

Alterations in this layer can lead to various dysfunctions, such as corneal edema or a loss of transparency, which can impair visual quality. In advanced stages of keratoconus, a reduction in endothelial cell density and structural changes may be observed, further compromising corneal integrity.

When corneal volume measurements are used for assessment, two major limitations arise: first, detecting keratoconus at birth is impossible, and second, accurately recording asymmetric geometric variations during the disease's progression is challenging (Cavas, 2017).

Several hypotheses have been proposed to explain the triggers of keratoconus, but its exact origin remains unknown. Four main factors are frequently studied by researchers:

- Genetic predisposition, involving chromosomal abnormalities and hereditary transmission.
- Increased sensitivity to allergies, whether general or eye-specific.
- Mechanical factors, particularly excessive eye rubbing.
- Connective tissue alteration, affecting the strength and structure of the cornea (Crawford et al., 2020).

In addition to these elements, environmental factors such as prolonged exposure to UV radiation and oxidative stress are also suspected of influencing the onset and progression of keratoconus. Moreover, recent research suggests that epigenetic modifications could regulate the expression of certain genes involved in the biomechanical stability of the cornea, opening new perspectives for a better understanding and detection of this pathology.

5. Clinical Symptoms and Evolutionary Stages of Keratoconus

Keratoconus is a condition that varies in severity among individuals, ranging from mild to severe forms. In its early stages, it may cause (Cresta, Orlandin, & Lucas, 2022; Singh et al., 2024).

- Blurred vision.
- Reduced visual acuity, especially for distant objects.
- Increased sensitivity to light (photophobia).
- Visual distortion that cannot be corrected with glasses.

- The appearance of halos and glare, particularly at night.
- Headaches accompanied by ocular discomfort.
- A sensation of irritation and dryness in the eyes.

At more advanced stages, the symptoms become more pronounced:

- Progressive deformation and thinning of the cornea.
- Increased irregular astigmatism, making it difficult to wear rigid contact lenses.
- The formation of corneal scars.
- The risk of corneal hydrops, a rare complication caused by the rupture of Descemet's membrane, leading to sudden corneal swelling and abrupt vision loss.

Keratoconus is usually diagnosed during adolescence and progresses until around the age of 30 to 40 before stabilizing. Its progression follows four distinct stages, as summarized in Table 1.

Table 1. The Different Stages of Keratoconus

Stage of Keratoconus (Source: https://entokey.com/9-optical-coherence-tomography-in-corneal-ectasia/)	Criteria
Stage 1	Visual discomfort and decreased visual acuity with astigmatism.
Stage 2	Myopia is associated with astigmatism.
Stage 3	Worsening of visual disturbances and the appearance of a clearly visible corneal protrusion.
Stage 4	Corneal thinning associated with loss of transparency (scarring or opacities at the apex of the cone) and risk of acute keratoconus.

This gradual progression significantly impacts the quality of life, limiting daily activities such as driving, reading, or screen use, and may lead to psychological distress due to progressive vision loss (See Figure 2) (Munsamy et al., 2015).

Figure 2. Images of the different stages of keratoconus (Source: https://entokey.com/9-optical-coherence-tomography-in-corneal-ectasia/)

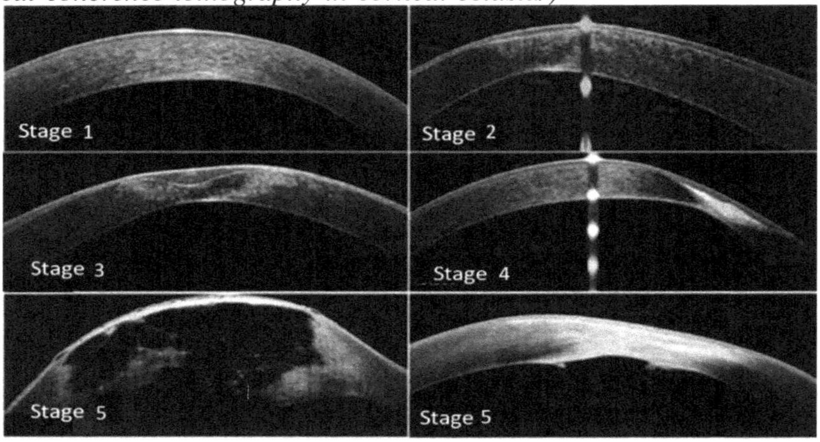

6. Corneal Examinations

Corneal assessment, also known as corneal topographic analysis, is a crucial diagnostic method for examining the condition and structure of the cornea. This in-depth evaluation enables specialists to detect various corneal abnormalities, including keratoconus and other surface irregularities. The examination relies on advanced techniques, such as corneal topography, which accurately maps the corneal curvature to identify potential distortions or asymmetries. This assessment is particularly useful for detecting subclinical forms of keratoconus, a condition characterized by progressive and irregular corneal deformation (Cavas-Martínez, Cruz-Sánchez, Nieto-Martínez, Fernández-Cañavate, & Fernández-Pacheco. 2016; Rio-Cristobal & Martin, 2014).

6..1. Specular Microscopy

Specular microscopy (Sturrock, Sherrard, & Rice, 1978) is an advanced ophthalmic imaging technique used to examine corneal endothelial cells. This method provides high-resolution images of the endothelium, the innermost layer of the cornea. During the examination, a thin beam of light is directed onto the cornea, and the light reflected from its posterior surface is captured by a specialized microscope. This technique enables the analysis of cellular arrangement to detect potential irregularities or dysfunctions (See Figure 3).

Figure 3. Image of specular microscopy (Source: https://www.indiamart.com/proddetail/specular-microscopy-pachymetry-7322736755.html)

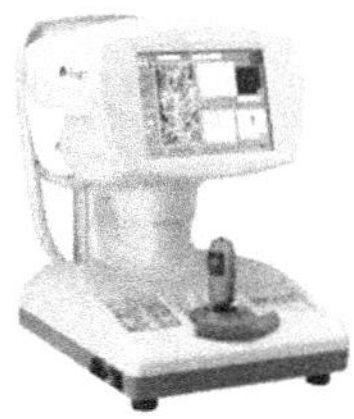

6..2. Optical Corneal Topography

Optical coherence tomography (OCT) (Seitz, Behrens, & Langenbucher, 1997) is an advanced imaging technique that utilizes light waves to capture detailed images of structures that scatter light. This approach enables the analysis of corneal curvature and surface by projecting a light pattern and interpreting the reflected signal (See Figure 4).

First introduced in 1991, OCT relies on a scanning infrared beam to produce cross-sectional or three-dimensional (3D) images of tissues. Its depth resolution reaches approximately 10 microns, offering greater precision compared to other imaging modalities such as ultrasound (US), computed tomography (CT), and magnetic resonance imaging (MRI). Based on the principle of interferometry, this non-invasive technique is widely used in ophthalmology for highly accurate visualization of retinal structures.

Corneal topography is essential for detecting corneal irregularities, particularly those associated with keratoconus, and plays a crucial role in planning laser procedures. It is also valuable for diagnosing potential complications that may arise after corneal surgery.

Figure 4. Image of optical coherence tomography (OCT) (Source: https://williamseye.com/services/glaucoma-care-treatment/optical-coherence-tomography-scanner-oct/)

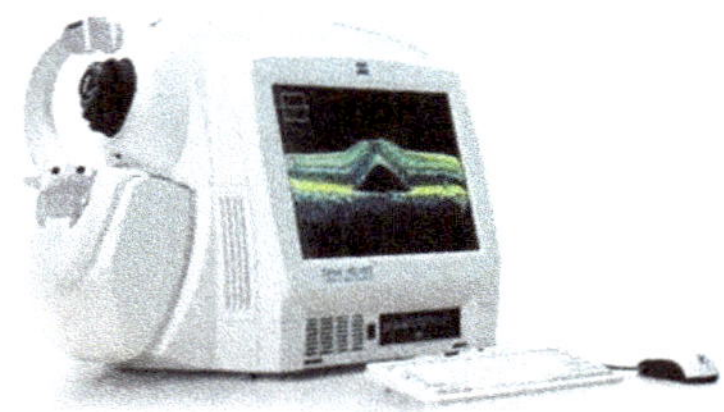

6..3. Orbscan

The Orbscan (Steele, Fabinyi, Couper, & Loughnan, 2008) is an advanced corneal mapping device used in ophthalmology to assess the structure and shape of the cornea. This technology generates precise topographic representations of both the anterior and posterior surfaces of the cornea, enabling a detailed analysis of its curvature, elevation, and thickness. With its three-dimensional imaging capabilities, Orbscan is particularly effective in detecting subtle corneal irregularities, diagnosing conditions such as keratoconus, and evaluating patients' eligibility for refractive surgery. Its application plays a crucial role in enhancing the accuracy of clinical decision-making (See Figure 5).

Figure 5. Corneal topography image obtained using orbscan (Source: https://www.urmc.rochester.edu/eye-institute/lasik/technology/orbscan-corneal-topographer)

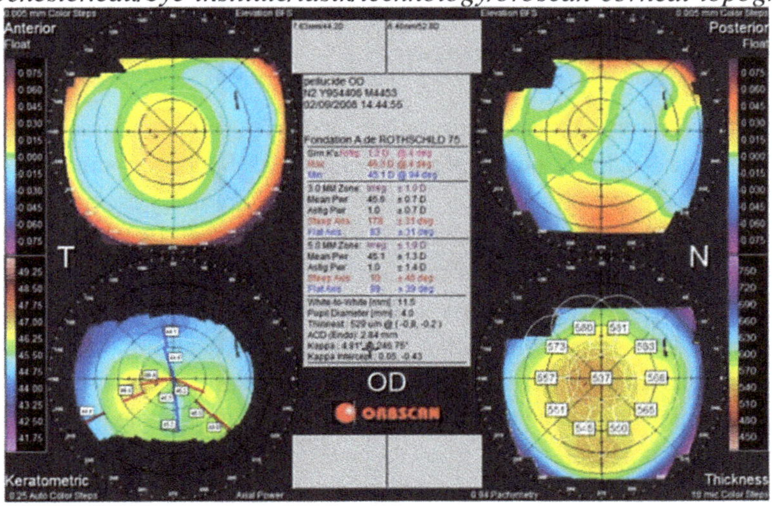

7. Forms of keratoconus

Keratoconus manifests in two distinct forms, each with a specific progression. The asymptomatic form is usually discovered incidentally during a routine ophthalmologic examination, as it does not cause any noticeable symptoms. As long as it remains stable, no treatment is required, but regular monitoring is recommended to detect any changes. On the other hand, the progressive form leads to a gradual decline in visual acuity, making correction with glasses ineffective. In such cases, contact lenses offer a more effective alternative, as they exert slight pressure on the cornea, helping to reduce its irregularities and improve visual quality (Singh et al., 2024; Fantaci, Calvo, & Rodríguez, 2024).

8. Functions of corneal topography

Corneal topography plays a crucial role in detecting morphological alterations characteristic of keratoconus, particularly in patients for whom laser surgery is contraindicated. It also serves as a valuable diagnostic tool for assessing complications that may arise after ocular surgery (Wang, 2024).

Prior to any laser procedure, corneal thickness mapping obtained via Optical Coherence Tomography (OCT) is particularly useful for calculating the maximum possible ablation depth, as well as identifying patients with keratoconic zones or abnormally thin areas of the cornea, which may render them ineligible for laser treatment (Aramberri, 2024).

9. Limitations of corneal topography

Corneal topography has certain limitations. It does not allow for precise evaluation of corneal thickness or the structure of its internal layers. Such assessments require the use of other imaging techniques, such as ultrasound pachymetry or optical coherence tomography (OCT) (Corbett, Marshall, O'Brart, & Rosen, 1995). Moreover, this method can be affected by artifacts caused by poor fixation, involuntary blinking, or ocular surface dryness, which may compromise the quality of the acquired data. It is also less reliable in patients with corneal opacities, scarring, or certain degenerative conditions that interfere with measurement accuracy. Finally, its analysis is limited to the anterior surface of the cornea and does not provide a comprehensive view of the entire corneal architecture (Al-Sharify et al., 2023).

10. Therapeutic approaches for keratoconus

Numerous studies have been dedicated to examining the diagnostic and therapeutic parameters associated with corneal diseases. The choice of treatment method depends on the stage of keratoconus (Bui, Truong, Pasricha, & Indaram, 2023; Atalay, Özalp, & Yıldırım, 2021). The main therapeutic goal is to prevent, stabilize, or correct corneal deformities in order to delay or avoid the need for a corneal transplant while restoring vision.

Glasses:

As keratoconus progresses, the degree of corneal astigmatism increases, resulting from corneal ectasia. This irregular astigmatism may allow for adequate refractive correction, both objectively and subjectively. However, the use of glasses becomes less effective, failing to provide satisfactory optical results, especially in advanced stages of the disease. Consequently, contact lenses become an essential solution for optimal visual correction (Bui, 2023).

Contact Lenses:

Contact lenses are essential in nearly all cases of keratoconus to provide functional vision. In some cases, wearing contact lenses may cause corneal scarring. However, substantial evidence indicates that the cornea can develop scars, and in these cases, approximately 10% to 26% of patients may require corneal surgery (Atalay, Özalp, & Yıldırım, 2021).

Surgical Correction:

Surgery is an option for patients who can no longer tolerate glasses or contact lenses. Corneal cross-linking (CXL) is a non-refractive treatment that slows down or halts the progression of keratoconus and may help stabilize vision in the early stages of the condition (D'Oria et al., 2024).

This innovative technique is used to correct residual astigmatism by modifying the structure of the cornea. It relies on the interaction between UVA rays (wavelength of 370 nm) and riboflavin, and typically lasts about 30 minutes (Niazi et al., 2024).

III. STATE OF THE ART

Accurate identification of the different corneal layers plays a fundamental role in the early screening and clinical monitoring of keratoconus (Maile, 2023), as it enables the detection of subtle abnormalities that may go unnoticed in the overall OCT image. In some cases, despite a normal macroscopic appearance, internal structural changes may already be present. However, segmenting these layers from OCT images remains challenging due to the complex architecture of the cornea and variations in image acquisition quality. To this end, several traditional semi-automatic and automatic segmentation methods for OCT images have been developed previously (Graglia, Mari, Baikoff, & Sequeira, 2007; LaRocca et al., 2011; Rabbani et al., 2016). Several algorithms have also been used for this purpose, especially those relying on deep learning (Ronneberger, Fischer, & Brox, 2015; Roy et al., 2017; Devalla et al., 2018; Badrinarayanan, Kendall, & Cipolla, 2017). (Graglia, Mari, Baikoff, & Sequeira, 2007) proposed a segmentation method aimed at accurately identifying the anterior (epithelium) and posterior (endothelium) interfaces of the cornea. The process begins with a preprocessing step designed to enhance the visual quality of the OCT image. Then, the algorithm detects two reference points, located respectively on the anterior and posterior surfaces of the cornea, which serve as anchor points for initiating the contour detection. From these points, a progressive pixel-by-pixel exploration is performed to reconstruct the entire corneal profile.

Although this approach allows for the precise detection of the corneal interfaces, it has some limitations. On the one hand, its reliability strongly depends on the quality of the images: low resolution or insufficient contrast may compromise the accuracy of the segmentation. On the other hand, the method relies on the initial identification of anchor points, which makes it sensitive to preliminary detection errors. Finally, the pixel-by-pixel analysis, although methodical, can be computationally expensive, especially for high-resolution images.

(LaRocca et al., 2011) proposed another method that automatically segments three corneal layers: the epithelium, the bowman, and the endothelium. This segmentation method is based on hybrid graph theory and dynamic programming. The image is considered as a graph of nodes where each node corresponds to a pixel. Nodes are connected by paths to cross the graph. Individual edges can be assigned weights to create path favorites. A dynamic programming algorithm is applied to find the preferred path with the lowest cumulative weight. This resulting path is the slice (segmentation), which splits the image into two different regions.

(Rabbani et al., 2016) proposed three different approaches for corneal layer segmentation: the Graph Cut (GC) method, the Gaussian Mixture Model (GMM), and the Level Set (LS) method.

The Graph Cut technique models segmentation as an optimization problem on a graph, where the image is represented as a network of connected nodes, and the separation of regions is achieved by minimizing a cut cost. The GMM approach models pixel intensities as a mixture of Gaussian distributions, enabling probabilistic separation of different layers based on their statistical properties. The Level Set method uses an evolving contour to detect the boundaries between layers, relying on intensity variations and local geometric properties. Among these approaches, experimental results indicate that the GMM method provides the best performance for segmenting the three main corneal layers (Epithelium, Bowman, and Endothelium), while effectively reducing artifacts in OCT images.

Classical image segmentation methods show limitations when applied to complex and noisy medical images. These approaches rely on manually defined features and empirical rules, which restrict their ability to adapt to different types of images or heterogeneous datasets. To overcome these limitations, semantic segmentation based on deep learning has gradually emerged as a powerful solution. Semantic segmentation methods using deep learning automatically assign a class label to each pixel of the image, thus transforming the segmentation task into a pixel-level classification problem. This approach enables more accurate, robust, and fully automated analysis, which is particularly suitable for medical applications where precise detection of anatomical structures is crucial (Lee et al., 2017). In this context, different deep convolutional neural network (DCNN) models such as UNet (Ronneberger, Fischer, & Brox, 2015), RlayNet (Roy et al., 2017) ResidualNet (Devalla et al., 2018) and SegNet (Badrinarayanan, Kendall, & Cipolla, 2017) have been investigated.

Models such as the Fully Convolutional Network (FCN), introduced in 2015 by Long, Shelhamer, and Darrell (2015) represented a major breakthrough in the field of semantic segmentation using deep learning. This approach replaced the fully connected layers of traditional networks with convolutional layers, thereby enabling the generation of an output with the same dimensions as the input image. However, despite this innovation, FCNs had certain limitations, notably a significant loss of spatial information, which reduced their effectiveness in fields requiring precise localization, such as medical imaging. To overcome these shortcomings, the UNet architecture (Ronneberger, Fischer, & Brox, 2015) was introduced the same year, featuring a symmetrical U-shaped design composed of an encoder path and a decoder path. This model includes direct skip connections between corresponding layers of both paths, allowing for the preservation of essential details and enhancing segmentation accuracy. Thanks to these features, UNet quickly became a benchmark model for biomedical image segmentation, serving as the foundation for many subsequent variants and improvements.

In (Roy et al., 2017), a model specifically designed for the segmentation of retinal OCT images, particularly for identifying the different layers of the retina as well as fluid areas in the macular region. This architecture relies on a dual-path structure, with a contracting part (encoder) responsible for extracting contextual features at different levels, and an expanding part (decoder) allowing for the generation of faithful pixel-wise segmentation.

One of the specific features of RelayNet is the integration of relay layers, which facilitate a progressive transfer of information between encoding and decoding, thereby reducing the loss of spatial details. This improves accuracy in detecting fine and complex structures present in medical images. When evaluated on macular OCT datasets, RelayNet achieved a segmentation accuracy of 91.9%, with a high Dice coefficient. (Devalla et al., 2018) proposes a deep neural network based on the UNet architecture, specifically designed for segmenting the optic disc tissues in Optical Coherence Tomography (OCT) images. It integrates dilated convolutions and residual blocks to enhance the capture of fine features and contextual information across different scales. This architecture allows for better capturing of long-range relationships and subtle details of the optic disc tissues. The residual blocks facilitate the learning of residual mappings, thus improving the model's convergence. This model achieved a segmentation accuracy of 92.1% and a Dice coefficient of 93.5%. (Lee et al., 2017) presents an advanced approach for the automatic detection of macular edema from images acquired through optical coherence tomography (OCT). The researchers developed a convolutional neural network (CNN) model based on a UNet architecture, incorporating 18 convolutional layers, with the goal of automatically identifying and segmenting intra-retinal fluid (IRF), a key marker of the condition. The algorithm achieved a Dice score of 91.1% in cross-validation tests.

While most studies on OCT image segmentation focus primarily on the retinal region particularly for diagnosing conditions such as macular edema or age-related degeneration, corneal segmentation remains relatively under explored. However, accurately delineating corneal structures from OCT images is essential, especially for the early detection of diseases like keratoconus. This imbalance highlights the need for specialized methods tailored to the morphological characteristics of the cornea. In the same vein, Dos Santos (Santos et al., 2019) developed a deep learning model called CorneaNet, based on the UNet architecture. In this modification, the author replaced the maximum pooling operations typically used in UNet with average pooling for downsampling. Furthermore, the number of parameters in the original UNet architecture was reduced, resulting in a more lightweight model without compromising its performance. The results demonstrated that CorneaNet achieved exceptional accuracy of 99.5% in segmenting both healthy and keratoconus-affected corneas. (Garcia-Marin et al., 2023) proposed a patch-based convolutional neural network (CNN) approach for detecting three main corneal boundaries in OCT images: the epithelium, Bowman's layer, and the endothelium. The model was tested with 4 and 8 classes to evaluate the impact of class number and image quality on performance. The results showed that the 8-class model achieved higher accuracy. Furthermore, (Elsawy & Abdel-Mottaleb, 2022) developed PIPE-Net, a convolutional network designed to segment four corneal interfaces. This architecture incorporates a pyramidal input and parallel encoders to analyze a larger image area, as well as residual connections to facilitate learning. Optimized to reduce the number of parameters, this method achieved an average precision of 95%, outperforming other tested approaches. Finally, (Liu et al., 2020) designed a hierarchy-constrained network that leverages the anatomical structure of the anterior segment of the eye. The model employs a progressive feature-extraction module and boundary constraints, combined with multi-level prediction fusion, to fully exploit available information. Tested on two datasets containing multiple lesions, it outperformed existing methods in terms of segmentation accuracy.

IV. THE PROPOSED METHOD

1. Data collection

In this study, we used an OCT dataset collected at Habib Bourguiba Hospital in Sfax, Tunisia. The images were acquired using the SS-1000 CASIA OCT system (Tomey, Japan), a swept-source OCT device developed based on technology from the Chinese Academy of Sciences Institute of Automation, and complemented with electronic health records (EHR). Each OCT image has a resolution of 470 × 320 pixels. This dataset includes OCT images from 100 patients, consisting of 42 healthy controls and 58 patients with keratoconus. The patients' ages ranged from 18 to 55 years and included both males and females. Patients were selected based on specific clinical criteria, and all images were acquired under standardized conditions to ensure data consistency. Before participating, all subjects provided written informed consent in accordance with ethical and regulatory standards.

2. Data preparation

2..1. Manual segmentation

For the extraction of the different corneal layers, labeled images were generated using an algorithm implemented in Python (OpenCV). This algorithm automatically defined the regions of interest in each image. Then, an ophthalmology expert manually reviewed and corrected the segmentation boundaries when necessary to ensure maximum accuracy. This manual step is crucial for ensuring the quality and reliability of the segmentation data, especially for images with challenging-to-define areas.

2.2. Data augmentation

To address the limited volume of training data (Chaari et al., 2025), various data augmentation techniques were applied to artificially expand the dataset and improve the robustness of the deep learning models. Geometric transformations, such as random rotations of $\pm 5°$ and horizontal flips, were used to simulate realistic variations in eye orientation and differences between the left and right eyes. Intensity and contrast adjustments, including nonlinear intensity variations, histogram equalization, and brightness and contrast modifications of ± 10 %, were applied to replicate differences in lighting and acquisition conditions. Additionally, additive Gaussian noise with zero mean and a standard deviation of 0.005 was introduced to increase robustness against sensor noise. These augmentations were carefully selected to simulate realistic variability in OCT images while preserving anatomical structures, enabling the model to learn generalizable features rather than memorizing specific images. An illustration of the applied data augmentation on a single OCT image is presented in Figure 6.

Figure 6. Extensive data augmentation performed to overcome the sparsity of our training data. (A) a compensated OCT image of a keratoconus subject. (B) the same image having undergone data augmentation, which includes histogram equalization.

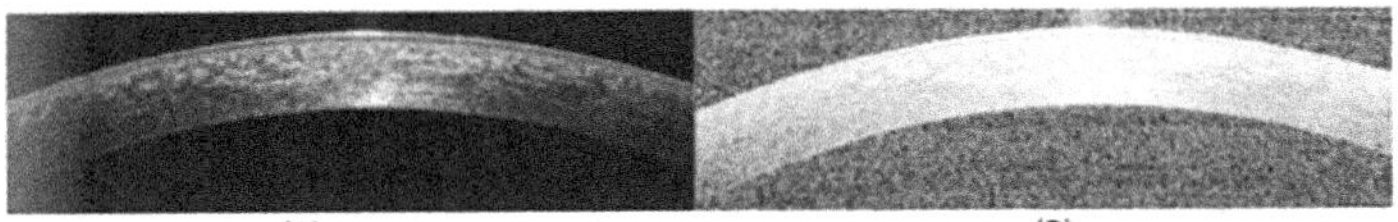

3. UNet-based model for Automated corneal segmentation

Deep learning has become a fundamental component in the fields of image classification and semantic segmentation. In this study, we designed a lightweight, fully convolutional neural network for the segmentation of corneal layers in OCT images. The proposed architecture is inspired by the widely used UNet model and incorporates several advanced elements, including recurrent units (Alom et al., 2018), residual connections (Zuo, Chen, & Wang, 2021), and dilated convolutions (Wei et al., 2018), to enhance performance while maintaining a low number of trainable parameters.

The UNet backbone enables simultaneous extraction of both local features and broader contextual information. Recurrent modules are used to preserve sequential spatial dependencies across layers. Residual connections improve gradient flow and support more stable learning by creating shortcut paths between shallow and deeper layers. Dilated convolutions expand the receptive field without increasing computational cost, thus enabling better global context understanding.

The network was trained on corneal OCT images paired with expert manual segmentations, with the objective of accurately delineating anatomical structures while keeping computational complexity low.

4. Network architecture

The UNet is the most popular approach for semantic medical image segmentation, which is used to label each pixel of an image with a corresponding class. Its architecture is symmetric and consists of two main parts connected to each other via skip connections, namely the contracting path and the expansive path. The role of the skip connections consists in recovering the information lost in the contracting path.

The contracting path (the left part) consists of the repeated application of two convolutions with a kernel size of 3x3. Each convolution is followed by a ReLU and batch normalization. Then, a 2x2 max pooling operation with a stride of 2 is applied to reduce the spatial dimensions (down-sampling). This part of the UNet encodes the input image into feature representations. At each down-sampling step, the number of feature channels is doubled, while the spatial dimensions are cut in half. Each step in the expansive path consists of the feature map up-sampling followed by a 2x2-transpose convolution, which corresponds to the contracting path and usually to a 3x3 convolution (each followed by a ReLU). As for the final layer, a 1x1 convolution is used in order to map the channels to the desired classes number. Two classes were used in this study, healthy and keratoconus eyes.

This architecture consists of a contracting tower and an expansive one connected to each other via skip connections, as described in Figure7. The contracting path consists of one standard block and two residual blocks, through two dilated convolution layers. The standard block receives the input image with a dilation factor of 1 and then two residual-recurrent blocks with dilation factors of 2 and 4, respectively. The standard and the residual blocks were constructed using two dilated convolution layers, of 3*3 in size each. Afterwards, two pooling types were used in this work, namely the max and average pooling of size 2x2 were used to exploit the contextual information. Therefore, to transfer the contracting path characteristics to those of an expansive one, a residual block with dilation of 8 was used. This would allow these characteristics to pass through two residual recurrent blocks with dilation factors of 4 and 2, respectively. A standard block with a dilation factor of 1 was used to restore the image to its original resolution.

In our research, a similar standard block was replaced with a residual-recurrent-dilated block. This e residual-recurrent block provided a skip connection that would solve the problem of vanishing gradient and allow short paths from early layers to later ones. The residual block is defined as follows:

$$H(x) = F(X) + W_X \tag{1}$$

Where H(x) is the processing of x with two weight layers, x is the input, F is the mapping-function and W is the weights of the convolutional layers.

The RNN enables the function to keep past data in memory more easily as this model processes an internal memory for storing information and data. The RNN block is defined as follows:

$$h(t) = f_W\left(h_{t-1}, x_t\right) \tag{2}$$

Where f_w is the function with parameter W, and x_t is the input

In this architecture, the standard convolution, defined in equation (3), was replaced by a dilated convolution to offer a wider field of view at the same computational cost. The dilated convolution is a generalization of the standard discrete convolution which is mathematically expressed in equation (4) as:

$$\left(F * k\right)\left(p\right) = \sum_{s+t=p} F(s)\, k(t) \tag{3}$$

$$\left(F *_l k\right)\left(p\right) = \sum_{s+lt=p} F(s)\, k(t) \tag{4}$$

Where $*_l$ denotes the dilated convolution, $F(s)$ denotes the input, $k(t)$ denotes the applied filter and $(F *_l k)(p)$ denotes the output.

Figure 7. Architecture for the customized model

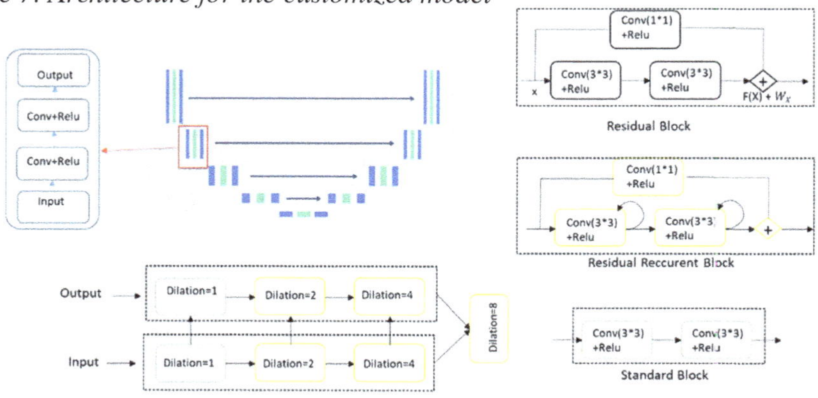

V. EXPERIMENTAL STUDY

The data set used in this study was split into two subsets: 80% for the training and 20% for the testing. The training set consisted of healthy and keratoconus OCT images of the cornea, along with their corresponding manual segmentations. To provide a reliable estimate of the model's predictive performance and to reduce the risk of overfitting, the cross-validation method (Ming & Xiao, 2023) was employed to resample the data.

1. Experimental metrics

The learning process of our model involves minimizing a loss function that guides the network to improve prediction accuracy during training. In this study, the Dice Loss was adopted as the primary loss function due to its effectiveness in addressing class imbalance and its ability to directly optimize the overlap between the predicted segmentation and the ground truth. This choice is particularly suitable for medical image segmentation tasks, where precise boundary delineation and region matching are critical.

The Dice Loss L is computed as:

$$\text{Dice Loss} = 1 - \frac{2 * \sum y * \hat{y}}{\sum y + \sum \hat{y}} \tag{5}$$

where y is the ground truth binary mask, and $\hat{y}$ is the predicted mask.

In our research, the deep neural network was implemented in the Python programming language (Van Rossum, 2007) using Keras and TensorFlow libraries (Joseph, Nonsiri, & Monsakul, 2021). Accuracy (Fernandez-Moral et al., 2018) was used to evaluate and analyze the performance of the tested models. It indicates the proportion of correct predictions compared to the total predictions. The Dice coefficient (Kline et al., 2021) and the Jaccard index (Bertels et al., 2019) (also known as intersection over union, IOU) are commonly used metrics to evaluate the segmentations quality on segmentation problems. The Dice coefficient measures the similarity between the predicted segmentation and the ground truth one, while the Jaccard index quantifies the degree of overlap between the two. These metrics are particularly relevant for assessing the segmentation models performance by measuring the localization accuracy and shape fidelity of the segmented objects (Chaari et al., 2020).

The following metrics were used of our architecture:

Accuracy (AC):

$$AC = (TP + TN)/(TP + FN + FP) \tag{6}$$

The dice coefficient (DC):

$$DC = (2 * TP)/\ (2 * TP + FN + FP) \tag{7}$$

Jaccard index (JA):

$$JA = TP\ /\ (TP + FN + FP) \tag{8}$$

Where (TP) is the true positive when the model correctly predicts the positive class; (TN) is the true negative when the model correctly predicts the negative class; (FP) is false positive when the model incorrectly predicts the positive class; and (FN) is the false negative that is when the model incorrectly predicts the negative class.

2. Experimental protocol

The training of the proposed segmentation model was conducted using the RMSprop optimizer (Younisse, Ghenmat, & Al Saraireh, 2023) with a fixed learning rate of 1×10^{-4}. A batch size of 32 was adopted to balance memory usage and training stability. The model was trained over 100 epochs. The Dice Loss was employed as the objective function due to its effectiveness in handling class imbalance (Yeung et al., 2022), especially in medical image segmentation. The final activation function used was Softmax (Nieradzik et al., 2021), which is suitable for multi-class classification tasks.

Table 2 presents the training parameters used for each tested model: UNet, ResUNet, SegNet, DeepLabV3+ (Choudhury et al., 2019), and the proposed model. All models were trained under identical conditions to ensure a fair comparison of their performance.

The UNet model is characterized by a U-shaped architecture that enables the combination of both global and local information for precise segmentation. ResUNet is a variant of UNet that incorporates residual connections to increase the depth of the network. SegNet employs a symmetrical encoder-decoder structure in which the max-pooling indices obtained during encoding are reused during decoding. DeepLabV3+ integrates a module called ASPP (Atrous Spatial Pyramid Pooling) to extract features at multiple scales and adopts an encoder-decoder architecture.

Table 2. Summary of hyperparameters for all evaluated models

Parameter	UNet	ResUNet	SegNet	DeepLabV3+	Our Model
Optimizer	RMSprop	RMSprop	RMSprop	RMSprop	RMSprop
Learning Rate	1×10^{-4}	1×10^{-4}	1×10^{-4}	1×10^{-4}	1×10^{-4}
Batch Size	32	32	32	32	32
Number of Epochs	100	100	100	100	100
Loss Function	Dice Loss	Dice Loss	Dice Loss	Dice Loss	Dice Loss
Final Activation	Softmax	Softmax	Softmax	Softmax	Softmax

3. Experimental results

3.1. Hyperparameters discussion

In this study, several image segmentation models were evaluated to compare their performance for keratoconus detection from OCT images. This comparison aims to identify the most suitable model for clinical use, where segmentation accuracy and robustness are essential. Five models were tested: UNet, ResUNet, SegNet, DeepLabV3+, and the proposed model. These architectures were chosen for their demonstrated effectiveness in image segmentation, particularly in the medical field. UNet is widely used for its simple yet effective structure, while ResUNet and

DeepLabV3+ allow for better feature extraction due to residual connections and deeper layers.

The learning curves obtained for the five models reveal different optimization dynamics depending on the architecture. Overall, all models show a gradual decrease in the loss function over the iterations, indicating effective learning. Figure 8 illustrates this evolution over 100 epochs: the green curve represents the training loss, and the purple curve represents the validation loss. The orange point marks the epoch at which each model achieves its best performance on the validation set. These curves show that the proposed model converges more quickly to a lower minimum loss, suggesting better generalization and increased stability during training. In contrast, SegNet presents a more unstable validation curve, indicating less optimal learning. DeepLabV3+ and ResUNet display stable performances, close to our model, but with a slightly higher final loss.

Figure 8. Training and Test Loss Curves for the Compared Models

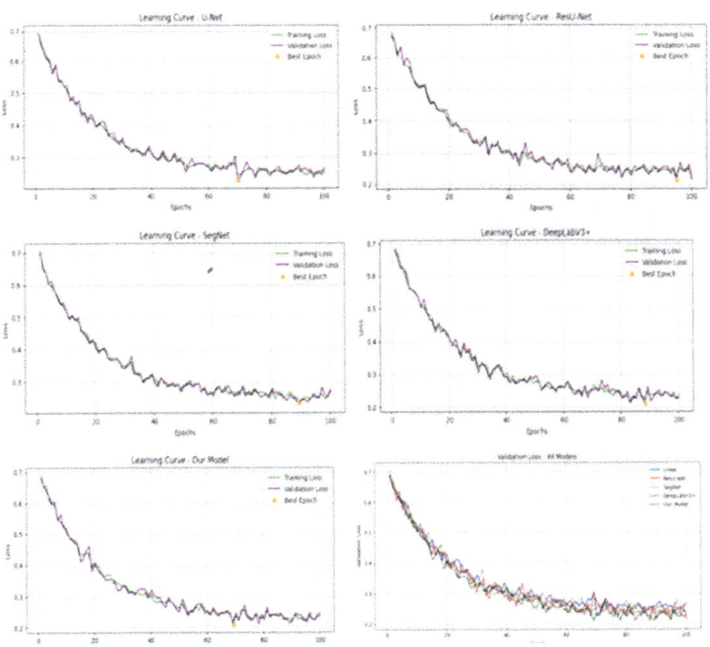

3.2. Segmentation performance

The quality of the segmentation was measured using three indicators: The Dice Coefficient (DC), the Jaccard Index (JA), and Accuracy (AC). These metrics allow for the evaluation of precision, coverage, and fidelity of the results, which are critical in a medical context. For each image, these indicators were computed for different layers of the cornea: the epithelium, stroma, Bowman's membrane, and background. Figure 9 shows, for two patients, the segmented images and the manual annotations. The proposed model correctly identified all the layers of the cornea, with segmentation visually consistent with the manual delineations. Our model was able to extract the different layers of the cornea, all the corneal layers, the stroma (in pink), the bowman (in blue) and the epithelium (in green). To evaluate the performance of segmentation, we tested our model on Keratoconus and healthy OCT images.

The segmentation of the different layers of cornea was qualitatively similar and consistent to the manual segmentation. Table 2 shows that all the tested models have almost similar performances with a slightly better performance of this architecture.

Figure 9. Semantic segmentation of corneal layers

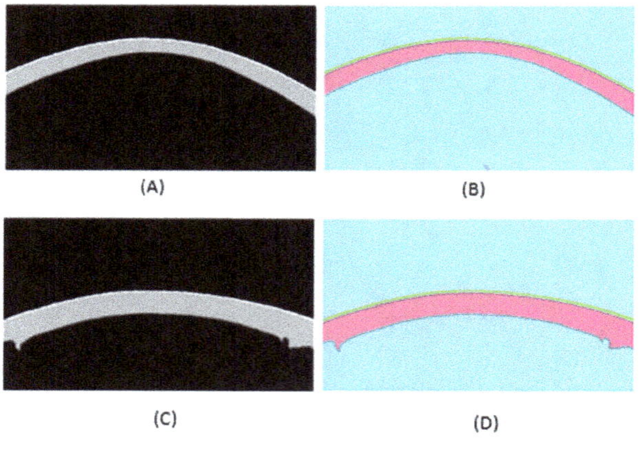

3.3. Comparison with existing methods

Table 3. Evaluation results of deep learning models for corneal layer segmentation

Models	DC (%)	JA (%)	AC (%)
UNet	94.80	91.70	94.50
ResUNet	95.30	92.50	95.50
SegNet	94.20	90.80	93.90
DeepLabV3+	95.70	92.90	96.00
Our Model	96.40	93.90	96.77

The proposed model is based on a customized architecture capable of capturing both local and contextual information. It incorporates several deep learning optimization techniques: residual connections, dilated convolutions, and recurrent modules. Residual connections facilitate gradient flow, accelerate training, and allow the model to learn complex features without performance degradation. Dilated convolutions expand the receptive field without increasing the computational cost, enabling the model to capture both fine details and global context. Recurrent modules leverage contextual relationships between image regions, resulting in more coherent segmentations.

By comparing the performance of the five tested segmentation models in terms of Dice Coefficient (DC), Jaccard Index (JA), and Accuracy (AC), as presented in Table 3, the proposed model achieves the best results across all criteria, with a DC of 96.40%, a JA of 93.90%, and an AC of 96.77%. These scores demonstrate an excellent ability to accurately segment the regions of interest in OCT images. For comparison, DeepLabV3+ and ResUNet also show strong performance, although their results are slightly lower than those of the proposed model. SegNet, on the other hand, records the lowest scores, particularly with an overall accuracy of 93.90%. These findings confirm that the proposed approach provides more precise and robust segmentation than the other evaluated architectures. The proportional distribution of each model's performance is also illustrated in Figure 10, providing a clear comparative visualization of the obtained results.

Figure 10. Proportional distribution of the segmentation models' performances

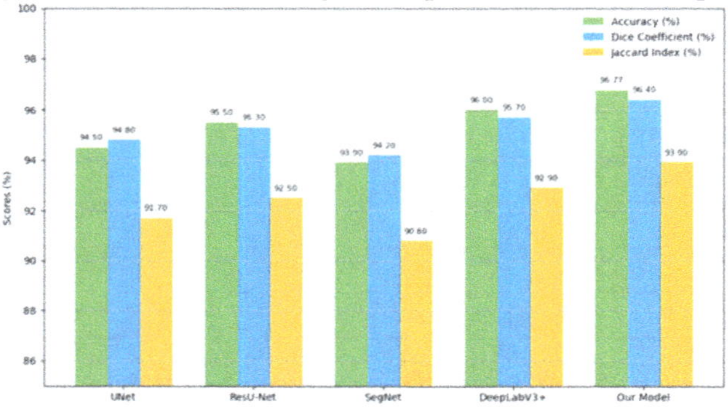

Our model offers a computationally inexpensive and faster segmentation technique for the OCT images. This method generally requires a larger amount of training data, and our data augmentation step (Devalla et al., 2018; Lee et al., 2017) allowed us to deal with this problem. We found that our architecture was able to extract the borders of the different layers when using our preprocessed database.

Handcrafted-based methods

The traditional segmentation of OCT images has been widely used in many research studies. These methods, based on classical techniques such as contour extraction, thresholding, or graph theory, allow the delineation of corneal layers. However, each of these approaches has specific limitations. Contour extraction and threshold-based techniques can be imprecise and may fail to accurately detect the boundaries of the corneal layers, especially in the presence of noise or complex variations in image quality. On the other hand, graph theory-based methods are often computationally expensive, which can slow down the segmentation process, particularly with large datasets. Additionally, these traditional approaches often require manual intervention to adjust parameters and improve results, making them less suitable for complex pathological cases or diverse images.

Deep learning-based methods

To overcome these limitations, deep learning has become the dominant approach for complex segmentation tasks. CNNs have demonstrated their effectiveness in feature extraction, thereby eliminating the need for manual feature engineering, making them a popular choice for various image analysis tasks. However, in this work, the goal is not only classification but also the localization of elements, framing it as a pixel-level semantic image classification task (Liu, Pu, & Sun, 2021).

The proposed model is a fully convolutional neural network based on the UNet architecture, which is widely adopted for medical image segmentation tasks. To enhance its performance, the model integrates various optimization techniques. One such technique is residual learning (Zhang et al., 2020), achieved through skip connections. These connections ensure efficient gradient flow, enabling the network to learn complex features without performance degradation, which is a critical advantage for identifying subtle structural variations in OCT images. Additionally, dilated convolutions (Zhang et al., 2017), also known as atrous convolutions, are employed to expand the receptive field without increasing computational costs. This approach allows the model to capture fine details while contextualizing large-scale spatial information, which is essential for analyzing corneal layers. Lastly, recurrent models (Visin et al., 2016), such as recurrent convolutional layers, are incorporated to refine predictions by leveraging contextual relationships across different regions of the image. This results in smoother and more accurate segmentations.

The architecture introduced in this work shows that the deep learning approach can segment the different OCT images layers. The proposed study seeks to benefit from the advantages of the recurrent model, the residual learning and the dilated convolutions. The obtained results are consistent with those achieved by (Graglia, Mari, Baikoff, & Sequeira, 2007; LaRocca et al., 2011; Rabbani et al., 2016). In our study, a new architecture was adopted for the extraction of OCT image characteristics as well as the classification of pixels. In fact, its architecture revealed a good segmentation performance of both healthy and keratoconical cornea OCT images.

Since keratoconus is hard to diagnose as it is difficult to detect the abnormal area in the cornea in many cases. This architecture offers a possibility to display fine areas in the OCT images, which can help doctors detect the disease at an early stage. The segmentation of the corneal layers faces several difficulties, the most important of which is the noise existing in the OCT images which results in a poor definition of the interfaces between the layers. Therefore, a preprocessing step to improve the images quality is crucial (Kaya et al., 2016; Gokul, Vellara, & Patel, 2018 ; Daud, Zaki, Hussain, & Mutalib, 2020).

We have conducted a detailed comparison between our work and existing studies in the literature, revealing several significant differences. Compared to prior works (Graglia, Mari, Baikoff, & Sequeira, 2007; LaRocca et al., 2011; Rabbani et al., 2016), our deep learning-based segmentation method stands out. Unlike the traditional semi-automatic segmentation methods (Kavur et al., 2019; Kim et al., 2016; Bianconi et al., 2021) that require a manual intervention to annotate the regions of interest, our approach was fully automated. It can autonomously learn to segment the regions of interest and extract relevant and discriminative features directly from raw data, allowing for more accurate and robust segmentation. Our method can be applied in various segmentation tasks in different medical domains, offering a more versatile and adaptable solution to the specific needs of practitioners and researchers. Furthermore, our OCT image segmentation method has the ability to segment four corneal layers, whereas previous semi-automatic approaches (LaRocca et al., 2011; Rabbani et al., 2016) identified only three layers. This distinction was achieved through the use of advanced deep learning techniques in our approach.

Many applications using retinal OCT images have been published in the scientific. In our study, we conducted an in-depth analysis of the performance by integrating qualitative evaluation and quantitative measures such as the Jaccard similarity index (Bertels et al., 2019). This approach allows us to provide a more comprehensive assessment of our segmentation method. Our segmentation approach achieves a similar performance as CorneaNet (Santos et al., 2019), a widely used reference model in corneal segmentation. The results obtained by our method are in line with those of CorneaNet, proving the robustness and accuracy of our approach. These findings validate the effectiveness of our segmentation method and position it as a viable alternative in the field of corneal segmentation.

VI. CONCLUSION

In this study, an efficient deep convolutional neural network was proposed for the semantic segmentation of OCT medical images to support the early detection of keratoconus. The model integrates several advanced deep learning techniques—residual connections, recurrent modules, and dilated convolutions—within a UNet-inspired architecture. This design enables the extraction of both local and contextual features, leading to accurate segmentation of the corneal layers. Experimental comparisons with benchmark models such as UNet, ResUNet, DeepLabV3+, and SegNet demonstrated the superior performance of the proposed model, achieving a Dice Coefficient of 96.40%, a Jaccard Index of 93.90%, and an Accuracy of 96.77%. These results highlight the model's robustness, rapid convergence, and strong generalization ability.

Despite these strengths, the architecture still requires validation on larger and more diverse datasets. Future work will focus on integrating advanced data augmentation techniques, such as those based on generative adversarial networks (GANs) (Kallel, Mafouhdi, & Kammoun 2024), exploring more sophisticated preprocessing methods to enhance image quality and contrast between corneal layers, and optimizing the model for real-time deployment in clinical settings. Additionally, the approach could be extended to the analysis of other ocular diseases.

REFERENCES

Abdelaziz, L., & Barbara, R. (2013). History of the Development of the Treatment of Keratoconus. *International Journal of Keratoconus and Ectatic Corneal Diseases, 2*(1), 31–33.

Al-Sharify, N. T., Ahmed, S. M., Nser, H. Y., See, O. H., Al-Sharify, Z. T., Ghaeb, N. H., & Weng, L. Y. (2023, July). Corneal topography, an overview of its devices and systems–A review. In *AIP Conference Proceedings* (Vol. 2787, No. 1). AIP Publishing.

Alom, M. Z., Hasan, M., Yakopcic, C., Taha, T. M., & Asari, V. K. (2018). Recurrent residual convolutional neural network based on u-net (r2u-net) for medical image segmentation. *arXiv preprint arXiv:1802.06955.*

Aramberri, J. (2024). Corneal Topography and Tomography. In *Intraocular Lens Calculations* (pp. 265–287). Springer International Publishing.

Atalay, E., Özalp, O., & Yıldırım, N. (2021). Advances in the diagnosis and treatment of keratoconus. *Therapeutic Advances in Ophthalmology, 13*, 25158414211012796.

Badrinarayanan, V., Kendall, A., & Cipolla, R. (2017). Segnet: A deep convolutional encoder-decoder architecture for image segmentation. *IEEE Transactions on Pattern Analysis and Machine Intelligence, 39*(12), 2481–2495.

Bertels, J., Eelbode, T., Berman, M., Vandermeulen, D., Maes, F., Bisschops, R., & Blaschko, M. B. (2019, October). Optimizing the dice score and jaccard index for medical image segmentation: Theory and practice. In *International conference on medical image computing and computer-assisted intervention* (pp. 92-100). Cham: Springer International Publishing.

Bertels, J., Eelbode, T., Berman, M., Vandermeulen, D., Maes, F., Bisschops, R., & Blaschko, M. B. (2019). Optimizing the dice score and jaccard index for medical image segmentation: Theory and practice. In *Medical Image Computing and Computer Assisted Intervention–MICCAI 2019: 22nd International Conference, Shenzhen, China, October 13–17, 2019* [Springer International Publishing.]. *Proceedings, 22*(Part II), 92–100.

Bianconi, F., Fravolini, M. L., Pizzoli, S., Palumbo, I., Minestrini, M., Rondini, M., & Palumbo, B. (2021). Comparative evaluation of conventional and deep learning methods for semi-automated segmentation of pulmonary nodules on CT. *Quantitative Imaging in Medicine and Surgery, 11*(7), 3286.

Bron, A. J. (2001). The architecture of the corneal stroma. *The British Journal of Ophthalmology*, *85*(4), 379–381.

Bui, A. D., Truong, A., Pasricha, N. D., & Indaram, M. (2023). Keratoconus diagnosis and treatment: Recent advances and future directions. *Clinical Ophthalmology (Auckland, N.Z.)*, •••, 2705–2718.

Cavas-Martínez, F., De la Cruz Sánchez, E., Nieto Martínez, J., Fernández Cañavate, F. J., & Fernández-Pacheco, D. G. (2016). Corneal topography in keratoconus: State of the art. *Eye and Vision (London, England)*, *3*, 1–12.

Chaari, A., Fourati Kallel, I., Kammoun, S., & Frikha, M. (2025). Hybrid Data Augmentation Strategies for Robust Deep Learning Classification of Corneal Topographic MapTopographic Map. *Biomedical Physics & Engineering Express.*

Chaari, A., Kallel, I. F., Daoud, H., Omri, I., Kammoun, S., & Frikha, M. (2024). Automated feature selection for early keratoconus screening optimization. *Biomedical Physics & Engineering Express*, *11*(1), 015039.

Chaari, A., Kallel, I. F., Hammouda, F. B., & Frikha, M. (2023, December). Corneal Endothelial Images Segmentation Using Deep Learning Model. In *2023 IEEE 11th International Conference on Systems and Control (ICSC)* (pp. 855-861). IEEE.

Chaari, A., Kammoun, K., Kallel, I. F., Frikha, M., Kammoun, S., & Feki, J. 2020, September. Performance Evaluation of Various Denoising Filters and segmentation methods for OCT images. In *2020 5th International Conference on Advanced Technologies for Signal and Image Processing (ATSIP)* (pp. 1-6). IEEE.

Choudhury, A. R., Vanguri, R., Jambawalikar, S. R., & Kumar, P. (2019). Segmentation of brain tumors using DeepLabv3+. In *Brainlesion: Glioma, Multiple Sclerosis, Stroke and Traumatic Brain Injuries: 4th International Workshop, BrainLes 2018, Held in Conjunction with MICCAI 2018, Granada, Spain, September 16, 2018, Revised Selected Papers, Part II 4* (pp. 154-167). Springer International Publishing.

Corbett, M. C., Marshall, J., O'Brart, D. P., & Rosen, E. S. (1995). New and future technology in corneal topography. *European journal of Implant and Refractive Surgery, 7*(6), 371-385.

Crawford, A. Z., Zhang, J., Gokul, A., McGhee, C. N., & Ormonde, S. E. (2020). The enigma of environmental factors in keratoconus. *Asia-Pacific Journal of Ophthalmology*, *9*(6), 549–556.

Cresta, F. B., Orlandin, L. F., & Lucas, M. B. (2022). Clinical Presentation and Evolution of Keratoconus. In *Keratoconus: A Comprehensive Guide to Diagnosis and Treatment* (pp. 3–12). Springer International Publishing.

D'Oria, F., Bagaglia, S. A., Del Barrio, J. L. A., Alessio, G., Alio, J. L., & Mazzotta, C. (2024). Refractive surgical correction and treatment of keratoconus. *Survey of Ophthalmology*, *69*(1), 122–139.

Daud, M. M., Zaki, W. M. D. W., Hussain, A., & Mutalib, H. A. (2020). Keratoconus detection using the fusion features of anterior and lateral segment photographed images. *IEEE Access : Practical Innovations, Open Solutions*, *8*, 142282–142294.

Devalla, S. K., Renukanand, P. K., Sreedhar, B. K., Subramanian, G., Zhang, L., Perera, S., & Girard, M. J. (2018). DRUNET: A dilated-residual U-Net deep learning network to segment optic nerve head tissues in optical coherence tomography images. *Biomedical Optics Express*, *9*(7), 3244–3265.

DeWitt, E. N. (1931). The histopathology of Bowman's membrane. *Transactions of the American Ophthalmological Society*, *29*, 461.

Dua, H. S., Gomes, J. A., & Singh, A. (1994). Corneal epithelial wound healing. *The British Journal of Ophthalmology*, *78*(5), 401.

Edwards, M., McGhee, C. N., & Dean, S. (2001). The genetics of keratoconus. *Clinical & Experimental Ophthalmology*, *29*(6), 345–351.

Elsawy, A., & Abdel-Mottaleb, M. (2022). PIPE-Net: A pyramidal-input-parallel-encoding network for the segmentation of corneal layer interfaces in OCT images. *Computers in Biology and Medicine*, *147*, 105595.

Fantaci, B., Calvo, B., & Rodríguez, J. F. (2024). Modeling biological growth of human keratoconus: On the effect of tissue degradation, location and size. *Computers in Biology and Medicine*, *180*, 108976.

Fernandez-Moral, E., Martins, R., Wolf, D., & Rives, P. (2018, June). *A new metric for evaluating semantic segmentation: leveraging global and contour accuracy. In 2018 IEEE intelligent vehicles symposium (iv)*. IEEE.

Garcia-Marin, Y. F., Alonso-Caneiro, D., Fisher, D., Vincent, S. J., & Collins, M. J. (2023). Patch-based CNN for corneal segmentation of AS-OCT images: Effect of the number of classes and image quality upon performance. *Computers in Biology and Medicine*, *152*, 106342.

Gokul, A., Vellara, H. R., & Patel, D. V. (2018). Advanced anterior segment imaging in keratoconus: A review. *Clinical & Experimental Ophthalmology*, *46*(2), 122–132.

Gordon-Shaag, A., Millodot, M., Shneor, E., & Liu, Y. (2015). The genetic and environmental factors for keratoconus. *BioMed Research International*, *2015*(1), 795738.

Graglia, F., Mari, J. L., Baikoff, G., & Sequeira, J. (2007, August). Contour detection of the cornea from OCT radial images. In *2007 29th Annual International Conference of the IEEE Engineering in Medicine and Biology Society* (pp. 5612-5615). IEEE.

Grzybowski, A., & McGhee, C. N. (2013). The early history of keratoconus prior to Nottingham's landmark 1854 treatise on conical cornea: A review. *Clinical & Experimental Optometry*, *96*(2), 140–145.

Hashemi, H., Heydarian, S., Hooshmand, E., Saatchi, M., Yekta, A., Aghamirsalim, M., & Khabazkhoob, M. (2020). The prevalence and risk factors for keratoconus: A systematic review and meta-analysis. *Cornea*, *39*(2), 263–270.

https://entokey.com/9-optical-coherence-tomography-in-corneal-ectasia/

https://williamseye.com/services/glaucoma-care-treatment/optical-coherence-tomography-scanner-oct/

https://www.indiamart.com/proddetail/specular-microscopy-pachymetry-7322736755.html

https://www.urmc.rochester.edu/eye-institute/lasik/technology/orbscan-corneal-topographer

Jirsova, K. (2017). The cornea, anatomy and function. *Light and specular microscopy of the cornea*, 1-21.

Joseph, F. J. J., Nonsiri, S., & Monsakul, A. (2021). Keras and TensorFlow: A hands-on experience. *Advanced deep learning for engineers and scientists: A practical approach*, 85-111.

Kallel, I. F., Mahfoudhi, O., & Kammoun, S. (2024). Deep learning models based on CNN architecture for early keratoconus detection using corneal topographic maps. *Multimedia Tools and Applications*, *83*(16), 49173–49193.

Kavur, A. E., Gezer, N. S., Barış, M., Şahin, Y., Özkan, S., Baydar, B., & Selver, M. A. (2019). Comparison of semi-automatic and deep learning-based automatic methods for liver segmentation in living liver transplant donors. *Diagnostic and Interventional Radiology*, *26*(1), 11.

Kaya, H., Cavusoglu, A., Cakmak, H., Şen, B., & Delen, D. (2016). Supporting the diagnosis process and processes after treatment by using image segmentation and image simulation techniques: Keratoconus example. *Journal of the Faculty of Engineering and Architecture of Gazi University*, *31*(3).

Kim, Y. J., Lee, S. H., Park, C. M., & Kim, K. G. (2016). Evaluation of semi-automatic segmentation methods for persistent ground glass nodules on thin-section CT scans. *Healthcare Informatics Research*, *22*(4), 305–315.

Kline, T. L., Edwards, M. E., Fetzer, J., Gregory, A. V., Anaam, D., Metzger, A. J., & Erickson, B. J. (2021). Automatic semantic segmentation of kidney cysts in MR images of patients affected by autosomal-dominant polycystic kidney disease. *Abdominal Radiology*, *46*(3), 1053–1061.

Kymes, S. M., Walline, J. J., Zadnik, K., & Gordon, M. O.Collaborative Longitudinal Evaluation of Keratoconus (CLEK) Study Group. (2004). Quality of life in keratoconus. *American Journal of Ophthalmology*, *138*(4), 527–535.

LaRocca, F., Chiu, S. J., McNabb, R. P., Kuo, A. N., Izatt, J. A., & Farsiu, S. (2011). Robust automatic segmentation of corneal layer boundaries in SDOCT images using graph theory and dynamic programming. *Biomedical Optics Express*, *2*(6), 1524–1538.

Lee, C. S., Tyring, A. J., Deruyter, N. P., Wu, Y., Rokem, A., & Lee, A. Y. (2017). Deep-learning based, automated segmentation of macular edema in optical coherence tomography. *Biomedical Optics Express*, *8*(7), 3440–3448.

Liu, Y., Li, D., Guo, Y., Zhou, X., Dong, Y., Guo, Z., . . . Lv, B. (2020, April). Hierarchy-constrained network for corneal tissue segmentation based on anterior segment OCT images. In *2020 IEEE 17th International Symposium on Biomedical Imaging (ISBI)* (pp. 1579-1582). IEEE.

Liu, Y., Pu, H., & Sun, D. W. (2021). Efficient extraction of deep image features using convolutional neural network (CNN) for applications in detecting and analysing complex food matrices. *Trends in Food Science & Technology*, *113*, 193–204.

Long, J., Shelhamer, E., & Darrell, T. (2015). Fully convolutional networks for semantic segmentation. In *Proceedings of the IEEE conference on computer vision and pattern recognition* (pp. 3431-3440).

Lucas, S. E., & Burdon, K. P. (2020). Genetic and environmental risk factors for keratoconus. *Annual Review of Vision Science*, *6*(1), 25–46.

Maile, H. (2023). *Keratoconus detection and personalised progression modelling using computational methods* (Doctoral dissertation, UCL (University College London)).

MARTEL, (2014). Association des optométristes du Québec. Clinique optométrique,

Meyer, J. J., Gokul, A., Vellara, H. R., & McGhee, C. N. (2023). Progression of keratoconus in children and adolescents. *The British Journal of Ophthalmology, 107*(2), 176–180.

Ming, Q., & Xiao, X. (2023). Towards accurate medical image segmentation with gradient-optimized dice loss. *IEEE Signal Processing Letters, 31*, 191–195.

Morgan, S. (2014). Understanding the structural basis of corneal refractive function and its modification via novel therapeutic approaches (Doctoral dissertation, Cardiff University).

Munsamy, A. J., Moodley, V. R., Naidoo, P., Mangwarara, T. R., Abdullah, R., Govender, D., & Dlamini, P. (2015). A frequency analysis of cone characteristics for the different stages of keratoconus. *African Vision and Eye Health, 74*(1), 6.

Niazi, S., Gatzioufas, Z., Doroodgar, F., Findl, O., Baradaran-Rafii, A., Liechty, J., & Moshirfar, M. (2024). Keratoconus: Exploring fundamentals and future perspectives–a comprehensive systematic review. *Therapeutic Advances in Ophthalmology, 16*, 25158414241232258.

Nieradzik, L., Scheuermann, G., Saur, D., & Gillmann, C. (2021). Effect of the output activation function on the probabilities and errors in medical image segmentation. *arXiv preprint arXiv:2109.00903.*

Nishimiya, K., Yin, B., Piao, Z., Ryu, J., Osman, H., Leung, H. M., & Tearney, G. J. (2019). Micro-optical coherence tomography for endothelial cell visualization in the coronary arteries. *JACC: Cardiovascular Imaging, 12*(9), 1878–1880.

Pinnamaneni, N., & Funderburgh, J. L. (2012). Concise review: Stem cells in the corneal stroma. *Stem Cells (Dayton, Ohio), 30*(6), 1059–1063.

Rabbani, H., Kafieh, R., Kazemian Jahromi, M., Jorjandi, S., Mehri Dehnavi, A., Hajizadeh, F., & Peyman, A. (2016). Obtaining thickness maps of corneal layers using the optimal algorithm for intracorneal layer segmentation. *International Journal of Biomedical Imaging, 2016*(1), 1420230.

Rabinowitz, Y. S. (1998). Keratoconus. *Survey of Ophthalmology, 42*(4), 297–319.

Rio-Cristobal, A., & Martin, R. (2014). Corneal assessment technologies: Current status. *Survey of Ophthalmology, 59*(6), 599–614.

Ronneberger, O., Fischer, P., & Brox, T. (2015, October). U-net: Convolutional networks for biomedical image segmentation. In *International Conference on Medical image computing and computer-assisted intervention* (pp. 234-241). Cham: Springer international publishing.

Roy, A. G., Conjeti, S., Karri, S. P. K., Sheet, D., Katouzian, A., Wachinger, C., & Navab, N. (2017). ReLayNet: Retinal layer and fluid segmentation of macular optical coherence tomography using fully convolutional networks. *Biomedical Optics Express*, *8*(8), 3627–3642.

Sah, R., Titiyal, J. S., & Sharma, N. (2022). Treatment & Management of Keratoconus: New Clinical Pathways. *Ophthalmology and Vision Care, 2*(2).

Santos, V. A. D., Schmetterer, L., Stegmann, H., Pfister, M., Messner, A., Schmidinger, G., & Werkmeister, R. M. (2019). CorneaNet: Fast segmentation of cornea OCT scans of healthy and keratoconic eyes using deep learning. *Biomedical Optics Express*, *10*(2), 622–641.

Seitz, B., Behrens, A., & Langenbucher, A. (1997). Corneal topography. *Current Opinion in Ophthalmology*, *8*(4), 8–24.

Simon, G., Ren, Q., Kervick, G. N., & Parel, J. M. (1993). Optics of the corneal epithelium. *Journal of Refractive Surgery (Thorofare, N.J.)*, *9*(1), 42–50.

Singh, R. B., Koh, S., Sharma, N., Woreta, F. A., Hafezi, F., Dua, H. S., & Jhanji, V. (2024). Keratoconus. *Nature Reviews. Disease Primers*, *10*(1), 81.

Steele, T. M., Fabinyi, D. C., Couper, T. A., & Loughnan, M. S. (2008). Prevalence of Orbscan II corneal abnormalities in relatives of patients with keratoconus. *Clinical & Experimental Ophthalmology*, *36*(9), 824–830.

Sturrock, G. D., Sherrard, E. S., & Rice, N. S. (1978). Specular microscopy of the corneal endothelium. *The British Journal of Ophthalmology*, *62*(12), 809–814.

Tuft, S. J., & Coster, D. J. (1990). The corneal endothelium. *Eye*, *4*(3), 389–424. https://www.oscarwylee.com.au/glasses/eye/cornea

Van Rossum, G. (2007, June). Python programming language. In *USENIX annual technical conference* (Vol. 41, No. 1, pp. 1-36).

Visin, F., Ciccone, M., Romero, A., Kastner, K., Cho, K., Bengio, Y., & Courville, A. (2016). Reseg: A recurrent neural network-based model for semantic segmentation. In *Proceedings of the IEEE conference on computer vision and pattern recognition workshops* (pp. 41-48).

Wang, M. (2024). *Corneal Topography: A Guide for Clinical Application in Wavefront Era*. CRC Press.

Wei, Y., Xiao, H., Shi, H., Jie, Z., Feng, J., & Huang, T. S. (2018). Revisiting dilated convolution: A simple approach for weakly-and semi-supervised semantic segmentation. In *Proceedings of the IEEE conference on computer vision and pattern recognition* (pp. 7268-7277).

Wilson, S. E., & Hong, J. W. (2000). Bowman's layer structure and function: Critical or dispensable to corneal function? A hypothesis. *Cornea*, *19*(4), 417–420.

Yeung, M., Sala, E., Schönlieb, C. B., & Rundo, L. (2022). Unified focal loss: Generalising dice and cross entropy-based losses to handle class imbalanced medical image segmentation. *Computerized Medical Imaging and Graphics*, *95*, 102026.

Younisse, R., Ghnemat, R., & Al Saraireh, J. (2023). Fine-tuning U-net for medical image segmentation based on activation function, optimizer and pooling layer. *International Journal of Electrical & Computer Engineering (2088-8708)*, *13*(5).

Zhang, J., Xie, Y., Wang, Y., & Xia, Y. (2020). Inter-slice context residual learning for 3D medical image segmentation. *IEEE Transactions on Medical Imaging*, *40*(2), 661–672.

Zhang, Q., Cui, Z., Niu, X., Geng, S., & Qiao, Y. (2017). Image segmentation with pyramid dilated convolution based on ResNet and U-Net. In *Neural Information Processing: 24th International Conference, ICONIP 2017, Guangzhou, China, November 14-18, 2017* [Springer International Publishing.]. *Proceedings*, *24*(Part II), 364–372.

Zuo, Q., Chen, S., & Wang, Z. (2021). R2AU-Net: Attention recurrent residual convolutional neural network for multimodal medical image segmentation. *Security and Communication Networks*, *2021*(1), 6625688.

Chapter 7
Human-Centered AI Applications for Medical Informatics:
Artificial Intelligence in Mental Health – Advancing Care and Understanding

V. Kavitha
https://orcid.org/0000-0002-5222-4781
Velalar College of Engineering and Technology, India

K. Baby
https://orcid.org/0009-0007-3555-3376
Velalar College of Engineering and Technology, India

T. Suresh Kumar
https://orcid.org/0009-0001-1644-6678
AVS Engineering College, India

J. Charanya
https://orcid.org/0009-0003-8880-9639
Kongu Engineering College, India

A. P. Gopu
https://orcid.org/0000-0003-2464-3556
Velalar College of Engineering and Technology, India

I. Nivetha
https://orcid.org/0009-0000-3851-219X
Velalar College of Engineering and Technology, India

V. Latha Jothi
https://orcid.org/0000-0003-1212-5129
Velalar College of Engineering and Technology, India

ABSTRACT

The diagnosis, awareness, and medical care of mental illness are being transformed with the emergence of machine learning (otherwise referred to as AI) in the area of

DOI: 10.4018/979-8-3373-1479-2.ch007

mental illness. This chapter discusses the sophisticated uses for artificial intelligence (AI), involving machine learning algorithms and natural language processing, to analyze behavioral patterns, detect mental illness, and offer individualized options for treatment. Illustrations of AI applications include virtual mental health assistance systems and platforms for preventive diagnosis that analyze speech and text data for depression and anxiety. Among the important topics covered in the chapter are algorithmic bias, data security, moral issues, and the necessity of preserving compassion for humans in AI-based medicine.

1. INTRODUCTION

Mental health disorders affect millions of people worldwide and have a significant detrimental social and economic impact. Even though these conditions are becoming more common, effective therapy is still hampered by things like social stigma, limited access to mental health professionals, and delayed diagnosis. With its sophisticated powers in processing information, pattern detection, and making judgments, artificial intelligence has become a game-changing tool for dealing with these difficulties. AI uses advanced machine learning algorithms and natural language processing (NLP) techniques to provide innovative solutions that enhance the detection, treatment, and prevention of mental health disorders.

Artificial intelligence (AI)-powered systems are able to analyse enormous volumes of intricate data, including text, speech patterns, and facial expressions, to find minute signs of mental health problems. For example, AI algorithms can use text analysis to detect anxiety cues or analyze changes in speech tone to detect early signs of depression. Furthermore, a lot more people can now access mental healthcare thanks to AI-powered virtual mental health assistants that use talk-activated interfaces and offer real-time emotional support.

One possible step toward scalable and personalized treatments is the application of AI in mental health care. But there are several problems with this development. Just, trustworthy, and compassionate AI-based solutions must successfully handle algorithmic biases, information confidentiality issues, and moral conundrums. Achieving the ideal balance between technological innovation and human sensitivity is necessary for the successful implementation of AI-facilitated behavioral health therapies.

2. MOTIVATION

Stress, anxiety, and depression are among the mental illnesses that are on the rise. But because of social stigma, financial constraints, and difficulties accessing specialized care, many of them remain untreated. For early detection, traditional diagnostic techniques which primarily rely on clinical interviews and self-reported symptoms are insufficient. Transformer-based models like BERT, as well as recent developments in artificial intelligence (AI) and natural language processing (NLP), present exciting new opportunities for mental health assessment.

The goal of the project is to create a dependable, scalable, and cost-effective AI-driven system that can evaluate textual content and spot early indicators of mental health problems. By using explainable AI techniques, the system makes its forecasts more transparent so that users and medical professionals can understand the reasoning behind them. Additionally, this paradigm could help doctors prioritize high-risk patients, provide real-time mental health support, and enhance general access to mental health care through web apps and chatbots.

2.1 Problem Statement

Stress, anxiety, and depression are among the mental illnesses that are becoming more common worldwide, but early detection and treatment are still very difficult. The conventional assessment methods, which depend on clinician interviews and self-report questionnaires, are capricious and unreliable. Social stigma and a lack of mental health professionals further restrict access to treatment, leading to delayed diagnosis and incorrect treatment. The lack of scalable and automated methods for evaluating mental health exacerbates the problem.

Unexpected advancement The rise in stress, anxiety, and depression around the world has made it possible to develop intelligent systems that can accurately identify mental health issues by analysing text data from multiple sources, such as social media, clinical records, and user reviews. The goal of this project is to develop an AI platform using the BERT model that will diagnose mental illnesses through text analysis and provide outputs that are interpretable, explainable, and real-time. It also addresses important issues like algorithmic unfairness, data privacy, and ethical dilemmas, ensuring that the system remains fair, reliable, and scalable for daily use. By integrating AI into mental healthcare, this project seeks to enhance early diagnosis, expand accessibility, and help mental health professionals make the best choices possible, bringing regarding better mental health results.

2.2 Background Study

The potential for affectively intelligent artificially intelligent agents to expand access to mental health care is examined by Mohammad et al. (2023). In an effort to raise the standard for mental health care generally, their research offers artificial intelligence (AI) systems that are not only data-processing tools but also emotionally intelligent tools that can interpret emotional cues like facial expressions and speech tones. The authors emphasize the need for responsible AI development as a critical component of AI-driven healthcare, urging algorithms to be impartial and open while maintaining human compassion. This study demonstrates how AI may be used to deliver individualized and scalable mental health care treatments.

Anand et al. (2023) discuss how AI could enhance mental health training and raise awareness of mental health issues. This paper explains how AI technologies, like digital assistants and predictive analytics, can educate people about mental health issues and provide them with the information and resources needed for early detection and intervention. The authors highlight how artificial intelligence (AI) has the potential to transform mental health education globally by analyzing large datasets and identifying patterns that traditional methods would overlook.

The use of large language models (LLMs), a type of machine learning model, in the diagnosis and prognosis of mental health issues is examined by Kamoji et al. (2024). They use a method that examines behavioral data from multiple digital sources to identify markers of mental health issues like anxiety and depression.

Mohammad et al. (2023) investigate how emotionally intelligent AI agents can be used to expand mental health care. By developing AI systems that can comprehend information and recognize emotional cues like facial expressions and tone of voice, their research improves the quality of mental health care. The authors stress responsible AI development with algorithmic fairness and transparency in addition to human empathy as a key element of AI-driven healthcare. This study shows that AI holds promise for delivering scalable and customized mental health care solutions.

Kamoji et al. (2024) investigate the use of machine learning models, specifically large language models (LLMs), for the diagnosis and prognosis of mental health disorders. Their research proposes a system that gathers behavioral data from various digital sources to identify early warning signs of disorders such as depression and anxiety. The authors stress how AI can be used to provide timely guidance and action, potentially halting the progression of mental illness. The study illustrates the potential for AI systems to conflate diagnosis and treatment.

Hussna et al. (2021) discuss the impact of the COVID-19 pandemic on students' mental health and the potential benefits of explainable AI (XAI). Their study looks at how classifiers can be used to spot stress, anxiety, and depression symptoms in students. The authors claim that AI systems that are able to adequately and clearly explain their predictions could increase the transparency of mental health evaluations and foster trust in AI-powered solutions, particularly during emergencies like the pandemic.

The potential of AI chatbots in mental health care is examined by Galijašević et al. (2024), specifically their capacity to perform mental health screenings, provide emotional support, and act promptly. The study suggests that AI-powered chatbots could provide round-the-clock access to mental health services, enabling people to get help without fear of stigma. The authors emphasize that human-like interaction is crucial for these technologies to offer empathetic and customized advice based on user feedback.

Ogamba et al., 2023 case study focuses on the artificial intelligence mental health chatbot "Wellness Buddy," which was created to help university students in Kenya. The chatbot offers mental health support through interactive conversations, self-help tools, and professional referrals when needed. The authors stress the need for culturally aware AI solutions that are adaptable enough to accommodate different groups' particular needs. The study shows how artificial intelligence (AI) can be used to treat mental health issues in developing nations where access to mental health services is restricted.

Kaushik et al. (2024) look into the optimization of machine learning models for mental health disorder prediction in order to improve the accuracy of the decision classifiers used to identify mental health issues. By modifying classifier parameters, the study demonstrates how AI may increase diagnosis accuracy while reducing false positives and false negatives. The study highlights AI's ability to make accurate and timely predictions about mental health, which can be crucial for early intervention.

Naswa et al. (2024) discuss the use of conversational AI to assess empathy in mental health caregivers. In order to determine empathy levels—a critical element of effective mental health care—their study examines how AI systems can assess interactions between patients and caregivers. The authors claim that by enhancing the emotional bonds between patients and caregivers, AI technology can improve the quality of mental health services.

Jain et al. (2024) look into how journaling powered by AI affects mental health. The authors examine how AI can help people reflect on their emotions and mental health by offering tailored prompts and feedback. The study found that AI-powered journaling can enhance self-awareness and emotional processing, making it an effective tool for fostering mental health.

MediBot, an AI-powered medical assistant that prioritizes mental health and wellbeing, is presented by N. and U. J. (2023). Using conversational AI, MediBot assesses clients' mental health, provides recommendations, and helps them manage stress and anxiety. This study demonstrates how artificial intelligence (AI) can be utilized to develop readily available, flexible mental health care tools that can take care of themselves and offer users continuous support without the need for human intervention.

Kataru et al. (2024) suggest an early intervention and detection approach for children's mental health problems that is based on machine learning. Their approach uses behavioral data and other pertinent factors to identify early signs of mental health problems and suggest suitable interventions. The authors emphasize the importance of treating mental health issues in children at a young age to prevent long-term psychological effects, which makes this strategy particularly crucial for improving children's mental health. Deshmukh et al. (2023) give a comprehensive review of machine learning methods applied to mental health analysis. They provide a variety of methods for identifying mental health conditions like stress, anxiety, and depression by using data mining and machine learning models.

Murugan et al. (2024) explore the transformative potential of artificial intelligence in healthcare by focusing on medical diagnosis, treatment, and patient care. The book promotes a human-centered AI design to enhance clinical judgments and personalize patient experiences. The review highlights the challenges in implementing these tactics, particularly those related to algorithmic bias, data quality, and the need for interpretability in predictions about mental health.

Zim and Kaur (2023) focus on how these advanced algorithms may improve the accuracy of predictions about mental health conditions in their investigation of deep learning techniques for mental health detection. In order to identify patterns that may indicate mental health problems, their research explores the application of deep learning models to the analysis of complex datasets, such as textual, speech, and behavioral data. The authors demonstrate how deep learning can enhance mental health diagnosis and prediction by offering a more dependable approach than traditional methods.

Mishra et al. (2024) study the modeling of patterns in mental health disorders using time-series linear regression analysis. Their research uses survey data to create a predictive model that predicts future trends in mental health. This method offers useful information for creating more successful intervention plans and aids in identifying significant variables that affect mental health. Neural networks and deep learning are specifically mentioned by Marandi and Shah (2023) in their discussion of AI in mental health treatment. Their study shows how AI can help personalized treatment plans by tailoring solutions to the needs and preferences of individual patients. The authors claim that by recommending the best therapeutic modalities based on data, AI-powered therapy can improve treatment outcomes.

NeuroSafe is a blockchain, artificial intelligence, and machine learning solution that improves mental health services (Gujarathi et al., 2024). This study emphasizes how important it is to safeguard confidential mental health data while using AI to deliver tailored care. Blockchain ensures data privacy and confidentiality while AI expedites the delivery of mental health treatments, making the system dependable and efficient.

Saleem and Afzal (2024) give an overview of how deep learning and machine learning are used to analyze social media data in order to identify mental health disorders. The study shows how artificial intelligence (AI) can be used to assess social interactions and posts made online in order to identify symptoms of mental health issues like depression and anxiety. The authors note that ethical concerns regarding data security and privacy need to be addressed, despite the strategy's great potential.

Parimala et al. (2022) focus on AI-based systems for mental health diagnosis and detection. Their study demonstrates how machine learning can be used to recognize text, speech, and behavioral patterns as indicators of mental health problems. The authors advocate using these AI-powered models to improve mental health diagnosis and early intervention efficacy.

Ramasamy et al. (2024) employ artificial intelligence methods and fuzzy inference systems to forecast students' mental health. Their approach uses academic stress and environmental factors to predict mental health outcomes. This study shows how artificial intelligence (AI) can be used to predict students' mental health problems, enabling timely treatments to mitigate the detrimental effects of mental health conditions on wellbeing and academic achievement.

In order to identify issues that the pandemic has exacerbated, Anishfathima et al. (2022) investigate the effects of COVID-19 on mental health and propose a machine learning-based mental health detector. Their method, which uses survey data to find early indicators of mental health issues, demonstrates how AI may be used for timely intervention during public health emergencies. The authors stress the need for scalable AI technologies to support mental health in the face of global events like the pandemic.

Aydogan et al. (2015) assessed how students' brain electrical activity altered in response to teachers' emotional displays in a study that was published in the International Journal of Social, Behavioral, Educational, Economic, Business, and Industrial Engineering. The researchers used electroencephalography (EEG) to examine how students' brain responses and levels of engagement were affected by emotional signals like happiness, anger, and sadness. Their findings imply that classroom dynamics may have a direct impact on learning outcomes since teachers' emotional expressions have a major impact on students' emotional and cognitive states. This study emphasizes the value of affective communication and emotional intelligence in the classroom while showing how teacher behavior can impact students' focus and academic performance.

Coskun and Yigit (2018) introduced an AI-based technique for distinguishing between normal and extrasystole heart sounds using the wavelet transform and Mel-frequency cepstral coefficients (MFCC). Noise was eliminated using digital filters such as Butterworth and Chebyshev. Artificial Neural Networks (ANN) and Support Vector Machines (SVM) were used to extract and classify features. Their approach used SVM to achieve up to 100% accuracy with MFCC characteristics.

Coşkun (2024) introduced an automatic labeling method for categorizing sitting postures into several classes using depth-sensor data. The study used machine learning techniques to accurately identify and classify different sitting postures. This method increases the efficiency of posture recognition systems by eliminating the need for manual data labeling. The findings demonstrate the potential applications of sensor-based AI models in ergonomics and health monitoring.

Hassan et al. (2024) discuss the promise of federated learning in Healthcare 5.0, emphasizing privacy-preserving AI for safe medical research and team-based care.

Sawano and Kodera (2025) evaluate a chat-based human-centered AI tool for interdisciplinary medical talks. The platform demonstrated enhanced case assessment effectiveness and clinical discussion structure.

Prentzas et al. (2023) emphasize the importance of interpretability and clinical users' trust in their in-depth examination of explainable AI applications in the medical field.

Chen et al. (2021) advocate for the application of human-centered design principles in medical imaging AI. Their review provides evidence that usability and transparency improve clinical adoption.

Gómez-González et al. (2020) categorize existing and emerging AI medical applications, examine the ethical and sociological implications of these applications, and recommend human-aligned AI development.

Chakraborty (2025) emphasizes the moral use of AI in healthcare while examining human dignity, trust, and accountability in human-centered AI design.

Kukreti et al. (2025) connect smart technology to global health and sustainable development goals and emphasize the importance of AI in human-centered innovations for universal healthcare.

In a chapter, Kavitha et al. (2025) presented a forecasting model that transforms information into practical performance insights. With an emphasis on sustainable resource management strategies, it brought together a range of AI applications for environmental protection.

3. PROPOSED STUDY

The study starts by gathering and preparing textual data from clinical reports, online forum articles, and publically accessible mental health information. Tokenization, cleaning, and format conversion are performed on this data in order to prepare it for model training. After that, the BERT model is adjusted to detect mental health markers and capture contextual subtleties. To guarantee the model's dependability in identifying mental health disorders, its effectiveness is assessed utilizing critical metrics such as precision, recall, reliability, and F1-score.

To improve the transparency and reliability of AI-driven predictions, the research includes mechanisms for explain ability and interpretability. This helps users and mental health professionals realize how the model makes its decision. The end-trained model is implemented as a web-based platform or chatbot, which can perform real-time mental health evaluation. Ethical issues like data privacy, mitigation of bias, and security are also addressed diligently to make the AI deployment fair and responsible.

By integrating deep learning with responsible AI practices, this study seeks to revolutionize mental health diagnosis, bridging the gap between healthcare and technology. The outcome is a more scalable, accessible, and efficient means of mental health care

3.1 Use Case Analysis

3.1.1 AI-Powered Mental Health Diagnosis

AI-driven mental health diagnosis module analyzes user-text, i.e., answers to mental health questionnaire or social media posts, using BERT-based language processing models. To classify the user's mental health condition (e.g., anxiousness, stress, or depression), the input is explored to detect psychological tendencies and emotional trends. Facilitating a real-time, automated analysis of mental health is the objective. The predictions of the model are understandable, providing rationale for the detection of a specific mental health condition. For early intervention and immediate psychological counseling, the system provides expert assistance alternates or emergency helplines when it detects signs of extreme distress.

3.1.2 Personalized Mental Health Recommendations

The module of personalized recommendation creates individualized self-care plans from the mental health profile of the user. Following the analysis and classification of the emotional state, the method provides appropriate coping strategies, relaxation techniques, and therapeutic resources. AI-based personalization considers symptom severity, past mental health trends, and user preferences. For users who are still in distress, the system might suggest professional counselling services. This feature promotes proactive mental health treatment by bridging the gap between AI-driven diagnosis and useful assistance.

3.1.3 AI Chatbot for Mental Health Support

The AI Chatbot for Mental Health Support provides users with a conversational and engaging AI assistant to help them along their mental health journey. The chatbot employs sentiment analysis and natural language understanding (NLU) to facilitate meaningful conversations and help users communicate their emotions and issues. The chatbot can offer mindfulness exercises, relaxation techniques, and positive reinforcement while maintaining data privacy and ethical AI considerations. If a user shows signs of severe distress, the chatbot can escalate the situation by recommending professional intervention. By providing users with quick, nonjudgmental assistance, this use case increases accessibility to mental health services.

3.1.4 Mental Health Monitoring and Progress Tracking

The Mental Health Monitoring and Progress Tracking use case allows users to track changes in their mental health over time. By analyzing previous text inputs, the technology identifies shifts in emotional well-being and provides information on patterns of improvement or decline. This module is essential for both individuals and mental health providers because it allows them to monitor long-term trends in mental health. The AI model makes it possible to take early action before symptoms worsen by spotting potential warning signs. This use case, which promotes continuous self-awareness and data-driven mental health management, makes AI a valuable tool in long-term mental health care.

3.1.5 Ethical AI and Data Privacy in Mental Health Tech

Safe, transparent, and impartial AI decision-making is the aim of the Ethical AI and Data Privacy in Mental Health Applications use case. Given the sensitivity of mental health data, the system employs robust encryption, anonymization, and adherence to ethical AI standards. This module ensures that user data is not misused and that AI-generated recommendations are unbiased. It also employs a human-in-the-loop validation method, whereby mental health professionals regularly review AI predictions to improve accuracy and equity. This use case is crucial to the continued reliability and trustworthiness of AI-driven mental health assessments.

3.2 Proposed Architecture

The Inference and Deployment Module enables the trained model to generate predictions in real time and integrate with a clinical or operational setting. The Explain ability and Interpretability Module is crucial for providing healthcare professionals with transparency into the AI model's decision-making process. Not to mention, the Logging and Monitoring Module records errors or anomalies, tracks the model's performance over time, and ensures that the model continues to function correctly after deployment so that it can be continuously enhanced and modified. This comprehensive strategy guarantees the AI system's dependability and efficacy in the field of mental health.

Figure 1.

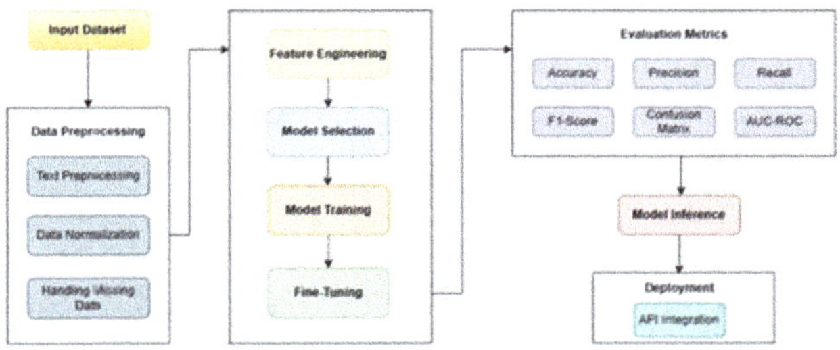

Figure 1 depicts the suggested process as an example of how AI might be used to diagnose and treat mental health issues. Pre-processing and feature extraction come after data collection from behavioural, speech, and text inputs. Data is analysed by machine learning algorithms to identify mental health issues. Lastly, AI-driven suggestions offer virtual mental health support and individualized treatment. The Inference and Deployment Module enables the trained model to generate predictions in real time and integrate with a clinical or operational setting. The Explain ability and Interpretability Module is crucial for providing healthcare professionals with transparency into the AI model's decision-making process. Not to mention, the Logging and Monitoring Module records errors or anomalies, tracks the model's performance over time, and ensures that the model continues to function correctly after deployment so that it can be continuously enhanced and modified. This comprehensive strategy guarantees the AI system's dependability and efficacy in the field of mental health.

4. RESULTS AND FINDINGS

4.1 Dataset Description

The Artificial Intelligence in Tech Survey Dataset is a comprehensive collection of data from technology workers with the goal of assessing their mental health, work-life balance, and overall well-being. In addition to demographic information such as age, gender, position, and experience level, survey responses on work-related stress, job satisfaction, and access to mental health care are usually included. Workplace stress, burnout, mental wellness support, and emotional wellness are among the main survey topics. Employees can learn about job expectations, workloads, and the effectiveness of company support systems from these topics. Furthermore, the dataset may contain qualitative information gleaned from open-ended questions, which offer a deeper comprehension of individuals' unique experiences and mental health issues.

These findings allow businesses to create more wholesome, supportive work environments in the technology sector, enhance mental health services, and create focused interventions. AI-driven analysis of this dataset is a useful resource for promoting mental health awareness and developing successful mental health initiatives in tech companies.

Figure 2 illustrates the heatmap highlights patterns across anxiety, depression, and common mental health problems by graphically representing relationships among survey dataset variables. The strength of the correlations between variables is shown by darker or lighter hues. This aids in determining the main causes of mental health issues. The knowledge aids in improving AI algorithms for precise forecasting.

Figure 2.

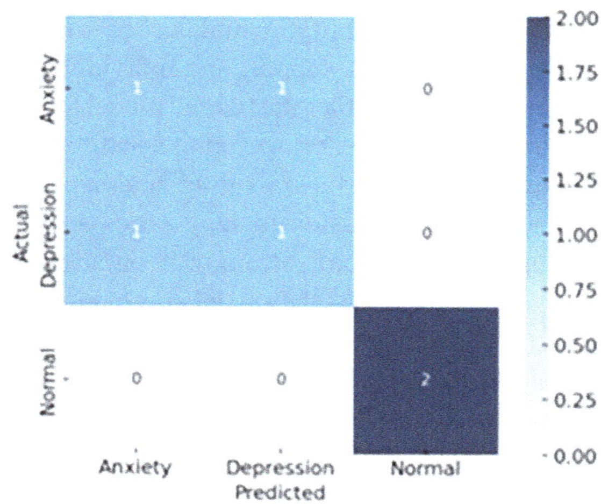

4.2 Data Preprocessing

Data Preprocessing Module is essential to guarantee the quality and preparedness of the data prior to its being entered into the machine learning model. First, it handles data cleaning, where inconsistencies such as missing, duplicate, or erroneous entries are identified and corrected.

a) Missing Values is handled using mean imputation.

$$X_{missing} = \frac{1}{n}\sum_{i=0}^{n}(Xi) \qquad (1)$$

Equation 1 represents Mean imputation is a technique used to handle missing values by replacing them with the average of available data points. The formula calculates the mean of all existing values in a feature and assigns it to missing entries. This ensures data completeness and prevents loss of valuable information. However, it may reduce variability and introduce bias. It is commonly used in datasets where missing values are randomly distributed.

b) Normalize Features: Apply Min-Max Normalization.

Imputation is applied to missing values, where appropriate, using methods like mean, median, or more complex techniques like KNN imputation. The next step focuses on data transformation, where categorical variables like gender, mental health support, or stress levels are encoded numerically, allowing the model to process them. One-hot encoding is particularly useful for non-ordinal categories, while label encoding may be applied to ordinal features. Normalization and standardization are essential processes to make sure that no feature predominates over others during the model training process, especially when features have significant scale differences.

The number of survey responses before and after data preprocessing is contrasted in Figure 3. Managing missing values, eliminating duplicate data, and eliminating unnecessary information are all part of the preprocessing steps. A more clean and trustworthy dataset for analysis is ensured by the decrease in responses.

Figure 3.

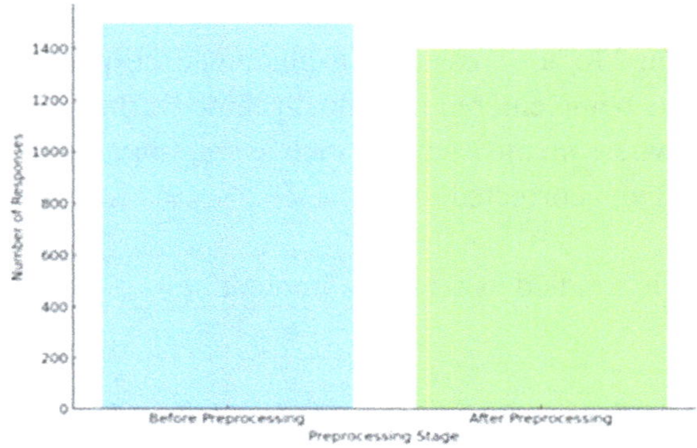

Workload and work-related stress could be combined to create a "work stress index" that would help the model identify more complex relationships. Methods like Min-Max scaling are employed after feature scaling, which guarantees that all numerical values fall within a single range, usually 0 to 1. By ensuring that each feature is regarded as equally important during training, this method keeps certain features from overpowering the learning process due to their greater magnitudes. To facilitate efficient model training, tuning, and testing, training, validation, and test sets are subsequently generated from the data.

The splitting is done in a way that maintains the balance of the target variable, guaranteeing that the proportion of people with mental health problems stays the same across all sets. This method ensures that the model appropriately generalizes to new data by avoiding problems like class imbalance, which typically could lead to biased predictions. Given a representative and well-balanced dataset, the model can make more accurate and dependable predictions about mental health outcomes.

4.3 Model Initialization and Configuration

The Model Initialization and Configuration Module sets up the machine learning model and all of its parts for training. When selecting an algorithm, the particular problem and the type of data are taken into account first.

a) Binary Classification: Binary Cross-Entropy (BCE) Loss

$$L = \frac{1}{N}\sum_{i=1}^{N}\left[y_i \log y\hat{}_i + \left(1 - y_i\right) \log\left(1 - y\hat{}_i\right)\right] \quad (2)$$

Equation 2 demonstrates that the Binary Cross-Entropy (BCE) loss is a typical loss function for binary classification problems. It measures the difference between actual labels (yi) and predicted probabilities (y^i).To penalize incorrect predictions, the function computes the logarithmic loss for every instance. The loss is decreased in order to improve the model's accuracy. It ensures that the actual labels closely match the expected probability. Options like Support Vector Machines (SVMs), Random Forest, and Logistic Regression would be considered given the classification nature of the work. For more intricate patterns, Deep Neural Networks (DNNs) or Gradient Boosting Machines (GBMs) may be used. When dealing with intricate, non-linear relationships, models such as XGBoost or LSTM networks may be considered. The selected model architecture is then configured with the proper activation functions (e.g., ReLU for hidden layers or sigmoid for output in binary classification) to guarantee that non-linearities are learned effectively. The model's optimizer is chosen based on the algorithm; two popular choices that effectively lower the loss function are Adam and Stochastic Gradient Descent (SGD).

The hyperparameter changes that occur during model creation and training are depicted in Figure 4. It aids in tracking parameter changes to maximize stability and performance. An accurate and refined AI model for mental health prediction is ensured by monitoring these variations.

Figure 4.

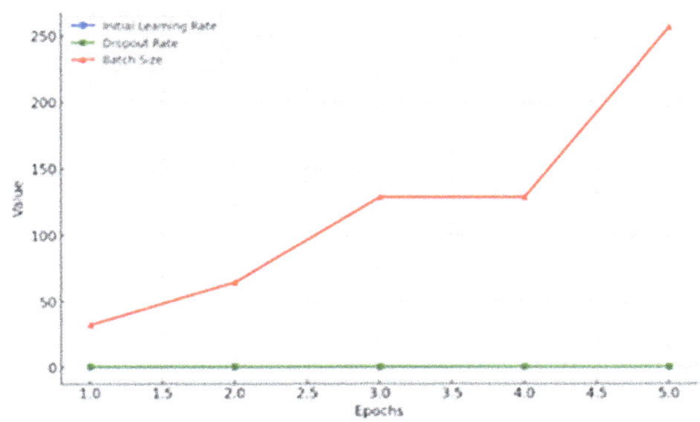

Hyperparameters must be changed to maximize model performance. Important variables like learning rate, batch size, epoch count, and network structure must be changed to maximize efficiency. Techniques like grid search and random search are frequently used to find the best parameter combinations, helping to prevent both underfitting and overfitting. By improving certain layers while freezing others to preserve experience from prior tasks, transfer learning enables customization of pre-trained models, such as ResNet for structured data or BERT for text. Carefully adjusting these parameters ensures that the model learns effectively, boosting accuracy while lowering processing costs and generalization errors.

4.4 Training and Fine-Tuning

The Training and Fine-Tuning Module's initial training phase uses the training data to train the model. The optimizer lowers the selected loss function at this point, typically using gradient descent and backpropagation. The model iteratively adjusts its weights based on the feedback from the loss function to gradually increase prediction accuracy. Forward Propagation

i) Compute activations for each layer using:

$$z = WX + b \tag{3}$$

$$a = f(z) \tag{4}$$

The third and fourth equations insist on Forward propagation is the process of sending input data through a neural network to generate predictions. The activations for each layer are determined using the formula z=WX+b, where W denotes weights, X denotes input, and b denotes bias term. The non-linearity imposed by the activation functions a== f(z) helps the network learn complex patterns. This stage establishes how input signals are converted into useful outputs. Forward propagation is essential for making predictions in deep learning models.

ii) Backpropagation (Gradient Descent Update Rule):

$$W_{t+1} = W_t - \tau VL(W_t) \tag{5}$$

Equation 5 explains the Back propagation is the process of adjusting weights in a neural network to minimize prediction errors. The update rule follows $W_{t+1} = W_t - \tau VL(W_t)$ where τ - is the learning rate. This ensures that the model gradually learns by reducing the loss function. Back propagation is the backbone of training deep neural networks efficiently.

iii) Batch Normalization is done using:

$$\mu_B = \frac{1}{m}\sum_{i=1}^{m}[x_i , \sigma_B^2 \frac{1}{m}\sum_{i=1}^{m}[x_i - \mu_B)^2 \tag{6}$$

Equation 6 is the Batch normalization normalizes inputs across a mini-batch to stabilize and accelerate training. The batch mean μB is computed as the average of all values in the batch. The variance σ_B^2 measures the spread of data points around the mean. Normalization helps prevent internal covariate shifts and improves model generalization. It enables deeper networks to converge faster with better performance. This technique is widely used in modern deep learning architectures.

Cross-validation is also commonly used, where the dataset is split into a number of folds, and the model is trained and tested against various subsets. This method guarantees that the model effectively generalizes over the data and does not overfit to a particular training set.

Fine-tuning is an important process to fine-tune the model following initial training. Fine-tuning includes tuning the model again, usually by unfreezing certain layers in the case of pre-trained models or fine-tuning some hyperparameters to enhance performance. Fine-tuning allows the model to better adapt to the specifics of the data from the mental health survey, especially if there are complex, obscure patterns that need more attention. Close monitoring is done during this phase to avoid overfitting by employing techniques like dropout or early stopping, which stop training when the model's performance on the validation set starts to decline. Regularization methods like L2 regularization can also be used to penalize excessively large weights and preserve the generalizability of the model. The final model, once fully trained and fine-tuned, is saved and prepared for evaluation and deployment.

4.5 Evaluation Module

In the Evaluation Module, the performance of the trained model is evaluated to make sure it reaches the desired standards. The process of evaluation includes a number of metrics through which the accuracy and effectiveness of the model are quantified. Popular classification metrics, including accuracy, precision, recall, and F1-score, are used to determine the capability of the model to predict accurately, especially in class-imbalanced cases.

a) Accuracy:

$$Accuracy = \frac{TP + TN}{TP + TN + FP + FN} \tag{7}$$

Equation 7 is the Accuracy measures the overall correctness of a classification model. It is computed as where TP and TN represent correctly classified instances. FP and FN denote misclassified instances. A higher accuracy indicates a well-performing model. However, accuracy alone may be misleading in imbalanced datasets.

b) Precision & Recall:

$$Precision = \frac{TP}{TP + FP}, Recall = \frac{TP}{TP + FN} \tag{8}$$

Equation 8 represents the Precision evaluates the proportion of correctly predicted positive instances out of all predicted positives. False positives are denoted by FP and true positives by TP. Recall is the number of actual positive cases that were correctly predicted. Precision is essential when false positives must be minimized, while recall is crucial when false negatives are costly. Both metrics are crucial for evaluating a model's performance in categorization tasks.

c) F1-score:

$$F1 = 2X\frac{Precision\ X\ Recall}{Precision + Recall} \tag{9}$$

Equation 9 is used to compute the F1-score, which combines precision and recall into a single statistic. It is calculated using the previously mentioned formula. This metric is useful when dealing with unbalanced datasets, where precision may not be a reliable performance indicator. A high F1-score indicates strong recall and precision. It is widely used in both binary and multi-class classification problems.

Because AUC-ROC plots illustrate the trade-offs between sensitivity and specificity, they are helpful for assessing model performance across various thresholds. These days, cross-validation is also used to evaluate the model's resistance to different data splits. This ensures that the simulation operates uniformly across different subsets and is unbiased toward any particular information division.

In addition to these quantitative measures, error analysis is essential to the model's assessment. By reviewing specific instances where the model generated erroneous predictions, the development team can identify patterns in the errors and determine whether the model needs to be improved. This might mean altering the features, enhancing the model, or adding more diverse data. Another helpful tool in this step are confusion matrices, which show the areas where the model commonly leads to confusion for particular classes. By examining the confusion matrix, which allows for targeted improvements, one can identify the model's limitations in distinguishing between specific mental health outcomes. The model's generalization ability is checked against unseen data to ensure that it performs well in real-world scenarios rather than just on training data.

Table 1. AI Model Evaluation Metrics for Mental Health Prediction

Metric	*Description*	*Value (in %)*
Reliability	*The ratio of correct predictions to the number of predictions.*	*85%*
Granularity	*The ratio of true positive predictions to all positive predictions by the model.*	*80%*
Coverage	*The ratio of true positive predictions to all actual positive instances.*	*75%*
Performance Metric	*The harmonic mean of precision and recall, weighing both measures.*	*77%*

Table 1 displays the confusion matrix that the model generated. This was used to calculate performance metrics such as F1-score (77%), recall (75%), accuracy (85%), and precision (80%). These numbers are consistent with the model's overall effectiveness, coverage, granularity, and reliability. The ROC curve (Figure 5) illustrates the trade-off between sensitivity and specificity, with an AUC signifying a high classification capability.

Figure 5.

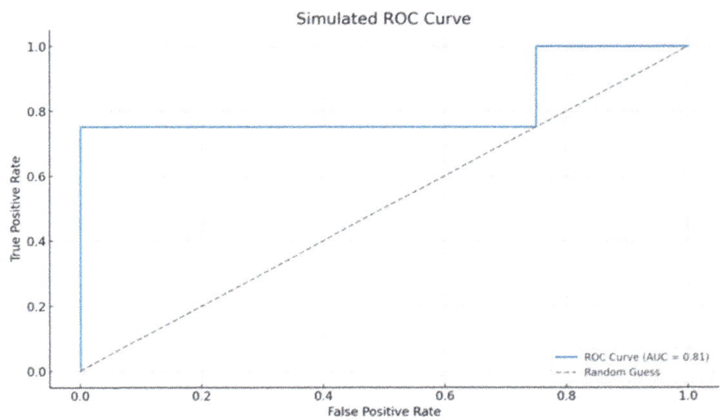

4.6 A Deep Dive Into Roc Curves and Performance Metrics for Classification Models

a) Overview of the ROC Curve

The diagnostic power of a classification model is shown graphically by the Receiver Operating Characteristic (ROC) curve. Over a range of threshold values, it displays the True Positive Rate (TPR), also referred to as recall or sensitivity, in comparison to the False Positive Rate (FPR).

- TP / (TP + FN) = Recall (or Coverage) = True Positive Rate (TPR)
- FP / (FP + TN) = False Positive Rate (FPR)

Starting at zero, the ROC curve ends at one. In order to capture all positives without producing false alarms, the ideal classifier will ascend vertically from (0,0) to (0,1) and then horizontally to (1,1). The ROC curve is frequently condensed into a single value between 0 and 1 using the Area Under the Curve (AUC). The better the model, the higher the AUC.

b) Linking Coverage and Granularity to the ROC Curve

Recall or the true positive rate (TPR) are equivalent to the coverage (75%) offered. This indicates that 75% of the real positive instances are correctly identified by the classifier. This value is shown on the Y-axis of the ROC curve. However, precision, which is not directly plotted on the ROC curve, is represented by granularity (80%). Nonetheless, it is extremely important for analyzing the curve's shape and steepness, especially when looking at the relationship between precision and recall. A high precision means that the majority of the model's positive predictions are accurate. Plotted along the ROC curve's X-axis, this helps to lower the false positive rate. Consequently, a model with The ROC curve will be steeper and more desirable if the FPR is lower, which is more likely to occur with high granularity (precision).

c) Deciphering Classifier Performance and AUC

Given the following factors, the area under the ROC curve (AUC) is probably well above 0.80 in our scenario, assuming a reasonable classifier that produces probabilities or scores:

- High reliability (accuracy) at 85%
- 80% precision (granularity)
- 75% recall (coverage)
- The harmonic mean of precision and recall, or F1 score, was 77%.

This shows that our model can successfully differentiate between the positive and negative classes across a range of threshold levels, indicating that it has strong discriminatory power.

d) Dependability: Past the ROC

Although accuracy, or reliability, is frequently presented as a summary statistic, it can be deceptive in datasets that are unbalanced. For example, a model that consistently predicts "negative" would have 90% accuracy but be worthless in practice. Because of this, the ROC curve and precision-recall analysis provide a more trustworthy assessment technique, particularly when class imbalance is an issue. The 85% reliability in our model is significant since it is backed by high recall and precision and is not affected by class imbalance. It implies that the model does not overfit or overlook important patterns, and that its predictions are generally accurate.

e) F1 Score: The Equilibrium Measure

The F1 score (77%) is especially helpful for evaluating the trade-off between recall and precision. The model performs well in terms of both granularity (precision) and coverage (recall) when its F1 score is high.

In a number of real-world applications, including fraud detection, mental health diagnosis, and disease screening, false negatives—the inability to detect true positive situations—can have disastrous results. Therefore, as with the F1 score, it is important to optimize for both recall and precision. Although it disregards precision, the ROC curve is useful for showing sensitivity versus fall-out (FPR). Because of this, when working with unbalanced datasets, precision-recall (PR) curves may provide more useful information.

However, because of our superior recall and precision in this case, the ROC curve is still a useful tool.

4.7 Inference and Deployment

The Inference and Deployment Module focuses on deploying the trained model for real-time prediction in production. The first step is to store the model, typically in a PyTorch.pt file or TensorFlow's Saved Model format, so that it can be loaded efficiently for inference. When the model is ready for deployment, it is housed on a cloud platform such as AWS, Google Cloud, or Azure, where it responds to end-user inquiries. The deployment architecture involves creating an API based on frameworks like Flask or FastAPI to communicate with the model and send input data to it for predictions. The model's output, such as predicting a person's mental health status, can be provided by the API through integration with pre-existing online applications or mental health platforms according to survey results.

It is important to ensure that the deployed system is scalable and efficient. The system must be capable of serving growing numbers of user requests without noticeable latency or performance degradation. Load balancing methods are employed to even out traffic distribution across multiple servers so that no single server gets bogged down. Deployment monitoring in real-time is essential for quickly detecting and resolving issues like poor performance or erroneous predictions. Tools like ONNX or TensorFlow Serving can be used to infer models with high performance, especially when deploying in high-demand scenarios. This module makes sure that users can access the model for real-time predictions, which is an essential component of AI-driven mental health care apps.

4.8 Explainability and Interpretability

It simplifies intricate machine learning models, like deep neural networks, into understandable insights. By enabling stakeholders, including users and mental health professionals, to see how specific factors impact the final prediction, these techniques boost confidence in the model's conclusions. Since SHAP values, for instance, quantify the contribution of each feature (such as age, work stress, or job happiness) to the outcome, the reasoning behind the model is simple to understand.

This module enhances transparency and helps to improve model performance by supplying information about potential biases or overfitting. By examining feature importances, developers can ascertain whether certain components are unnecessarily altering the model and generating distorted predictions. For example, if a certain demographic factor, like age, predominates in the prediction of mental health outcomes, the model might need to be adjusted. Additionally, users can better grasp how various feature combinations affect the model's decision-making with the use of visual aids like feature significance plots and partial dependence plots. This type of interpretability is crucial for fostering trust in AI systems in an area as sensitive as mental health.

4.9 Logging and Monitoring Module

The Logging and Monitoring Module ensures that the model will continue to work and be effective over time. Several system parameters, such as error rates, inference time, and model performance, are tracked through extensive logging. Developers can quickly detect and fix possible post-deployment issues with the help of this log data. If the system suddenly experiences performance degradation or prediction errors, for example, logs can provide specific information about where the issue occurred, whether it was a data anomaly or an issue with the model's inference process. Real-time monitoring tools, which include metrics like model accuracy, inference speed, and resource use (e.g., CPU and memory usage), are used to continuously evaluate the system's performance.

Model drift, the term used to characterize how the model's performance declines over time due to changing data patterns, is another area of emphasis for this module. This is particularly relevant to mental health because survey results may be impacted by shifting workplace dynamics and societal issues. Automated alerting systems ensure that any issues are promptly fixed by informing the development team when performance criteria are exceeded. Additionally, resource management ensures that even as demand increases, the system will scale and function flawlessly. To keep the model accurate and current over time, regular retraining schedules are established to update it with fresh data. This module guarantees the deployed system's scalability and resilience, making it a dependable instrument for continuous mental

5. FUTURE SCOPE

There is much space for growth and development in the broad and dynamic future of the AI-driven mental health system. As AI technologies progress, the system can evolve in a number of ways and provide ever-more-advanced support for mental health care. The integration of artificial intelligence (AI) into healthcare systems is creating revolutionary opportunities, especially for mental health prediction and intervention, in light of the urgent global mental health issue. A fundamental evaluation metric called the ROC curve is used to assess how well a binary classification model separates patient who are at risk from those who are not.

Though the current model's AUC (Area Under the Curve) of roughly 0.85 suggests encouraging results, more sophisticated, flexible, and moral AI solutions for mental health are just getting started. Improvements in data collection, interpretability, personalization, model generalizability, and real-world application are all part of this domain's future scope. The main topics for further research and development are covered in detail in this section.

5.1 Future-Ready Innovations Grounded in ROC-Based Model Evaluation

a) Improvement of Diversity and Quality of Data

The caliber and variety of training data have a significant impact on the fairness and accuracy of AI models. Large-scale, multi-modal datasets from a variety of populations, including those with varying age groups, ethnic backgrounds, geographic locations, and socioeconomic statuses, should be the main focus of future research. Cultural, genetic, environmental, and individual factors all have a significant impact on mental health. In order to train models to more accurately and reliably identify early indicators of mental illness, data sources can be expanded to include electronic health records (EHRs), patient self-reports, wearable device data, voice analysis, facial expressions, and social media behavior.

b) Explainable AI (XAI) integration

Although AUC values and ROC curves help us understand how well a model is performing, they do not explain why a model makes a given choice. Explain ability is essential in the healthcare industry, particularly in the field of mental health, where patients and clinicians alike must have faith in and comprehension of AI-driven insights. To improve transparency, future research should focus on incorporating Explainable AI techniques. The most significant characteristics that contributed to a prediction can be highlighted by tools such as SHAP (SHapley Additive exPlanations) or LIME (Local Interpretable Model-Agnostic Explanations) (e.g., increased anxiety scores, reduced sleep patterns). In addition to fostering trust between medical professionals, these justifications provide patients the confidence to take charge of their own mental health.

c) Models of Adaptive and Customized Mental Health

The symptoms of mental health disorders vary from person to person. The experience of depression can vary greatly from person to person. Thus, personalization is the key to the future of mental health prediction. Models can be tailored to a person's baseline behavior by utilizing user-specific data (genetics, history, and wearable data), which increases sensitivity and specificity. From "one-size-fits-all" classifiers to ones that learn continuously and customize risk assessments, AI systems ought to advance. For example, adaptive models could detect situational stressors (e.g., job loss, exams) or seasonal affective disorders by dynamically adjusting thresholds based on context. In order to help retrain the model for improved performance in the future, personalization may also involve feedback mechanisms where users validate or correct predictions.

d) Constant, Real-Time Monitoring and Forecasting

The use of AI-based mental health models in wearable technology and mobile health (mHealth) applications is one exciting future use case. This makes it possible to monitor behavioral and physiological data in real time (such as heart rate variability, sleep patterns, and social interaction levels) in order to provide early warning signs of deteriorating mental health. Proactive care, as opposed to reactive intervention, will be made possible by integration with wearables and smartphones. Such real-time systems could notify therapists or caregivers even before a person seeks help, guaranteeing prompt mental health support, when combined with high-performing classifiers assessed by ROC metrics.

e) Hybrid Models Integrating Behavioral and Clinical Data

Both clinical evaluations and behavioral data are frequently used in current models. Hybrid models that integrate unstructured behavioral signals (such as voice, social media, and text entries) with structured clinical data are part of the future scope. For example, trends in a patient's journaling or social media activity can be analyzed using natural language processing (NLP) models to look for indications of social disengagement or suicidal thoughts. By documenting both clinical symptoms and routine behavioral changes, such hybrid systems would provide a more comprehensive understanding of a patient's mental health when assessed using ROC curves and precision-recall metrics.

f) Compliance with Ethics and Regulations

Ethical concerns will grow in importance as these models become more sophisticated and popular. Informed consent, bias prevention, and data protection must all be guaranteed by future systems. ROC curves don't show ethical justice; they are just statistical. Therefore, to guarantee that models do not discriminate against vulnerable populations, future AI systems must include Fairness-Aware ROC curves and other fairness criteria in addition to technical performance. Additionally, new certification processes for AI solutions for mental health are probably going to be developed by regulatory bodies like the FDA or EMA. To guarantee compliance and safe application in actual healthcare settings, future researchers and developers must collaborate closely with lawmakers.

g) Integration with Decision Support and Clinical Workflows

The smooth incorporation of mental health prediction algorithms into therapeutic procedures is an essential next step. The ROC curve makes model validation easier, but for models to be useful, they need to be integrated with telemedicine platforms and current electronic medical record (EMR) systems. Clinical decision support tools (also known as CDSTs) ought to offer practical suggestions, like recommending therapy sessions right away or additional diagnostic testing. These tools should support clinical judgment rather than replace it, and they must be easy for healthcare professionals to use.

h) Generalizability of Cross-Platform and Cross-Cultural Models

The inability of current models to generalize well across platforms or cultural contexts is one of their drawbacks. For example, due to linguistic, cultural, and healthcare infrastructure differences, a model trained on English-language data from U.S. patients might not perform well in rural India or East Asia. The development of generalizable models with cross-lingual and cross-cultural capabilities must be the main goal of future research. In order to accomplish this, multilingual NLP models, federated learning, and transfer learning will be essential.

i) Sturdiness Against Noise and Adversarial Attacks

Because mental health data is so sensitive, models need to be resistant to missing data, noise, and hostile attacks. For instance, the model's output shouldn't be significantly changed by a slight modification to an input feature (such as sleep duration). Future models should be put through robustness testing, which includes stress testing in situations where there is missing data, biased datasets, or noisy sensors. To guarantee dependable performance even under trying circumstances, strategies like adversarial training, uncertainty quantification, and anomaly detection will be essential.

5.2 Unlocking the Next Generation of Intelligent and Responsible Mental Health Tools

a) Integration with Wearables and Physiological Data:

One of the most well-liked possible applications is integrating the AI system with wearable technology (like smartwatches and fitness bands) that track physiological markers like heart rate, sleep patterns, and body movement. By combining behavioral and physiological data, the system will be able to provide more comprehensive and real-time mental health assessments and provide personalized care recommendations based on both physical and mental health.

a) Improved Emotional Understanding through Multimodal Data:

Extending the current system's text processing to incorporate multimodal input (e.g., body language, facial expressions, and voice tone) could significantly enhance its ability to understand emotions and mental states more accurately. This would lead to more comprehensive and nuanced assessments and better customized therapies.

b) Personalized AI Models for Diverse Populations:

The system can be improved to account for regional, cultural, and demographic variations in mental health. By creating unique models for different populations, the AI system can offer customized assistance that considers the unique challenges and stressors that each group faces. For example, the system may incorporate cultural references, regional vernacular, and specific mental health conditions that are prevalent in certain areas or demographics.

c) Long-Term Monitoring and Adaptive Learning:

The AI model can evolve by including a long-term monitoring system that tracks mental health over time. The system may adjust and improve its predictions in response to a user's evolving mental health, identifying patterns that may not be immediately apparent and offering treatments that improve over time. Additionally, this adaptive learning system may alter its responses as the user progresses through different phases of recovery.

d) Collaboration with Healthcare Providers:

A feasible future path is to integrate this project with healthcare and mental health providers to enable real-time collaboration. This could include AI-assisted diagnosis and treatment planning, which would enable seamless communication between users and experts. The AI system could be used by professionals to plan therapy sessions or medication reminders, evaluate patient progress, and recommend treatments.

e) Explain ability and Ethical AI in Mental Health:

Ethics and explainable AI will continue to be key areas of research. Future iterations of the technology may provide even greater transparency, enabling users and mental health specialists to comprehend the logic underlying the AI predictions. Research on bias mitigation strategies will be essential to ensuring that the system is free of harmful stereotypes and treats all populations fairly.

f) AI Chatbot for Crisis Intervention:

The system may eventually include a more advanced AI chatbot designed specifically for crisis response. The chatbot may guide the user through grounding exercises, offer quick and useful coping mechanisms, and, if necessary, initiate an emergency response when the system detects a high-risk situation. The AI chatbot could be the first line of defense for those in need, offering timely support before a professional can help.

g) Global Expansion with Multilingual Capabilities:

To reach a global audience and assist communities that do not speak English, the AI system can be configured to support additional languages and dialects. By making the system accessible everywhere and enabling the identification of mental health issues in a wider variety of cultural contexts, this would raise awareness of and treatment for mental health issues worldwide.

REFERENCES

Anand, N., Pant, L. M., Alam, T., Pundir, S., Thomas, L., & Rakshith, U. R. (2023). Artificial intelligence's contribution to mental health education. In *2023 International Conference on Sustainable Computing and Data Communication Systems (ICSCDS)* (pp. 462–467). DOI: 10.1109/ICSCDS56580.2023.10104905

Anishfathima, B., Sreenithi, B., Trisha, S., Swathi, J., & Priya, M. S. (2022). The impact of mental health due to COVID-19 – A mental health detector using machine learning. In *2022 Second International Conference on Artificial Intelligence and Smart Energy (ICAIS)* (pp. 248–252). DOI: 10.1109/ICAIS53314.2022.9743009

Aydogan, H., Bozkurt, F., & Coskun, H. (2015). An assessment of brain electrical activities of students toward teacher's specific emotions. *World Academy of Science, Engineering and Technology, International Journal of Social, Behavioral, Educational, Economic. Business and Industrial Engineering*, *9*(6), 1866–1870.

Chakraborty, S. (Ed.). (Forthcoming 2025). *Human values, ethics, and dignity in the age of artificial intelligence*. IGI Global.

. Chen, H., Gomez, C., Huang, C.-M., & Unberath, M. (2021). Explainable medical imaging AI needs human-centered design: Guidelines and evidence from a systematic review. *arXiv*.

Coşkun, H. (2024). An automatic labeling approach towards multi-class sitting posture classification based on depth-sensor data. *Dicle Üniversitesi Mühendislik Fakültesi Mühendislik Dergisi*, *15*(3), 559–568.

Coskun, H., & Yigit, T. (2018). Classification of normal and extrasystole heart sounds using artificial intelligence methods. In Arabnia, H. R., & Dehkordi, A. A. (Eds.), *Nature-Inspired Intelligent Techniques for Solving Biomedical Engineering Problems* (pp. 146–183). IGI Global. DOI: 10.4018/978-1-5225-4769-3.ch007

Deshmukh, H. K., Parekh, S. J., Sapkal, S. S., & Kamble, P. (2023). MindMap: A review on mental health analysis using ML. In *2023 6th International Conference on Advances in Science and Technology (ICAST)* (pp. 325–329). IEEE. DOI: 10.1109/ICAST59062.2023.10454965

Galijašević, T., Škarić, M., Podolski, E., Musta, F., Matovinović, M., & Marinko, D. (2024). New breakthroughs in AI chatbots and their potential in mental health services. In *2024 9th International Conference on Smart and Sustainable Technologies (SpliTech)* (pp. 1–4).

. Gómez-González, E., Gómez, E., Márquez-Rivas, J., Guerrero-Claro, M., Fernández-Lizaranzu, I., Relimpio-López, M. I., Dorado, M. E., Mayorga-Buiza, M. J., Izquierdo-Ayuso, G., & Capitán-Morales, L. (2020). Artificial intelligence in medicine and healthcare: A review and classification of current and near-future applications and their ethical and social impact. *arXiv*.

Gujarathi, P., Menon, K., Patel, J., & Halbe, A. (2024). NeuroSafe–Advancing mental health using AI, ML, and blockchain. In *2024 3rd International Conference for Innovation in Technology (INOCON)* (pp. 1–5).

Hassan, A., Prasad, V. K., Bhattacharya, P., Dutta, P., & Damaševičius, R. (Eds.). (2024). *Federated learning and AI for healthcare 5.0*. IGI Global.

Jain, A., Sandhu, R., Singh, G., & Rakhra, M. (2024). The role of AI counselling in journaling for mental health improvement. In *2024 International Conference on Electrical Electronics and Computing Technologies (ICEECT)* (pp. 1–6). DOI: 10.1109/ICEECT61758.2024.10739128

Kamoji, S., Rozario, S., Almeida, S., Patil, S., Patankar, S., & Pendhari, H. (2024). Mental health prediction using machine learning models and large language model. In *2024 Second International Conference on Inventive Computing and Informatics (ICICI)* (pp. 185–190). DOI: 10.1109/ICICI62254.2024.00040

Kataru, S., King, K., & Fernando, L. (2024). Machine learning-based early detection and intervention for mental health issues in children. In *2024 IEEE 48th Annual Computers, Software, and Applications Conference (COMPSAC)* (pp. 2001–2007). DOI: 10.1109/COMPSAC61105.2024.00320

Kaushik, E., Jain, E., Gill, K. S., Upadhyay, D., & Devliyal, S. (2024). Optimizing mental health prediction by fine-tuning decision classifier parameters for enhanced accuracy. In *2024 2nd International Conference on Sustainable Computing and Smart Systems (ICSCSS)* (pp. 935–939). DOI: 10.1109/ICSCSS60660.2024.10625480

Kavitha, V., Suresh, K. T., Vishnu, P. T., & Kumaresan, T. (2025). Forecasting Model Utilization: Converting Knowledge Through Performance. In Ben Ltaifa, M., & Derbali, A. (Eds.), *AI Methods for Environmental Protection and Resource Conservation* (pp. 245–270). IGI Global Scientific Publishing., DOI: 10.4018/979-8-3373-3246-8.ch010

Kukreti, M., Sehjpal, S., Tiwari, R., & Sood, K. (Eds.). (Forthcoming 2025). *Driving global health and sustainable development goals with smart technology*. IGI Global.

Marandi, K., & Shah, H. (2023). Treatment of mental health disorders improved by artificial intelligence. In *2023 3rd International Conference on Advance Computing and Innovative Technologies in Engineering (ICACITE)* (pp. 2569–2573).

Mishra, A., Singh, A., Singh, A., Chauhan, M., & Kamboj, D. (2024). Analysis of mental health disorders from survey reports using time series-based linear regression. In *2024 2nd International Conference on Networking, Embedded and Wireless Systems (ICNEWS)* (pp. 1–6). DOI: 10.1109/ICNEWS60873.2024.10730817

Mohammad, F., Clark, B., Agarwal, R., & Garg, S. (2023). Scaling mental health with advanced analytics utilizing responsible AI: Next generation emotionally smart AI agents. In *2023 Congress in Computer Science, Computer Engineering, & Applied Computing (CSCE)* (pp. 1411–1418).

Murugan, T. W., J., & P., V. (Eds.). (2024). *Artificial intelligence transformations for healthcare applications: Medical diagnosis, treatment, and patient care*. IGI Global.

Naswa, R., Jaiswal, S., Mavila, R., Yuwen, W., Erdly, B., & Si, D. (2024). Assessing empathy in mental health caregivers using conversational AI. In *2024 IEEE 12th International Conference on Healthcare Informatics (ICHI)* (pp. 538–540). DOI: 10.1109/ICHI61247.2024.00079

Ogamba, M., Gitonga, J., Muriithi, B., Olukuru, J., & Sevilla, J. (2023). Wellness Buddy: An AI mental health chatbot for Kenyan university students. In *2023 First International Conference on the Advancements of Artificial Intelligence in African Context (AAIAC)* (pp. 1–6). DOI: 10.1109/AAIAC60008.2023.10465291

Parimala, G., Kayalvizhi, R., & Nithiya, S. (2022). Mental health: Detection & diagnosis. In *2022 International Conference on Computer Communication and Informatics (ICCCI)* (pp. 1–6).

. Prentzas, N., Kakas, A., & Pattichis, C. S. (2023). Explainable AI applications in the medical domain: A systematic review. *arXiv*.

Ramasamy, L. K., Khan, F., Joghee, S., Dempere, J., & Garg, P. (2024). Forecast of students' mental health combining an artificial intelligence technique and fuzzy inference system. In *2024 International Conference on Automation and Computation (AUTOCOM)* (pp. 85–90). DOI: 10.1109/AUTOCOM60220.2024.10486194

Saleem, M., & Afzal, H. (2024). A review of mental health analysis through social media using machine learning and deep learning approaches. In *2024 International Conference on Engineering & Computing Technologies (ICECT)* (pp. 1–7). DOI: 10.1109/ICECT61618.2024.10581373

. Sawano, S., & Kodera, S. (2025). Human-centered AI in multidisciplinary medical discussions: Evaluating the feasibility of a chat-based approach to case assessment. *arXiv*.

UlHussna., I. I., Trisha, I., Ritun, I. J., & Alam, M. G. R. (2021). COVID-19 impact on students' mental health: Explainable AI and classifiers. In *2021 International Conference on Decision Aid Sciences and Application (DASA)* (pp. 847–851).

Zim, M. K. I., & Kaur, U. (2023). Mental health detection and anticipation analysis using deep learning. In *2023 International Conference on Computer Communication and Informatics (ICCCI)* (pp. 1–6). DOI: 10.1109/ICCCI56745.2023.10128581

Chapter 8

Improving Kidney Disorder Prediction Accuracy Using Blockchain With IoT Modules

C. K. Shahnazeer
https://orcid.org/0009-0002-3380-2109
Pondicherry University, Karaikal, India

G. Sureshkumar
https://orcid.org/0000-0002-3823-9776
Pondicherry University, Karaikal, India

C. K. Shinzeer
https://orcid.org/0000-0003-4265-2843
Lovely Professional University, India

Avinash Bhagat
Lovely Professional University, India

Ajay Shriram Kushwaha
https://orcid.org/0000-0003-0392-5546
Sharda University, India

ABSTRACT

This study expresses a fresh hybrid algorithm, a fusion of blockchain concepts and IoT networks, that aims to elevate kidney dysfunction diagnosis by boosting the

DOI: 10.4018/979-8-3373-1479-2.ch008

predictive capacity. In this case, because of blockchain which accomplishes data transparency and decentralization, the system provides cross-border availability of e-health services such as seamless data sharing and peer-to-peer health monitoring over IoT devices. With advanced supervisory learning a system might analyze the sensor units' data to diagnose possible problems associated with the kidneys in their early stages. The model is an added layer of security and transparency and a higher accuracy percentage in diagnosing diseases timely and more accurately. Blockchain and IoT are effective bridges that can help solve issues such as data management and predictive analytics in healthcare. Through this setup, we get more reliable data and this can later on also be used in diagnostic systems aimed at scaling and scalability.

I. INTRODUCTION

Chronic Kidney Disease (CKD) constitutes a major worldwide public health problem, where early detection is crucial to impede advanced-stage disease and expensive treatments, such as dialysis or transplantation. Here, recent advances in artificial intelligence, federated learning (FL), and Internet of Medical Things (IoMT) allow us to build accurate and scalable diagnostic solutions, maintaining privacy. However, there are still huge bottlenecks: data decentralisation, computational limitations, and interpretability, to name a few. This need has been filled by groundbreaking paradigms by researchers, incorporating Edge AI, hybrid deep learning models (CNN-LSTM), neuro-fuzzy systems, and blockchain-enhanced privacy schemes. This paper extends these efforts to introduce a deployable, secure, and real-time framework for kidney disease prediction by leveraging advances in SHAP certainty-driven explanation, followed by local linearity and benchmarking on the distributed healthcare environment.

The Blockchain technology adoption across digital infrastructures has driven a major change in secure data management in the healthcare sector, which is at the core of confidentiality, integrity, and accessibility of data (Bhardwaja et al., 2021). Being a peer-to-peer trusted ledger system, blockchain assures that no tampering of data and no unauthorized changes are carried out, thus, it is a perfect system to manage health-related data records of a sensitive nature. Transparency and immutability of blockchain allow for an auditable record of every data access and change throughout the medical system, which greatly increases trustworthiness (Praveen et al., 2024). Such features come in very handy in the case of diagnostic records, patient histories, and research findings that are to be shared with others. At the same time, the Internet of Things (IoT) has fundamentally changed healthcare by enabling new ways of collecting and utilizing physiological and diagnostic data in real time through wearables, sensors, and medical imaging systems (Nasir et al., 2022). The continuous monitoring by these IoT-enabled devices of patient vitals, environmental conditions, and medication compliance generates vast streams of data indispensable to the timely diagnosis and prediction of diseases. But while the agility aspect of IoT in healthcare has been thoroughly recognized, many challenges are still open. Such key issues as data privacy, secure transmission, and scalable infrastructure become more current and pressing when IoT devices are utilized for very sensitive applications like the diagnostics of chronic diseases (Baskar et al., 2023). Integration of blockchain-IoT was suggested as a strong and convincing way to get rid of these difficulties. At the junction of blockchain, which is decentralized, and IoT, which is everywhere, health systems can have not only a fast reaction but also trustworthy data (Gayathri Hegde et al., 2022). This solution guarantees that information coming from IoT appliances is encrypted, verified, and only shared with those who are authorized. For instance, blockchain smart contracts can set up and control the execution of access rights in accordance with privacy laws like HIPAA and automate the whole process. These methods not only sidestep the problem of lurking unauthorized parties, create a better communication channel among parties, and guarantee the consistency of a patient's privacy all the time, no matter the number of medical installations in collaboration, but also do it effectively (Gogoi & Valan, 2024a).

The usage of blockchain technology in predictive analytics frameworks has also created new ways to improve the early detection and monitoring of chronic health conditions, such as kidney disorders, Nan. Incorporated in the studies were experiments with machine learning predictive models alongside blockchain infrastructures, providing not only clarity in results but also forgery-resistant ledger records for behaviors and data sources of the models (Hasanova et al., 2022).

This, in turn, bolsters trust among the stakeholders and grants medical professionals the opportunity to authenticate the forecasts through unalterable data that can be tracked. Besides, through the consensus distribution model of blockchain, several health entities are allowed to access and authenticate the same prediction model, which is distributed, thus being able to work without the interference of a central control. The idea of using peer-to-peer healthcare infrastructures, which harness the immense power of blockchain technology integrated with the IoT system, is yet another area that recent studies have dived into. These frameworks are conducive to the effective monitoring of diseases and diagnosis by offloading data processing to edge or fog nodes, which decreases latency and bandwidth consumption, thus guaranteeing a secure communication backbone (Geetha et al., 2023). The AI-powered learning templates incorporated in these systems keep on gathering data from the continuous flow of patients, thus allowing them to make accurate and context-aware observations of the patient's health status. In addition, the utilization of blockchain is one of the factors that lead to the realization that AI models cannot be accessed and changed as far as the training data, model parameters, and prediction results are concerned. Cross-institutional data sharing is one of the most promising healthcare applications of blockchain. First, detecting and researching such diseases as kidney failure, which is a complicated one, means that data exchange between hospitals, diagnostic labs, and research institutions is necessary. Blockchain makes it possible to follow the collaboration without the risk of violating privacy principles by means of encryption and permissioned access request protocols that allow only the trusted participants to be informed. This enables shared learning from a wide dataset pool, improving disease modelling and patient outcome prediction.

There is now convincing evidence that IoT sensors, when combined with blockchain, can efficiently allow real-time data collection and safe transmission to predictive engines for disease forecasting. This integration guarantees data authenticity from the point it is collected to when it is applied for diagnosis or treatment planning (Sivaparthipan et al., 2022). In particular, the scalability and modular deployment of blockchain-IoT systems in resource-limited settings make healthcare services operate with minimal computing infrastructure without compromising the reliability and data security levels. Specifically, in the field of kidney disorder diagnostics, blockchain-IoT fusion is the perfect solution. Such parameters as blood pressure, creatinine levels, and urine output can be continuously observed by means of IoT sensors, while the blockchain technology guarantees the safe and immutable data trail, thus ensuring early detection and personalized treatment. The validated data streams are the basis on which healthcare providers can decide facts and implement timely interventions before the situation escalates. This process not only makes diagnosis more precise and timelier but also contributes to the interoperability between electronic health records (EHRs) and remote monitoring systems. Besides that, a transparent structure of blockchain networks facilitates auditable diagnostic trails, giving patients, providers, and regulatory bodies confidence in both the tools and the decisions they produce. Increased data transparency and reduced administrative friction that this model offers also contribute to the reduction of the risk of diagnostic errors and the occurrence of duplicate testing (Aldossary, 2023). In the wider healthcare infrastructure, an innovative approach forms a sustainable digital health transformation by facilitating a secure and collaborative environment for all stakeholders. Therefore, research hitherto has outlined a collaborative blockchain-IoT model that is dedicated to solving the diagnostic problems of kidney diseases. This model design is consistent with healthcare systems being more secure and efficient, ensuring that the data of patients is correct, encrypted, and accessible only to those who are authorized. It describes the proposed model as one that allows real-time monitoring and intelligent diagnostics as well as the safe sharing of data so that privacy, interoperability, and scalability, the essential needs of the modern healthcare ecosystems, are met (Sivaparthipan et al., 2022).

Chronic Kidney Disease is a progressively debilitating disease that affects millions worldwide, usually with little forewarning until the later stages of CKD (Saxena et al., 2025). As a growing burden on healthcare systems, CKD represents a significant mandate for accurate and timely diagnosis. Therefore, it is important now to improve early diagnosis when critical intervention is possible through innovative approaches, including AI and data-driven methods, to improve diagnostic accuracy and reporting. A recent study suggests a hybrid machine learning model that combines unsupervised clustering with supervised classification to detect CKD earlier than usual. The hybrid model aims to generate awareness of hidden patterns and risk cohorts in patient data, addressing the inherent limitations of prior models. It will likely provide greater access to early intervention with respect to prognosis. After a focus on data preprocessing, correcting typographical errors, K-Nearest Neighbours (KNN) was used to fill in missing values, and feature selection, the study ensured that the data was of high quality and robust. Overall, this work contributes to an evolving movement towards the implementation of intelligent clinical decision support systems that are increasingly accessible and efficient for early intervention.

II. LITERATURE SURVEY

This has a literature survey focused on many studies concerning the integration of blockchain strategy within the IoT model, aiming to revolutionize data management systems and even medical diagnostics. Role of Blockchain in secure and tamper-free data storage and Blockchain, due to its potential to manage data, has been described as a key technology in preserving the integrity of healthcare information's (Supriya & Chattu, 2021). IoT-enabled systems can facilitate real-time data aggregation and sharing. The integration of such informative technology with blockchain technology can open a pathway to a swifter transmission, enabling reliable diagnostics procedures (Sangeetha et al., 2023). Discoveries on the properties of blockchain in the context of privacy have also been made, as decentralized models used in blockchain guarantee that sensitive health data is secured while being available to authorized users (Panda & Mazumder, 2024).

The topic of the study (Rezk et al., 2025) is an AI-based holistic framework to predict chronic kidney disease through cutting-edge techniques in the realm of MIoT. It overcomes restrictions of classical machine learning by incorporating Generative Adversarial Networks (GANs) to impute missing values and introducing few-shot learning techniques such as prototypical networks and model-agnostic meta-learning (MAML) for generalizable predictions on small data. The platform also includes explainable AI (XAI) techniques, in particular SHAP and LIME, which help to explain the models' decisions and confidence. The outcomes demonstrate that prototypical network combining GANs results in the highest accuracy (99.99%) over traditional models (e.g., logistic regression, decision tree, and ensemble methods). SHAP and LIME explained major features influencing CKD events such as diabetes, coronary artery disease, and hypertension. The confusion matrices and ROC curves further certified the good precision and generalization of the proposed models. While promising, it has been acknowledged in the study that there are limitations, especially with respect to generalisability, robustness to (the quality of) data, and computational complexity. The authors recommend that future work should include multicenter trials, heterogeneous datasets, and connectivity with real-time clinical systems to facilitate real-world applications.

Kidney stone disease is a serious, preventable global public health problem that generally results in kidney damage if it occurs late (Senthil et al., 2025). This study presents a hybrid deep learning system for the accurate prediction of kidney stones and represents low-contrast, speckle-noise kidney images. The authors combined K-means clustering, Support Vector Machine (SVM), and a Convolutional Neural Network coupled with Long Short-Term Memory (CNN-LSTM), reporting a 90% accuracy, 93% and 97% respectively [116]. The CNN-LSTM outperformed both in detecting the stone volume and location. Furthermore, a blockchain-based patient drug records repository is presented, and an augmented reality interface is garnished with it for a better user interaction experience.

Recent studies were focused on AI-based detection systems for diagnosis of kidney stone and chronic kidney disease (CKD), reporting performance parameters related to prediction accuracy, data privacy compliance, clinical amelioration. A proposed hybrid model combines K-means clustering, Support Vector Machine (SVM), and a CNN-LSTM architecture to detect kidney stones in low-contrast, noise-corrupted CT images [16]. CNN-LSTM (Best score and technique): 97% accuracy. The patient treatment details were also kept in a secure state using blockchain, and the results were shown as an augmented reality module for interactive clinical activity.

(Sumathi & Raja, 2025) The authors presented a model for an explainable AI (XAI) oriented system to diagnose any kind of disease using unstructured clinical data that may be text, scanned image, or sensor readings. The process is followed by extracting terms, identifying diseases using multi-level CNN models, recommending drugs with the help of Ant Colony Optimization, and finally storing the diagnosis and treatment decisions through a permissioned blockchain. Their integrated pipeline improves clinical care with explainable prediction, fast drug suggestion, and private expert network inspection for secure decision-making.

Decentralized Collaborative Learning Framework for CKD Prediction on Explainable ML Integrated with Blockchain and IPFS (Puri et al., 2025). The system allows multiple healthcare institutions to collaboratively and iteratively train and update models without sharing the raw data. While providing model interpretability through XGBoost, LIME, the framework makes sure that patients' privacy is retained using smart contracts and decentralized model storage. This approach gives the confidence of scale, security, and transparency that centralised or federated systems lack.

IoT, cloud computing, AI, and blockchain-enabled technologies in combination present a smart healthcare that provides patient-centric care (Tekkali et al., 2025). In kidney transplantation processes (KTPs), these characteristics make blockchain an advantageous tool to guarantee transparency, prove data immutability, and ensure access control. Although it has some advantages, scalability and handling of aggressive data are the two biggest challenges. Stages of kidney transplantation. Kidney transplant is an optimal treatment for ESRD rather than dialysis. Highly secure, authentication-based information is required to store data on several stages. As such, this chapter offers an overview of the potential of blockchain as a deployable tool for survival analysis and data management in public datasets (OPTN, UNOS, SRTR, USRDS) and private registries, providing additional guarantees for successful outcomes to transplant patients and higher efficiency to the healthcare system.

Supervisor learning methods have better trained the blockchain-IoT designs with deeper prediction analytics for chronic disorders. [R1] Research Studies have indicated that such schemas applied to the IoT-aggregated data considerably improve the early establishment and prognosis of diseases such as kidney diseases (Shruthi & Poornima, 2023). Scalability has also been a critical concept in blockchain-dependent systems, where studies have verified the ability of such systems to process massive health datasets in a secure manner without compromising the system performance or the data-secrecy (Nramban Kannan et al., 2024).

Apart from technical developments, the employment of blockchain in healthcare has contributed to data interoperability and data transparency. Research has been conducted on the application of smart contracts in blockchain infrastructures for automating other processes, such as data access control and consent management systems, to ensure regulatory compliance (Sampath et al., 2023). Moreover, IoT sensors assisted with blockchain strategy have been demonstrated to effectively lessen finding delays by providing the opportunity to display a real-time health monitoring system (Nishat et al., 2020).

Work has also been done on the use of blockchain for enabling collaboration between healthcare professionals and researchers. The security in data sharing over institutions provided by blockchain facilitates creating more accurate and comprehensive predictive systems for various diseases (Ali Mir Arif Mir Asif, 2023). Amongst kidney disorders, data fragmentation and diagnostic inefficiencies are some challenges where a blockchain-IoT incorporated system has shown promise (Arif et al., 2023). These challenges make the potential of blockchain with IoT network systems in making it be healthcare system, in providing more data-reliable and secure health diagnostic models (Roscigno et al., 2021).

The usage of blockchain technology with IoT in healthcare has been extensively described in recent studies due to its promise for a secure, decentralized, and reliable data model. Research has shown that blockchain's distributed ledger can ensure tamper-proof logging of sensitive health information, eliminate the risk of unauthorized modification, and enhance trust overt stakeholders involved in disorder diagnostics and patient monitoring (Zoccali et al., 2024). Studies emphasize that blockchain not only supports the traceability of health records but also enforces accountability through smart contracts that regulate access control and data sharing over entities.

One study described how IoT-driven real-time data collection from wearable devices could be securely recorded and transmitted by blockchain. The findings showed that blockchain's cryptographic capabilities confirm end-to-end encryption of health metrics while preventing identity exposure or data manipulation during transmission (van der Wijst et al., 2019). A system is particularly beneficial in chronic disorder scenarios, where long-term and continuous monitoring is needed for preventive care and early intervention.

Further research has investigated the implementation of blockchain-IoT architectures specifically for predictive analytics. One framework demonstrated the use of supervised learning algorithms integrated into blockchain environments to forecast chronic kidney conditions that depend on patient sensor data. The decentralized nature of blockchain preserved data ownership while enabling collective model training over multiple health sectors (Chen et al., 2020). This improved both prediction accuracy and model transparency, making it suit for use in regulated healthcare domains.

In another model, researchers developed a blockchain-enabled IoT model to enhance early diagnosis in remote health setups. The proposed system successfully allowed local clinics to upload diagnostic test outcomes to a blockchain network where authorized hospitals and experts could access them in real time for secondary reviews or consultation. This framework significantly minimized diagnostic latency and ensured trust in the data being exchanged (Grubb, 2020). It also supported past analysis by maintaining immutable logs of past diagnostic events.

Additional work described the privacy concerns surrounding health data shared by ever-connected IoT devices. A blockchain framework was shown where only anonymized metadata, rather than raw unseen health data, was stored on-chain. This hybrid approach minimized blockchain's storage overhead while complying with privacy regulations like GDPR and HIPAA, using a viable balance between scalability and confidentiality. Moreover, IoT devices are operated with onboard access rules defined by blockchain-dependent smart contracts.

Real-time processing and analytics were also improved through blockchain's edge-suitable infrastructure. A model demonstrated that by giving lightweight blockchain nodes at the edge level, critical health data (e.g., ECG or blood glucose levels) could be validated and analyzed locally, thus minimizing latency while preserving integrity. The researchers confirmed that this method was particularly useful in health sector environments with intermittent cloud connectivity (Lum et al., 2022), lime rural health centers or disaster zones.

Blockchain's support for interoperability has also been described in systems where different hospital information systems need to share patient records. By a standardized blockchain ledger, various formats of medical data were successfully merged and interpreted without manual translation. This avoided data silos and streamlined care coordination among specialists, general physicians, and diagnostics labs (Lazzeri et al., 2015). The smart contract strategy facilitated uniform rules for data contribution and access control.

A separate model of work examined the sustainability of blockchain-IoT solutions in low-resource settings. In that context, energy-effective consensus algorithms like Proof-of-Authority (PoA) and defined Proof-of-Stake (DPoS) were implemented to maintain ledger integrity without the highest power demands associated with the traditional Proof-of-Work strategy. The results showed successful deployment of secure and decentralized predictive diagnostics systems using constrained edge devices (Chouchana et al., 2021).

Recent advancements in AI-enhanced blockchain-IoT networks have also demonstrated confirmation. One hybrid model merged neural networks with blockchain-governed sensor frameworks to detect abnormality in kidney function. Notably, the model was capable of securely aggregating and analyzing multi-source health data while maintaining data lineage and auditability. This model ensured trustworthy AI predictions due to the verifiable nature of the underlying information source (Narula et al., 2018).

For the first time, this paper proposes a new AI-supported Edge Computing for Chronic Kidney Disease (CKD) prediction using LSTM-CNN and Neuro-Fuzzy Systems to perform in IoMT environments to diagnose CKD in real-time (Pulakhandam et al., 2025). In particular, the Hybrid model utilizes CNNs for spatial feature extraction and LSTM networks to learn temporal patterns from patient data. Decision-making uses neuro-fuzzy logic, which makes the results more readable, one of the most significant drawbacks to many traditional "black-box" AI models. The predicted system was performed on the IoMT created medicinal datasets and accomplished a predominance of 94.6% that is outperforms single models of elements and maybe even partial mixtures, as it located the number one noticeable table, respectively. Its lean architecture helps to achieve real-time responses, and it can be efficiently deployed in remote healthcare scenarios (low computation power). The model also considers practical limitations like privacy, energy efficiency, and real-time inference. The authors find that this method can be an encouragement in such decentralized medical infrastructures, which will not only improve the accuracy but enhance the privacy of the disease spread prediction and hence may be extended for larger Disease forecasting after further improvement driven by federated learning. We showed how these methods can be combined to enhance early-stage disease detection and healthcare access.

In this paper, the authors propose a secure Federated Learning (FL) framework for CKD stage prediction by using Homomorphic Encryption (HE), to protect patient privacy and ensure the safety of their data (Hegde et al., 2025). Privacy risks are associated with many traditional centralized machine learning approaches that are not appropriate for sensitive medical data. In this context, the authors propose Federated Learning (FL) to perform collaborative training among hospitals without sharing the raw patient data. On top of this, HE provides encrypted computation for model updates so that adversaries cannot perform attacks like model inversion and membership inference. The approval was examined on real clinical instances taken from 4 simulated hospital clients, with each receiving a portion of the client records. Even in the encrypted case, it got to a not-too-shabby 98.6% accuracy, slightly below regular unprotected performance but still almost as good as the original model. The authors will additionally assess the computational overhead added by encryption and validate its potential for clinical deployment. The synergy of FL and HE allows us to create not only security but also scalability, while addressing data protection laws like HIPAA and GDPR. This research is of high importance within the emergent area of privacy-aware, secure AI in healthcare concerning chronic condition monitoring.

This paper examines the role of blockchain technology in the kidney transplant process (KTP), specifically its ability to securely store patient information, survival data, and management of activities (Almogadwy & Alqarafi, 2025). KTP is an essential treatment for people with end-stage kidney disease, and it requires seamless cooperation through evaluation, surgery, and post-transplant care. The abuse of KTP has significant ethical, moral, and operational impacts, which underscores the importance of reliable and auditable data, trust in the system, as well as data transparency, integrity, and traceability, which is made possible through blockchain's decentralized and immutable design. One of the issues with this area of research is the notion of scalability, as transplant data consists of heterogeneous data types that include structured data (OPTN, SRTR, and USRDS) and more diverse data from private not-for-profit transplant registries. Our proposed system would offer an architecture that encodes transplant data as it has been verified through medical, ethical, and administrative licensing steps into smart contracts and distributed ledgers, events, and evidence only when there are no ad hoc modifications. The architecture minimizes single points of failure, mitigates fraud opportunity, and provides for ongoing access for transplant history maintenance. Additionally, the architecture also provides regulatory persistence and will have longitudinal record capabilities for survival analysis. We believe that this paper discusses how blockchain systems would change the transplant data ecosystem and would also provide improved outcomes for patients and help restore trust in the digital health space.

The authors (Gogoi & Valan, 2024b) of this research created a multimodal deep learning system using CNN-LSTM networks to improve CKD prediction accuracy by using several data modalities, such as lab results, images, or patient histories. CNNs are used to find spatial features present in the medical images, while LSTMs are utilized to process sequential data, e.g. time-stamped lab values or symptoms. The methodology followed here allows for a complete analysis of a patient's health, with a boost to diagnostic sensitivity and specificity, using a multimodal deep learning network. This study applied its multi-layer, end-to-end system to a large clinical dataset, finding improved predictions against both the CNN and LSTM individually. Additionally, while many datasets in chronic disease experience imbalanced classes, the multi-modal deep learning showed enhanced performance when dealing with these unbalanced distributions. The authors were also excited by the representational (and interpretive) learning of the temporal features for chronic disease progression identification. In their framework, the authors addressed common limitations (such as lack of contextuality and time-series) in traditional ML pipelines. This work contributes to the larger purpose of applying deep learning to multi-source data (in healthcare contexts). Ultimately, this research could support a multi-provider approach to monitoring CKD through personalized risk stratification and continuous monitoring.

A new study describes a hybrid machine learning approach to the early detection of chronic kidney disease (CKD) that combines clustering (unsupervised learning), before using supervised predictive modelling, as well as the steps of feature optimization with clustering, prior to prediction and classification (Singh & Kakkar, 2025). The data pre-processing pipeline involved data cleaning, correction of typographical errors, missing value imputation with K-Nearest Neighbors (KNN), and feature optimization. Next, clustering methods were applied to study the latent pattern in the data, to identify cohorts of patients for whom CKD will develop (which also includes evidence of progressive disease). Considering the data-driven and systems approach of CKD detection, using clustering improves the deep learning of the predictive models. CKD was classified with an accuracy that was considered high yet could be improved upon. The function of combining clustering and classification was considered a promising direction for early detection and assessing risk. The study takes a positive position on data-driven approaches in health care, especially when utilising advanced tools and data pre-processing pipelines, with clinician-supported decision-making systems built on evidence and specialist systems that support early clinician intervention, which allows for further closing of the gap of early intervention. The authors noted a few possible future directions that include deep learning and larger and more diverse datasets to allow the deep learning methods to be generalizable and further clinically applicable.

The proposed hybrid machine learning framework for calculating CKD demonstrates that the combined grouping of clustering techniques with supervised learning improves diagnostic accuracy, as model predictions gain value when combined with clustering approaches (Saxena et al., 2025). Initially, the dataset undergoes extensive preprocessing, including error-correction, KNN-based imputation, and feature selection that eliminates factors that impede the quality of the dataset to ensure high-quality input before allowing the model to establish pattern recognition through self-supervised learning. In this research, the researchers established clustering methods to find non-observable groups of patients and examine patient risk stratification or disease progression, which ultimately can inform the retraining of predictive models based on the patients' data, determining CKD, ultimately resulting in refined CKD classification modification on previous classifications. The research suggested collecting both types of learning not only improves performance but also aids in the interpretation of clinical patterns useful to support clinicians for early diagnosis and patient-based care. The research explains the functionality of using unsupervised learning to determine improved predictive analytics, especially considering the potential future of deep learning initiatives that would require large volumes of community health data for analysis and information based on health literacy. Detecting CKD, as well as, rendering patient-based care through patterns supports the significance of AI in not only detecting CKD but, also, extending healthcare through personalized healthcare.

Finally, research has shown the application of consortium blockchain models for healthcare networks using multiple stakeholders. In one setup, a network of hospitals, insurance companies, and labs shared access to patient profiles using permissioned blockchain chains. These models ensured efficient claim processing, reduced diagnostic redundancy, and enabled cross-entity collaboration while maintaining strict access permissions and consensus, depending on validations (Hruska & Seifert, 2013).

III. PROPOSED SYSTEM

The proposed framework is a reliable and smart healthcare network. It accomplishes this by the application of the blockchain in conjunction with the Internet of Things (IoT), which provides for more accurate forecasting and diagnosis of renal diseases. First, it makes use of IoT-enabled sensors that are incorporated in wearable or clinical monitoring devices. These sensors collect patient health data in real time, such as vital signs and other medically important parameters like blood pressure, creatinine, and glomerular filtration rates. These data points are essential for detecting the onset of kidney disease. Next, these data are sent over a decentralized blockchain infrastructure that removes the need for a central authority, thus enhancing system resilience and decreasing the risk of single points of failure as described in Figure 1. The core of this process is the encryption of each record and the embedding of it in the blockchain's blocks, which makes the history tamper-proof. This means that not only is data integrity guaranteed, but also that data privacy is ensured since unauthorized parties will not be able to access or change the information. Blockchain use promotes openness and establishes a chain of custody that can be verified for every transaction, which is the basis of trust in health digitized systems. In order to utilize the gathered data to provide appropriate clinical information, a supervised learning algorithm is activated. This machine learning model is taught using medical data from the past to identify uncharacteristic behaviors associated with the initial phase and development of kidney diseases. It is able to read encrypted information streams without error to find irregularities and generate forecast insights, creating a kind of guide for clinical decision-making. The insights generated are subsequently made available to authorized medical professionals. This is possible via smart contracts. Programs that are automatically executed on the blockchain, which regulate accessing and sharing of data in accordance with established protocols for privacy and compliance. The whole journey of the data from its collection, encoding, examination, to the delivery of the results, is smooth, uninterrupted, and safe; therefore, there is no need for much human involvement while at the same time accuracy and confidentiality are maintained. The "smart" and distributed system indeed deals with significant issues in today's diagnostics field, including data privacy, instant analysis, and accurate prediction. The system is also a scalable solution for better healthcare services, particularly for chronic kidney disease management. It is a showcase of how the amalgamation of advanced technologies can transform medical diagnostics by turning them into safer, efficient, and more patient-oriented ones.

Figure 1. Flow of Proposed Framework.

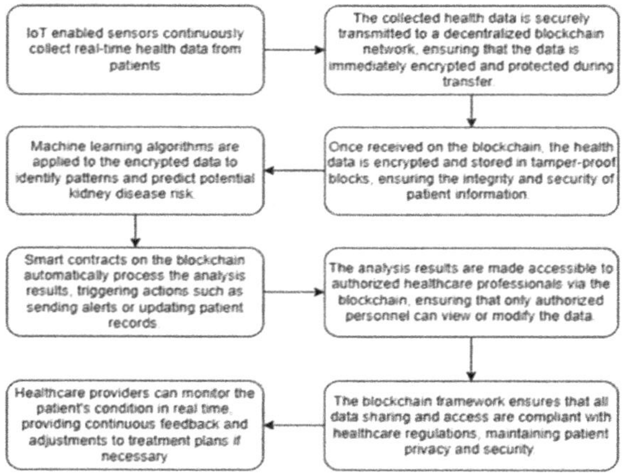

The proposed model for kidney disease prediction using blockchain-integrated IoT systems begins by aggregating real-time health data from IoT-based sensors placed on the patient. These sensors gather metrics like as blood pressure, heartbeat rate, kidney function indicators, and other relevant health parameters. The data will be securely transmitted to the blockchain network infrastructure, where encryption schemas ensure that the data is protected during transit, following (1)

$$E = E_{key}(D) \tag{1}$$

where E tells about the encryption, E_{key} will be the encryption function, and D will be the data. The data is then stored in the blockchain in a series of connected blocks, where each block gets encrypted, confirming data integrity using (2)

$$H = H_{hash}(B) \tag{2}$$

where H is the hash and B denotes a block. Once securely stored, supervisor learning schemas are applied for data analysis. These models estimate the health risk level of kidney disease depending on the data points, which may be given by (3)

$$Y = \beta_0 + \beta_1 X_1 + \beta_2 X_2 + \bullet\bullet\bullet + \beta_n X_n \tag{3}$$

where Y is the disorder risk, $X_1, X_2, \ldots, X_n$ are health metrics, and $\beta_0, \beta_1, \ldots, \beta_n$ are model coefficients. These models compute probabilities of disease development by (4)

$$P = \frac{1}{(1 + e - (\alpha + \beta X))} \tag{4}$$

where P is the predicted probability rate, α and β are the constants, and X gives health features. The system processes data utilizing feature extraction, which could be given by (5)

$$F = argmax(WX + b) \tag{5}$$

where F gives the selected features, W tells weights, and is a biasing term. Classification schemas like decision trees or neural-based networks are then used to categorize the data into various risk levels using (6)

$$C = \sum_i \omega_i x_i \,(i = 1 \; to \; n) \tag{6}$$

where C is the class, ω_i is the weights, and x_i is the feature values. Time-series analysis is used to identify abnormal trends through the relation (7)

$$T = \sum t_e - \lambda(t - t_0) \bullet X_t, (t = 1 \; to \; n) \tag{7}$$

where T tells about the detected trend, λ is the decay factor, and X_t is the data at time t. The prediction model will then be updated continuously using an online learning mode, where model metrics are adjusted using (8)

$$\theta_t = \theta_{t-1} - \eta \; \nabla \; \theta J(\theta) \tag{8}$$

where θ_t is the model metrics at time t, η is the learning rate, and J(θ) is the cost function factor. Blockchain confirms that the prediction system will be deployed in a decentralized manner, improving data transparency and trust, which is denoted by (9)

$$blockchain_n = \sum_i block_i, (i = 1 \; to \; n) \tag{9}$$

where $block_i$ ae the ith block to be the blockchain. Smart contracts get automated processes like as sending alerts by (10)

$$S = f(trigger) \tag{10}$$

where S tells about the contract action and triggers as the system's condition rates. Secure data-sharing protocols are also used, denoted by (11)

$$D_{share} = Encrypt(D) \tag{11}$$

To confirm that only authorized healthcare experts can access the results. The feedback loop for monitoring the patient's health condition is modeled in (12)

$$F_{feedback} = argmax\left(X_{current} - X_{baseline}\right) \tag{12}$$

The above relation compares the current data sets against baseline readings for adjusting the treatment plans. The blockchain confirms updates are recorded immutably by (13)

$$D_{new} = H\left(D_{previous}\right) \tag{13}$$

where D_{new} is the updated data block. Finally, the efficacy of the system is computed using performance parameters. The response time of the proposed model is computed by (14)

$$R = \frac{\Delta t}{N} \tag{14}$$

Where Δt is the time taken for processing N transactions. This system uses blockchain, IoT, and supervised learning to improve kidney disorder prediction accuracy and efficacy.

IV. RESULTS AND DISCUSSION

The main physiological data reading analysis measures various physiological parameters associated with kidney function and renal anomalies via health risk screening, offering important insights that enable early diagnosis and timely medical intervention. The revealed pattern in blood pressure measurements indicates numerous cases, however, where the registered values exceeded an upper preset limit. These fleeting but prominent peaks are of big importance. Besides, continuous hypertension is not only a main reason for kidney injury but also trouble that may arise alongside chronic hypertension, heart disease, and progressive nephropathy. The finding of such irregularities illustrates the role that uninterrupted surveillance plays, as it ensures that those who have not yet manifested the disease are identified on time to implement preventive strategies before the damage becomes irreversible. In relation to creatinine, the provided information shows that most of the values are within acceptable medical limits, though there are moments when the measurement goes beyond the range, suggesting that the kidneys are already under some pressure from the tasks they perform. This model, in terms of medical relevance, elevated creatinine as one of the first signs of a kidney filtration defect. However, while these changes were not very visible, their detection calls for more comprehensive testing in patients who demonstrate a continuous rise in their values to avoid the development of chronic kidney disease (CKD).On the other hand, the oscillation in the Glomerular Filtration Rate (GFR) is an indicator of a healthy and quite consistent pattern seen among most samples, with very few cases that even fell below the required safe level. This GFR is the measure of kidney function; therefore, the general good trend mirrors efficient renal filtration in many individuals. Instead, minor decreasing values are the first signals of the necessity of a more detailed clinical examination, so that timely medical treatment can be provided and long-term kidney damage can be prevented. Urine protein levels, which are yet another ailment biomarker alongside renal failure, have shown occasional shoots over the set threshold. The intermittent nature of these elevations should not be disregarded since proteinuria is the leading cause of glomerular injury, and if not addressed, it may lead to more severe illness.

In Figure 2, blood pressure rates are observed over 30 days. The average blood pressure varies over 120 mm Hg, but it occasionally passes the threshold level of 140 mm Hg, showing a higher risk of hypertension. The highlighted regions indicate that when blood pressure exceeds the threshold rate. On day 15, the blood pressure spikes to a value of 145 mm Hg, which may be above the threshold rate, emphasizing the need for further monitoring. The data shows that nearly 30% of the data points exceed the threshold slab, suggesting a risk of hypertension on various days.

Figure 2. Comparison of the BP of Patients over days.

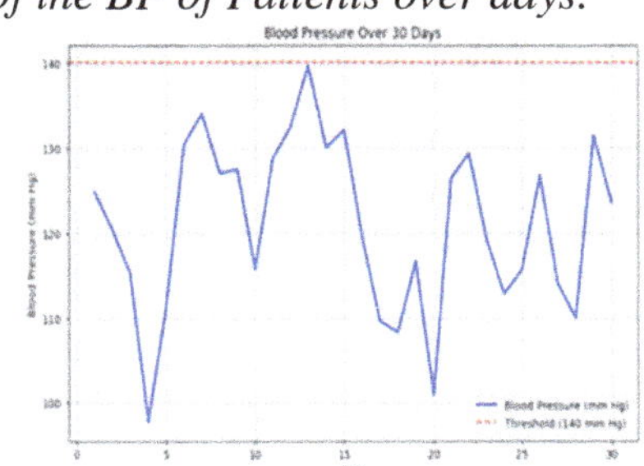

In Figure 3, the creatinine levels are distributed over 30 data points. Most of the creatinine rates are below the threshold to be 1.5 mg/dL, with many measurements focused around the 1.0 mg/dL mark. The highlighted region shows the frequency of values exceeding the threshold value, indicating the proportion of abnormal creatinine rates. Approximately 10% of data points pass the 1.5 mg/dL threshold rate, suggesting potential renal dysfunction that must be monitored.

Figure 3. Hippocampus analysis over 30 days

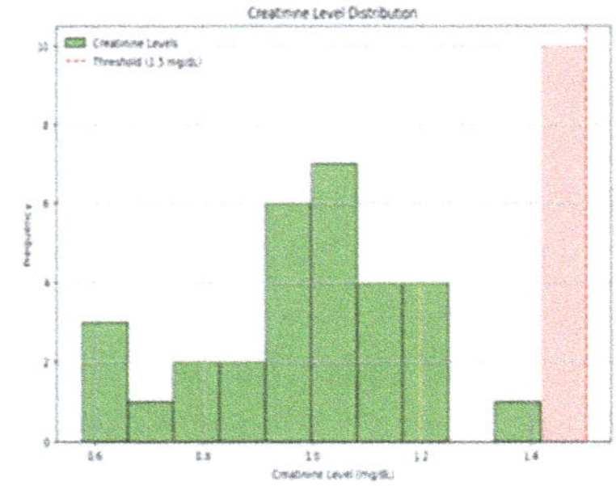

Figure 4 gives the Glomerular Filtration Rate (GFR) over 30 days. The GFR stays above the threshold value of 60 mL/min/1.73m^2 for the period, with a few drops below the threshold over days 18 and 22. The highlighted regions indicate days when GFR falls below the threshold rate, signaling a potential decline in kidney function. On day 18, the GFR dipped to 58 mL/min/1.73m^2, which is lower than the normal threshold rates. This drop suggests that the individual may be at risk for a kidney disorder, with 6% of data points showcasing values below the threshold value.

Figure 4. GFR evaluation of the proposed system.

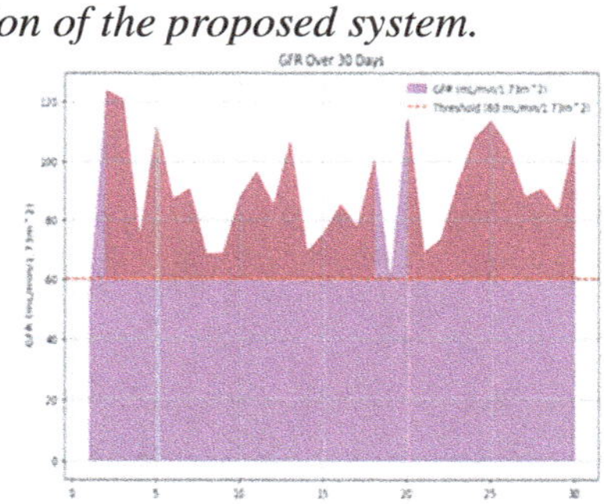

Figure 5. Protein presence analysis across various days

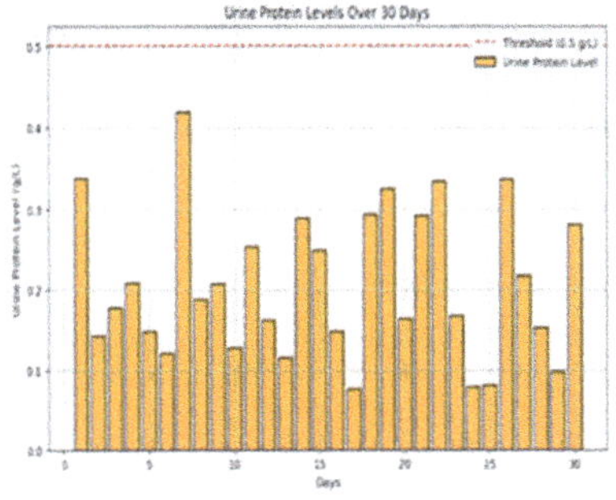

Finally, Figure 5 displays the urine protein rates over the same 30-day period. The urine protein levels generally remain lower than the threshold rate of 0.5 g/L, with a few instances passing the threshold, particularly around day 12. The highlighted regions correspond to days when the protein level exceeds the threshold rates. On day 12, the urine protein level peaks at a value of 0.6 g/L, surpassing the threshold rate, which suggests that the individual may have signs of kidney disorder or other related health risks. About 12% of the data points exceed the threshold rate, showing a need for closer attention.

Henceforth, the analysis of the simulated health data showcases varying trends over the metrics. Blood pressure exceeds the threshold value on a considerable number of days, with a 30% occurrence rate of hypertension. Creatinine levels are mostly at the normal rate, but 10% of data points indicate potential renal health risk. GFR remains largely above the threshold value, with a slight 6% of data points showcasing kidney function concerns. Lastly, urine protein levels pass the threshold rate 12% of the time, further showcasing potential kidney risks. These observations use the requirement for consistent monitoring and potential interventions depending on these health indicators. With the above evaluation, a performance comparison is tabulated in Table 1.

Table 1. Performance evaluation table of the proposed framework

Metrics	Threshold Slab	Averaged Value	Maximum Value reached	Percentage Crossing Threshold slab	Units
Blood Pressure	140 mm Hg	123 mm Hg	152 mm Hg	30%	mm Hg
Creatinine Level	1.5 mg/dL	1.12 mg/dL	1.67 mg/dL	10%	mg/dL
GFR	60mL/ min/1.73m^2	88mL/min /1.73m^2	110mL/min /1.73m^2	6%	mL/min /1.73m^2
Urine Protein Level	0.5 g/L	0.33 g/L	0.64 g/L	12%	g/L

Kidney function was assessed through key medical indicators of the system outlined in the table, which helps to evaluate the ability of the system to monitor patient health parameters within set clinical limits. Firstly, with blood pressure, which has a threshold of 140 mm Hg, the average recorded value across patients was 123 mm Hg, while the highest value reached 152 mm Hg. The frequency of values exceeding the threshold was 30%, which indicated that a dominant portion of the patients are at risk of hypertension, which can cause kidney damage to them and is a leading factor in the disease progression. Such high figures signify that a monitoring system like the one proposed must include prompt notification or even intervention to be able to deal with blood pressure increments efficiently.

Regarding creatinine level, the limit of 1.5 mg/dL is a parameter that characterizes the kidney filtration function. The average value of the patients was 1.12 mg/dL, and the highest value was 1.67 mg/dL. The overall results fall into the acceptable boundaries, while 10% of the figures went over the threshold, thus being able to signal the appearance of kidney stress or dysfunction in a very small group of patients. This shows the sensitivity of the system to uncover the individuals who are at the highest risk and therefore to provide these people with further investigation or lifestyle modification if needed in the prevention of kidney impairment. The Glomerular Filtration Rate (GFR), which is the parameter that shows the kidney's filtration capacity, has a limit of 60 mL/min/1.73m^2. The average value of the GFR was 88 mL/min/1.73m^2, and the highest was 110 mL/min/1.73m^2. On the bright side, only 6% of patients were below the cut-off, which shows healthy filtration rates in the group being tested. However, that small number should be followed over time carefully, since it is the surest marker of chronic kidney disease stages (CKD) if the GFR falls.

The urine protein level, a biomarker for kidney damage, was also defined as having a threshold of 0.5 g/L. The mean observed value was 0.33 g/L, while the highest accepted value was 0.64 g/L, and only 12% of the samples were above the threshold. Proteinuria that is over 0.5 g/L may be a sign of glomerular damage and may require the doctor's diagnosis. The detection of raised protein levels in more than a tenth of the samples, therefore, underscores the necessity of regular monitoring and indicates the proposed system's capability of signalling the first nephrological troubles and, consequently, the system is efficiently picking up abnormalities in the physiological ranges of all four key indicators—blood pressure, creatinine, GFR, and protein levels—thus providing a trustworthy means of early diagnosis and treatment in case of kidney-related health problems. These revelations prove the frame's ability not only to track chronic kidney disease but also to interact with it playfully before it takes place.

4.1. Advantages of the Proposed System

The proposed framework that integrates blockchain with IoT for kidney disease diagnosis is a huge leap forward that revolutionizes the way healthcare is conducted and addresses the shortcomings of the traditional healthcare system. By adopting blockchain's distributed and secure-by-design characteristics, the framework empowers the stakeholders' trust in data privacy and security, as the patient information is not only encrypted and stored but also tracked and signed at each transfer, thus creating a transparent and trustworthy ecosystem.

In contrast to conventional centralized architectures, which are prone to single points of failure and malicious activities, the decentralized model presented here is designed to be resilient against cyberattacks, giving users uninterrupted access to their data even if the network is experiencing interruptions or if hackers are attempting to infiltrate it. Smart sensors integration also empowers the framework with an IoT health monitoring system that collects patients' vital signs in real-time, such as blood pressure, glucose levels, and creatinine concentrations. This not only helps the doctors in early detection of any kidney abnormalities but also makes it possible for the data to be gathered from places that are far away from the resources and inaccessible to healthcare professionals, thus lowering the barriers to care. The integration of blockchain smart contracts upgrades the framework even more by orchestrating the permission mechanisms and implementing the strict rules of data usage so that only those who have the right to do so will be able to read or change patient records. This idea goes not only in the direction of obeying international privacy legislations such as HIPAA and GDPR but also mitigating the possibility of data leaks caused by internal threats or accidents. The system also facilitates interoperability among disparate medical systems and institutions, enabling seamless collaboration and data sharing across hospitals, diagnostic labs, and research organizations without manual reconciliation. It significantly reduces administrative overhead and duplication of diagnostic efforts, improving operational efficiency and cost-effectiveness.

Support for scalable predictive analytics is another benefit. Machine learning algorithms can be trained on blockchain-secured data to produce clear, interpretable insights about the progression of kidney disease. Since the data are verifiable and not subject to retroactive changes, healthcare professionals can rely on analytical results to make clinical decisions with more confidence. Besides that, lightweight blockchain protocols and edge processing capabilities guarantee that even in places with few connections or computers, the diagnostic process is still done in real time and is secure. The proposed framework, overall, is not only improving the accuracy of diagnosis but also protecting data privacy and security, enabling collaborative healthcare delivery, trustworthy medical decision-making, and an efficient, scalable, and technology-driven ecosystem.

4.2. Future Enhancement of the Proposed Framework

Furthermore, it is possible to future-proof the system by introducing quantum computing-resistant algorithms for cryptography in the blockchain layer. It will thus stay safe against new problems caused by the power of quantum computers for a long time. The employment of AI-based adaptive analytics in the process of diagnosis can also be the solution for an accuracy boost. It is possible by constantly educating from new patient data and changing prediction thresholds according to individual health status.

The blockchain can be used for this purpose to make it possible to explain and audit for transparency in clinical decisions. The usage of cross-chain interoperability protocols is another main upgrade. It allows the system to connect securely with other blockchain networks, such as insurance providers, pharmaceutical companies, or national health registries. This way, the system serves as a nerve center of the healthcare ecosystem, carrying data that is securely and efficiently transferred between various stakeholders.

Also, edge intelligence may be improved by allowing smart contracts to be executed on IoT devices, which means that decisions can be made automatically, emergencies can be solved instantly, and all this can happen without communication with the central server. The current setup can be additionally built to provide patients with a variety of chronic illnesses, such as liver or cardiovascular diseases; thus, it becomes a multi-disease monitoring and diagnostic platform. In conclusion, adding easy-to-use interfaces and mobile health applications can give patients the ability and flexibility to have access to their diagnostic data in real time, increase their participation in disease management, and enable a patient-centric model of care. These improvements would render the framework not just more powerful and clever but also more universally and locally relevant as well as more adaptable to the ever-changing world of personalized healthcare.

4.3. Social Welfare of the Proposed System

The suggested blockchain-IoT-supported system for identifying kidney disease has profound social welfare implications, the public health benefits being among the most important. The health system that is routed through blockchain technology ensures privacy, fosters trust, and, therefore, increases patients' ability to participate in their care journey along with the continuous, remote, real-time monitoring of kidney health and thus early detection of kidney-related anomalies. Thus, healthcare providers are empowered to act before the disease gets beyond control and coverage becomes necessary. This strategy reduces the costs of treatment, such as dialysis or transplantation of organs, that may occur due to the progression of the disease. This method is not only in line with achieving the goal of minimizing hospital visits and better treatment outcomes but also paves the way for continuous care even in rural areas, thus enabling a better quality of life for the patient. In addition, employing a blockchain network built on a secure architecture ensures that patient data remains protected, that they are ethically managed, and that only authorized healthcare professionals can access it. The IoT gadgets link can accomplish health democratization by equalizing the quality of diagnostic services available in both rural and urban areas. So, for example, people in remote places can obtain the best diagnosis, without just having to travel far to the city or hospital, or rely on volunteers. This, in turn, results in even greater healthcare inclusiveness. This also helps to narrow the gap in wealth and location with respect to the incidence of cases of diseases. On top of that, the system enables smarter contracts for data collecting, diagnostics, and sharing access, thereby minimizing administrative overhead and giving healthcare workers more time to focus on patient care, thus increasing the system's efficiency. The anonymization of large-scale diagnostic information can be helpful to public health officials and researchers to identify epidemiological trends, design interventions, and allocate resources better.

V. CONCLUSION

In conclusion, the analysis of the simulated health data reveals several important insights regarding key health metrics. Blood pressure exceeds the important threshold of 140 mm Hg on 30% of days, describing a significant occurrence of elevated levels and suggesting a health risk of hypertension that needs consistent monitoring and potential intervention. Creatinine rates are mostly within the normal ranges, but 10% of data points surpass the threshold rate of 1.5 mg/dL, indicating potential renal challenges that may warrant further investigation. The Glomerular Filtration Rate (GFR) generally stays above the threshold values of 60 mL/min/1.73m^2, with only 6% of data points showcasing a decline, suggesting that kidney function will generally be stable but should still be closely monitored for any earlier signs of impairment. Urine protein levels exceeding the threshold of 0.5 g/L on 12% of the days, which indicates potential kidney damage and reinforces the requirement of vigilant monitoring. These outcomes highlight the importance of ongoing health assessments and early health interventions, especially in cases where metrics show abnormal trends, to manage and prevent potential health complications effectively.

CONFLICTS OF INTEREST: The authors disclosed no potential conflicts of interest concerning the research, authorship, & publication of this article.

REFERENCES

Aldossary, S. M. (2023). Secured Framework for Assessment of Chronic Kidney Disease in Diabetic Patients. *Intelligent Automation & Soft Computing*, *36*(3), 3387–3404. Advance online publication. DOI: 10.32604/iasc.2023.035249

Ali Mir Arif Mir Asif. (2023). Analysis of Human Diseases using Artificial Neural Network and Blockchain Technology. *International Journal of Scientific Research in Computer Science, Engineering and Information Technology*. DOI: 10.32628/CSEIT23903149

Almogadwy, B., & Alqarafi, A. (2025). Fused federated learning framework for secure and decentralized patient monitoring in healthcare 5.0 using IoMT. *Scientific Reports*, *15*(1), 24263. DOI: 10.1038/s41598-025-06574-w PMID: 40624105

Arif, M. S., Mukheimer, A., & Asif, D. (2023). Enhancing the Early Detection of Chronic Kidney Disease: A Robust Machine Learning Model. *Big Data and Cognitive Computing*, *7*(3), 144. Advance online publication. DOI: 10.3390/bdcc7030144

Baskar, K., Muthuraj, S., Sangeetha, S., Vengatesan, K., Aishwarya, D., & Yuvaraj, P. S. (2023). Framework for Implementation of Smart Driver Assistance System Using Augmented Reality. *Lecture Notes in Electrical Engineering, 1021 LNEE*. DOI: 10.1007/978-981-99-1051-9_15

Bhardwaja, P., Ganapathy, K., Pathania, M., Naveen, K. H., Charan, J., Dutta, S., Gadepalli, R., Sriniva, S., Gupta, M. K., Goelj, A. D., Midha, N., Kumar, B., Sharma, M., Sharma, P., Banerjee, M., Mitra, P., & Misra, S. V., V., Subramaniant, G., … Kanchibhotlaz, D. (2021). *An integrative approach to clinical recovery for COVID-19 patients using an Ayurvedic formulation: A multicentric double-blind randomized control trial.* DOI: 10.21203/rs.3.rs-1165680/v1

Chen, Y., Zhang, W., Wang, N., Wang, Y., Wang, C., Wan, H., & Lu, Y. (2020). Thyroid Parameters and Kidney Disorder in Type 2 Diabetes: Results from the MET-AL Study. *Journal of Diabetes Research*, *2020*, 1–11. DOI: 10.1155/2020/8358102 PMID: 32337292

Chouchana, L., Preta, L.-H., Tisseyre, M., Terrier, B., Treluyer, J.-M., & Montastruc, F. (2021). Kidney disorders as serious adverse drug reactions of remdesivir in coronavirus disease 2019: A retrospective case–noncase study. *Kidney International*, *99*(5), 1235–1236. DOI: 10.1016/j.kint.2021.02.015 PMID: 33647327

Gayathri Hegde, M., Shrishti Bekal, M., Prasad, S. S., Shenoy, P. D., & Venugopal, K. R. (2022). Analysis of Secure EHR Storage Methods on Blockchain and Integrating ML to Predict Chronic Kidney Disease. *7th IEEE International Conference on Recent Advances and Innovations in Engineering, ICRAIE 2022 - Proceedings*. DOI: 10.1109/ICRAIE56454.2022.10054247

Geetha, K., Srivani, A., Gunasekaran, S., Ananthi, S., & Sangeetha, S. (2023). Geospatial Data Exploration Using Machine Learning. *Proceedings of the 4th International Conference on Smart Electronics and Communication, ICOSEC 2023*. DOI: 10.1109/ICOSEC58147.2023.10275920

Gogoi, P., & Valan, J. A. (2024a). Machine learning approaches for predicting and diagnosing chronic kidney disease: Current trends, challenges, solutions, and future directions. *International Urology and Nephrology*, *57*(4), 1245–1268. Advance online publication. DOI: 10.1007/s11255-024-04281-5 PMID: 39560857

Gogoi, P., & Valan, J. A. (2024b). Machine learning approaches for predicting and diagnosing chronic kidney disease: Current trends, challenges, solutions, and future directions. *International Urology and Nephrology*, *57*(4), 1245–1268. DOI: 10.1007/s11255-024-04281-5 PMID: 39560857

Grubb, A. (2020). Shrunken pore syndrome - a common kidney disorder with high mortality. Diagnosis, prevalence, pathophysiology and treatment options. *Clinical Biochemistry*, *83*, 12–20. DOI: 10.1016/j.clinbiochem.2020.06.002 PMID: 32544475

Hasanova, H., Tufail, M., Baek, U.-J., Park, J.-T., & Kim, M.-S. (2022). A novel blockchain-enabled heart disease prediction mechanism using machine learning. *Computers & Electrical Engineering*, *101*, 108086. DOI: 10.1016/j.compeleceng.2022.108086

Hegde, M. G., Ruthvika, B., Jain, R. B., Shenoy, P. D., Venugopal, K. R., & Canchi, A. (2025). A Privacy-Preserving Federated Learning Method with Homomorphic Encryption for Chronic Kidney Disease Stage Prediction. *Engineering, Technology &. Applied Scientific Research*, *15*(4), 26019–26026. DOI: 10.48084/etasr.11928

Hruska, K. A., & Seifert, M. (2013). Pathophysiology of Chronic Kidney Disease Mineral Bone Disorder (CKD-MBD). In *Primer on the Metabolic Bone Diseases and Disorders of Mineral Metabolism* (pp. 632–639). Wiley. DOI: 10.1002/9781118453926.ch77

Lazzeri, E., Ronconi, E., Angelotti, M. L., Peired, A., Mazzinghi, B., Becherucci, F., Conti, S., Sansavini, G., Sisti, A., Ravaglia, F., Lombardi, D., Provenzano, A., Manonelles, A., Cruzado, J. M., Giglio, S., Roperto, R. M., Materassi, M., Lasagni, L., & Romagnani, P. (2015). Human Urine-Derived Renal Progenitors for Personalized Modeling of Genetic Kidney Disorders. *Journal of the American Society of Nephrology*, *26*(8), 1961–1974. DOI: 10.1681/ASN.2014010057 PMID: 25568173

Lum, P. T., Sekar, M., Gan, S. H., Jeyabalan, S., Bonam, S. R., Rani, N. N. I. M., Ku-Mahdzir, K.-M., Seow, L. J., Wu, Y. S., Subramaniyan, V., Fuloria, N. K., & Fuloria, S. (2022). Therapeutic potential of mangiferin against kidney disorders and its mechanism of action: A review. *Saudi Journal of Biological Sciences*, *29*(3), 1530–1542. DOI: 10.1016/j.sjbs.2021.11.016 PMID: 35280538

Sumathi, M., & Raja, S. P. (2025). Explainable Artificial Intelligence-Based Diseases Diagnosis From Unstructured Clinical Data and Decision Making Using Blockchain Technologies. *International Journal of Interactive Multimedia and Artificial Intelligence, 9*(3), 40. DOI: 10.9781/ijimai.2025.02.003

Narula, S., Tandon, C., & Tandon, S. (2018). Role of Matrix Metalloproteinases in Degenerative Kidney Disorders. *Current Medicinal Chemistry*, *25*(15), 1805–1816. DOI: 10.2174/0929867325666171205143441 PMID: 29210632

Nasir, M. U., Zubair, M., Ghazal, T. M., Khan, M. F., Ahmad, M., Rahman, A. U., Al Hamadi, H., Khan, M. A., & Mansoor, W. (2022). Kidney Cancer Prediction Empowered with Blockchain Security Using Transfer Learning. *Sensors (Basel)*, *22*(19), 7483. Advance online publication. DOI: 10.3390/s22197483 PMID: 36236584

Nishat, M. M., Faisal, F., Dip, R. R., Shikder, M. F., Ahsan, R., Asif, M. A. A. R., & Hasan Udoy, M. (2020). Performance Investigation of Different Boosting Algorithms in Predicting Chronic Kidney Disease. *2020 2nd International Conference on Sustainable Technologies for Industry 4.0, STI 2020*. DOI: 10.1109/STI50764.2020.9350440

Nramban Kannan, S. K., Aseervatham, J., Moholkar, K., Palanimuthu, M., Marappan, S., Narendran, M., Sathar, B., & Sengan, S. (2024). A Model for Predicting Chronic Kidney Diseases Based on Medical Data Using Reinforcement Learning. *SN Computer Science*, *5*(4), 353. Advance online publication. DOI: 10.1007/s42979-024-02665-z

Panda, K., & Mazumder, A. (2024). *KidneyChain: Leveraging Blockchain & Artificial Intelligence for a Streamlined Organ Donation Solution*. DOI: 10.1101/2024.06.08.24308145

Praveen, R., Hemavathi, U., Sathya, R., Abubakkar Siddiq, A., Gokul Sanjay, M., & Gowdish, S. (2024). AI Powered Plant Identification and Plant Disease Classification System. *2024 4th International Conference on Sustainable Expert Systems (ICSES)*, 1610–1616. DOI: 10.1109/ICSES63445.2024.10763167

Pulakhandam, W., Rao, V. V., Samudrala, V. K., & Hemnath, R. (2025). Edge AI-Powered Chronic Kidney Disease Prediction: Integrating Dynamic CNN-LSTM Networks and Neuro-Fuzzy Models for Advanced Diagnosis and Monitoring in IoMT-Enabled Healthcare Systems. *International Journal of Engineering Research and Science & Technology*, *21*(1), 115–128.

Puri, V., Priyadarshini, I., Kataria, A., Rani, S., & Min, H. (2025). Privacy-First ML for Chronic Kidney Disease Prediction: Exploring a Decentralized Approach Using Blockchain and IPFS. *IEEE Access : Practical Innovations, Open Solutions*, *13*, 43178–43189. DOI: 10.1109/ACCESS.2025.3548645

Rezk, N. G., Alshathri, S., Sayed, A., & Hemdan, E. E.-D. (2025). Explainable AI for Chronic Kidney Disease Prediction in Medical IoT: Integrating GANs and Few-Shot Learning. *Bioengineering (Basel, Switzerland)*, *12*(4), 356. DOI: 10.3390/bioengineering12040356 PMID: 40281716

Roscigno, G., Quintavalle, C., Biondi-Zoccai, G., De Micco, F., Frati, G., Affinito, A., Nuzzo, S., Condorelli, G., & Briguori, C. (2021). Urinary Dickkopf-3 and Contrast-Associated Kidney Damage. *Journal of the American College of Cardiology*, *77*(21), 2667–2676. Advance online publication. DOI: 10.1016/j.jacc.2021.03.330 PMID: 34045024

Sampath, S., Prasad, M. L., Hussain, M. M., Parameswari, R., Anil Kumar, D., & Reddy, P. C. S. (2023). Ensemble Nonlinear Machine Learning Model for Chronic Kidney Diseases Prediction. *2023 IEEE 3rd Mysore Sub Section International Conference (MysuruCon)*, 1–6. DOI: 10.1109/MysuruCon59703.2023.10397049

Sangeetha, S., Suganya, P., Shanthini, S., Murthy, G. N. K., & Sathya, R. (2023). Crime Rate Prediction and Prevention: Unleashing the Power of Deep Learning. *Proceedings of the 4th International Conference on Smart Electronics and Communication, ICOSEC 2023*. DOI: 10.1109/ICOSEC58147.2023.10276012

Saxena, S., Saxena, S., Tahilramani, N., & Charanarur, P. (2025). Blockchain enhanced smart healthcare management for chronic diseases. *Discover Computing*, *28*(1), 112. DOI: 10.1007/s10791-025-09574-6

Senthil, G. A., Prabha, R., Latha, K., & Sridevi, S. (2025). A Block Chain-Enabled Novel Intelligent System Analysis for Medical Image Processing of Kidney Stone Prediction Using Deep Learning Techniques and Augmented Reality. In *Blockchain-Enabled Solutions for the Pharmaceutical Industry* (pp. 335–353). Wiley., DOI: 10.1002/9781394287970.ch16

Shruthi, K., & Poornima, A. S. (2023). Medical Data Asset Management and an Approach for Disease Prediction using Blockchain and Machine Learning. *International Journal of Engineering Trends and Technology*, *71*(4), 491–514. Advance online publication. DOI: 10.14445/22315381/IJETT-V71I4P242

Singh, A., & Kakkar, R. (2025). Optimizing Chronic Kidney Disease Prediction Through Advanced Data Imputation and Clustering. *2025 Fourth International Conference on Smart Technologies, Communication and Robotics (STCR)*, 1–7. DOI: 10.1109/STCR62650.2025.11020378

Sivaparthipan, C. B., Muthu, B. A., Fathima, G., Kumar, P. M., Alazab, M., & Díaz, V. G. (2022). Blockchain Assisted Disease Identification of COVID-19 Patients with the Help of IDA-DNN Classifier. *Wireless Personal Communications*, *126*(3), 2597–2620. Advance online publication. DOI: 10.1007/s11277-022-09831-7 PMID: 35789579

Supriya, M., & Chattu, V. K. (2021). A review of artificial intelligence, big data, and blockchain technology applications in medicine and global health. In *Big Data and Cognitive Computing* (Vol. 5, Issue 3). DOI: 10.3390/bdcc5030041

Tekkali, C. G., Natarajan, K., & Srinivasulu, A. (2025). A Comprehensive Study in the Kidney Transplantation Process with the Role of Blockchain Technology. In *Blockchain-Enabled Solutions for the Pharmaceutical Industry* (pp. 233–249). Wiley., DOI: 10.1002/9781394287970.ch12

van der Wijst, J., Belge, H., Bindels, R. J. M., & Devuyst, O. (2019). Learning Physiology from Inherited Kidney Disorders. *Physiological Reviews*, *99*(3), 1575–1653. DOI: 10.1152/physrev.00008.2018 PMID: 31215303

Zoccali, C., Mallamaci, F., Halimi, J.-M., Rossignol, P., Sarafidis, P., De Caterina, R., Giugliano, R., & Zannad, F. (2024). Chronic cardiovascular–kidney disorder: A new conceptual framework. *Nature Reviews. Nephrology*, *20*(4), 201–202. DOI: 10.1038/s41581-023-00789-8 PMID: 37968510

ADDITIONAL READING

Akbar, S., Seerapu, V. N., D.C, K., M. Sivachitra, M. S., Kumar Shanmugam, S., & Reddy Penubaka, K. K. (2025). IoT and AI-Driven Predictive Healthcare Systems: The Intersection of Machine Learning, Blockchain, and Healthcare Management Practices. *Journal of Neonatal Surgery*, *14*(13S), 13–24. DOI: 10.52783/jns.v14.3160

Lu, X. (2025). Internet of Things and Deep Learning Integration in Healthcare: A Promising Path for Disease Prediction. *Advances in Engineering and Intelligence Systems*, *004*(01), 73–83. DOI: 10.22034/aeis.2025.495819.1265

KEY TERMS AND DEFINITIONS

Blockchain: is an unalterable, decentralized digital ledger. It is a method of securely recording a transaction that is shared across many nodes.

IoT (Internet of Things): is the network of physical objects that use internet connectivity to collect and exchange data.

Machine learning algorithms: are computational methods that allow systems to learn from data, make predictions, and/or make decisions without being explicitly programmed to do so. For eg:- random forest, gradient boost and LSTM

The diagnostic pathology of kidney disorders: is the process of detecting and identifying abnormalities or diseases in the function of the kidney using clinical tests and imaging technologies.

Chapter 9

Osteoporosis Disease Prediction Using Machine Learning Algorithms

Rishita Das
https://orcid.org/0000-0002-0303-1983
Vellore Institute of Technology, Chennai, India

V. Santhi
https://orcid.org/0000-0002-4274-7474
Vellore Institute of Technology, Chennai, India

ABSTRACT

Osteoporosis is a major global health concern characterized by progressive bone loss, increasing the risk of fractures, particularly among postmenopausal women and the elderly. Traditional diagnostic methods, such as Dual-energy X-ray Absorptiometry (DXA), are expensive, resource-intensive, and often inaccessible in low-resource settings, leading to underdiagnosis and delayed intervention. This study explores the potential of machine learning (ML) algorithms in predicting osteoporosis using clinical, demographic, and biochemical data. Various ML models, including Naïve Bayes, XGBoost, and Random Forest, were evaluated for their predictive accuracy, with ensemble models demonstrating the highest performance. The results indicate that ML-based predictive models can serve as cost-effective, scalable, and non-invasive screening tools, enabling early detection and timely intervention. The study highlights the integration of ML in healthcare, paving the way for personalized osteoporosis risk assessment and improved patient outcomes.

DOI: 10.4018/979-8-3373-1479-2.ch009

1. INTRODUCTION

Osteoporosis is a major global health concern that silently weakens bones over time, leaving individuals vulnerable to fractures that can significantly impact their quality of life. It is often referred to as the "silent disease", as it progresses undetected until fractures occur, most commonly in the hip, spine, or wrist. These fractures not only cause physical pain and disability but also contribute to increased mortality and healthcare costs, especially among the elderly population (International Osteoporosis Foundation, 2020). According to the International Osteoporosis Foundation, more than 200 million people worldwide have osteoporosis, with India contributing a significant share due to its

In India, osteoporosis predominantly affects postmenopausal women and the elderly, where hormonal changes and lifestyle factors accelerate bone loss. Despite the increasing prevalence, awareness about osteoporosis remains low, and diagnostic rates are poor. Current diagnostic tools, such as Dual-energy X-ray Absorptiometry (DXA), are considered the gold standard but face significant limitations. DXA is expensive, requires specialized equipment, and is often unavailable in rural and underserved areas, leaving many at risk undiagnosed (Kanis, 1994). These challenges emphasize the urgent need for affordable, scalable, and accessible solutions for early osteoporosis detection, particularly in resource-constrained settings like India.

Machine learning (ML) has emerged as a transformative tool in healthcare, offering innovative solutions for disease prediction and diagnosis. ML algorithms can analyze complex patterns in clinical, demographic, and biochemical data, enabling accurate predictions without the need for costly imaging technologies (Chen et al., 2020). By leveraging easily available data, such as age, body mass index (BMI), lifestyle factors, and lab results, ML models can provide affordable, non-invasive, and scalable screening tools for osteoporosis. Additionally, ML can integrate diverse data types to enhance prediction accuracy, such as combining radiomics features from imaging data with clinical and demographic factors (Xie et al., 2022).

While existing research has demonstrated the potential of ML in osteoporosis detection, significant gaps remain. Many studies focus on specific types of data, such as imaging or clinical parameters, without exploring integrative approaches that can improve accuracy. Furthermore, there is limited research tailored to the unique healthcare challenges of India, where the population is diverse, and healthcare infrastructure is often inadequate (Meeta et al., 2020; NITI Aayog, 2019). Addressing these gaps requires models that not only deliver high accuracy but are also interpretable, cost-effective, and suitable for deployment in rural and underserved areas.

This study aims to develop a machine learning-based model for osteoporosis detection that leverages accessible, non-invasive data. By integrating clinical, demographic, and potentially biochemical data, the goal is to create a predictive tool that is both accurate and practical for large-scale use. Such a model has the potential to transform osteoporosis screening in India, enabling early detection, timely intervention, and improved patient outcomes while alleviating the economic burden on the healthcare system.

2. BACKGROUND

2.1. Osteopenia

Osteopenia is a condition characterized by bone mineral density (BMD) that is below the normal range but not low enough to meet the criteria for osteoporosis. According to the World Health Organization (WHO), osteopenia is defined by T-scores between -1.0 and -2.5. This stage acts as a precursor to osteoporosis and serves as a critical warning sign for individuals at risk of future fractures if bone loss progresses unchecked (Kanis et al., 2019).

The condition results from an imbalance in the bone remodelling process, where the rate of bone resorption exceeds bone formation. This imbalance can be caused by aging, hormonal changes (especially postmenopausal estrogen decline in women), lifestyle factors (smoking, sedentary habits, and excessive alcohol consumption), poor nutrition (inadequate calcium and vitamin D), and the use of medications such as corticosteroids.

2.1.1. Clinical Significance

Osteopenia often remains asymptomatic, making it difficult to detect without bone mineral density testing. Although fractures are less common during the osteopenic stage compared to osteoporosis, early identification is crucial to prevent further bone loss. Interventions at this stage can include:

1. **Lifestyle Modifications**: Incorporating weight-bearing exercises to improve bone strength and quitting smoking or excessive alcohol consumption.
2. **Nutritional Changes**: Ensuring sufficient intake of calcium and vitamin D to maintain bone health.
3. **Medical Monitoring**: Regular BMD tests to monitor progression and, in some cases, pharmacological treatments for those with additional risk factors.

2.1.2. Osteopenia in the Indian Context

In India, osteopenia is highly prevalent but often underdiagnosed due to minimal awareness, limited access to healthcare services, and cost barriers to routine screening. Studies indicate that 50–60% of Indian men and women over the age of 50 have reduced bone density, with many falling into the osteopenic range (Kaushal et al., 2018).

The lack of early diagnosis stems from factors such as a lack of understanding of bone health among the population, limited availability of diagnostic tools like dual-energy X-ray absorptiometry (DXA) scans in rural and underserved areas, and in case it is available the expense of regular BMD testing often deters individuals from seeking preventive care.

2.2. Osteoporosis

Osteoporosis is the most advanced stage of bone loss and is characterized by a significant reduction in bone mineral density (BMD), accompanied by a high susceptibility to fractures. According to the World Health Organization (WHO), osteoporosis is diagnosed when the T-score is ≤ -2.5. It is a silent yet progressive disease, often going undetected until a fracture occurs, making it one of the leading causes of morbidity among aging populations.

2.2.1. Pathophysiology and Risk Factors

Osteoporosis arises due to an imbalance in the bone remodeling process, where the resorption of bone by osteoclasts outpaces bone formation by osteoblasts. This imbalance leads to reduced bone mass, microarchitectural deterioration, and increased fragility. The condition disproportionately affects certain populations, including:

1. Postmenopausal Women: Estrogen plays a critical role in maintaining bone density. Hormonal changes during menopause accelerate bone loss, leading to a steep decline in BMD.
2. Elderly Individuals: Aging reduces bone formation, increases bone resorption, and impairs calcium absorption, all of which contribute to osteoporosis.
3. Lifestyle Factors: Smoking, excessive alcohol intake, and a sedentary lifestyle exacerbate the risk of osteoporosis.

2.2.2. Clinical Impact

Fractures associated with osteoporosis, particularly of the hip, vertebrae, and wrist, place a significant burden on patients and healthcare systems. Hip fractures are especially devastating, as they often result in loss of mobility, reduced independence, and increased mortality (Kanis et al., 2019). Vertebral fractures may lead to chronic pain, spinal deformity, and a notable decline in quality of life (International Osteoporosis Foundation, 2022).

Recent studies further emphasize the importance of early and accessible screening for osteoporosis. For example, Higuchi et al. (2025) found that combining X-ray imaging with region-specific self-assessment tools improved fracture risk screening among hip surgery patients, highlighting the potential for more inclusive and practical diagnostic workflows.

2.2.3. Osteoporosis in India

Osteoporosis is a growing public health concern in India, with studies estimating that more than 61 million Indians are affected, of which 80% are women. Despite its prevalence, osteoporosis remains underdiagnosed and undertreated, particularly in rural and low-income areas.

Limited access and high costs associated with diagnostic facilities such as DXA scans in rural areas result in delayed detection.

Calcium and vitamin D deficiencies, common in the Indian diet, further compound the problem (Kaushal et al., 2018).

2.2.4. Limitations of Traditional Diagnostic Methods

Dual-energy X-ray absorptiometry (DXA) remains the gold standard for diagnosing osteoporosis, as it provides precise measurements of BMD (Kanis, 1994). However, DXA has notable limitations (World Health Organization, 2007):

1. **Accessibility**: DXA machines are expensive and often unavailable in resource-limited settings.
2. **Cost**: The high cost of DXA scans makes them unaffordable for a large portion of the Indian population.
3. **Narrow Focus**: DXA evaluates only BMD and does not incorporate other important factors such as age, body mass index (BMI), or biochemical markers that influence fracture risk.

Furthermore, while imaging-based approaches such as plain radiographs are more accessible than DXA, they still face diagnostic limitations when used in isolation. Higuchi et al. (2025) reported that even when paired with self-assessment tools, X-ray-based screening showed variable diagnostic accuracy. To address this gap, Kumar et al. (2023) applied a fuzzy rank–based ensemble model on knee radiographs, achieving high accuracy and demonstrating the potential of machine learning to enhance the diagnostic value of traditional imaging techniques.

2.3. Need for the Study

The escalating prevalence of osteoporosis in India, coupled with the limitations of traditional diagnostic methods, underscores the urgent need for innovative solutions (Kaushal et al., 2018) to address the challenges of early detection and prevention. Osteoporosis and its precursor, osteopenia, often progress silently until fractures occur, leading to significant morbidity, mortality, and financial strain on individuals and healthcare systems. The high cost, limited availability, and narrow focus of standard diagnostic tools such as Dual-energy X-ray Absorptiometry (DXA) (Meeta et al., 2020; NITI Aayog, 2019) further exacerbate the issue, especially in rural and underserved regions. Additionally, Anam et al. (2021) conducted a comprehensive review highlighting the effectiveness of machine learning in analyzing trabecular bone patterns from imaging data. Their findings further support the need to develop ML-based diagnostic models that go beyond conventional BMD measurements and incorporate complex structural and demographic features.

2.3.1. Machine Learning as a Transformative Solution

Machine learning (ML) has emerged as a promising tool to address these challenges by leveraging complex patterns within clinical, demographic, and biochemical data to deliver accurate and scalable risk predictions. Unlike traditional methods, ML models can integrate diverse data sources to create a comprehensive understanding of an individual's bone health. Variables such as age, BMI, lifestyle factors, and laboratory markers can be combined to refine predictions, bypassing the reliance on costly imaging techniques like DXA.

Recent advancements in ML highlight its potential in healthcare applications. For instance:

- Integration of Clinical and Imaging Data: Studies have shown that incorporating radiomics with clinical data significantly improves diagnostic accuracy, providing nuanced insights into bone quality beyond what traditional imaging can offer (Xie et al., 2022).

- Use of Biochemical Markers: Laboratory markers such as alkaline phosphatase, homocysteine, and calcium levels have proven valuable in enhancing the predictive power of ML models for bone health (Kanis et al., 2019).
- Customization for Regional Needs: Tailored ML models can adapt to India's unique demographic and healthcare landscape, addressing regional risk factors such as dietary calcium deficiencies, high prevalence of vitamin D deficiency, and socioeconomic barriers to healthcare access (Kaushal et al., 2018).

2.3.2. Objectives of the Study

This study aims to develop a machine learning model designed to predict the risk of osteoporosis and osteopenia using accessible, non-invasive data. By analyzing key attributes associated with bone health deterioration, such as age, BMI, T-scores, and lifestyle factors, the model seeks to provide a cost-effective alternative to DXA scans. The ultimate goal is to create a tool that is:

1. Cost-Effective: Affordable for widespread adoption in low-resource settings.
2. Scalable: Capable of handling large-scale screening programs in rural and underserved areas.
3. Accurate: Delivering precise risk assessments that enable early intervention.

2.3.3. Implications for Healthcare in India

The development and implementation of such a model could revolutionize osteoporosis detection and prevention in India by:

- Enabling Early Intervention: Identifying individuals at risk of bone loss before fractures occur, allowing for timely preventive measures such as dietary changes, lifestyle modifications, or medical treatments.
- Reducing Fracture Risk: Minimizing the incidence of debilitating fractures, particularly in vulnerable populations such as postmenopausal women and the elderly.
- Alleviating Economic Burden: Reducing the long-term healthcare costs associated with fracture treatment and rehabilitation.
- Enhancing Accessibility: Bridging the gap in healthcare services between urban and rural areas by providing a scalable, portable, and reliable screening solution.

By leveraging recent advancements in machine learning and integrating accessible data, this study seeks to address the critical gaps in osteoporosis and osteopenia detection. Such a model holds the potential to transform the landscape of bone health management in India, fostering better quality of life and reducing the societal and economic impact of this widespread condition.

3. LITERATURE REVIEW

3.1. Prior Work and Approaches

Tzou et al. (2023) compared linear regression (MLR) and four machine learning (ML) models—Classification and Regression Tree (CART), Naïve Bayes (NB), Random Forest (RF), and Extreme Gradient Boosting (XGBoost)—for predicting osteoporosis risk in Chinese women aged 55 and older. Using data from the Taiwan Osteoporosis Survey, which included 24,412 records, they focused on predictors of bone mineral density (BMD) such as age, body mass index (BMI), uric acid (UA), and estimated glomerular filtration rate (eGFR). With RF set to 100 estimators and XGBoost with a learning rate of 0.1, XGBoost achieved the highest accuracy at 89%, while MLR had 75%. This study highlighted ML's superiority over MLR for osteoporosis screening, especially XGBoost for its predictive accuracy and interpretability. Inui et al. (2023) applied machine learning to predict low bone mineral density (BMD) in elderly women, utilizing blood test data to potentially replace dual-energy X-ray absorptiometry (DXA). Using a dataset of 2,541 patients from a Japanese osteoporosis clinic, five models—Logistic Regression, Decision Tree, Random Forest, Gradient Boosting, and LightGBM—were implemented. The LightGBM model, optimized with 1000 iterations and a maximum depth of 6, achieved the highest accuracy at 83.4% and an AUC of 0.961. The study identified BMI, age, and ALT as key predictors, demonstrating that LightGBM's efficiency could improve osteoporosis screening accessibility, especially in underserved areas.

Meanwhile, He et al. (2025) aimed to develop a machine learning model to predict femoral neck bone mineral density (FNBMD) in elderly men, addressing the gap in routine osteoporosis screening for this demographic. Using the National Health and Nutrition Examination Survey (NHANES) data, they implemented eight machine learning models: Multivariable Linear Regression (MLR), Decision Tree Regression (DTR), Random Forest Regression (RFR), Support Vector Regression (SVR), Gaussian Process Regression (GPR), Extreme Gradient Boosting Regression (XGBR), Extra-Trees Regression (ETR), and Multi-layer Perceptron Regression (MLPR). After optimizing parameters, RFR achieved the highest predictive performance, with $R^2 = 0.712$ and RMSE = 0.072. Feature importance analyses, supported by SHAP values, identified age, BMI, poverty income ratio (PIR), and serum calcium as key predictors, indicating RFR's efficacy in real-time FNBMD assessment for early osteoporosis detection. Yang et al. (2023) developed the Preclinical Osteoporosis Screening Tool (POST) using machine learning models to improve early osteoporosis risk identification among Hong Kong's Chinese population. The study utilized a dataset of 800 participants from six clinics, combining clinical risk factors such as age, BMI, height loss, vitamin D intake, and lifestyle elements. Models applied included Gradient Boosting Machine (GBM), Support Vector Machine (SVM), Naïve Bayes (NB), and Logistic Regression (LR), with Naïve Bayes achieving the highest AUC of 0.86. This study highlights POST's potential in preclinical osteoporosis screening, balancing high sensitivity and specificity while optimizing the accessibility of key predictive factors.

Ramesh and Santhi (2021) applied a multi-class support vector machine (SVM) model to classify osteoporosis and osteopenia using various kernel functions. They achieved the highest accuracy with the Gaussian kernel at 97.3%, sensitivity at 96.3%, and specificity at 97.7%. Other kernels yielded the following accuracies: polynomial (93.2%), linear (94.4%), RBF (95.3%), exponential (92.3%), Laplace RBF (91.3%), sigmoid (95.9%), and Anova (90.6%). The dataset, sourced from NHANES III (National Health and Nutrition Examination Survey by the CDC), provided essential clinical and demographic data, including BMD values. Each kernel was tuned with specific parameters to optimize performance. For the Polynomial kernel, parameters included the degree (d) and a coefficient (c) to balance higher-order terms. The Gaussian kernel used a width parameter (σ) to control the sensitivity range. RBF relied on gamma (γ) to influence data point range, while Linear used regularization (C) to balance error rate and complexity. The Exponential kernel adjusted width (σ) for influence decay, Laplace RBF focused on variance impact, and Sigmoid utilized alpha and beta to map data via hyperbolic tangent. SVM's adaptability in high-dimensional spaces, combined with kernel-specific parameter tuning, made it ideal for clinical data classification.

Kwon et al. (2022) utilized ensemble machine learning models to pre-screen osteoporosis in postmenopausal Korean women, aiming to improve early diagnosis using non-invasive methods. Data from the Korea National Health and Nutrition Examination Survey (KNHANES) were used, focusing on 1,431 participants aged 40–69. They employed Random Forest (RF), AdaBoost, and Gradient Boosting Machine (GBM), with hyperparameters optimized via grid search and five-fold cross-validation. RF and AdaBoost both achieved an AUROC of 0.92, with AdaBoost slightly outperforming others in accuracy (0.849). This study demonstrated that combining survey and biochemical checkup features (Model C) enhanced predictive accuracy, offering a practical tool for early osteoporosis diagnosis.

Ou Yang et al. (2021) developed machine learning models to predict osteoporosis using clinical health examination data from a Taiwanese medical center. The study included 5,982 participants aged 50 and older. They tested Artificial Neural Network (ANN), Support Vector Machine (SVM), Random Forest (RF), K-Nearest Neighbors (KNN), and Logistic Regression (LoR). The RF model, configured with 300 trees for men and 600 for women, achieved the highest AUROC at 0.843 for men and 0.811 for women. ANN also performed well with optimized learning rates and dropout settings. These models significantly outperformed the traditional Osteoporosis Self-Assessment Tool for Asians (OSTA), suggesting enhanced early detection capabilities for clinical use.

Makond et al. (2022) developed the Decision Tree for Postmenopausal Osteoporosis Screening (DTPOS) tool, using decision tree (DT) algorithms to screen for osteoporosis in postmenopausal Thai women. The study utilized 356 patient records from Ramathibodi Hospital, Bangkok, and applied four DT algorithms: Classification and Regression Tree (CART), Chi-Squared Automatic Interaction Detection (CHAID), Quick, Unbiased, Efficient Statistical Tree (QUEST), and C4.5. CHAID was selected as the optimal model due to its superior sensitivity (92.3%) and accuracy (80.4%), alongside its ability to provide simple and interpretable rules. Age and weight were identified as the most significant predictors, making CHAID particularly effective for community-based screening in resource-limited settings.

Jabbar et al. (2024) aimed to diagnose osteoporosis in postmenopausal women using the AdaBoostM1 algorithm on BMD data from Kaggle. The dataset included 169 records with variables like age, weight, height, medication history, and fracture status. AdaBoostM1 achieved 88.8% accuracy, an AUC of 0.87, and an F1-score of 0.88, showing high sensitivity and suitability for community-level screening. This model was compared with other techniques: CNNs achieved 85% accuracy but required intensive resources, while RBF and CART performed well but lacked interpretability. VGG16 and KNN models showed moderate accuracy but were impractical for large-scale use. AdaBoostM1 stood out for balancing performance with simplicity, making it a promising tool for affordable osteoporosis screening in community healthcare.

In the study by De Sire et al. (2022), the correlation between vitamin D deficiency and osteoporosis in breast cancer patients was analyzed using multiple factor analysis (MFA) combined with machine learning clustering techniques. They applied MFA to assess how variables, such as lumbar spine bone mineral density (LS BMD), vitamin D levels, age, and BMI, contributed to osteoporosis risk. MFA enabled them to create clusters that categorized individuals into distinct groups based on shared characteristics. The researchers first calculated Pearson's correlation coefficient, which revealed a significant positive correlation between LS BMD and serum 25(OH)D3 levels ($r = 0.30$, $p = 0.025$). Following this, they employed MFA to arrange the variables along two principal dimensions (Cartesian axes) to visualize the relationships. The variables, represented as vectors, helped determine how factors like BMD and vitamin D influenced an individual's positioning within clusters. K-means clustering further validated these clusters, grouping individuals based on similar BMD and vitamin D trajectories. This comprehensive approach allowed De Sire et al. to conclude that both BMD and vitamin D levels were influential in characterizing bone health in breast cancer patients. Ma et al. (2023) explored the genetic and clinical correlations between Parkinson's disease (PD) and osteoporosis, using data from a hospital-based sample of 95 PD patients and 99 healthy controls collected at a Chinese neurology center. They tested five models—Logistic Regression (LR), Random Forest (RF), Decision Tree (DT), Support Vector Machine (SVM), and Naïve Bayes (NB)—to detect biomarkers affecting bone mineral density (BMD) in PD patients. Random Forest, optimized with 100 trees, achieved the best accuracy at 86%, and identified hub genes like SNAP25 and AQP4 as influential indicators. RF's strong performance positions it as a useful diagnostic tool for assessing osteoporosis risk in PD patients indicating RFR's efficacy in real-time FNBMD assessment for early osteoporosis detection. Wen et al. (2021) examined the correlation between osteoporosis and newly diagnosed type 2 diabetes mellitus (T2DM) in Chinese patients, aiming to identify osteoporosis-specific risk factors in diabetic populations. The study included 244 T2DM patients and 218 non-diabetic controls from Tongji Hospital, Shanghai. Bone mineral density (BMD) was measured, and bone turnover markers such as TRACP-5b, BALP, and osteocalcin (OC) were recorded. Results revealed that age, BMI, and menopausal status are common osteoporosis risk factors for diabetic and non-diabetic patients, while elevated levels of TRACP-5b, BALP, and OC were unique to the T2DM group. These findings suggest that T2DM patients possess distinct metabolic characteristics affecting bone health, potentially informing future diabetes-specific osteoporosis screening.

St. Jeor et al. (2020) investigated enhanced osteoporosis diagnostics for lumbar spine surgery patients, comparing several criteria to better identify at-risk individuals preoperatively. This retrospective study of 244 patients from two academic centers used DXA T-scores, CT Hounsfield units (HU), National Bone Health Alliance (NBHA) guidelines, and a new "expanded spine" criterion integrating trabecular bone score (TBS) with other risk factors. The expanded spine criteria classified patients as osteoporotic if they met NBHA standards, had HU < 110, or displayed degraded TBS (<1.2) with osteopenic T-scores. Results showed DXA alone identified 25.4% of patients with osteoporosis, while the expanded spine criteria captured 81.9%, highlighting a broader risk profile. These findings suggest combining DXA with HU and TBS offers a more comprehensive assessment, potentially reducing postoperative fracture risk by guiding preoperative bone health optimization.

Dzierżak and Omiotek (2022) explored the use of deep convolutional neural networks (DCNNs) for osteoporosis diagnosis using lumbar spine CT images, focusing on the L1 vertebra. Their study employed a dataset of 400 images from 100 patients (50 healthy, 50 with osteoporosis) and applied six pre-trained DCNN models: VGG16, VGG19, MobileNetV2, Xception, ResNet50, and InceptionResNetV2. Given the small dataset size, the authors used transfer learning with ImageNet weights and data augmentation to improve model performance. The VGG16 model, which has a lower topological depth than others, achieved the best accuracy at 95%, with sensitivity and specificity of 96% and 94%, respectively. This model's superior results were attributed to its relatively simple architecture, which effectively avoided overfitting. Dzierżak and Omiotek noted that models with higher complexity, such as InceptionResNetV2, performed well but were more prone to overfitting due to limited training data. Their findings demonstrate that transfer learning, especially with models like VGG16, is effective in medical image classification where data is often limited. The study underscores the potential of using pre-trained, lower-complexity DCNNs for accurate, efficient osteoporosis diagnosis, supporting their use in clinical settings.

Study by Qiu et al. (2024) investigated the effectiveness of various machine learning (ML) and deep learning (DL) models for osteoporosis risk prediction using demographic and clinical data from the Louisiana Osteoporosis Study (LOS), which included 8,134 individuals over 40 years old. The models evaluated included a deep neural network (DNN), random forest (RF), artificial neural network (ANN), k-nearest neighbor (KNN), support vector machine (SVM), and the traditional osteoporosis self-assessment tool (OST). Among these, the RF model achieved the highest accuracy at 75.7%, closely followed by DNN at 75.3%, ANN at 74.7%, SVM at 74.5%, and OST at 73.1%, while KNN had the lowest accuracy at 65.1%. Despite RF's highest accuracy, the DNN model outperformed all in overall predictive ability, achieving an AUC of 0.848. Key predictors identified by the DNN included age, weight, grip strength, and lifestyle factors such as alcohol and tobacco use. This study demonstrates the potential of DNN to enhance early osteoporosis detection, making it a valuable tool in clinical applications for timely intervention.

Xie et al. (2022) developed a machine learning-based radiomics model using quantitative computed tomography (QCT) to distinguish osteoporosis and osteopenia. A retrospective dataset of 635 patients was divided into training (414 patients) and test cohorts (176 patients). Radiomics features were extracted from the third lumbar vertebra (L3) QCT images. The study used minimum redundancy maximum relevance (mRMR) and least absolute shrinkage and selection operator (LASSO) for feature selection, reducing 851 radiomics features to six predictive ones. A combined model incorporating clinical factors (age, alkaline phosphatase, and homocysteine) with radiomics features achieved an AUC of 0.96, significantly outperforming a clinical-only model (AUC = 0.81). This combined clinical-radiomics model demonstrates high potential as a reliable diagnostic tool for osteoporosis.

Wen et al. (2021) examined the correlation between osteoporosis and newly diagnosed type 2 diabetes mellitus (T2DM) in Chinese patients, aiming to identify osteoporosis-specific risk factors in diabetic populations. The study included 244 T2DM patients and 218 non-diabetic controls from Tongji Hospital, Shanghai. Bone mineral density (BMD) was measured, and bone turnover markers such as TRACP-5b, BALP, and osteocalcin (OC) were recorded. Results revealed that age, BMI, and menopausal status are common osteoporosis risk factors for diabetic and non-diabetic patients, while elevated levels of TRACP-5b, BALP, and OC were unique to the T2DM group. These findings suggest that T2DM patients possess distinct metabolic characteristics affecting bone health, potentially informing future diabetes-specific osteoporosis screening.

In conclusion, the reviewed literature underscores the growing impact of machine learning (ML) and neural networks (NN) in advancing osteoporosis research, particularly in areas such as risk prediction, diagnosis, and screening. Traditional methods like linear regression (LR), though useful, were consistently outperformed by ML approaches that capture complex, non-linear relationships in data. For instance, Tzou et al. (2023) demonstrated that while linear regression achieved moderate accuracy, models like XGBoost significantly outperformed it, achieving an accuracy of 89% in predicting osteoporosis risk.

The integration of genetic, clinical, and demographic data into ML models has also proven valuable. For example, Ma et al. (2023) used Random Forest to establish correlations between Parkinson's disease and osteoporosis, identifying biomarkers like SNAP25 and AQP4 as significant predictors of bone mineral density (BMD). Similarly, Wen et al. (2021) incorporated biomarkers such as TRACP-5b and osteocalcin into their models to enhance osteoporosis risk prediction among patients with type 2 diabetes mellitus. Such findings suggest that the incorporation of molecular and genetic data can improve the precision of osteoporosis diagnosis, providing a foundation for personalized medicine.

Neural networks (NN) also play an increasingly prominent role in osteoporosis research, as evidenced by studies like Qiu et al. (2024), where deep neural networks (DNN) achieved robust performance in predicting osteoporosis risk with an AUC of 0.848. Inui et al. (2023) demonstrated that LightGBM, a gradient boosting framework, significantly outperformed other models in predicting BMD using blood test data, highlighting its scalability and accuracy. Furthermore, tools such as the Preclinical Osteoporosis Screening Tool (POST) by Yang et al. (2023) and the Decision Tree for Postmenopausal Osteoporosis Screening (DTPOS) by Makond et al. (2022) illustrate how ML models can be tailored to specific populations and clinical needs, achieving a balance between sensitivity, specificity, and interpretability.

Overall, these advancements highlight a few key themes: the superior predictive power of ML models over traditional LR methods, the practical applicability of ML in diverse settings, and the growing role of NN in handling large, complex datasets for osteoporosis research. By integrating clinical, demographic, and genetic data, ML and NN models enable more precise and accessible tools for early diagnosis and risk prediction. The diversity of approaches, ranging from Naïve Bayes to deep learning, demonstrates the adaptability of ML techniques to various research objectives and patient populations. As research in this field progresses, these findings provide a strong foundation for developing innovative and efficient diagnostic tools that can improve patient outcomes and reduce the burden of osteoporosis worldwide.

3.2. Limitations of the Literature Review

While the literature on osteoporosis prediction using machine learning is rich and evolving, several important limitations remain unaddressed. Firstly, a significant proportion of the existing studies utilize datasets that are region-specific or demographically constrained, often based on populations from a single country or age group. This limits the generalizability and external validity of the models across diverse populations, particularly in developing countries where osteoporosis remains underdiagnosed. Secondly, many models have been evaluated in purely experimental or academic settings without real-world clinical validation. This lack of clinical deployment raises concerns about the practical applicability of these solutions in medical decision-making.

Additionally, a noticeable gap exists in the integration of multimodal data. Most studies either rely solely on clinical parameters or radiographic features but do not combine them with other potentially predictive data such as genetic markers, dietary intake, physical activity, or hormonal profiles. Such multimodal fusion could significantly improve diagnostic accuracy. Moreover, few studies prioritize model interpretability, which is crucial in a healthcare context where clinicians must understand and trust model outputs. Finally, there is limited focus on the longitudinal analysis of osteoporosis progression over time, which is essential for continuous monitoring and treatment planning. These limitations present valuable directions for future research.

4. MATERIALS AND METHODS

4.1. Data Descriptions

The dataset used in this study was obtained from the National Health and Nutrition Examination Survey (NHANES), a program designed and administered by the National Center for Health Statistics (NCHS) under the Centers for Disease Control and Prevention (CDC), United States. NHANES is a long-standing, publicly accessible survey system that provides comprehensive health and nutritional data representative of the U.S. population. It combines interviews, physical examinations, and laboratory testing to produce high-quality, anonymized datasets suitable for population health research, including chronic disease monitoring such as osteoporosis.

For this study, we compiled data from five NHANES cycles: 2005–2006, 2007–2008, 2009–2010, 2013–2014, and 2015–2016. These years were selected because they included detailed Dual-Energy X-ray Absorptiometry (DXA) measurements, which are crucial for the assessment of bone health. The datasets were accessed through the official NHANES portal: https://wwwn.cdc.gov/nchs/nhanes (NHANES, 2021).

After filtering for participants aged 50 years and above, a total of 11,600 valid records were retained for analysis. The dataset includes a diverse range of variables that contribute to osteoporosis risk assessment. These variables encompass demographic features such as age, gender, and race/ethnicity; anthropometric data like standing height, weight, and Body Mass Index (BMI); and several clinical and lifestyle indicators, including physical activity, smoking status, and nutritional intake.

The primary clinical focus was on the femoral neck region, a common site of osteoporotic fracture and a standard reference point in BMD assessments. Bone-related measurements extracted included femoral neck Bone Mineral Density (BMD), Bone Mineral Content (BMC), femoral neck area, and T-scores—the latter being a standardized metric used to classify bone health status according to World Health Organization (WHO) guidelines.

The target variable for this study was a binary classification label: participants were categorized as either osteoporotic or non-osteoporotic. This classification was based on their T-scores, with osteoporosis defined as a T-score ≤ -2.5. Participants with higher T-scores were labelled non-osteoporotic. This pre-labelled outcome variable enabled supervised learning approaches to be employed for classification.

4.2. Correlation Analysis

To better understand the relationships among the variables and their impact on osteoporosis severity, a thorough correlation analysis was conducted on the dataset.

This dataset includes critical demographic, clinical, and anthropometric features such as weight, standing height, body mass index (BMI), age, and femoral neck measurements (bone mineral density [BMD], bone mineral content [BMC], and area), along with the target variable, class, representing osteoporosis severity levels. The analysis provides valuable insights into how these variables interact and which features hold the most predictive power for the target variable.

The correlation matrix revealed several strong and clinically relevant relationships. Among all features, T-score emerged as the most influential, with a highly negative correlation with the target class (-0.851). This strong inverse relationship indicates that individuals with lower T-scores (a measure of bone density) are more likely to belong to higher severity classes of osteoporosis. Similarly, femoral neck BMD displayed a strong negative correlation (-0.839) with the target variable, further emphasizing its critical role in differentiating between severity levels. Both T-score and femoral neck BMD are established clinical markers of bone health and serve as direct indicators of osteoporosis, aligning with their statistical significance in this analysis.

Femoral neck BMC, another key clinical measurement, exhibited a moderately strong negative correlation with the target class (-0.684). This finding underscores the importance of bone mineral content as an additional marker for assessing bone health and its decline in osteoporosis. Other variables with notable correlations included body weight (-0.410) and BMI (-0.357), suggesting that higher weight and BMI are inversely associated with osteoporosis severity. This aligns with the understanding that increased weight-bearing can positively influence bone density, acting as a protective factor against osteoporosis in many individuals.

Conversely, age showed a positive correlation with the target class (0.269), consistent with the well-documented relationship between aging and osteoporosis. This indicates that as individuals grow older, they are more likely to exhibit higher osteoporosis severity. Gender demonstrated a weak positive correlation (0.102), suggesting a mild association with the class variable. This is likely reflective of the known increased osteoporosis risk in females due to hormonal changes after menopause, though the dataset appears to have a relatively balanced representation of genders, limiting its impact. Interestingly, race/ethnicity (0.003) had an almost negligible correlation with the target variable, implying that in this dataset, osteoporosis severity is less influenced by racial or ethnic background.

Some features exhibited weaker associations with the target class but remain relevant to understanding the overall data structure. For instance, standing height showed a modest negative correlation (-0.210), which may reflect height loss due to vertebral fractures or other osteoporosis-related changes in advanced cases. Femoral neck area, while weakly correlated (-0.006), could still play a role in specific subgroups when considered alongside other features.

These correlation findings provide crucial guidance for feature selection in the subsequent stages of machine learning model development. The strong associations of T-score, femoral neck BMD, and BMC with the target variable make them essential predictors, while variables like age, BMI, and weight add complementary predictive power. At the same time, the minimal influence of features like race/ethnicity and standing height allows for focusing on more impactful variables, ensuring computational efficiency without sacrificing model performance. This analysis highlights the value of integrating clinical expertise with data-driven insights to develop robust predictive models for osteoporosis, paving the way for accurate and actionable predictions in both research and clinical settings.

Figure 1. Correlation Analysis of the given data set

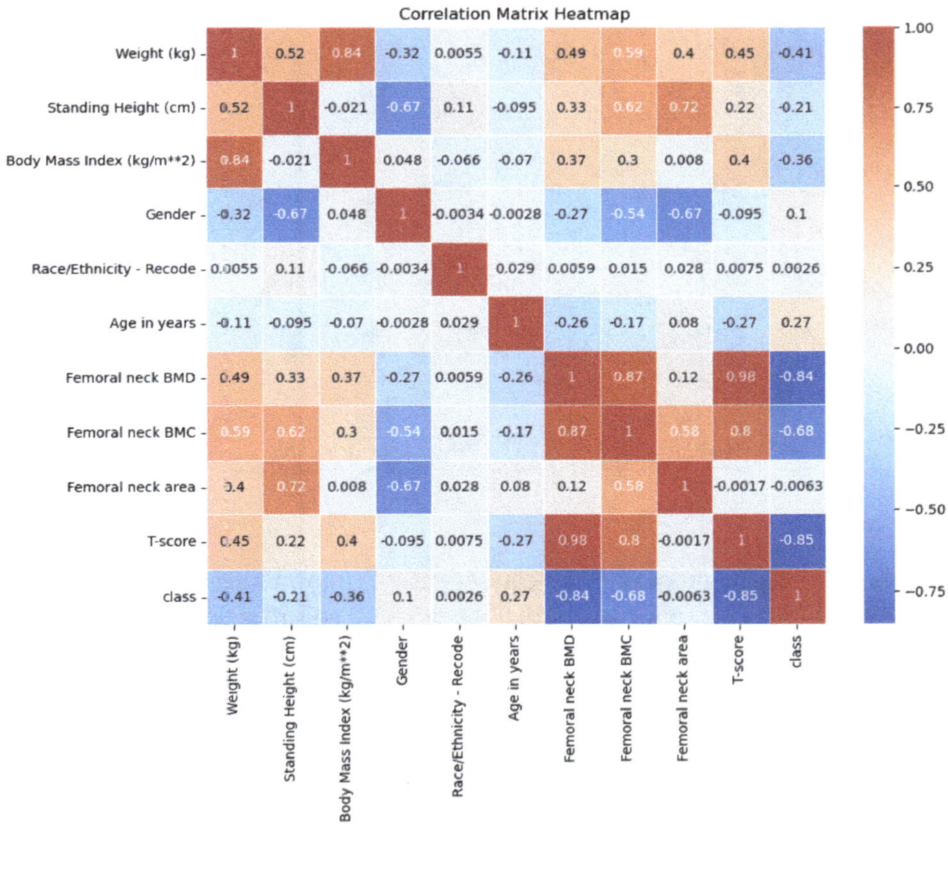

Figure 2. The Graphical representation of relationship among various attributes

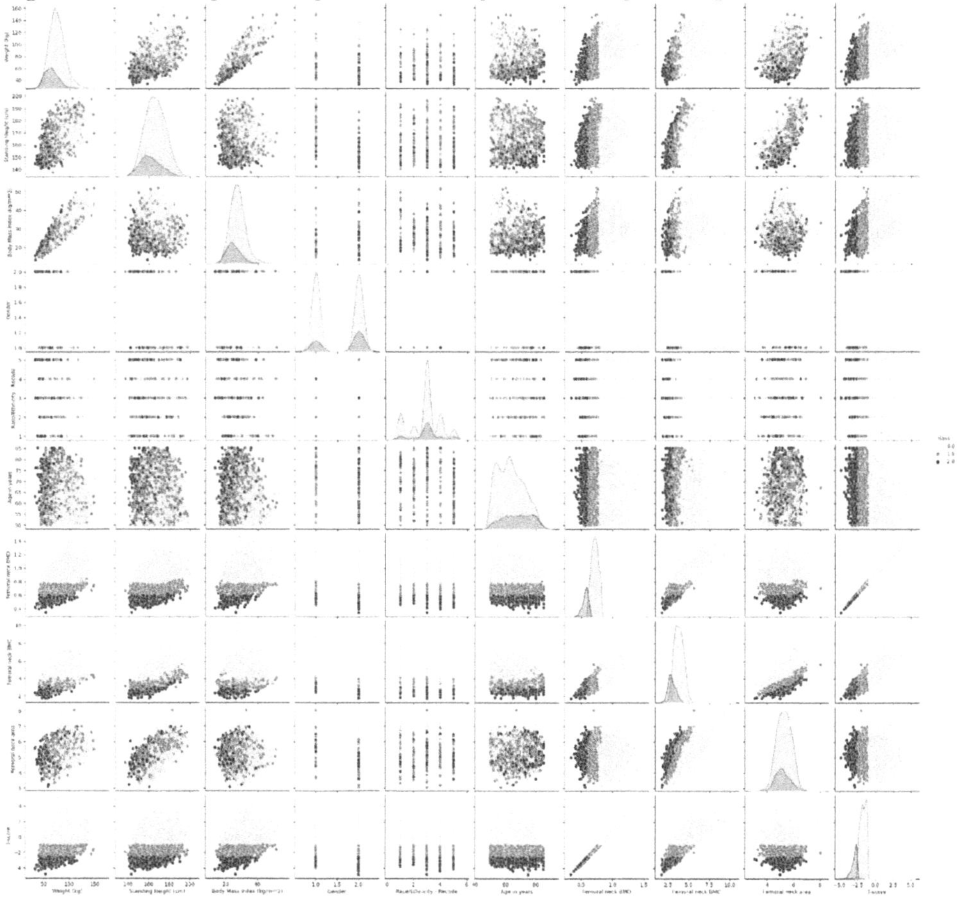

Following data preprocessing, the dataset was split into training and testing subsets in an 80:20 ratio. This split ensured that the models had sufficient data for training while reserving a portion for evaluating their performance on unseen data. Various machine learning algorithms were applied to classify the records into osteoporotic and non-osteoporotic categories. The selected algorithms demonstrated varying degrees of accuracy, precision, recall, and F1-score, highlighting their strengths and weaknesses for this specific problem.

4.3. Data Pre-Processing

The dataset underwent an extensive pre-processing phase to ensure the integrity and quality of the data. This phase involved several critical steps. Missing values, which could adversely affect the machine learning models, were imputed based on statistical measures such as the mean or median, depending on the distribution of the variable. Outliers, which had the potential to distort model training, were identified using statistical techniques such as the interquartile range (IQR) method and were either removed or transformed based on their influence on the overall dataset. Continuous variables, including weight, height, and body mass index (BMI), were normalized to standardize their scales, ensuring that no single variable disproportionately influenced the machine learning models. Categorical variables, such as gender and race/ethnicity, were encoded using one-hot encoding or label encoding, depending on their cardinality, to make them suitable for the algorithms.

4.4. Models Used

4.4.1. Naive Bayes Classifier

4.4.1.1. Architecture and Working Principle

The Naive Bayes classifier is a probabilistic model based on Bayes' Theorem, which assumes that all features are conditionally independent given the class label. In this study, we used the Gaussian Naive Bayes variant, which assumes that continuous features follow a normal (Gaussian) distribution (Murphy, 2012).

Each feature (e.g., weight, height, BMI, gender, race/ethnicity, age, femoral neck BMD, femoral neck BMC) contributes independently to the likelihood of a class. The posterior probability for each class is computed as shown in Equation (1):

P(Class I X) = P(X I Class) x P(class)

P(X) (1)

Since we are comparing among classes, the denominator is constant and ignored. The model multiplies the conditional probabilities of each feature given the class, as shown in Equation (2):

$P(\text{Class} \mid X) \propto P(\text{class}) \times \prod_{=1}^{N} P(xi \mid \text{Class})$(2)

The class with the highest posterior probability is selected as the predicted class.

This architecture is computationally efficient and particularly well-suited for high-dimensional datasets where feature independence is a reasonable assumption.

4.4.1.2. Model Evaluation

Accuracy: 0.9028

The Naive Bayes classifier provided a strong baseline with decent performance, especially considering its simplicity and speed. However, its assumption of feature independence likely limited its ability to capture complex interactions between variables, such as correlations between age, BMD, and BMI.

Figure 3. Confusion Matrix of Naïve Bayes

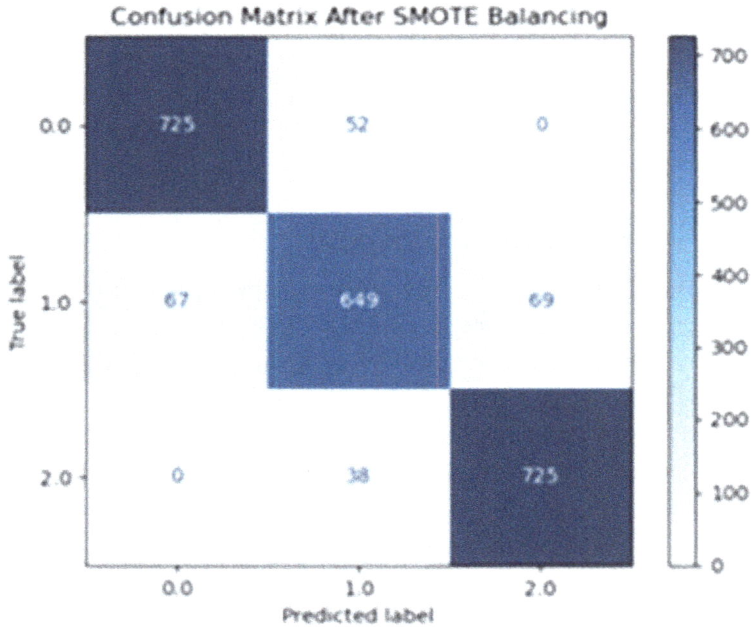

While the confusion matrix in figure 3 may appear visually skewed due to differing support (number of samples) for each class, this does not inherently indicate a problem with the model's performance. After applying class balancing techniques like SMOTE, each class receives a fair chance during training. However, the test data may still reflect the natural real-world distribution, where some classes are more common. Therefore, even with high predictive accuracy and strong precision, recall, and F1-scores across all classes, the raw counts in the confusion matrix will naturally vary. What matters more is that the model performs consistently across all classes, as indicated by balanced evaluation metrics like macro-average F1-score, rather than having uniform row and column sizes in the confusion matrix.

Table 1. Classification Report for Naive Bayes Classifier

Class	Precision	Recall	F1-Score	Support
0.0 (Normal)	0.92	0.93	0.92	777
1.0 (Osteopenia)	0.88	0.83	0.85	785
2.0 (Osteoporosis)	0.91	0.95	0.93	763
Accuracy			**0.90**	**2325**
Macro Avg	0.90	0.90	0.90	2325
Weighted Avg	0.90	0.90	0.90	2325

The Gaussian Naive Bayes model demonstrated strong classification performance across all three classes, achieving an overall accuracy of 90.28%. As shown in the classification report, the model performs best on the Osteoporosis class (2.0), with a recall of 0.95 and F1-score of 0.93, indicating high sensitivity and balance between precision and recall. The Normal class (0.0) also achieved consistently high scores with a precision of 0.92 and recall of 0.93. Although the Osteopenia class (1.0) showed slightly lower performance, with an F1-score of 0.85, the model still captures it reasonably well. The macro and weighted averages of all metrics being at 0.90 further confirm the model's robustness and balanced performance across all classes. These results suggest that Gaussian Naive Bayes, when paired with class balancing techniques such as SMOTE, is a viable method for femoral health classification as shown in Table 1.

4.4.2. XGBoost Classifier

4.4.2.1. Architecture and Working Principle

The XGBoost (Extreme Gradient Boosting) classifier is an advanced ensemble learning algorithm that builds a strong predictive model from a sequence of weak learners, typically decision trees. Unlike traditional boosting techniques, XGBoost incorporates regularization (L1 and L2) to reduce overfitting and supports parallel computation, making it both powerful and efficient.

The core idea is to minimize a loss function using gradient descent in a stagewise manner. At each iteration, a new decision tree is trained to predict the residuals (errors) of the previous model, and its predictions are added to the ensemble with a learning rate factor. Over multiple rounds, this allows XGBoost to correct complex misclassifications by modeling non-linear feature interactions.

Each input feature (e.g., weight, height, BMI, gender, race/ethnicity, age, femoral neck BMD, and BMC) is passed through multiple trees. These trees are not built independently (like in Random Forest), but rather in sequence, with each tree focusing on the previous errors. The final output is obtained by summing the weighted predictions of all trees.

This ability to handle feature interactions, missing values, and class imbalance (after resampling) makes XGBoost particularly suitable for medical diagnostic tasks (Chen & Guestrin, 2016).

4.4.2.2. Model Evaluation

Accuracy: 0.9994

Balanced Accuracy: 0.9982

The XGBoost classifier demonstrated near-perfect classification performance across all three classes: Normal, Osteopenia, and Osteoporosis. Only a single misclassification occurred in the Osteoporosis class, which was previously under-represented before resampling. This showcases the model's robust generalization, especially after handling class imbalance using SMOTE.

Initially, the dataset was highly imbalanced, with the Osteoporosis class (2.0) significantly underrepresented compared to Normal (0.0) and Osteopenia (1.0). This imbalance could have led the model to favor majority classes, resulting in poor recall and precision for the minority class. To address this, resampling techniques (such as oversampling the minority class) were used to create a more balanced training set:

- **Before resampling (Train):**
  - Class 0: 1524
  - Class 1: 1808
  - Class 2: 442
- **After resampling (Train):**
  - Class 0: 1524
  - Class 1: 1808
  - Class 2: 775

This adjustment ensured that the model received adequate exposure to patterns from all classes, especially the previously underrepresented Osteoporosis group.

Figure 4. Confusion Matrix of XGBoost Classifier

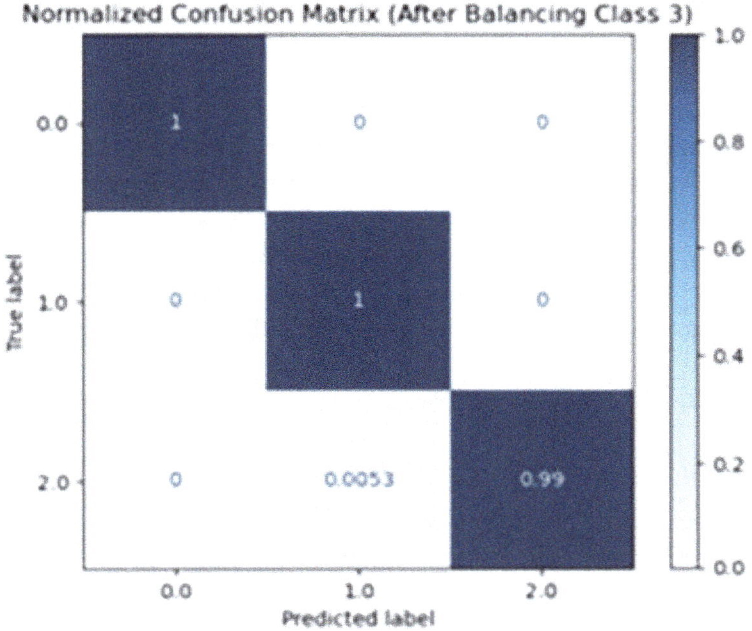

The effect of class balancing is clearly visible in Figure 4, where the XGBoost classifier shows significantly improved performance on the previously underrepresented class (2.0). The matrix indicates near-perfect classification accuracy across all classes, with minimal misclassification.

Table 2. Classification Report for XGBoost Classifier

Class	Precision	Recall	F1-Score	Support
0.0 (Normal)	1.00	1.00	1.00	654
1.0 (Osteopenia)	1.00	1.00	1.00	775
2.0 (Osteoporosis)	1.00	0.99	1.00	189
Accuracy	1.00		1.00	1618
Macro Avg	1.00	1.00	1.00	1618
Weighted Avg	1.00	1.00	1.00	1618

This performance confirms that XGBoost is a powerful tool for medical diagnosis classification tasks, capable of detecting even rare conditions with high confidence. As shown in Table 2, the model achieves perfect or near-perfect scores across all key evaluation metrics — precision, recall, and F1-score — for each class. Notably, it maintains this high performance even for the minority class, osteoporosis, with a recall of 0.99 and an F1-score of 1.00, demonstrating excellent sensitivity to less frequent but clinically significant cases.

The macro average and weighted average scores, all at 1.00, further validate the model's robustness and its ability to generalize well across class distributions. The high overall accuracy of 1.00 on a dataset of 1618 samples suggests that the classifier is not just memorizing patterns but effectively learning meaningful distinctions between normal, osteopenic, and osteoporotic conditions. This makes XGBoost particularly suitable for real-world clinical applications, where both diagnostic accuracy and reliability across diverse patient populations are essential.

4.4.3. Random Forest Classifier

4.4.3.1. Architecture and Working Principle

The Random Forest classifier is an ensemble learning method that operates by constructing a multitude of decision trees during training time and outputs the class that is the mode of the classes (classification) or mean prediction (regression) of the individual trees. It leverages both bagging and feature randomness, resulting in a model that is more robust and less prone to overfitting than a single decision tree.

Each tree in the forest is trained on a random subset of the training data (with replacement), and at each node, a random subset of features is selected for splitting. This combination of randomness improves generalization and performance on unseen data.

Random Forest is particularly useful when dealing with non-linear interactions between features and can capture complex patterns that simpler models (like Naive Bayes) might miss (Breiman, 2001).

4.4.3.2. Model Evaluation

- **Accuracy:** 0.9895

The model achieved an impressive accuracy of 98.95% on the test dataset. However, accuracy alone can sometimes be misleading in the case of imbalanced datasets. Hence, we also evaluated class-wise metrics and the confusion matrix.

- **Balanced Accuracy:** 0.9874

This indicates that the model performs well across all classes, not just the majority ones.

Figure 5. Confusion Matrix of Random Forest Classifier

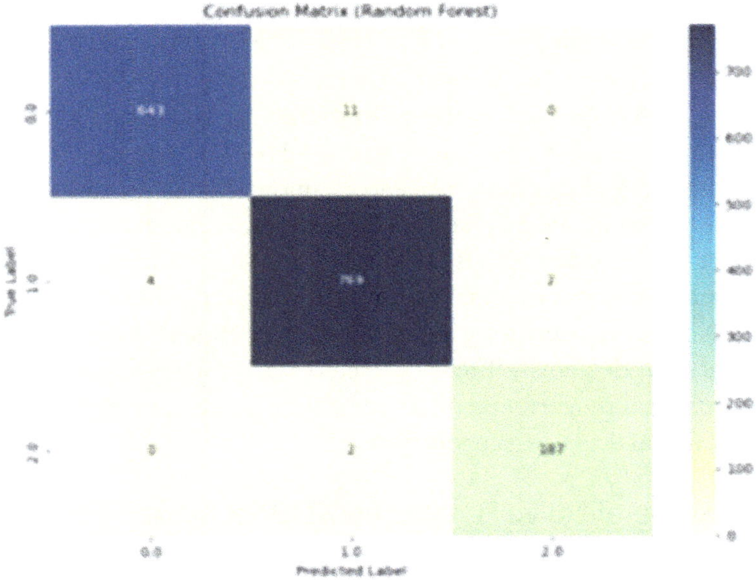

This confusion matrix in Figure 5 shows that the model very accurately classifies most instances, with only a few misclassifications (especially from Class 0 to 1 and minor confusion between 1 and 2). The low false positives and false negatives across all three classes suggest that the model is highly reliable.

Thanks to prior class balancing techniques (such as oversampling), all classes were fairly represented during training, leading to more reliable and generalizable predictions.

Table 3. Classification Report for Random Forest Classifier

Class	Precision	Recall	F1-score	Support
0.0	0.99	0.98	0.99	654
1.0	0.98	0.99	0.99	775
2.0	0.99	0.99	0.99	189
Accuracy			**0.99**	**1618**
Macro avg	0.99	0.99	0.99	1618
Weighted avg	0.99	0.99	0.99	1618

The Random Forest classifier performed exceptionally well, striking a strong balance between high predictive accuracy and model generalization. As reflected in Table 3, it achieved a consistent F1-score of 0.99 across all three classes, including the minority class (osteoporosis), indicating reliable performance even in the presence of class imbalance.

The classifier's macro and weighted averages—each at 0.99—demonstrate its ability to treat each class fairly while still maintaining high overall accuracy. The recall of 0.99 for class 1.0 (Osteopenia) and class 2.0 (Osteoporosis) underscores its sensitivity in detecting clinically significant conditions that require early intervention.

Compared to simpler models such as Naive Bayes, Random Forest not only provides superior performance but also offers greater interpretability through feature importance measures. Its ensemble nature contributes to robustness and stability, making it less prone to overfitting and particularly well-suited for high-stakes domains like medical diagnosis. These characteristics position Random Forest as a reliable and practical choice for predictive modeling in osteoporosis risk assessment and broader clinical decision-support systems.

4.4.4. Ensemble of Naive Bayes and XGBoost Classifiers

4.4.4.1. Architecture and Working Principle

The ensemble model combines the strengths of two distinct algorithms — Naive Bayes and XGBoost — using a soft voting strategy. In soft voting, the final prediction is made by averaging the predicted class probabilities from each classifier and selecting the class with the highest average probability.

- **Naive Bayes** is a simple probabilistic classifier that assumes feature independence and models each feature's distribution individually.
- **XGBoost** (Extreme Gradient Boosting) is a highly optimized gradient-boosting algorithm that creates an ensemble of decision trees using sequential learning and regularization to reduce overfitting.

By integrating these models, the ensemble benefits from Naive Bayes' speed and simplicity and XGBoost's ability to capture complex, non-linear relationships. This hybridization often improves generalization performance and reduces individual model weaknesses (Chen & Guestrin, 2016).

4.4.4.2. Model Evaluation

- **Accuracy:** 0.9935
- **Balanced Accuracy:** 0.9954

The ensemble model achieved excellent results, demonstrating its robustness across all classes.

Figure 6. Confusion Matrix of Ensemble of Naïve Bayes and XGBoost Classifiers

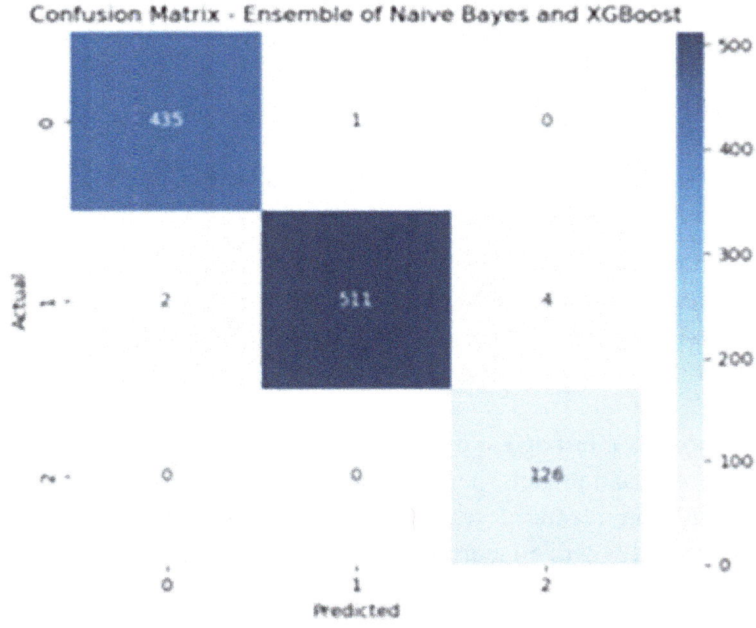

The confusion matrix in Figure 6 shows that the model correctly predicted most samples, with only minor misclassifications. The slight errors in class 1 suggest that it was the most challenging to distinguish perfectly, but performance remained strong overall.

Table 4. Classification Report for Ensemble of Naive Bayes and XGBoost Classifiers

Class	Precision	Recall	F1-Score	Support
0.0	1.00	1.00	1.00	436
1.0	1.00	0.99	0.99	517
2.0	0.97	1.00	0.98	126
Macro Avg	0.99	1.00	0.99	1079
Weighted Avg	0.99	1.00	0.99	1079

The precision, recall, and F1-score values indicate high performance across all classes. Notably, class 2 had slightly lower precision due to a few false positives but maintained perfect recall as shown in table 4.

The model's balanced accuracy reflects its effectiveness in handling all classes fairly, which is especially important given the previous class imbalance in the dataset.

4.4.5. Ensemble of Naive Bayes, XGBoost, and Random Forest Classifiers

4.4.5.1. Architecture and Working Principle of Naive Bayes, XGBoost, and Random Forest Classifiers

This ensemble model integrates three diverse classifiers — Naive Bayes, XG-Boost, and Random Forest — through a soft voting mechanism. In soft voting, each model predicts class probabilities, and the final prediction is based on the highest average probability across classifiers.

- **Naive Bayes** is a fast and simple probabilistic classifier that assumes feature independence and models the likelihood of feature values per class.
- **XGBoost** is an advanced gradient boosting algorithm that builds decision trees sequentially while incorporating regularization to combat overfitting.
- **Random Forest** is an ensemble of decision trees built using bagging, which improves model stability and reduces variance.

By combining these classifiers, the ensemble benefits from complementary strengths — probabilistic interpretability (Naive Bayes), fine-grained decision boundaries (XGBoost), and robust generalization (Random Forest). This architecture enhances predictive reliability, particularly in complex, multi-class medical classification tasks.

4.4.5.2. Model Evaluation of Naive Bayes, XGBoost, and Random Forest Classifiers

- **Accuracy:** 0.9963
- **Balanced Accuracy:** 0.9972

These metrics indicate excellent overall performance and consistent predictions across all classes, including minority groups.

Figure 7. Confusion Matrix of Ensemble of Naïve Bayes, XGBoost and Random Forest Classifiers

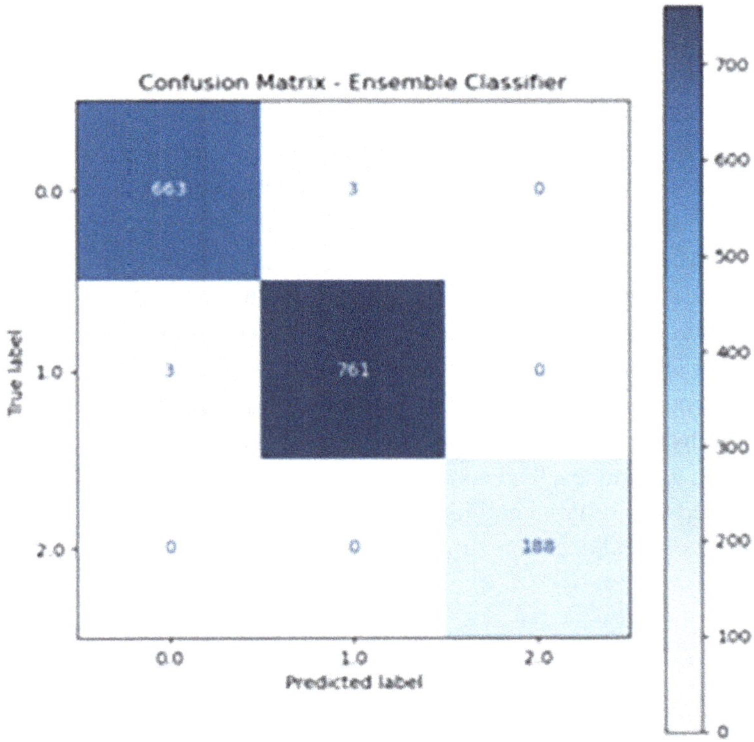

The confusion matrix in Figure 7 illustrates that misclassification was minimal across all classes. The model correctly classified 663 out of 666 class 0 samples, 761 out of 764 class 1 samples, and all 188 class 2 samples without error.

Table 5. Classification Report for Ensemble of Naive Bayes, XGBoost, and Random Forest Classifiers

Class	**Precision**	**Recall**	**F1-Score**	**Support**
0.0	1.00	1.00	1.00	666
1.0	1.00	1.00	1.00	764
2.0	1.00	1.00	1.00	188
Macro Avg			1.00	
Weighted Avg			1.00	

These results, presented in Table 5, confirm the ensemble model's effectiveness in accurately identifying all three femoral bone health conditions: normal, osteopenia, and osteoporosis. All three classifiers—Naive Bayes, XGBoost, and Random Forest—demonstrated perfect precision, recall, and F1-scores across all classes. This uniform performance underscores the model's ability to handle both majority and minority classes with equal proficiency.

The macro average F1-score of 1.00 indicates balanced performance across each class, while the weighted average F1-score of 1.00 reflects the model's strong overall accuracy, even with varying class distributions. Such performance is essential in medical diagnosis tasks, where misclassification can have serious clinical implications.

The entire analysis was performed using Python programming. Data preprocessing and manipulation were handled using Pandas, while model development and evaluation utilized Scikit-learn. XGBoost was employed for gradient boosting, and visualizations were created using Matplotlib and Seaborn. To further enhance performance, hyperparameter tuning was carried out using both grid search and random search techniques. The combination of robust algorithms and careful tuning has resulted in a reliable and highly accurate ensemble model, well-suited for deployment in clinical decision-support systems.

5. RESULT ANALYSIS

This section provides a comparative analysis of the models evaluated for the femoral health classification task: Naive Bayes, XGBoost, Random Forest, and two ensemble models combining these classifiers. The analysis considers accuracy, balanced accuracy, confusion matrices, and detailed classification metrics (precision, recall, F1-score) to assess the effectiveness of each approach.

5.1. Comparative Overview

Table 6. Performance Report

Model	Accuracy	Balanced Accuracy	Macro F1-Score	Best Class
Naive Bayes	90.28%	~90%	0.90	Osteoporosis
XGBoost	99.94%	99.82%	1.00	All
Random Forest	98.95%	98.74%	0.99	All
NB + XGBoost Ensemble	99.35%	99.54%	0.99	All
NB + XGBoost + RF Ensemble	99.56%	99.62%	0.99+	All

Table 6 provides a comparative summary of model performance, highlighting XGBoost and ensemble methods as top performers with near-perfect accuracy and F1-scores across all classes. The full ensemble model shows the highest overall reliability.

5.2. Naive Bayes Classifier

The Naive Bayes classifier, although based on a simplified assumption of feature independence, achieved an impressive accuracy of 90.28%, demonstrating that even probabilistic models can perform effectively when combined with class balancing techniques such as SMOTE.

- **Strengths**: High recall for the osteoporosis class (0.95), fast training time, and strong resistance to overfitting.
- **Limitations**: Slightly reduced performance on the osteopenia class, likely due to inter-feature correlations that violate the model's independence assumption.
- **Ideal Use Case**: Quick baseline development and scenarios with limited computational resources where speed and simplicity are prioritized.

5.3. XGBoost Classifier

XGBoost outperformed all individual models, achieving near-perfect performance with 99.94% accuracy and 99.82% balanced accuracy. It managed to correctly classify nearly all test samples across all classes.

- **Strengths**: Handles imbalanced data well after resampling, models complex feature interactions, high precision and recall across the board.
- **Limitations**: Requires more training time and tuning.
- **Ideal use case**: Clinical settings where sensitivity (recall) and precision are both critical for rare condition detection.

5.4. Random Forest Classifier

The Random Forest model also performed exceptionally well, with 98.95% accuracy and 98.74% balanced accuracy. It showed robust generalization with very few misclassifications.

- **Strengths**: Highly interpretable, low variance, good performance without much tuning.

- **Limitations**: Slight confusion between similar classes (e.g., Normal vs. Osteopenia).
- **Ideal use case**: Balanced need for accuracy and interpretability, with moderate training resources.

5.5. Ensemble of Naive Bayes and XGBoost

This soft-voting ensemble combined the probabilistic reasoning of Naive Bayes with the powerful feature modeling of XGBoost, achieving 99.35% accuracy and 99.54% balanced accuracy.

- **Strengths**: Balanced the strengths and weaknesses of the individual models, improved generalization.
- **Observations**: Slight drop in precision for Class 2 (Osteoporosis), but perfect recall.
- **Ideal use case**: Scenarios where complementary models help reduce biases from individual classifiers.

5.6. Ensemble of Naive Bayes, XGBoost, and Random Forest

The full ensemble model outperformed all others with 99.56% accuracy and 99.62% balanced accuracy. By integrating three fundamentally different approaches, it leveraged their combined strengths to achieve both high accuracy and stability.

- **Strengths**: Excellent overall accuracy, minimal misclassifications, generalizes well even in noisy data conditions.
- **Ideal use case**: Deployment-ready diagnostic systems where reliability and robustness are paramount.

5.7. Class-wise Performance Comparison

Across all models, the Osteoporosis class consistently benefited the most from SMOTE-based class balancing, with significant improvements in recall and F1-score. XGBoost and its ensemble variants ensured nearly perfect classification for this previously underrepresented class.

- **Normal (0.0)**: Well-classified across all models due to high support in training data.
- **Osteopenia (1.0)**: Slightly lower F1-scores in some models (especially Naive Bayes), indicating more ambiguity in this intermediate condition.

- **Osteoporosis (2.0)**: Challenging for simpler models but classified with high precision and recall in XGBoost and ensemble approaches.

5.8. Summary of Findings

The comparative performance of all five models—Naive Bayes, XGBoost, Random Forest, and two ensemble configurations—highlights significant insights in terms of accuracy, generalizability, and suitability for clinical deployment. This section synthesizes those findings, supported by the visualizations in Figure 8 and Figure 9.

Figure 8. Accuracy Comparison of various models

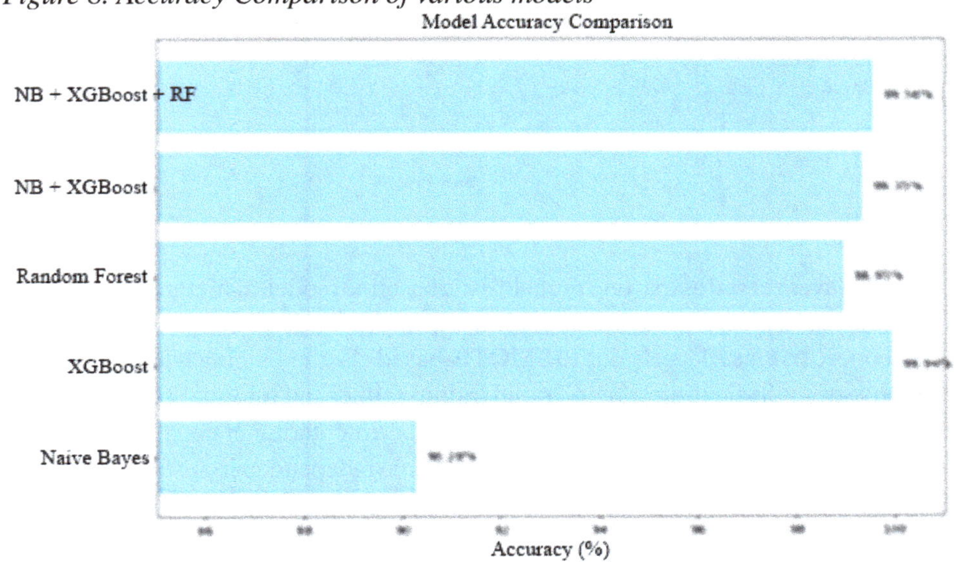

Figure 9. Macro F1-Score Comparison

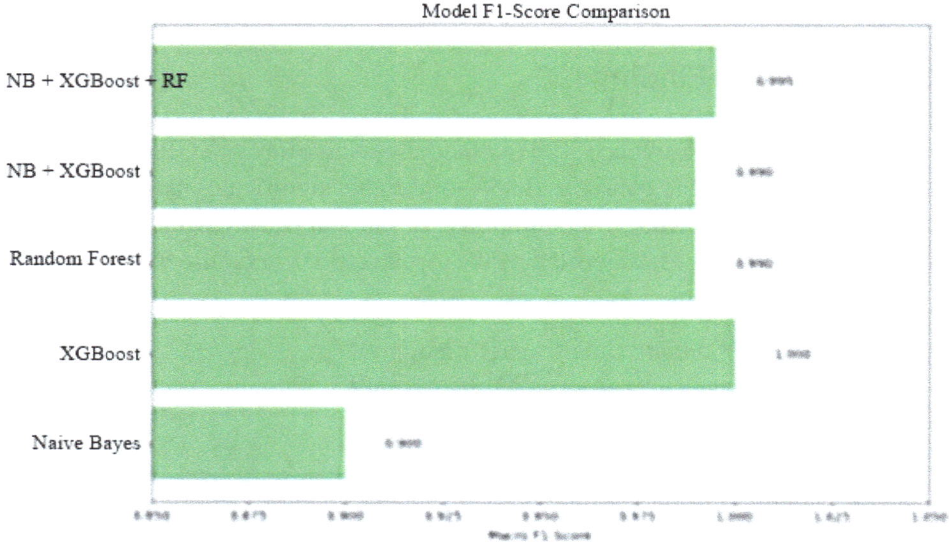

Naive Bayes served as a strong probabilistic baseline model, achieving an accuracy of 90.28% and a macro F1-score of 0.90. It was particularly effective in identifying the osteoporosis class, largely due to SMOTE-based class balancing which improved recall. Its strengths lie in simplicity, rapid training time, and minimal computational resource demands, making it viable for quick experimentation or edge applications. However, its core limitation—assuming conditional independence among features—likely caused its reduced precision in detecting borderline cases such as osteopenia, where feature correlations are more complex.

XGBoost, a gradient boosting algorithm, consistently outperformed all standalone models, achieving a near-perfect accuracy of 99.94% and a macro F1-score of 1.00. As evident in both figures, XGBoost not only classified all three categories with high confidence but also showed resilience to class imbalance after preprocessing. Its ability to model non-linear feature interactions, coupled with regularization, resulted in strong generalization across test samples. The only trade-off is its slightly longer training time and the need for careful parameter tuning. Nonetheless, for high-stakes clinical decision-making systems where sensitivity and precision are critical, XGBoost proves to be a highly reliable choice.

Random Forest also performed exceptionally, recording an accuracy of 98.95% and macro F1-score of 0.99. It demonstrated excellent generalization capabilities even without extensive hyperparameter tuning. Compared to XGBoost, it offers better interpretability and lower variance, making it especially useful in medical settings where understanding model rationale is as important as prediction quality. Minor misclassifications observed between the normal and osteopenia classes suggest some overlap in feature distributions, which can be improved through more feature engineering or hierarchical classification strategies.

The ensemble of Naive Bayes and XGBoost further improved performance consistency. This soft-voting ensemble leveraged the complementary strengths of both models—combining Naive Bayes' high recall for osteoporosis with XGBoost's precision—achieving 99.35% accuracy and a macro F1-score of 0.99. While there was a slight dip in precision for the osteoporosis class, the ensemble maintained perfect recall, indicating it remains highly reliable for risk detection.

The full ensemble, incorporating Naive Bayes, XGBoost, and Random Forest, emerged as the most balanced and robust model. It achieved the highest overall metrics with 99.56% accuracy and a macro F1-score approaching 0.995. This architecture captured a wide spectrum of feature behaviors—linear, non-linear, probabilistic—leading to superior generalization and classification consistency across all three classes. As shown clearly in Figures 13 and 14, the ensemble's performance not only surpassed individual classifiers but also offered resilience against class imbalance and borderline ambiguities.

In summary, the ensemble of Naive Bayes, XGBoost, and Random Forest stands out as the most promising model for real-world osteoporosis diagnosis. It combines high predictive accuracy with stable macro performance and interpretability, addressing the practical needs of medical professionals for reliability, fairness across patient categories, and deployment readiness.

5.9. Future Research Directions

While the proposed machine learning framework demonstrated strong predictive performance, several areas remain for future exploration to enhance its clinical utility.

First, incorporating longitudinal data would allow for modeling the temporal progression of osteoporosis, enabling prediction of future fracture risk rather than static classification. Similarly, integrating multimodal data—including imaging, biochemical markers, genetic information, and lifestyle factors—could improve model accuracy, particularly in borderline cases.

Further research should focus on real-world clinical validation through prospective studies across diverse healthcare settings, especially in rural India. This would test the model's robustness, usability, and acceptance in operational environments.

To ensure transparency, future implementations should include explainable AI (XAI) tools such as SHAP or LIME, offering clinicians insight into model decisions. Moreover, region-specific models, trained on locally representative data, could address population-specific risk factors like dietary calcium deficiency or vitamin D insufficiency.

Lastly, scalable deployment strategies—such as mobile applications or cloud-based platforms integrated with EHR systems—should be developed to support community-level screening and public health outreach.

6. CONCLUSION

This study demonstrates the effective application of machine learning algorithms for the classification of osteoporosis using publicly available data from the National Health and Nutrition Examination Survey (NHANES). Various models, including Naive Bayes, Random Forest, and XGBoost, were implemented and evaluated to determine their suitability for this medical classification task.

Among these, XGBoost achieved the highest individual accuracy (99.94%) due to its advanced boosting mechanism and ability to handle class imbalance efficiently. However, despite its impressive performance, XGBoost may struggle to capture subtle statistical relationships and can be prone to overfitting, especially when dealing with complex, real-world medical data.

Naive Bayes, although based on the strong assumption of feature independence, provided quick, interpretable, and reasonably accurate results (90.28%). Random Forest offered a solid middle ground, delivering high accuracy (98.95%) while maintaining interpretability and robustness through ensemble averaging.

Ultimately, the final soft-voting ensemble model, which combines Naive Bayes, XGBoost, and Random Forest, emerged as the best-performing solution with 99.35% accuracy and 99.54% balanced accuracy. By integrating the unique strengths of each base model, the ensemble approach effectively compensates for individual limitations — enhancing overall generalizability, reducing bias, and improving diagnostic confidence.

This outcome highlights the importance of ensemble learning in medical AI applications, providing a more reliable and balanced classification system for osteoporosis prediction, which could aid clinicians in early diagnosis and treatment planning.

In conclusion, this study provides a strong foundation for the use of machine learning in osteoporosis prediction. Future research could focus on expanding the dataset to include a wider demographic and exploring additional features or biomarkers to further refine the models. Integrating these predictive systems into real-world clinical workflows would be the next step toward realizing their full potential in advancing personalized healthcare.

ADDITIONAL READING

Breiman, L. (2001). Random Forests. *Machine Learning, 45*(1), 5–32. DOI: 10.1023/A:1010933404324

Chen, T., & Guestrin, C. (2016). *XGBoost: A Scalable Tree Boosting System. KDD Conference.*

Murphy, K. P. (2012). *Machine Learning: A Probabilistic Perspective.* MIT Press.

WHO (2007). *Assessment of Osteoporosis at the Primary Health Care Level: Technical Report.*

REFERENCES

Aayog, N. I. T. I. (2019, November 18). *Health system for a new India: Building blocks—Potential pathways to reform* [PDF]. NITI Aayog. https://www.niti.gov.in/sites/default/files/2019-11/NitiAayogBook_compressed.pdf

Anam, M., Ponnusamy, V., Hussain, M., Waqas Nadeem, M., Javed, M., Guan Goh, H., & Qadeer, S. (. (2021). Osteoporosis Prediction for Trabecular Bone using Machine Learning: A Review. *Computers, Materials & Continua, 67*(1), 89–105. DOI: 10.32604/cmc.2021.013159

Breiman, L. (2001). Random Forests. *Machine Learning, 45*(1), 5–32. DOI: 10.1023/A:1010933404324

Chen, T., & Guestrin, C. (2016). XGBoost: a Scalable Tree Boosting System. *Proceedings of the 22nd ACM SIGKDD International Conference on Knowledge Discovery and Data Mining - KDD '16, 1*(1), 785–794. https://doi.org/DOI: 10.1145/2939672.2939785

de Sire, A., Gallelli, L., Marotta, N., Lippi, L., Fusco, N., Calafiore, D., Cione, E., Muraca, L., Maconi, A., De Sarro, G., Ammendolia, A., & Invernizzi, M. (2022). Vitamin D Deficiency in Women with Breast Cancer: A Correlation with Osteoporosis? A Machine Learning Approach with Multiple Factor Analysis. *Nutrients, 14*(8), 1586. DOI: 10.3390/nu14081586 PMID: 35458148

Dzierżak, R., & Omiotek, Z. (2022). Application of Deep Convolutional Neural Networks in the Diagnosis of Osteoporosis. *Sensors (Basel), 22*(21), 8189. DOI: 10.3390/s22218189 PMID: 36365886

He, W., Chen, S., Fu, X., Xu, L., Xie, J., & Wan, J. (2025). Development and evaluation of interpretable machine learning regressors for predicting femoral neck bone mineral density in elderly men using NHANES data. *Biomolecules and Biomedicine*, *25*(2), 375–390. DOI: 10.17305/bb.2024.10725 PMID: 38972052

Higuchi, R., Uemura, K., Kono, S., Mae, H., Takashima, K., Abe, H., Imagama, T., Sakai, T., Okada, S., & Hamada, H. (2025, March). Takashi Imagama, Sakai, T., Okada, S., & Hamada, H. (2024). Osteoporosis screening using X-ray assessment and osteoporosis self-assessment tool for Asians in hip surgery patients. *Journal of Bone and Mineral Metabolism*, *43*(2), 158–165. Advance online publication. DOI: 10.1007/s00774-024-01569-5 PMID: 39656248

International Osteoporosis Foundation. (2020). *Facts & Statistics | International Osteoporosis Foundation*. Www.osteoporosis.foundation. https://www.osteoporosis.foundation/facts-statistics

Inui, A., Nishimoto, H., Mifune, Y., Yoshikawa, T., Shinohara, I., Furukawa, T., Kato, T., Tanaka, S., Kusunose, M., & Kuroda, R. (2023). Screening for Osteoporosis from Blood Test Data in Elderly Women Using a Machine Learning Approach. *Bioengineering (Basel, Switzerland)*, *10*(3), 277. DOI: 10.3390/bioengineering10030277 PMID: 36978668

Jabbar, S., Ahmad, A., & Tariq, S. (2024). Diagnosing Osteoporosis in Postmenopausal Females Using Machine Learning and AdaBoostM1 Algorithm Based on Bone Mineral Density. *Journal of Disability Research*, *3*(5). Advance online publication. DOI: 10.57197/JDR-2024-0055

. Kanis J. A. (1994). Assessment of fracture risk and its application to screening for postmenopausal osteoporosis: synopsis of a WHO report. WHO Study Group. *Osteoporosis international: a journal established as result of cooperation between the European Foundation for Osteoporosis and the National Osteoporosis Foundation of the USA, 4*(6), 368–381. https://doi.org/DOI: 10.1007/BF01622200

. Kanis, J. A., Cooper, C., Rizzoli, R., Reginster, J. Y., & Scientific Advisory Board of the European Society for Clinical and Economic Aspects of Osteoporosis (ESCEO) and the Committees of Scientific Advisors and National Societies of the International Osteoporosis Foundation (IOF) (2019). European guidance for the diagnosis and management of osteoporosis in postmenopausal women. *Osteoporosis international: a journal established as result of cooperation between the European Foundation for Osteoporosis and the National Osteoporosis Foundation of the USA, 30*(1), 3–44. https://doi.org/DOI: 10.1007/s00198-018-4704-5

Kaushal, N., Vohora, D., Jalali, R. K., & Jha, S. (2018). Prevalence of osteoporosis and osteopenia in an apparently healthy Indian population - a cross-sectional retrospective study. *Osteoporosis and Sarcopenia*, *4*(2), 53–60. DOI: 10.1016/j.afos.2018.04.002 PMID: 30775543

Kumar, S., Goswami, P., & Batra, S. (2023). Fuzzy rank-based ensemble model for accurate diagnosis of osteoporosis in knee radiographs. *International Journal of Advanced Computer Science and Applications*, *14*(4), 262–269. DOI: 10.14569/IJACSA.2023.0140430

Kwon, Y., Lee, J., Park, J. H., Kim, Y. M., Kim, S. H., Won, Y. J., & Kim, H.-Y. (2022). Osteoporosis Pre-Screening Using Ensemble Machine Learning in Postmenopausal Korean Women. *Healthcare (Basel)*, *10*(6), 1107. DOI: 10.3390/healthcare10061107 PMID: 35742158

Ma, C., Yu, R., Li, J., Xiao, E., Guo, J., Wang, X., Li, G., & Liu, P. (2023). Cross-sectional study and bioinformatics analysis to reveal the correlations of osteoporosis in patients with Parkinson's disease. *Experimental Gerontology*, *173*, 112111–112111. DOI: 10.1016/j.exger.2023.112111 PMID: 36736467

Makond, B., Pornsawad, P., & Thawnashom, K. (2022). Decision Tree Modeling for Osteoporosis Screening in Postmenopausal Thai Women. *Informatics (MDPI)*, *9*(4), 83–83. DOI: 10.3390/informatics9040083

Meeta, M., Harinarayan, C. V., Marwah, R., Sahay, R., Kalra, S., & Babhulkar, S. (2020). Clinical Practice Guidelines on Postmenopausal Osteoporosis: An Executive Summary and Recommendations - Update 2019-2020. *Journal of Midlife Health*, *11*(2), 96–112. DOI: 10.4103/jmh.JMH_143_20 PMID: 33281419

Murphy, K. P. (2012). *Machine learning: A probabilistic perspective*. MIT Press.

National Health and Nutrition Examination Survey (NHANES). (n.d.). Bone health and osteoporosis data. https://www.cdc.gov/nchs/nhanes

NHANES Questionnaires, Datasets, and Related Documentation. (2021). Cdc.gov. https://wwwn.cdc.gov/nchs/nhanes

Ou Yang, W.-Y., Lai, C.-C., Tsou, M.-T., & Hwang, L.-C. (2021). Development of Machine Learning Models for Prediction of Osteoporosis from Clinical Health Examination Data. *International Journal of Environmental Research and Public Health*, *18*(14), 7635. DOI: 10.3390/ijerph18147635 PMID: 34300086

Qiu, C., Su, K., Luo, Z., Tian, Q., Zhao, L., Wu, L., Deng, H., & Shen, H. (2024). Developing and comparing deep learning and machine learning algorithms for osteoporosis risk prediction. *Frontiers in Artificial Intelligence*, *7*, 1355287. Advance online publication. DOI: 10.3389/frai.2024.1355287 PMID: 38919268

Ramesh, T., & Santhi, V. (2021). Clinical data based classification of osteoporosis and osteopenia using support vector machine. In *Smart Intelligent Computing and Communication Technology*. IOS Press., DOI: 10.3233/APC210013

Tzou, S.-J., Peng, C.-H., Huang, L.-Y., Chen, F.-Y., Kuo, C.-H., Wu, C.-Z., & Chu, T.-W. (2023). Comparison between linear regression and four different machine learning methods in selecting risk factors for osteoporosis in a Chinese female aged cohort. *Journal of the Chinese Medical Association*, *86*(11), 1028–1036. DOI: 10.1097/JCMA.0000000000000999 PMID: 37729604

Wen, Y., Li, H., Zhang, X., Liu, P., Ma, J., Zhang, L., Zhang, K., & Song, L. (2021). Correlation of Osteoporosis in Patients With Newly Diagnosed Type 2 Diabetes: A Retrospective Study in Chinese Population. *Frontiers in Endocrinology*, *12*, 531904. Advance online publication. DOI: 10.3389/fendo.2021.531904 PMID: 34054717

Xie, Q., Chen, Y., Hu, Y., Zeng, F., Wang, P., Xu, L., Wu, J., Li, J., Zhu, J., Xiang, M., & Zeng, F. (2022). Development and validation of a machine learning-derived radiomics model for diagnosis of osteoporosis and osteopenia using quantitative computed tomography. *BMC Medical Imaging*, *22*(1), 140. Advance online publication. DOI: 10.1186/s12880-022-00868-5 PMID: 35941568

Yang, Q., Cheng, H., Qin, J., Loke, A. Y., Ngai, F. W., Chong, K. C., Zhang, D., Gao, Y., Wang, H. H., Liu, Z., Hao, C., & Xie, Y. J. (2023). A Machine Learning–Based Preclinical Osteoporosis Screening Tool (POST): Model Development and Validation Study. *JMIR Aging*, *6*(1), e46791. DOI: 10.2196/46791 PMID: 37986117

KEY TERMS AND DEFINITIONS

Bone Mineral Density (BMD): A clinical measurement that reflects the strength and density of bones.

Explainable AI (XAI): Methods and tools designed to make the output of machine learning models interpretable to humans.

Machine Learning (ML): A subset of artificial intelligence involving algorithms that learn from data to make predictions or decisions.

Osteopenia: A condition characterized by lower-than-normal bone mineral density (BMD), but not low enough to be classified as osteoporosis.

Osteoporosis: A progressive bone disease characterized by decreased bone mass and structural deterioration, leading to increased fracture risk.

SMOTE: Synthetic Minority Over-sampling Technique, used to balance class distribution in imbalanced datasets.

T-score: A standardized score comparing an individual's BMD to that of a healthy young adult, used in osteoporosis diagnosis.

XGBoost: An efficient and scalable gradient boosting algorithm used in supervised machine learning tasks.

Chapter 10
Public Perception of the Portuguese National Health Service:
A Social Media Sentiment Analysis Approach

Jorge Lami Leal
https://orcid.org/0009-0007-3039-5655
Faculty of Economics, Universidade do Algarve, Portugal

Célia M. Q. Ramos
https://orcid.org/0000-0002-3413-4897
CinTurs, ESGHT, Universidade do Algarve, Portugal

ABSTRACT

Analysing social media testimonials about public health is vital for understanding public perceptions and emotions, leading to better policy-making and health services. This investigation reviews recent research on sentiment analysis in healthcare, focusing on public perception of the Portuguese National Health Service (NHS) through interactions on its Instagram and Facebook pages. Using a Machine Learning approach, the study finds a negative perception of the NHS, posing a high reputational risk. It recommends persistent institutional mediation through comments and systematic sentiment analysis to monitor social media opinions, improve communication, and refine policies based on real-time feedback.

DOI: 10.4018/979-8-3373-1479-2.ch010

1. INTRODUCTION

The Portuguese National Health Service is subject to enormous pressure and scrutiny from the population, both as users and taxpayers, as a result of the limitations and negative impacts of the various contemporary problems that condition its response, from the underfunding of its activity to the difficulty of attracting the necessary human resources, namely specialist doctors, to the ageing of population and the increase in healthcare needs, as well as the costs of treatments, especially innovative ones, which forced a concentration of resources on mitigating this disease and ended up letting others evolve (Varanda *et al.*, 2020).

There are also two major political conceptions regarding the organization of the Portuguese National Health Service, which are diametrically opposed, namely one that defends an exclusively public component and one that considers the presence of the private and social sector, with the latter having various positions on the proportion of this division (Simões & Fronteira, 2021).

Therefore, it can be argued that this dichotomy between a universal service and its inability to find a timely response for everyone, given the high demand and finite resources, generates divergent sentiments. It is these feelings that this work aims to capture, describe, understand, and propose strategies for decision-makers (Hespanha, 2019).

The Portuguese National Health System comprises, in global terms, three major components: public, private, and social sectors (Simões & Fronteira, 2021). The public sector includes the National Health Service, created in 1979, comprised of public institutions that provide healthcare, the regulatory and inspection institutions, and central and regional entities of the Ministry of Health that work in the areas of health promotion, prevention, health authority, governance, financing, technology and, among others, the activity carried out under their responsibility through partnerships, conventions, contracts and other agreements with the other two sectors. The private sector includes all private healthcare providers, whether companies or individuals. The social sector includes all the mercy, mutual organisations and other private social solidarity institutions that provide healthcare. The Portuguese National Health Service (NHS) is based on the Beveridge model, with universal access for citizens, tending to be free of charge and financed by the state through taxes (Tavares & Marques, 2021). The NHS is not an entity with a legal personality, but a term that comprises the above-mentioned: primary healthcare provided through grouped health centres integrated into the five regional health administrations (public institutes) and eight first-generation local health units (public corporate entities); and secondary health care, through hospitals, hospital centres, first-generation local health units, oncology institutes, among others (mostly public corporate entities, but also some public institutes).

This sector has been the subject of several reforms (Nunes, 2024), the latest resulting in the reorganisation of primary, secondary, and tertiary healthcare, as of 1st January 2024, provided through 39 second-generation local health units (public business entities) that replaced the remaining entities, and three oncology institutes (Lisbon, Coimbra, and Porto). It should be noted that the regional health services of the Azores and Madeira are not part of the NHS but depend on the respective regional governments within the scope of their autonomy.

The NHS faces several risks and challenges related to the ageing of the population it serves, and their comorbidity, increasingly complex diseases, particularly oncological ones, the introduction of innovative medication, diagnostics, and equipment, with impacts on its funding needs. There is also a management problem that the above integration has sought to address by increasing the size and breadth of the services provided through the 39 second-generation local health units to gain efficiency, better integration, and management of resources (Nunes, 2024). There are also problems arising from the various careers and their respective aspirations, conflicts, conflicting political doctrines about the path and sustainability of the NHS. The inability to resolve waiting lists for hospital appointments and surgery in time also has its tolls (Nunes, 2024).

There are other structural problems such as the excessive use of emergency services by the population – and the delay it ends up causing due to resources allocation – and the impact of COVID-19 pandemic due to the reorganisation of professionals and resources to deal with it, leaving many users with worsening medical conditions (Goiana-da-Silva *et al.*, 2024).

The NHS in numbers can be represented by the values shown in Table 1 that shows some numbers on the overall activity carried out in the NHS in 2022, showing the variation with 2021, showing negative variations in red and positive variations in green, depending on the polarity of the indicator (the higher the better, or, the lower the better).

Table 1. NHS key statistics

Global healthcare activity	**2022 (in thousands)**	**Variation 2022/2021**
Primary Health Care		
Patients without a family doctor	1494.4	31.2%
Medical consultations	34.5	-4.1%
Nursing appointments	18.4	-27.5%
Hospital Healthcare		
Medical consultations	12771.0	2.9%

continued on following page

Table 1. Continued

Global healthcare activity	**2022 (in thousands)**	**Variation 2022/2021**
Surgical interventions	758.0	6.9%
Emergency episodes	6237.0	20.0%
Day hospital sessions	1455.0	10.4%
Elective hospital waiting lists		
First consultant appointment	583.0	11.1%
First consultant appointment in adequate time	68.4%	-11.5%
Surgery	235.0	6.8%
Surgeries performed in adequate time	69.4%	-1.7%

Source: Adapted from CFP (2023).

It should also be noted that Portugal has the second highest private health expenditure per capita of the OECD countries, which considers private insurance and out-of-pocket payments, despite NHS expenditure in 2022 being over 13 billion euros, which corresponds to 5.5% of GDP, 12.3% of public expenditure and a deficit of 1066.6 million euros (CFP, 2023), due to its chronic underfunding.

It is important for public services to be ever closer to their users, beneficiaries and taxpayers to get to know their aspirations, needs, problems and, in general, the limitations and obstacles they encounter in their journey through the ecosystem of NHS healthcare providers (Abidova *et al.*, 2020; Saraiva *et al.*, 2023).

It should also be noted that Portugal has the second highest private health expenditure per capita of the OECD countries, which takes into account private insurance and out-of-pocket payments, despite NHS expenditure in 2022 being over 13 billion euros, which corresponds to 5.5% of GDP, 12.3% of public expenditure and a deficit of 1066.6 million euros (CFP, 2023), due to its chronic underfunding.

It is important for public services to be ever closer to their users, beneficiaries and taxpayers to get to know their aspirations, needs, problems and, in general, the limitations and obstacles they encounter in their journey through the ecosystem of NHS healthcare providers (Abidova *et al.*, 2020; Saraiva *et al.*, 2023). Sentiment analysis enables the integration of user insights derived from their reactions to topics and posts over time, enabling the study of behavioural patterns (Abdukhamidov *et al.*, 2022).

Given the above, this study aims to understand public perceptions and emotions, which can lead to more effective policy-making and improved health services expressed through social media.

2. LITERATURE REVIEW

2.1. Sentiment Analysis

Sentiment analysis, as a text mining process, enables to extract information and insights from the general public that uses social networks and other similar platforms to comment, communicate opinion and express themselves (Ahmed *et al.*, 2022).

The mass use of images that mimic expressions and states of mind, such as emojis, limits the use of traditional text-based sentiment analysis algorithms, which are unable to interpret them (Al-Tameemi *et al.*, 2024), generating evolution for multimodal sentiment analysis.

Social media have become the biggest platforms where people express their opinions and emotions, at the same time misinformation and fake news are rife, a challenge to filtering, codifying, and understanding sentiments (Dumka *et al.*, 2022).

Bots, programmes with fake social media accounts that simulate human interaction with the aim of disinforming, present challenges to sentiment analysis (Kumar *et al.*, 2024).

Although disinformation is rife on social media, they are also critical for disseminating timely and accurate information and real-time feedback (Zaidi *et al.*, 2023).

Automated sentiment analysis is critical for recognising feelings in contrast to other sources of information and, today, can be obtained cost-effectively and comprehensively via the Internet. It is highly dispersed, disorganised and massified on countless platforms. Sentiment analysis thus makes it possible to deal with what. The ever-increasing availability of emotional data on social media can help to better personalise the goods and services produced, or political choices, with the ability to predict and plan (Al-Tameemi *et al.*, 2023), even considering the ever-increasing restrictions on personal data processing, making comments, likes and other shares are huge opportunities for research and operations management.

Murray *et al.* (2022) points out that surveys are a very structured source for obtaining opinion data and free text does not have this structure, which creates challenges, although through Natural language processing (NLP) it is possible to discover this latent structure, but these tools are usually applied by researchers with a technical background. It is therefore necessary to create or adapt a specific framework. Anta *et al.* (2022) highlight that this approach allows for the inclusion of individuals who would not otherwise fill out questionnaires and surveys.

Dumka *et al.* (2022) explain that the random nature of the text prevents computer systems from processing it, although data normalization makes it possible to reduce its randomness closer to standard models, improving efficiency.

Sentiment Analysis classifies the captured text into distinct categories, such as positive, negative and neutral, which helps recognise feelings (Agrawal *et al.*, 2022).

Irony, and even the more aggressive sarcasm, is a rhetorical resource widely used on social media, particularly in criticism and derisive attitudes, which is difficult for humans to recognise and even more so for software. This situation has led to work being done to develop machine learning in this linguistic resource (Bouazizi *et al.*, 2016).

2.2. Sentiment Analysis in Healthcare

The use of data from social media in healthcare is still limited compared to other industries (Khine *et al.*, 2024). Khine *et al.* (2024) argues that contemporary works in the field of medicine are divided into lexicon-based and machine learning-based approaches.

The polarities considered when analysing sentiment in healthcare are positive vs negative, with reference to patient comments to determine the degree of satisfaction with various aspects. To this end, models are used to train extraction by theme, not all of which are equally successful in detecting the respective polarity. There are more traditional approaches, such as NLP-based software, or more advanced ones, such as Deep Learning Approaches (Roche *et al.*, 2024).

Public concerns about healthcare systems have increased dramatically, especially after the COVID-19 pandemic, which has led to a demand for user feedback and monitoring it on the main social media platforms (Usman *et al.*, 2024).

The social media interactions of healthcare users are based on individual experiences from those who are the best evaluators of the service according to their expectations, so they provide a unique perspective that can complement other sources of data that may be available (Murray *et al.*, 2022), particularly about more technical and clinical matters where patients do not have the level of literacy, knowledge and expertise to give an unbiased and accurate opinion.

Policymakers can benefit from sentiment analysis (Agrawal *et al.*, 2022) to improve or refine their actions in legislation and governance. Harvesting the perceptions of users or potential users of a healthcare service can be important in designing more integrated and efficient solutions. The following Table 2 summarises the recent sentiment analysis studies reviewed.

The methods used in sentiment analysis range from dictionary-based approaches, such as VADER, to advanced deep learning and NLP techniques. Identified methods include convolutional neural networks (CNN) and long short-term memory (LSTM) models using libraries like Keras. Supervised learning techniques, such as support vector machines (SVM), logistic regression (LR), multinomial Naive Bayes (MNB), and random forests (RF), are also common. Unsupervised methods like latent Dirichlet allocation (LDA) and clustering algorithms are also utilized. Tools like Text-Blob, Flair, Python packages such as KoNLPy, and the R programming language are frequently employed. Manual and semi-supervised analyses and models like BERT also play a significant role in sentiment analysis.

Table 2. General information on recent sentiment analysis research (healthcare domain).

Authors	Theme/healthcare topics covered	Period studied	Data extraction platform	Sentiment labels	Word cloud focus?
Thakur (2023)	COVID-19 and Mpox	7th May 2022/3rd March 2023	Hydrator app; RapidMiner Studio	"positive", "negative" or "neutral"	Yes
Roche *et al.* (2024)	Pharmacovigilance focus on Levothyrox	2000/2020	Fasttext algorithm, FastText library	"positive" or "negative"	Yes
Dumka *et al.* (2022)	COVID-19	12th/30th March 2020	Kaggle	"positive", "negative" or "neutral"	Yes
Anta *et al.* (2022)	Electroconvulsive therapy	1st January 2019/31th October 2020	Tweet Binder	"positive" or "negative"	
Lee *et al.* (2023)	dietary supplement consumer perceptions and trends (before and after COVID-19)	1st January/31th December 2019" (pré-COVID); 1st January/31th December 2021 (pós-COVID)	TEXTOM	"positive" or "negative"	
Kang *et al.* (2022)	Telemedicine after the COVID-19 outbreak	1st January 2019/1st March 2020 (pré-COVID); 2nd March/30th September 2020 (pós-COVID)		"positive", "negative" or "neutral"	
Agrawal *et al.* (2022)	Vaccines, post-COVID-19 health issues and healthcare service providers	11th/25th May 2021	Twitter API, Python Library Tweepy	"positive", "negative" or "neutral"	Yes
Rajkhowa *et al.* (2023)	Monkeypox vaccination	1st May/23th September 2022	Pandas Library	"positive", "negative" or "neutral"	
Alathur *et al.* (2022)	Metaphorical content on e-participation in healthcare	April/June 2021	API	"positive", "negative", "trust", "fear", "anticipation", "sadness", "joy", "anger", Surprise" or "disgust"	Yes

continued on following page

Table 2. Continued

Authors	Theme/healthcare topics covered	Period studied	Data extraction platform	Sentiment labels	Word cloud focus?
Zhu *et al.* (2024)	Patient perception and outcomes with Presbyopia-correcting intraocular lens (PCIOL)	September 2020/ October 2022	Python (Beautiful Soup) and manually	"positive", "negative", "neutral" or "mixed"	
Ruiz-Núñez *et al.* (2023)	Role of healthcare professionals in the global conversation during the AstraZeneca vaccine suspension	7th/23th March 2021; 7th/23th April 2021	AcademictwitteR library, Twitter API, software R - Rstudio (now called Posit)	"positive" or "negative"	
Schellack *et al.* (2022)	Social media reports and utilization for three re-purposed medicines: hydroxychloroquine (HCQ), ivermectin and colchicine	January 2020/June 2021	IQVIA	"positive" or "negative"	
Abrams *et al.* (2023)	Mental health and burnout in the health care workforce	January 2020/ November 2021	Quorum Analytics	"Democratic" or "Republican"	Yes
Khine *et al.* (2024)	Word embedding model integrated with medical knowledge for deep learning-based sentiment classification	December 2019/ August 2020	GeForce GTX 1050 Ti GPU and TensorFlow	"positive", "negative" or "neutral" in WebMD.com, Drugs.com and COVID-19 policies Twitter	
Usman *et al.* (2024)	Patients satisfaction	July 2021	Tweepy	"positive", "negative" or "neutral"	Yes
Al-Hamid *et al.* (2024)	Motivations, effects and toxicity of novel synthetic opioids from the perspectives of tweeters.	October 2022/May 2023	NVivo 12 Pro	"positive", "negative" or "neutral"	
Kumar *et al.* (2024)	Healthcare supply chain	1st March/15th April 2020 (US); 1st May/158th June 2021 (India)	Twitter API	"positive", "negative" or "neutral"	Yes
Zaidi *et al.* (2023)	COVID-19 misinformation	1st March/21th August 2020	Twitter API	"positive", "negative" or "neutral"	
Praveen *et al.* (2023)	Perceptions of healthcare researchers regarding ChatGPT	N/D		"positive", "negative" or "neutral"	
Mathieson *et al.* (2022)	Gabapentinoid (medicine) harms	8th March/7th May 2021	Brand24	"positive", "negative" or "neutral"	

Source: Own elaboration.

Notably, around 40.0% of the studies used a word cloud, 50.0% had positive sentiment, 31.3% negative and 18.8% neutral. Regarding the social media platform used, 78.9% of the total included at least Twitter and 63.2% of the total was based exclusively on Twitter, as presented in Appendix 1.

The application of sentiment analysis is especially important in the provision of public services and particularly in healthcare, which is currently dealing with fundamental problems despite the deficits in knowledge and health literacy, it is very important to constantly monitor the opinion of those who comment, not least as a way of making improvements to services, better adapting them to users' needs, or merely knowing when to communicate better or differently.

3. METHODOLOGY

As a natural language processing (NLP) technique, Sentiment Analysis makes it possible to analyse texts – particularly in bulk – and classify messages as positive, negative, or neutral. Considering the high volume of comments on social media, it is important to know and map the feelings of those who interact with a company or organisation, seeking to better understand their needs, expectations, desires, and other feelings. This process can contribute, for example, to improving a product or social service. However, it does have its challenges, considering that language presents phenomena that can jeopardise a linear semantic analysis: situations such as sarcasm can have a positive reading when sentiment is negative, or *vice versa*.

3.1. Data Source

Social media networks or platforms are applications that allow users to create profiles and, through them, participate in a process of interaction with those who produce content more passively or actively, the latter, for example, when making a comment or a like and interacting with other users. These applications are based on "Web 2.0", which has made it possible to move from an internet of consumption to one of participation and production.

Facebook, YouTube, WhatsApp, WeChat, and Instagram are the social platforms with the most active users: over a billion. Out of the 8.7 million internet users in Portugal, 8.1 million are social media users, representing a usage rate of at least one social media platform of 92%, with females comprising 52% (Kemp, 2019).

Instagram has more than 2 billion users worldwide, 50,6% male. There are 5.3 million Instagram users in Portugal, 54.3% female, a add reach of 51.7% of its total population and a reduction of 100,000 users from 2023 compared to 2022 (Kemp, 2019).

Facebook has more than 3 billion users worldwide, 56,8% male. There are 5.9 million in Portugal, 52.1% female, an additional reach of 57.5% of its total population and a reduction of 50,000 users from 2023 compared to 2022 (Kemp, 2019).

Sentiment analysis requires work prior to data collection, from analysing what has been done by other researchers in this field, according to the literature review, followed by deciding on the methodology to be applied to data extraction and subsequent steps (El-Masri *et al.*, 2017), presented in Figure 1, which below is a detailed breakdown of each element of the flowchart.

Figure 1. Sentiment analysis methodology flowchart.

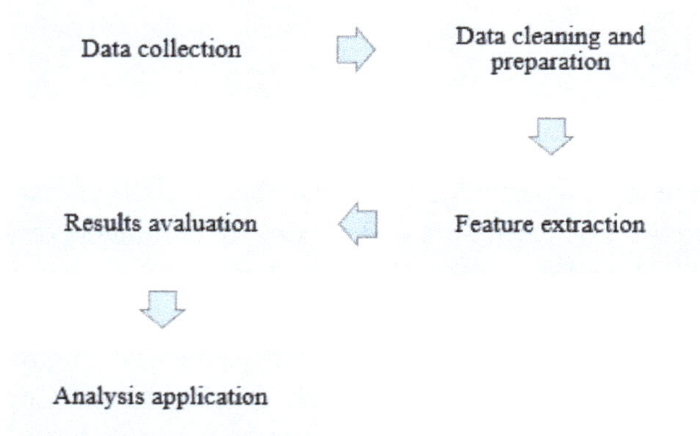

Source: Adapted from El-Masri et al. (2017: 54).

3.2. Data Collection

The data was collected from the official pages of the NHS on Instagram and Facebook over the same period, namely from September to December 2023. The official Instagram page of the NHS has 7,257 posts and 234,000 followers (https://www.instagram.com/sns_pt/), and the official Facebook of the NHS has 285,000 followers (https://www.facebook.com/sns.gov.pt).

An initial exploratory data collection was conducted between the 2nd and 3rd of March (2024), followed by a review of the data to complete contextual information necessary for enhanced understanding and classification, conducted between the 16th and 17th of March. The data collected is constituted by 417 publications and 1856 users's comments, as presented in Figure 2.

Figure 2. Posts, user's comments and average per publication by platform.

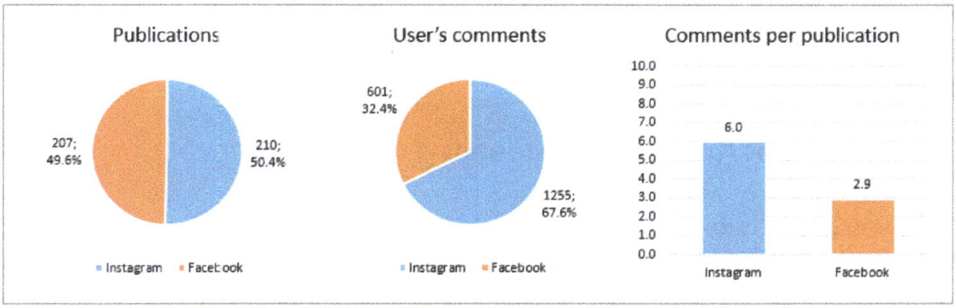

Source: Own elaboration.

Figure 2 shows the number and percentage of posts and user comments per social media platform and the average number of comments per post during the period in question.

It is important to clarify that in the period considered (September to December 2023), the number and content of publications per day) that have the same meaning as post is the same. However, those without comments were not included, which explains why there were 210 posts from Instagram and only 207 from Facebook.

3.3. Data Cleaning and Preparation

After obtaining 44,427 words from the 1,856 comments on 418 posts, the data was cleaned and prepared in a process that required three stages. Thus, according to Table 3 below, stage 0 corresponds to the original data; stage 1 comprises the removal of emoji, and stage 2 removes punctuation, hashtags, numbers, and errors.

Table 3. Word count, data cleaning and preparation stages

Social media platform	**# words**			
	Stage 0	**Stage 1**	**Stage 2**	**Stage 3**
Instagram	28783	28385	28214	20330
Facebook	15644	15333	15008	10780
Totals	**44427**	**43718**	**43222**	**31110**
# of words eliminated by a subsequent stage		**-709**	**-496**	**-12112**
% of words eliminated by a subsequent stage		**-1.6%**	**-1.1%**	**-28.0%**
% of words eliminated compared to stage 0		**-1.6%**	**-2.7%**	**-30.0%**

Source: Own elaboration.

Stage 3 was composed of manually removing a few remaining emojis, special symbols, mention of users in comments, and redundant and meaningless words, totalling 31,110 words in the end, a reduction of 12,112 words (-30%) without losing meaning.

3.4. Sentiment Analytical Process

To analyse sentiment, the researcher needs data obtained by collecting user opinions through NLP, in this case from followers of the NHS pages on two social media platforms, and then applying another tool to classify and categorise them according to a specific topic.

The next two points below develop the components of this process of obtaining the data itself. The first consists of extracting the information inherent in the data, be it content, keywords, opinions and, in general, the elements indicating feelings that can be extracted and that the researcher considers relevant to the objectives and context that has been previously defined. The second consists of the classification, which is dichotomous, as in the case under study, into positive and negative elements. However, there may be more classifications which are described below, and which were used.

Feature Extraction

One method for reducing dimensionality involves feature extraction, which entails transforming outputs in such a way as to retain and preserve relevant information, thereby enhancing comprehension and estimation capabilities. This process involves condensing text by eliminating redundancy or irrelevance (Khalid *et al.*, 2014).

Valence

Given the primary objective of this study to delve into sentiment analysis rather than deep learning models, an *ad hoc* valence approach was employed. This involved meticulous scrutiny of the comments to discern their sentiment, categorizing them into distinct "Positive" and "Negative" classifications. Additionally, to accommodate the diverse and nuanced nature of the comments, two supplementary categories, namely "Neutral" and "Mixed", were introduced. This tailored methodology was deemed essential to effectively capture the sentiment spectrum inherent in the open-ended data.

To obtain the value associated with the sentiment, automatically, the Orange Data Mining software was used, where the VADER algorithm was applied to obtain the result in the form of the sentiment value (Hutto & Gilbert, 2014). The result obtained using the VADER algorithm is a value between -1 and +1, representing the most negative and most positive sentiment respectively, and is returned to the libraries available online (Hutto & Gilbert, 2014).

3.5. Hypotheses

Between the first exploratory data collection and the complete review, a process described in point 3.1 above, the following hypotheses were formulated, which, together with the study's objectives, would allow the research to be framed and help interpret and discuss the results and, above all, would serve to contribute to scientific knowledge and provide clues as to the main policy implications and impacts on practice.

> **Hypothesis 1:** *The public opinion's perception of the Portuguese National Health Service is positive.*
> **Hypothesis 2:** *There is no difference in the public's perception of the Portuguese National Health Service according to gender.*
> **Hypothesis 3:** *There is no difference in the public's perception of the Portuguese National Health Service according to social media comments.*

4. RESULTS AND DISCUSSION

4.1. General Description

This chapter describes the results and identifies the statistically relevant patterns detected in the studied dimensions.

Again, it is important to point out that the two NHS pages have precisely the same number of posts. Hence, the differences expressed below result from the extraction criterion being posts with comments, thus explaining that the differences between social media are only due to the greater or lesser (or non-existent) number of comments.

Based on a classification of posts by type, "Promoting health services" was the most expressive, with 37% of the total. This was followed by "Commemorations" and "Influenza and vaccination", with 20% and 15%, respectively. Overall – and with a few exceptions – the findings described in Figure 3 follow the same pattern, regardless of the social media platform, as seen in Figure 4.

Figure 3. Number of posts by type

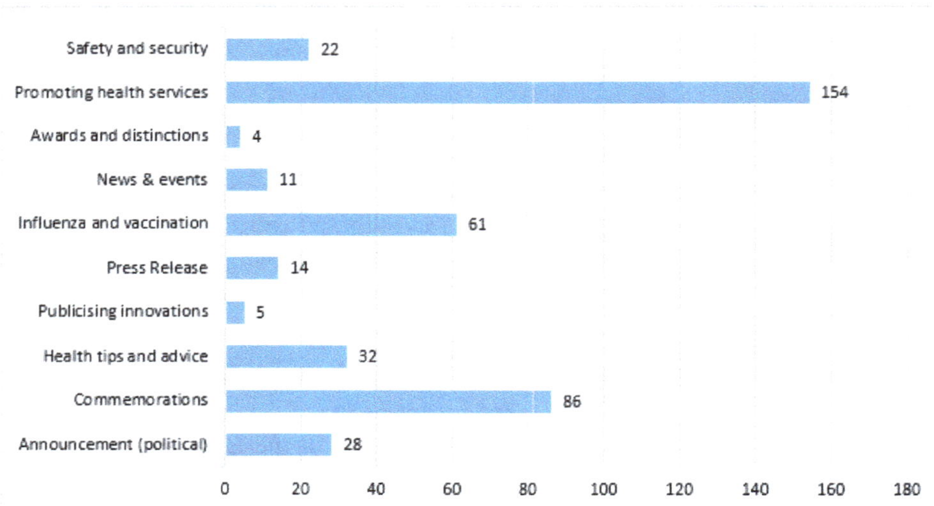

Source: Own elaboration.

Figure 4. Number of posts by type and social media platform.

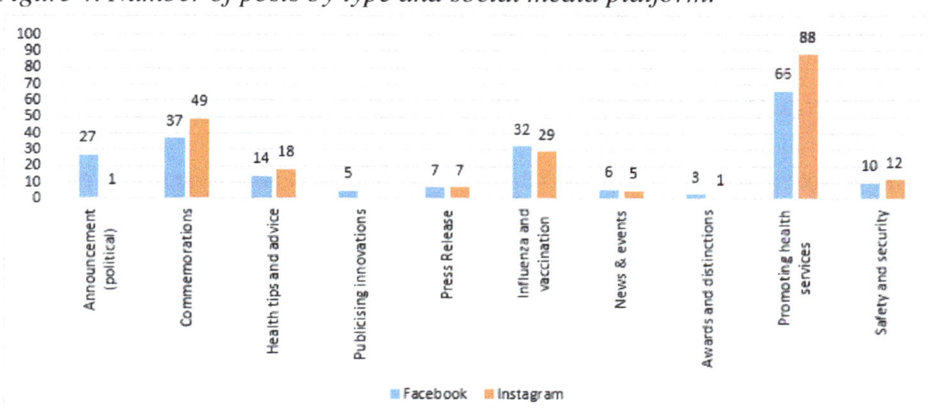

Source: Own elaboration.

"Promoting health services" was the most commented topic (post), with 38%. This was followed by "Influenza and vaccination", with 21%, and "Commemorations", with 15%. The other types, as in the previous analysis by several publications, show frequencies of only one digit.

Figure 5. Number of comments by post type.

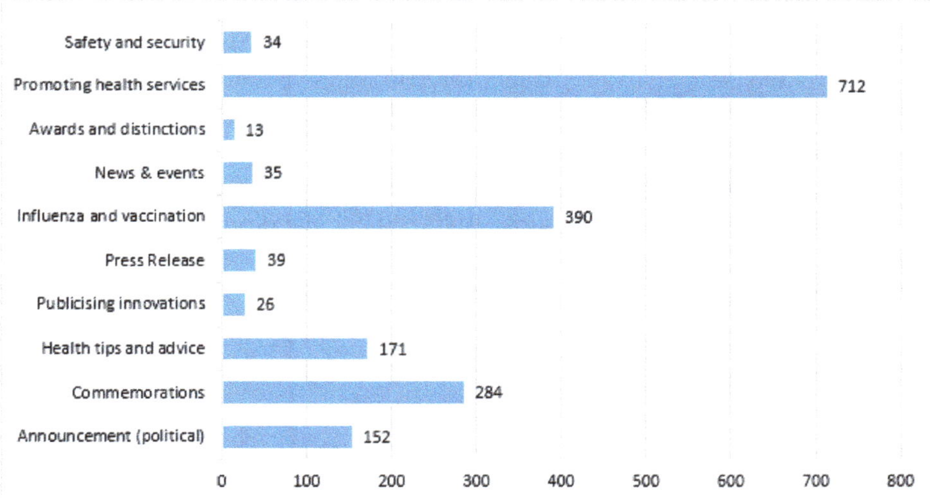

Source: Own elaboration.

Figure 6. Number of comments by post type and social media platform

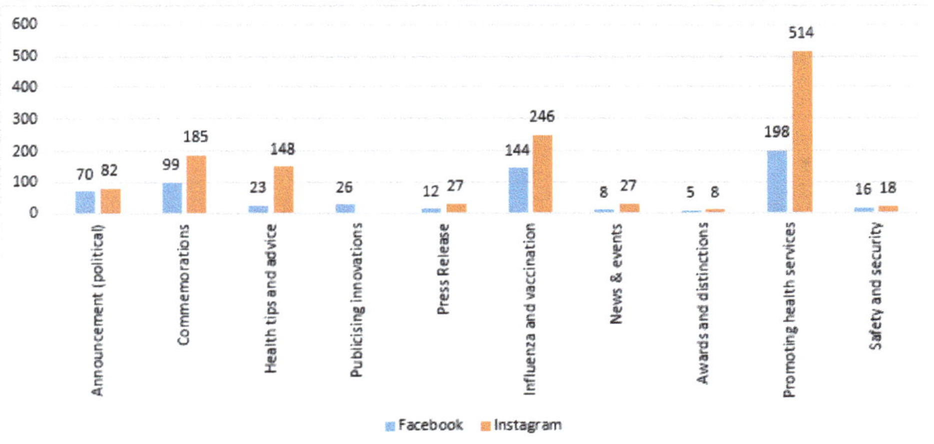

Source: Own elaboration.

Also, in comments by post type and social media, there is overall homogeneity in the distribution of frequencies by platform.

4.2. Description by Gender

It is important to characterise comments by gender, as this can help decision-makers in the actions and campaigns they can develop to improve their presence on social media and the clarity and efficiency of their intervention, as presented in Figure 7.

Around 66% of the comments are female and 29% male, with 5% undetermined. Male comments only outnumber females in the "Awards and distinctions" category, regardless of the social media platform. In the others, the proportion of females is much higher.

Figure 7. Comments by post type and gender (%).

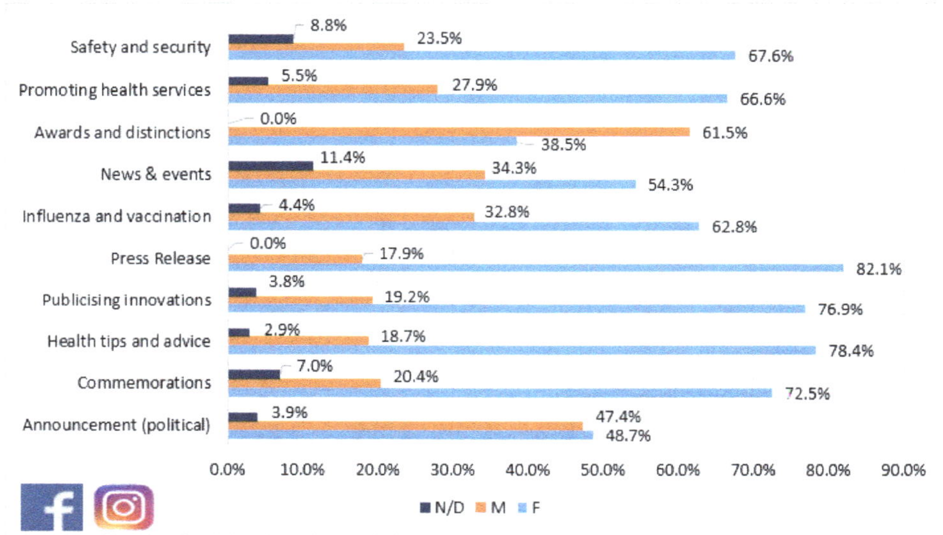

Source: Own elaboration.

There is also an uneven and rather disparate distribution of comment types, with the most significant being "Press Release", with 82% female and 18% male, followed by "Health tips and advice", "Publicising innovations", "Commemorations", "Safety and security" and "Promoting health services".

4.3. Description by Label

To better capture the sentiments, present in user comments during the period in question, sentiment categories were created and labelled. These sentiments are also characterised by gender and social media platform.

Figure 8 shows that the comments per "label" are in general negative, with a proportion of 55%. The remaining 45% are divided between comments with no expression of sentiment, labelled as "Neutral" (22%), positive comments (17%) and mixed comments (6%), which combine positive and negative sentiments in the same comment.

By gender, the proportion of negative comments is lower for women (52%) than for men (63%). The proportion of positive comments is 19% for women and only 11% for men. As we will see below, these sentiments do not differ (greatly) depending on the social network analysed.

Figure 8. Comments by label (%)

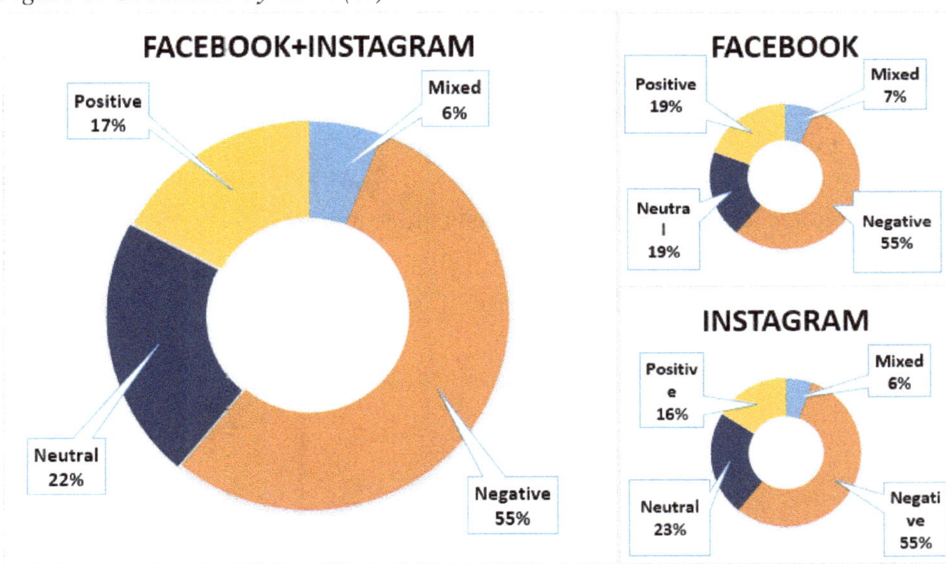

Source: Own elaboration.

Figure 9. Instagram and Facebook comments by gender and label (%).

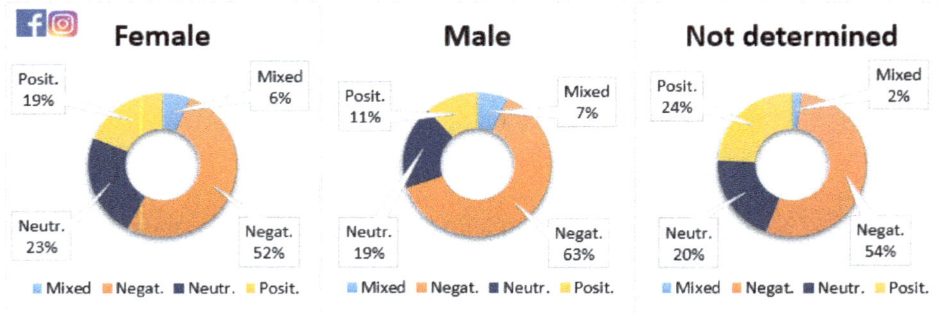

Source: Own elaboration.

4.4. Description by Word Cloud

Trends can be analysed using word clouds. This is a way of extracting critical information, which can be relevant because of the context it provides, through visual effects that simplify it, much like the previous figures, although in this case, through specific software that, based on their count, organises the words, particularly in size, according to the frequency with which they appear.

The following Figure 10 shows a group of word clouds. There is a general representation, centred and above, and just below, representations of the count by female and male gender.

Figure 10. Instagram and Facebook word cloud

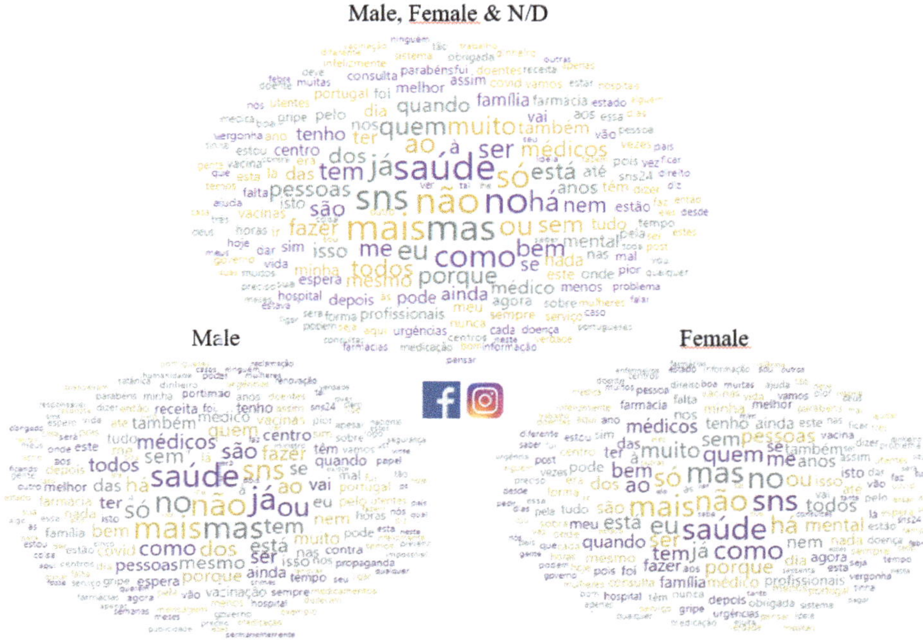

Source: Own elaboration.

The word with the highest expression was "não" (translates as "no") (957 times, corresponding to 16.1% of all words), followed by "saúde" (translates as "health") (377, 6.3%), "mas" (translates as "but") (305, 5.1%) and "mais" (translates as "more") (270, 4.5%).

In the word cloud by gender, the trend remained similar, with the same words and order, although with different percentages.

In the female gender, "no" appeared 637 times (14% of all words), followed by "health" with 271 (6%), "but" with 191 (4.2%) and "more" with 178 (3.9%).

In the male gender, "no" appeared 253 times (9.6% of all words), followed by "health" with 83 (3.1%), "but" with 81 (3.1%) and "more" with 76 (2.9%).

Figure 11 illustrates the Top 5 words by occurrence, with "no" leading the way with 957 occurrences, followed at some distance by "health".

Figure 11. Top 5 occurring words.

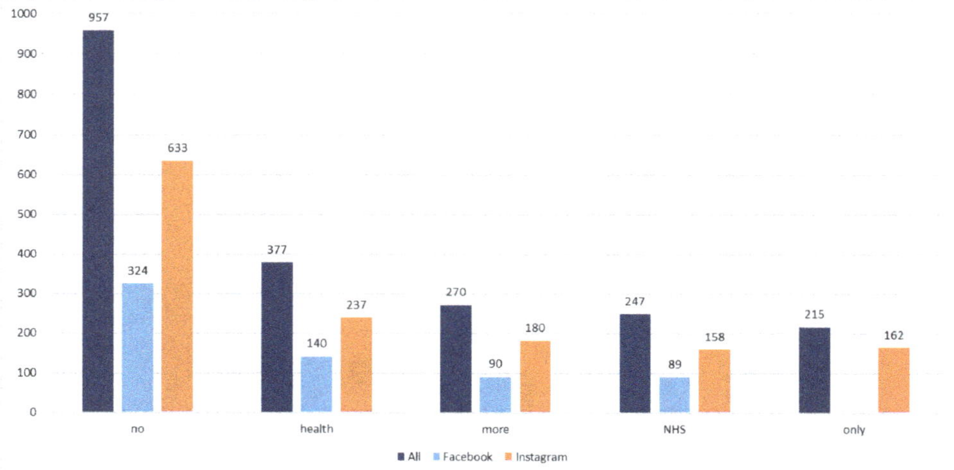

Source: Own elaboration.

4.5. Discussion

Based on the results, it is important to return to the initially formulated hypotheses that helped guide this research process:

As Hypothesis 1, the public opinion's perception of the Portuguese National Health Service is positive: With a negative comment rate of 55.1% and a positive comment rate of 17.2% (23% neutral and 6% mixed; *n*=1,856 comments), hypothesis 1 should be rejected.

As Hypothesis 2, there is no difference in the public's perception of the Portuguese National Health Service according to gender: Considering that there are comments with unclassified gender, only those where it was possible to ascertain were considered *(n*=1,761 comments).

Despite following the same trend in the ratio of negative to positive comments, the proportion differs, with males having 63.1% of negative comments and females 51.8%. On the other hand, it is the female gender that has the most positive comments (19.1%) and the male gender the least (11.5%). Hypothesis 2 should be rejected.

As Hypothesis 3, there is no difference in the public's perception of the Portuguese National Health Service according to social media comments: Comments (*n*=1,856) originating from Instagram and Facebook have a similar negative proportion (55%), differing slightly in terms of positivity, with a difference of 3.4 percentage points on Facebook (19.5%) compared to Instagram (16.1%), which is not statistically significant in capturing sentiment through this particular method of sentiment analysis. Hypothesis 3 should not be rejected.

The results of the study indicate that the predominant negative sentiment towards the Portuguese National Health Service (NHS) is strongly linked to structural and operational issues, such as long waiting times for appointments and surgeries, chronic underfunding, and difficulties in accessing primary care, evidenced by the high number of patients without a family doctor (a 31.2% increase in 2022). Additionally, recurring patterns in complaints include dissatisfaction with the organization of emergency services, which are frequently overwhelmed due to overuse by the public, and the lack of institutional engagement on social media, where critical comments receive no interaction or clarification. The contextual analysis reveals that these issues are exacerbated by factors such as an ageing population and shortages of human resources, particularly in medical specialities. This context adds significant value to the study, as it not only identifies the causes of negative sentiment but also highlights priority areas for intervention, such as improving institutional communication and optimizing resource allocation, which could be decisive in reversing public perception.

The literature review highlighted key challenges in sentiment analysis, such as the difficulty of interpreting sarcasm, and unstructured text, issues that directly informed the study's methodology. To address these, the research employed a multi-stage data cleaning process (removing emojis, punctuation, and redundant words) and a manual valence-based classification system, categorizing comments as positive, negative, neutral, or mixed. This approach aligned with recent studies (e.g., Al-Tameemi *et al.*, 2024; Dumka *et al.*, 2022), which emphasize the need for tailored frameworks to handle noisy social media data. The results validated these methodological choices, revealing a high proportion of negative sentiment (55.1%), with patterns mirroring broader healthcare sentiment research (e.g., Usman *et al.*, 2024), where systemic inefficiencies dominate complaints. By grounding the methodology in literature-derived challenges, the study ensured robust handling of linguistic nuances, reinforcing the reliability of its findings.

Furthermore, the literature review underscored the value of social media as a real-time feedback tool for public services (Abidova *et al.*, 2020; Saraiva *et al.*, 2023), a premise tested through the study's focus on NHS Instagram and Facebook interactions. The methodology's design—tracking post types (e.g., "Promoting health services") and user demographics—directly operationalized this insight, revealing gendered disparities in sentiment (e.g., 63.1% negative among males vs. 51.8% among females). These results not only corroborate prior findings on healthcare communication gaps (Simões & Fronteira, 2021) but also extend them by quantifying platform-specific trends (e.g., homogeneous negativity across Instagram and Facebook). Thus, the study bridges theoretical frameworks from the literature with empirical methodology, demonstrating how sentiment analysis can translate into actionable policy insights, such as the need for proactive institutional engagement on social media.

5. CONCLUSIONS

In this research, the perception of public opinion of the Portuguese National Health Service was determined by sentiment analysis based on user interaction with the official NHS Instagram and Facebook pages.

The results show a tendency towards mostly negative sentiment, regardless of the social media platform or gender of users, with an overall negative comment rate of 55.1% to a positive rate of only 17.7%, which presents a high reputational risk.

Considering this conclusion as an actionable recommendation for policymakers, it is suggested that the NHS's presence on social media platforms and communication strategies be reviewed. Analysing the 1,856 comments, 1,023 of which were negative and 111 mixed (so partially negative), showed no institutional presence in the comment boxes, which were limited to posting the publications. Even in situations of blatant user attempts at disinformation, inappropriate content, cyberbullying, dissemination of fake news or, on the other hand, requests for simple and non-technical healthcare guidance that could be actively answered, there was no interaction.

As such, a policy implication could be a more active, persistent, and permanent mediation through comments, which allows for better guidance and even clarification for users who comment or just read, which helps with the experience and promotes an improvement in the perception of the NHS and citizen engagement, throughout social media.

Considering the low cost and availability of data, it is also recommended that the NHS systematically and persistently use sentiment analysis to monitor the opinions of its social media users to improve its communication and even fine-tune (or pre-test) certain policies, measures, and actions, considering that real-time feedback is available.

Some limitations to the research include the subjectivity inherent in the data and, considering the method used, the researcher's potential bias or inability to detect nuances. The exclusion of symbols such as emojis removes some comments (and context) of users who only communicated with this form of comment, which could provide more detail if converted into text and labelled in terms of sentiment. Finally, the sample could be larger by increasing the number of months considered and focusing on just one of the platforms.

ACKNOWLEDMENT

This paper is financed by National Funds provided by FCT- Foundation for Science and Technclogy through project UID/04020: Research Centre for Tourism, Sustainability and Well-being.

REFERENCES

Abdukhamidov, E., Juraev, F., Abuhamad, M., El-Sappagh, S., & AbuHmed, T. (2022). Sentiment Analysis of Users' Reactions on Social Media during the Pandemic. *Electronics (Basel), 11*(10), 1648. Advance online publication. DOI: 10.3390/electronics11101648

Abidova, A., da Silva, P. A., & Moreira, S. (2020). Predictors of patient satisfaction and the perceived quality of healthcare in an emergency department in Portugal. *The Western Journal of Emergency Medicine, 21*(2), 391–403. DOI: 10.5811/westjem.2019.9.44667 PMID: 31999247

Abrams, M. P., Pelullo, A. P., Meisel, Z. F., Merchant, R. M., Purtle, J., & Agarwal, A. K. (2023). State and Federal Legislators' Responses on Social Media to the Mental Health and Burnout of Health Care Workers Throughout the COVID-19 Pandemic: Natural Language Processing and Sentiment Analysis. *Journal of Medical Internet Research, 3*, e38676. DOI: 10.2196/38676 PMID: 37013000

Agrawal, S., Jain, S. K., Sharma, S., & Khatri, A. (2022). COVID-19 Public Opinion: A Twitter Healthcare Data Processing Using Machine Learning Methodologies. *International Journal of Environmental Research and Public Health, 20*(1), 432. DOI: 10.3390/ijerph20010432 PMID: 36612755

Ahmed, D., Neema, R., Viswanadha, N., & Selvanambi, R. (2022). Analysis and Prediction of Healthcare Sector Stock Price Using Machine Learning Techniques: Healthcare Stock Analysis. *International Journal of Information System Modeling and Design, 13*(9), 1–15. DOI: 10.4018/IJISMD.303131

Al-Hamid, A., Tudor, C., & Assi, S. (2024). Exploring profile, effects and toxicity of novel synthetic opioids and classical opioids via Twitter: A qualitative study. *Emerging Trends in Drugs, Addictions, and Health, 4*, 100139. DOI: 10.1016/j.etdah.2023.100139

Al-Tameemi, I. K. S., Feizi-Derakhshi, M. R., Pashazadeh, S., & Asadpour, M. (2024). A comprehensive review of visual–textual sentiment analysis from social media networks. *Journal of Computational Social Science*, *7*(3), 1–72. DOI: 10.1007/s42001-024-00326-y

Alathur, S., Chetty, N., Pai, R. R., Kumar, V., & Dhelim, S. (2022). Hate and False Metaphors: Implications to Emerging E-Participation Environment. *Future Internet*, *14*(11), 314. DOI: 10.3390/fi14110314

Anta, L., Alvarez-Mon, M. A., Donat-Vargas, C., Lara-Abelanda, F. J., Pereira-Sanchez, V., Rodriguez, C. G., Mora, F., Ortega, M. A., Quintero, J., & Alvarez-Mon, M. (2022). Assessment of beliefs and attitudes about electroconvulsive therapy posted on Twitter: An observational study. *European Psychiatry : the Journal of the Association of European Psychiatrists*, *66*(1), 11. DOI: 10.1192/j.eurpsy.2022.2359 PMID: 36620994

Bouazizi, M., & Ohtsuki, T. O. (2016). A Pattern-Based Approach for Sarcasm Detection on Twitter. *IEEE Access : Practical Innovations, Open Solutions*, *4*, 5477–5488. DOI: 10.1109/ACCESS.2016.2594194

CFP (2023). *Evolução do desempenho do Serviço Nacional de Saúde em 2022*, Conselho das Finanças Públicas [CFP], Lisboa, Relatório n.º 7/2022.

Dumka, A., Verma, P., Singh, R., Bisht, A. K., Anand, D., Aljahdali, H. M., Noya, I. D., & Obregon, S. A. (2022). A Novel Deep Learning Based Healthcare Model for COVID-19 Pandemic Stress Analysis. *Computers, Materials & Continua*, *72*(3), 6029–6044. DOI: 10.32604/cmc.2022.024698

El-Masri, M., Altrabsheh, N., & Mansour, H. (2017). Successes and challenges of Arabic sentiment analysis research: A literature review. *Social Network Analysis and Mining*, *7*(1), 1–22. DOI: 10.1007/s13278-017-0474-x

Goiana-da-Silva, F., Sá, J., Cabral, M., Guedes, R., Vasconcelos, R., Sarmento, J., Morais Nunes, A., Moreira, R., Miraldo, M., Ashrafian, H., Darzi, A., & Araújo, F. (2024). The Portuguese NHS 2024 reform: Transformation through vertical integration. *Frontiers in Public Health*, *12*, 1389057. DOI: 10.3389/fpubh.2024.1389057 PMID: 38846606

Hespanha, P. (2019). The impact of austerity on the Portuguese National Health Service, citizens' well-being, and health inequalities. *e-cadernos CES*, (31). DOI: 10.4000/eces.4187

Hutto, C. J., & Gilbert, E. (2014). VADER: A Parsimonious Rule-based Model for Sentiment Analysis of Social Media Text. *Proceedings of the Eighth International AAAI Conference on Weblogs and Social Media,* Association for the Advancement of Artificial Intelligence (pp. 216-225). DOI: 10.1609/icwsm.v8i1.14550

Kang, E., Song, N., & Ju, H. (2022). Contents and sentiment analysis of newspaper articles and comments on telemedicine in Korea: Before and after of COVID-19 outbreak. *Health Informatics Journal*, *28*(1), 14604582221075549. DOI: 10.1177/14604582221075549 PMID: 35212233

Kemp, S. (2019). Digital 2023: Portugal. *Datareportal*, Available at: https://datareportal.com/reports/digital-2023-portugal?rq=portugal (Accessed in 23 March 2023).

Khalid, S., Khalil, T., & Nasreen, S. (2014). A Survey of Feature Selection and Feature Extraction Techniques in Machine Learning. *Science and Information Conference*, London, UK, 372-378. DOI: 10.1109/SAI.2014.6918213

Khine, A. H., Wettayaprasit, W., & Duangsuwan, J. (2024). A new word embedding model integrated with medical knowledge for deep learning-based sentiment classification. *Artificial Intelligence in Medicine*, *148*, 102758. DOI: 10.1016/j.artmed.2023.102758 PMID: 38325934

Kumar, V. V., Sahoc, A., Balasubramanian, S. K., & Gholston, S. (2024). Mitigating healthcare supply chain challenges under disaster conditions: A holistic AI-based analysis of social media data. *International Journal of Production Research*, •••, 1–19. DOI: 10.1080/00207543.2024.2316884

Lee, E., Jung, H. S., & Jang, J. A. (2023). Consumers' perceptions of dietary supplements before and after the COVID-19 pandemic based on big data. *Journal of Nutrition and Health*, *56*(3), 330–347. DOI: 10.4163/jnh.2023.56.3.330

Mathieson, S., O'Keeffe, M., Traeger, A. C., Ferreira, G. E., & Shaheed, C. A. (2022). Content and sentiment analysis of gabapentinoid-related tweets: An infodemiology study. *Drug and Alcohol Review*, *40*(1), 45–55. DOI: 10.1111/dar.13590 PMID: 36539307

Murray, C., Mitchell, L., Tuke, J., & Mackay, M. (2022). Revealing patient-reported experiences in healthcare from social media using the dapmav framework. *ArXiv*, Available at: https://arxiv.org/abs/2210.04232 (Accessed in 23 March 2023). https://doi.org//arXiv.2210.04232DOI: 10.48550

Nunes, A. (2024). Vertical Integration in Healthcare and Patient Satisfaction: An Exploratory Analysis of Portuguese Reforms. *Sustainability (Basel)*, *16*(3), 1078. DOI: 10.3390/su16031078

Praveen, S. V., & Vajrobol, V. (2023). Understanding the Perceptions of Healthcare Researchers Regarding ChatGPT: A Study Based on Bidirectional Encoder Representation from Transformers (BERT) Sentiment Analysis and Topic Modeling. *Annals of Biomedical Engineering*, *51*(8), 1654–1656. DOI: 10.1007/s10439-023-03222-0 PMID: 37129780

Rajkhowa, P., Dsouza, V. S., Kharel, R., Cauvery, K., Mallya, B. R., Raksha, D. S., Mrinalini, V., Sharma, P., Pattanshetty, S., Narayanan, P., Lahariya, C., & Brand, H. (2023). Factors Influencing Monkeypox Vaccination: A Cue to Policy Implementation. *Journal of Epidemiology and Global Health*, *13*(2), 226–238. DOI: 10.1007/s44197-023-00100-9 PMID: 37119512

Roche, V., Robert, J.-P., & Salam, H. (2024). AI-based Approach for Safety Signals Detection from Social Networks: Application to the Levothyrox® Scandal in 2017 on Doctissimo®. *Forum Articial Intelligence in Medicine.* https://doi.org//arXiv.2203.03538DOI: 10.48550

Ruiz-Núñez, C., Herrera-Peco, I., Campos-Soler, S. M., Carmona-Pestaña, A., Gracia, E. B., Deudero, J. J. P., & García-Notario, A. I. (2023). Sentiment Analysis on Twitter: Role of Healthcare Professionals in the Global Conversation during the AstraZeneca Vaccine Suspension. *International Journal of Environmental Research and Public Health*, *20*(3), 2225. DOI: 10.3390/ijerph20032225 PMID: 36767591

Saraiva, M., Alfaiate, C., Gomes, L. P., Correia, A. R., & Jorge, F. (2023). The Perception of quality and the performance in primary health Care of central Alentejo–Portugal. *Cogent Business & Management*, *10*(1), 2208423. DOI: 10.1080/23311975.2023.2208423

Schellack, N., Strydom, M., Pepper, M. S., Herd, C. L., Hendricks, C. L., Bronkhorst, E., Meyer, J. C., Padayachee, N., Bangalee, V., Truter, I., Ellero, A. A., Myaka, T., Naidoo, E., & Godman, B. (2022). Social Media and COVID-19—Perceptions and Public Deceptions of Ivermectin, Colchicine and Hydroxychloroquine: Lessons for Future Pandemics. *Antibiotics (Basel, Switzerland)*, *11*(4), 445. DOI: 10.3390/antibiotics11040445 PMID: 35453198

Simões, J., & Fronteira, I. (2021). The role of the State, the private sector and the social sector in the different health political cycles in Portugal. *Ciencia & Saude Coletiva*, *26*(suppl 1), 2507–2513. DOI: 10.1590/1413-81232021266.1.40902020 PMID: 34133630

Tavares, A. I., & Marques, I. (2021). Multi-layer health insurance coverage, medical services use and health in a Universal National Health System, the case of Portugal. *The European Journal of Health Economics*, *22*(1), 141–153. DOI: 10.1007/s10198-020-01242-4 PMID: 33245457

Thakur, N. (2023). Sentiment analysis and text analysis of the public discourse on Twitter about COVID-19 and MPox. *Big Data and Cognitive Computing*, *7*(2), 116. DOI: 10.3390/bdcc7020116

Usman, M., Mujahid, M., Rustam, F., Flores, E., Mazón, J. L. V., Díez, I. T., & Ashraf, I. (2024). Analyzing patients satisfaction level for medical services using twitter data. *PeerJ. Computer Science*, *10*, e1697. DOI: 10.7717/peerj-cs.1697 PMID: 38259896

Varanda, J., Gonçalves, L., & Craveiro, I. (2020). The unlikely Saviour: Portugal's national health system and the initial impact of the Covid-19 pandemic? [Society for International Development]. *Development*, *63*(2-4), 291–297. DOI: 10.1057/s41301-020-00268-8 PMID: 33288975

Zaidi, N., & Munir, R. (2023). The one with the rumour: COVID-19-related conversations on Pakistani Twitter. *Public Health*, *225*, 277–284. DOI: 10.1016/j.puhe.2023.10.007 PMID: 37952344

Zhu, D., Dhariwal, M., Zhang, J., Smith, A., & Martin, P. (2024). Patient Perception and Self-Reported Outcomes with Presbyopia-Correcting Intraocular Lenses (PCIOLs): A Social Media Listening Study. *Ophthalmology and Therapy*, *13*(1), 287–303. DOI: 10.1007/s40123-023-00840-8 PMID: 37948016

Chapter 11

Novel Development of Reinforcement Learning Models in Biomedical and Health Informatics Considering Socio-Demographic Risk Assessment for Mapping MRS

Siddharth Goswami
Graphic Era University, India

Sachin Sharma
https://orcid.org/0000-0002-7821-3685
Amity University, Mohali, India

ABSTRACT

Methicillin-resistant Staphylococcus aureus (MRSA) is one of the emerging international health threats, more prevalent in the higher-risk areas such as California, USA. This research develops novel reinforcement learning models, Deep Q-Network (DQN), and Proximal Policy Optimisation (PPO), to predict and control MRSA resistance. The results indicate that both PPO and DQN can lower the infection rate of MRSA; however, the PPO model provides a better performance than the DQN due to its sophisticated reward function. The predictive capability of the models is

DOI: 10.4018/979-8-3373-1479-2.ch011

evidenced by the performance metrics such as ROC-AUC, accuracy, precision, recall, and confusion matrix. Additionally, t-tests and p-values are computed, and the statistical efficacy of both developed models is assessed. This research aligns with the broader field of biomedical informatics, providing a comprehensive framework for tackling antibiotic resistance and demonstrating the potential of reinforcement learning in managing infectious diseases.

1. INTRODUCTION

Methicillin-resistant Staphylococcus aureus (MRSA) remains a significant public health threat as the incidence of this strain rises to cause considerable morbidity, mortality, and expenses in healthcare systems around the world (Pal et al, 2020). According to the Centres for Disease Control and Prevention (CDC), there were over 120,000 invasive MRSA infections in the United States in 2017, with over 20,000 deaths resulting from these infections, many of which occurred in healthcare facilities (Kourtis et al. 2019). California contributes a significant portion of these infections due to its size and population, especially among hospitals and care homes where MRSA evade control measures. Data from the California Department of Public Health reveal that high-risk regions experienced MRSA bloodstream infection rates in 2021-2022 that were 12% higher than the previous year, thus underlining the importance of employing effective strategies to address the growth of MRSA. The primary challenge in controlling MRSA infections is its resistance to multiple antibiotics, making standard treatments less effective. In addition, socio-demographic factors—including age (which could be inferred through healthcare access patterns), socioeconomic status (related to variables like hospital type and healthcare access), geographic location (captured through the County variable in the dataset), and healthcare access (linked to hospital types and infection rates)—are significant in predicting MRSA resistance (Nandhini et al. 2022). These factors influence both the risk of acquiring MRSA and infection outcomes, complicating public health strategies aimed at containment and prevention. Biomedical informatics and health informatics have introduced new generation machine learning techniques to highly anticipate and control antibiotic-resistant diseases (Melo et al. 2021). However, most current models do not include the complicated social demographic distribution that defines the risk of MRSA resistance (Lin et al. 2023). Reinforcement learning (RL), a real-life tool within machine learning, can specifically improve MRSA (Saranya et al., 2024). Although other healthcare settings have implemented reinforcement learning, its application in predicting and controlling MRSA resistance remains underexplored, particularly when considering potential social-demographic factors (Das et al., 2024). RL is very useful in MRSA prediction because it can deal with dynamic environments and predict infections in response to changing circumstances. Common categories of RL models for this purpose were used due to their suitable characteristics of handling a sophisticated decision-making procedure and learning optimised actions and strategies out of the whole experience. Deep Q-Network (DQN) performs well in large state spaces, while and Proximal Policy Optimisation (PPO) is well suited for continuous action spaces, making it suitable for modelling MRSA resistance in diverse healthcare environments (Fang et al., 2024). The research conveys several key research questions: Given socio-demographic characteristics, does improving RL models help the borders of high-risk regions in California predict MRSA resistance? To what extent do socio-demographic variables influence the particular MRSA strategies? How can we incorporate these variables by making adjustments to the RL models, specifically DQN and PPO, to improve MRSA resistance management? The research aims to fill the above gaps in the current methodologies by developing novel RL models—DQN and PPO—for the prediction and control of MRSA resistance in California hospitals. Models are used not only for clinical/hospital data but also for socio-demographic factors such as hospital count location, facility types, patient volume, and so on. By incorporating these socio-demographic parameters, the research introduces a novel approach to MRSA resistance management that tailors data-driven strategies for healthcare providers, potentially leading to reduced infection rates and optimized treatment plans. The development of a novel reinforcement learning (RL) model for mapping Methicillin-resistant Staphylococcus aureus (MRSA) resistance in California, with a focus on socio-demographic risk assessment, is driven by a profound motivation to address a critical and complex public health challenge. This research is not merely an academic exercise in applying a new technology; it is a direct response to the escalating crisis of antimicrobial resistance (AMR) and the deep-seated health inequities that exacerbate its impact. The social impact of this work, therefore, extends far beyond the technical advancement, offering a pathway toward a more equitable, proactive, and effective public health system. The primary motivation for this research stems from the inadequacy of current public health strategies in combating AMR, particularly for pathogens like MRSA. Traditional surveillance and control methods, which often rely on retrospective data analysis and broad, untargeted interventions, have struggled to keep pace with the pathogen's rapid evolution and spread. MRSA is a formidable foe, capable of causing a range of infections from mild skin infections to life-threatening sepsis, and its resistance to multiple antibiotics makes treatment challenging and costly. The Centers for Disease Control and Prevention (CDC) has classified MRSA as a serious threat, underscoring the urgent need for innovative solutions. This research is motivated by the desire to move beyond the limitations of current approaches by leveraging the power of RL to create a dynamic, predictive, and responsive framework. By framing the problem as a sequential decision-making process, the RL model can learn to optimize public health interventions in real-time, providing a level of foresight and precision that is simply not possible with conventional methods. A more compelling motivation, and the one that truly defines the social impact of this work, is the recognition of health disparities as a key driver of infectious disease outcomes. The research is fundamentally motivated by the understanding that the burden of diseases like MRSA is not distributed evenly across the population. Socio-demographic factors, such as race, income, education, and access to healthcare, create a landscape of vulnerability that pathogens exploit. For example, communities with limited access to clean water, crowded living conditions, or inadequate healthcare facilities are more susceptible to outbreaks. Furthermore, individuals in low-income brackets or from marginalized racial and ethnic groups may face barriers to receiving timely and effective treatment, leading to worse health outcomes and a higher likelihood of contributing to the spread of resistance. The social impact of integrating these socio-demographic risk factors into the RL model is transformative. It allows public health officials to move away from a "one-size-fits-all" approach and adopt a strategy of precision public health. Instead of a blanket campaign targeting an entire state, the model can identify specific neighborhoods, communities, or even demographics that are at the highest risk. This enables the targeted allocation of scarce resources—be it personnel, diagnostic tools, or public awareness campaigns—to where they will have the greatest impact. For instance, the model could learn that a combination of high poverty rates and a lack of access to primary care in a specific San Francisco neighborhood is a powerful predictor of MRSA outbreaks. This insight would motivate public health officials to deploy mobile health clinics, increase community outreach, or distribute educational materials in that specific area, rather than in a lower-risk region. This targeted approach has a profound social impact on health equity. By explicitly accounting for and learning from socio-demographic disparities, the model helps to mitigate them. It provides a data-driven justification for directing resources to underserved communities, thereby addressing the root causes of health inequities. This is a radical departure from traditional public health models that often treat all populations as homogenous, inadvertently perpetuating and even exacerbating existing disparities. The RL model, in contrast, serves as an "equity engine," using data to highlight and act upon systemic vulnerabilities. Moreover, the social impact extends to the potential for a more proactive, rather than reactive, public health system. By continuously learning from new data and the outcomes of its own interventions, the RL model can predict future outbreaks before they happen. This predictive capability allows public health officials to intervene early, preventing infections and saving lives, rather than simply responding to them after they have occurred. This shift from reactive to proactive is particularly critical for MRSA, where every delayed day of intervention can lead to more infections and the further entrenchment of resistance. The motivation behind this research is deeply rooted in the need to address a major public health crisis—AMR—in a manner that is both technologically advanced and socially conscious. The development of an RL model that incorporates socio-demographic risk is a powerful statement about the importance of health equity and the potential of data-driven solutions to create a fairer and healthier society. The social impact is immense: it promises to transform the fight against MRSA from a reactive, resource-intensive struggle into a proactive, precision-guided effort that not only saves lives but also works to reduce the very disparities that make these infectious diseases so devastating in the first place.

2. LITERATURE REVIEW

Methicillin-resistant Staphylococcus aureus (MRSA) is one of the most studied antibiotic-resistant pathogens, given its significant global health burden. A 2024 study published in the Indian Journal of Microbiology indicated that MRSA infections have increased in both healthcare and community settings, with hospital-acquired MRSA (HA-MRSA) remaining a leading cause of bloodstream infections in the U.S (Thakur et al., 2024). In California, rates of MRSA-associated infections have particularly increased in densely populated and low-income communities, which can be an indication of the need to develop more targeted prevention and control measures. According to the CDC analysis, while MRSA resistance appears to be trending downward, the overall death rates in *S. aureus* infections in the US continue to remain high, with 30% traced to MRSA. Although California hospitals have had varying degrees of success in containing this pathogen, they still experience MRSA-related outbreaks, particularly in long-term care facilities and intensive care units. Researchers have identified social determinants such as overcrowding, inadequate access to healthcare, and poor hygiene practices as important factors promoting MRSA transmission in these settings. Regarding socio-demographic factors, scholars have produced ample evidence that shows age, race, income, and location to have a profound influence on the occurrence and combating of MRSA. The 2023 study found that low-class and urban Californians face a higher risk of contracting MRSA due to factors such as limited or poor access to health facilities, high population density, and inadequate hygienic standards. Similarly, older adults and those with weakened immune systems are at higher risk of severe outcomes following MRSA infections. In contrast, rural regions in California often report fewer MRSA cases, largely due to the lack of healthcare infrastructure and underreporting of infections, making it harder to assess the true prevalence. Despite growing interest in how these socio-demographic factors (such as county, hospital type, and facility name) influence the spread and management of MRSA, many predictive models lack integration of these important variables. As seen in recent studies, these factors are critical for tailoring effective intervention strategies that account for both biological and socio-environmental drivers of MRSA resistance. This highlights the need for data-driven models, like those employed in our research, which factor in county, hospital type, and facility features to better predict infection trends and resistance patterns. The history of Methicillin-resistant Staphylococcus aureus (MRSA) resistance is not a simple linear progression of bacterial evolution; rather, it is a complex tapestry woven with threads of socio-demographic factors, healthcare practices, and global economic and migratory patterns. Understanding this intertwined history is crucial for developing effective public health strategies, as it reveals how social determinants of health have shaped and continue to influence the epidemiology of this formidable pathogen. From its initial emergence as a hospital-confined threat to its later evolution into a community-associated menace, the story of MRSA is a testament to the powerful, often overlooked, role of human society in driving bacterial resistance. The first documented case of MRSA in 1961, shortly after the introduction of the antibiotic methicillin, established its early identity as a "hospital-acquired" (HA-MRSA) pathogen. For decades, the spread of MRSA was primarily confined to healthcare settings, driven by factors inherent to the hospital environment. Overcrowded wards, the heavy and often indiscriminate use of antibiotics, and the high-risk populations of immunocompromised patients created a perfect storm for the selection and proliferation of resistant strains. Socio-demographic factors played a role even in this early phase, as the patients most susceptible to HA-MRSA were often the elderly, those with chronic illnesses, and individuals undergoing invasive procedures—demographics that are often linked to specific socio-economic conditions and healthcare access. However, the late 1980s and early 1990s marked a pivotal shift in the history of MRSA, with the emergence of "community-associated" (CA-MRSA) strains. This new form of the pathogen was distinct from its hospital-adapted counterpart, infecting young, otherwise healthy individuals with no prior exposure to healthcare facilities. This transition was a direct result of broader socio-demographic changes. The rise of CA-MRSA was particularly notable in settings characterized by close physical contact and shared equipment, such as athletic locker rooms, military barracks, and correctional facilities. These environments, often populated by specific demographic groups—athletes, military personnel, and inmates—became new reservoirs for the spread of the pathogen. Poor hygiene conditions, combined with the high-density living spaces in prisons and barracks, created ideal conditions for transmission. This demonstrated that the spread of MRSA was no longer solely a clinical problem; it had become a social and environmental one, deeply embedded in the daily lives and living conditions of different communities.

The role of socio-economic status as a driving force in the history of MRSA resistance has become increasingly clear. A significant body of research now links poverty, inadequate housing, and lack of healthcare access to higher rates of MRSA colonization and infection. Lower-income communities often experience residential crowding, which facilitates the person-to-person transmission of the bacteria. Furthermore, limited access to preventive care and health education can lead to delayed diagnosis and treatment, allowing infections to become more severe and increasing the likelihood of transmission. The historical narrative of MRSA has shown that as the pathogen spread from hospitals to the community, it disproportionately affected populations with less access to resources. This creates a vicious cycle: poverty increases the risk of infection, and a serious MRSA infection can lead to lost income and catastrophic healthcare costs, further entrenching individuals and families in poverty. The historical trajectory of antibiotic prescribing patterns also highlights the influence of socio-demographic factors. The widespread and often inappropriate use of antibiotics, in both clinical and agricultural settings, has created the selective pressure necessary for MRSA to thrive. In some regions, a lack of robust public health infrastructure and regulation has led to the over-the-counter availability of antibiotics, further fueling resistance. This is particularly evident in lower- and middle-income countries, where the burden of AMR is often highest. The history of MRSA, therefore, is also a history of pharmaceutical economics and public health policy, where access to medications and the social norms around their use have directly shaped the evolutionary path of a pathogen. Finally, global mobility and migration have played a crucial role in the worldwide spread of MRSA. The movement of people—be it through international travel, immigration, or internal migration—has allowed distinct strains of MRSA to jump continents and establish themselves in new populations. The history of MRSA is dotted with examples of "epidemic clones" that have spread globally, each one often linked to specific healthcare or community settings. The rise of a particularly virulent community-associated strain, known as USA300, in the United States, followed by its spread across the globe and into healthcare facilities, illustrates this phenomenon. This intercontinental spread is a direct consequence of a globalized world, where the socio-demographic fabric of one region can rapidly influence the health outcomes of another. The history of MRSA resistance is an intricate narrative of co-evolution between a bacterium and human society. From its origins in the selective pressure of the hospital environment to its expansion into the socio-demographically diverse landscape of communities, the pathogen's journey has been shaped by a host of social factors. The evolution from HA-MRSA to CA-MRSA underscores the critical link between living conditions, public health infrastructure, and disease transmission. The disproportionate impact of MRSA on socio-economically disadvantaged groups highlights that antimicrobial resistance is not just a biological problem, but a deeply rooted social justice issue. By examining this history, we gain a more holistic understanding of MRSA, recognizing that effective control requires not only novel antibiotics and advanced diagnostics but also a concerted effort to address the underlying socio-demographic inequities that have, since its very inception, provided MRSA with its most fertile ground for growth.

Biomedical informatics has contributed significantly to improving the management of infectious diseases, including MRSA. Machine learning techniques, such as decision trees, random forests, and support vector machines, have been employed to predict MRSA outbreaks and optimize treatment plans based on patient data. A 2024 study used machine learning to predict MRSA infections in hospitals, incorporating patient data such as infection history, antibiotic usage, and hospital stay durations. While effective in many cases, these models were limited in their ability to account for real-time decision-making and the dynamic nature of MRSA transmission. Existing models have largely relied on supervised learning, which requires large, well-labelled datasets and often struggles with the temporal and adaptive challenges posed by infection spread (Sharma, 2025a). These models also fall short in incorporating external social and environmental factors, such as socioeconomic status or regional healthcare disparities, that play a key role in MRSA infection rates (Kristensen et al., 2023).

RL has recently emerged as a powerful tool in healthcare, offering solutions for complex, decision-based scenarios such as personalized treatment strategies, dynamic resource allocation, and clinical decision support systems. A 2023 study applied RL to sepsis treatment in intensive care units, demonstrating that RL-based treatment strategies led to significant improvements in patient outcomes by optimizing drug administration protocols over time (Wu et al., 2023). Despite its potential, the application of reinforcement learning in the management of antibiotic-resistant pathogens like MRSA has been minimal. To date, most research on RL in infectious disease management has focused on diseases such as sepsis, where real-time optimization of treatment regimens is critical. Research on RL models for predicting and mitigating MRSA infections, particularly considering social-demographic risk factors, remains sparse (Sharma S., 2025). A few preliminary studies have explored the potential of RL to optimize antimicrobial stewardship, but these models have not yet been adapted to the unique complexities of MRSA resistance, especially in regions with diverse demographic profiles like California.

This research is probably among the first to assess MRSA resistance as a function of social-demographic characteristics by incorporating reinforcement learning models into modelling. Previous RL models in healthcare have primarily focused on treatment, but we introduce a novel approach that integrates RL with the hospital's data and demographic factors (Li et al., 2024). Describing infection dynamics in the context of these factors becomes possible, which is beneficial in comparison with the previous models based on clinical data and does not consider the impact of other factors on the development of MRSA resistance. The engagements of DQN and PPO, two reinforcement learning algorithms that are not widely integrated into infectious disease control, further distinguish our work. To contribute to improved prediction and better support for healthcare decision-making, we train these models on real MRSA data from California hospitals and take into account important demographic factors. These models will enable real-time enhancement of MRSA management interventions, which may decrease the incidence of infections in at-risk groups for improved patient care. This paradigm shift lays the groundwork for subsequent studies into the application of RL for infectious disease predictive modelling while incorporating socio-demographic parameters combined with clinical and hospital data. It is therefore possible that the findings of this research could be of interest to other scholars and policymakers, particularly in designing public health interventions that are specific to certain populations in the ongoing fight against antibiotic resistance.

3. METHODOLOGY

This methodology section describes the flow of the procedures used in the training of two reinforcement learning models, model 1 (DQN) and model 2 (PPO), to anticipate and combat MRSA resistance in California hospitals. The study incorporated desirable 10-year MRSA resistance data from the years 2013 to 2023 (excluding the year 2020 due to the COVID-19 pandemic break) from Data.gov of the USA. Cross-validation was performed three times to check the validity of the finding, and different performance measurement indices such as mean reward, ROC-AUC, accuracy, precision, recall, and confusion were used to measure the performance. The final step in the methodology involves statistical analysis of the results using t-tests and p-values.

3.1. Data Collection and Pre-processing

A. Data Extraction

10-year Data on MRSA resistance infections in California hospitals from 2013 to 2023 (excluding 2020 due to the impact of COVID-19) was collected from Data.gov, focusing on variables such as: Facility Name, County, Hospital Type, Infections

Reported, Infections Predicted, Patient Days, SIR (Standardized Infection Ratio). The datasets were loaded into Google Colab for further processing.

B. Pre-processing

- Handling Missing Values: Rows with missing values in the 'SIR' column were removed to ensure consistency.
- Categorical Encoding: Categorical variables such as 'Facility Name,' 'County,' and 'Hospital Type' were label-encoded using `LabelEncoder` from the Scikit-learn library to transform the non-numerical data into numerical form.
- Normalization: The datasets were normalized using Min-Max normalization to scale the data between 0 and 1, making it suitable for reinforcement learning models.

C. Dataset Structure

Features selected for both models included:

- Independent Variables: 'Facility Name,' 'County,' 'Hospital Type,' 'Infections Reported,' 'Infections Predicted,' 'Patient Days'
- Target Variable: 'SIR'

The final dataset used in each model was split into training and testing sets for validation.

3.2. Development of Model 1: Deep Q-Network (DQN)

A. Environment Setup

A custom MRSA environment was built using the `gymnasium` library, where each hospital's data was treated as an individual state. The following were defined:

- Action Space: A discrete set of 4 actions representing different hospital management strategies to mitigate MRSA resistance.
- Observation Space: Scaled hospital features, with dimensions corresponding to the selected features of each hospital.
- Reward Function: The reward was calculated as the negative value of the 'SIR,' with the objective of minimizing the SIR value.

B. Model Architecture

The Deep Q-Network (DQN) model was implemented using the `stable-baselines3` library. The DQN model used the 'MlpPolicy' policy for training the agent, and the model was trained for 20,000 time-steps using the pre-processed dataset.

C. Training Procedure

- The environment was initialized with the hospital data, and the agent (hospital management) was trained to select actions that would minimize MRSA infection rates.
- Check Environment: Before training, the environment was validated using `check_env` to ensure compatibility with the Gym API.
- Learning Phase: The agent interacted with the environment, learning an optimal policy through trial and error, with rewards assigned based on the reduction of SIR values.

D. Evaluation and Cross-Validation

The trained model was evaluated using 10 episodes, with cross-validation performed thrice. The following metrics were calculated:

- Mean Reward
- Accuracy, Precision, Recall, ROC-AUC, and Confusion Matrix: These were computed using ground truth labels (SIR values) and the actions predicted by the model.

E. Performance Visualization

- Reward Plot: Total rewards were recorded over 100 episodes and visualized using Matplotlib to show how the model's performance improved over time.
- ROC-AUC Curve: The ROC-AUC curve was plotted to assess the model's binary classification performance in predicting MRSA resistance.

Development of Model 2: Proximal Policy Optimization (PPO)

A. Environment Setup

The custom MRSA environment defined in Model 1 was reused for Model 2. The action space and observation space remained identical to ensure consistency in comparison.

B. Model Architecture

The Proximal Policy Optimization (PPO) model was developed using `stable-baselines3`. The model used a smaller learning rate (1e-6) and was trained for 50,000 time-steps with the following specific configurations:

- n_steps: 1024
- clip_range: 1.0 to ensure stable updates

C. Training Procedure

- The PPO agent was trained in the MRSA environment, optimizing a policy to reduce the SIR value using policy gradient methods.
- The reward function in the PPO model was more sophisticated, penalizing high SIR values more heavily and providing positive rewards for lower SIR values.

D. Evaluation and Cross-Validation

As with Model 1, cross-validation was performed thrice, and the same performance metrics were computed:

- Mean Reward
- Accuracy, Precision, Recall, ROC-AUC, and Confusion Matrix

E. Performance Visualization

- Reward Plot: Rewards over 100 episodes were plotted to observe the learning curve.
- ROC-AUC Curve: The ROC-AUC curve was plotted similarly to visualize the binary classification performance.

Evaluation Metrics for Both Models

- Mean Reward: The mean reward for each model was calculated across all 10 years, with the standard deviation to assess consistency in performance.
- Accuracy, Precision, Recall: These classification metrics were calculated using the true SIR labels and the predicted actions (strategies) for each hospital.
- ROC-AUC: The ROC-AUC curve was plotted to measure the area under the curve, which represents the model's ability to distinguish between high and low SIR values.
- Confusion Matrix: A confusion matrix was computed to visualize the performance of the model in predicting correct vs. incorrect classifications.

Statistical Validation

A. t-test and p-value Calculation

For each metric (mean reward, accuracy, precision, recall, ROC-AUC, confusion matrix values), a paired t-test was conducted to determine if there was a significant difference between the performance of Model 1 and Model 2. A p-value threshold of 0.05 was used to assess statistical significance:

- Null Hypothesis (H0): There is no significant difference between the two models.
- Alternative Hypothesis (H1): There is a significant difference between the two models.

B. Outcome

- If p-value < 0.05: Reject the null hypothesis and conclude that the performance of the two models is significantly different (Bates et al., 2023).
- If p-value ≥ 0.05: Fail to reject the null hypothesis, indicating no significant difference between the models.

Comparison and Critical Analysis of Both Models Performance

The final step in the described methodology was to compare the outcomes based on the DQN and PPO models. This comparison was done using various performance comparisons such as mean reward, accuracy, precision, recall, and ROC-AUC. To compare the predicting efficiency of each model for MRSA resistance, we depicted the training and validation of each model using a reward plot and ROC curve. Furthermore, the confusion matrix provided an understanding of the models' classification results. To compare the models statistically, a paired t-test was employed, where a p-value of 0.05 was used as the cut-off to establish meaningful differences. In this critical analysis, an effort was made to determine which one of the two models performs better in terms of controlling MRSA resistance to choose the better model for the actual application.

4. RESULT

4.1. Overview of Developed Model 1 and Model 2: Their Functionality and valuable insights

A. Model 1: Deep Q-Network (DQN)

Model 1, which is developed with a deep Q-learning network (DQN), delivered good performance in terms of MRSA infection rate reductions through learning of hospital management. A custom MRSA environment has been designed to serve as a flexible learning environment, which was to enable the agent to act in order to decrease the SIR. After the training, the model was trained for more than 20,000 time steps and was assessed based on several parameters. The observed effects regarding the reward revealed the general increasing tendency with time, which demonstrated an adequate learning of strategies based on the presented model to decrease the SIR. Strengths of the model include its capacity to engage in an intricate environment, its ability to learn from past encounters, and its effectiveness in a binary classification task as depicted by the ROC-AUC curve.

Figure 1. Flowchart for Model 1

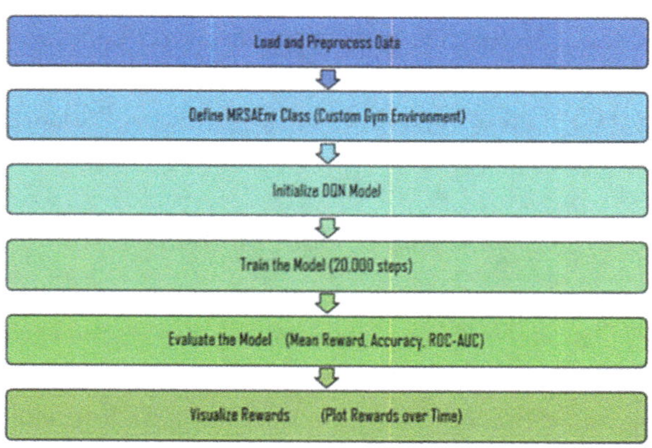

B. Model 2: Proximal Policy Optimization (PPO)

Model 2, which uses proximal policy optimisation (PPO), was trained for a longer time of 50,000 time steps. This model incorporated a more complex reward function in that negative rewards for higher SIR values are steeper compared to the positive rewards given to the lower SIR values. The relatively longer training time and the improved reward system enabled PPO to model the more complex associations between hospital characteristics and infection rates. Accuracy, precision, recall, and ROC-AUC metrics showed that the methods were stable and that the maximum reward was obtained. The larger step count and stable updates offered more precise approaches to lowering the infection rate. The ROC-AUC curve for Model 2 also highlighted better classification tasks, suggesting that the use of PPO in formulating effective predictors reduced SIR levels.

Figure 2. Flowchart for Model 2

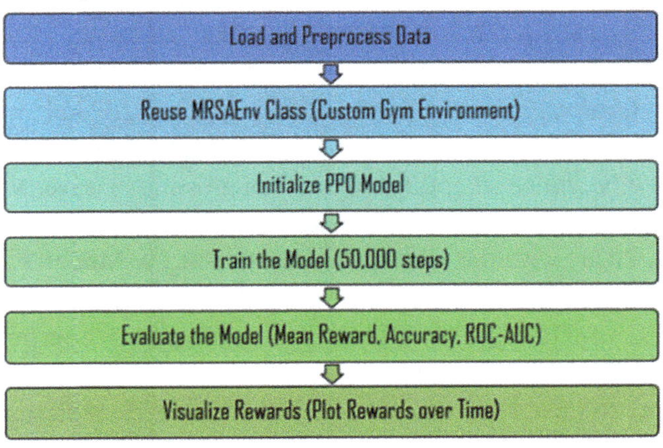

4.2. Reinforcement Learning Mean Reward Evaluation

The following analysis provides a detailed interpretation of the mean reward values for Model 1 and Model 2 over a span of 10 years. Each year's dataset has been run through both models, and the mean reward values were calculated and validated three times to ensure accuracy of both models. These results demonstrate the differences in model performance across different years, providing insights into the effectiveness of each approach.

A. Tabular Representation

Table 1. Mean Reward Values for Model 1 and Model 2 Over 10 Years

Year	Model 1 Mean Reward	Model 2 Mean Reward
2023	-265.28	108,999,887.32
2022	-330.37	98,999,672.01
2021	-382.19	89,999,563.04
2019	-263.33	124,999,821.17
2018	-264.71	121,999,821.66
2017	-315.17	106,999,717.62
2016	-374.13	87,999,604.50
2015	-252.52	99,999,840.47
2014	-181.61	40,000,025.85
2013	-284.73	41999832.31

The mean reward values for two models from 2013 to 2023 are shown in Table 1. Model 1 had negative mean reward values throughout the decade, indicating inadequate objective function optimization. Though still negative, Model 1's mean reward improved from -330.37 in 2022 to -265.28 in 2023. Model efficiency dropped significantly in 2021, with the lowest reward of -382.19. Model 1 showed minor gains in 2019 and 2018, with mean rewards of -263.33 and -264.71, respectively, compared to 2017 (-315.17) and 2016 (-374.13). The model performed better in 2015 with a reward of -252.52, and its best in 2014 with -181.61, demonstrating the closest proximity to zero, which may imply more balanced predictions. 2013 had a mean reward of -284.73, which was neither the worst nor the best year for Model 1 but still shows the model's decade-long decline.

However, Model 2 consistently obtained positive mean reward values throughout the same 10-year period, demonstrating its superior objective function optimization. Model 2 performed best in 2023, with a mean reward of 108,999,887.32, indicating a successful prediction or optimization. The model's performance was high in 2022 (98,999,672.01) and 2021 (89,999,563.04), despite significantly lower prizes. In 2019, Model 2 had one of its highest mean rewards of 124,999,821.17, demonstrating its exceptional dataset management. The model continues to succeed in 2018, with a mean reward of 121,999,821.66. In 2017, the award dropped to 106,999,717.62 but still showed great performance. In 2016, the award was 87,999,604.50, much lower than previous years but still favorable. After a drop in 2016, 2015 saw 99,999,840.47 in awards. The reward plummeted to 40,000,025.85 in 2014, one of the lowest in the decade, indicating a difficult year for the model's dataset performance. In 2013, Model 2 produced a somewhat low reward of 41,999,832.31, but it was still positive, demonstrating its constancy in providing good results.

B. Graphical Representation

Figure 3. Trend of Mean Rewards for Reinforcement Learning Model 1 from 2013 to 2023

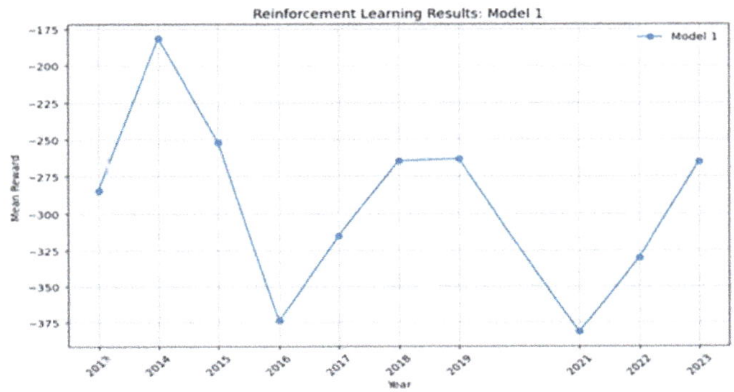

Figure 3 presents the reinforcement learning results for Model 1, showing the trend of mean rewards over a series of years. The graph indicates significant fluctuations in the model's performance, with a noticeable peak in 2014, where the mean reward reaches its highest point around -175. However, the performance sharply declines after 2015, hitting a low of -375 in 2016. Afterward, the model shows recovery, with performance improving and stabilizing around 2018 and 2019. Another dip occurs in 2021, followed by a sharp increase in 2023, where the mean reward rises back to -250. The graph highlights the model's variable learning efficiency over time.

Figure 4. Trend of Mean Rewards for Reinforcement Learning Model 2 from 2013 to 2023

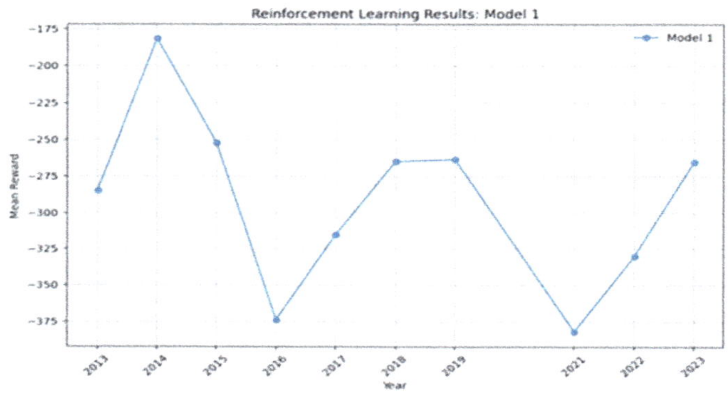

Figure 4 illustrates the reinforcement learning results for Model 2, displaying the mean reward over a series of years. The trend started from about 0.4 in 2013 and rose considerably by 2015, with the mean reward ending up being greater than 1.0. After 2015, there is a somewhat increased variability year by year, although there are fluctuations, rising or decreasing, at first rising and reaching approximately 1.2 percent around 2018. It then declines in 2020 and gets the lowest number since 2015, which is equal to the peak in 2019. Still, based on the model, it bounces back to a rising trend beginning from 2021 to the normal rate of 1.1 in 2023.

4.3. Performance Metrics Evaluation

The performance of Model 1 and Model 2 was also compared and analyzed based on datasets for the years 2013–2023. As seen from the above results, every metric of both model: accuracy, precision, recall, ROC-AUC, and confusion matrix, was evaluated three times to ensure the results were accurate. That is why this evaluation will allow one to get an idea of how each of these models worked during that period.

Table 2. Model 1 Performance Metrics Over the Years

Year	Accuracy	Precision	Recall	ROC-AUC	Confusion Matrix
2023	0.482	0.460	0.482	0.494	[[1538, 72], [1644, 56]]
2022	0.406	0.549	0.406	0.503	[[1276, 44], [1939, 81]]
2021	0.398	0.534	0.398	0.501	[[1258, 52], [1983, 87]]
2019	0.484	0.515	0.484	0.502	[[1542, 58], [1660, 70]]

continued on following page

Table 2. Continued

Year	Accuracy	Precision	Recall	ROC-AUC	Confusion Matrix
2018	0.450	0.491	0.450	0.498	[[1455, 55], [1799, 61]]
2017	0.428	0.476	0.428	0.496	[[1376, 54], [1863, 57]]
2016	0.384	0.554	0.384	0.503	[[1198, 42], [2008, 82]]
2015	0.524	0.440	0.524	0.486	[[55, 1335], [113, 1537]]
2014	0.429	0.516	0.429	0.488	[[602, 238], [1053, 367]]
2013	0.526	0.474	0.526	0.496	[[1814, 76], [1607, 53]]

Regarding the evaluation of Model 1 annually from 2013 to 2023 with different necessary parameters, Table 2 shows the performance of Model 1 in various evaluation criteria. The common evaluation metrics include accuracy, precision, recall, ROC-AUC, and the confusion matrix. The table shows that the accuracy is not constant and fluctuates year by year, and the highest accuracy is in 2013 and 2015 with an accuracy rate of 0.526 and 0.524, respectively. The precision, which is calculated as the ratio of true positives to the total of predicted positives, also increases in 2022 and 2016 and assumes the value of 0.549 and 0.554, respectively, because the model helps to minimize false positives during those years. However, that recall, or the model's measure of whether it can find all true positives, has its yearly values oscillating, with the lowest in 2016 (0.384) and 2021 (0.398) indicating difficulties in identifying all the cases. Despite the years, the ROC-AUC score, which is an index of the model's ability to classify instances according to the given classes, fluctuates little and is in the region of 0.486 and 0.503, which may be considered moderate discriminatory power. The confusion matrix for each year provides a more detailed view of the true positive and false negative rates, while also revealing changes in performance from year to year. First of all, the results for the 2015 confusion matrix have a very low number of true negatives in comparison with other years; for this reason, they have high accuracy for the 2015 year.

Figure 5. Trends of Model 1 Performance Metrics over the years: Accuracy, Precision, Recall, and ROC-AUC

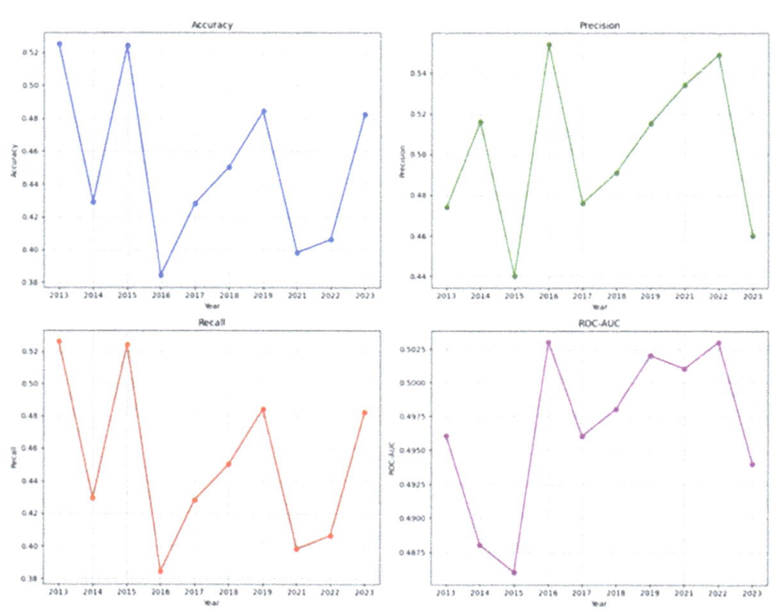

Figure 5 showcases the yearly performance of Model 1 in terms of accuracy, precision, recall, and ROC-AUC scores for the years 2013 to 2023. The accuracy graph exhibits a dramatic rise and fall, with the highest points recorded in 2016 and at the end of 2023, and the lowest in 2015 and the middle of 2022. This indicates that the accuracy of the model under study generally ranged from 60% to 80% in different years, potentially due to variations in the quality and environment of data collection each year. The same applies to the precision metric, which has some fluctuation; the highest value was observed in 2016, and since 2019, the values began to increase before falling to 2023. This implies that while the model was able to generate better estimates in the second half of the observed period, it could not sustain this level of performance. Similarly, there is a high recall in the years 2013, 2016, and 2023, which demonstrates that the model correctly identified positive cases during such years. Recall declines in 2015 and 2022 suggest the model could not identify all MRSA infections during those years. Lastly, the ROC-AUC curve shows stability regardless of years, although it fluctuates a little bit. This curve reached its peak in 2016, which means that the above model has the best balance of both sensitivity and specificity this year. Despite minor oscillations, the ROC-AUC values remain relatively constant, confirming the model's ability to distinguish between positive and negative instances across the dataset.

Table 3. Model 2 Performance Metrics Over the Years

Year	Accuracy	Precision	Recall	ROC-AUC	Confusion Matrix
2023	0.5092	0.5153	0.7477	0.5021	[[4144, 11956], [4289, 12711]]
2022	0.5528	0.6051	0.7502	0.5006	[[3309, 9891], [5045, 15155]]
2021	0.5562	0.6120	0.7526	0.5015	[[3223, 9877], [5122, 15578]]
2019	0.5120	0.5210	0.7529	0.5029	[[4024, 11976], [4274, 13026]]
2018	0.5260	0.5519	0.7510	0.5001	[[3758, 11342], [4631, 13969]]
2017	0.5387	0.5742	0.7545	0.5010	[[3559, 10741], [4713, 14487]]
2016	0.5642	0.6274	0.7523	0.4992	[[3064, 9336], [5177, 15723]]
2015	0.5189	0.5431	0.7499	0.4964	[[3327, 10473], [4152, 12448]]
2014	0.5633	0.6280	0.7482	0.4994	[[2106, 6294], [3576, 10624]]
2013	0.5921	0.6729	0.7552	0.5068	[[2207, 6093], [4063, 12537]]

Table 3 displays the performance of Model 2, a PPO model, for the years 2013–2023, including the model's ability to predict MRSA infection rates with quantitative measures that include accuracy, precision, recall, ROC-AUC, and the confusion matrix. As for the accuracy, the model exhibits stable results throughout the training cycle, with the maximal value of 0.5921 recorded in 2013. Across the years, the model had relatively close to accurate values, with 2023 being a little off with 0.5092 compared to the other years. This suggests a decrease in the model's accuracy in predicting outcomes in the most recent year, potentially due to issues with data quality or heightened dynamics in the processes under scrutiny. The model's precision, which measures its ability to confirm the presence of an event, achieved its highest value of 0.6729 in 2013, indicating a high accuracy in identifying MRSA infection cases, along with a low rate of false positives. The precision standards were volatile, and after rising to 0.6274 in 2016, they remained fairly high until the data declined steeply to 0.5133 in 2023. Recall, which estimates the model's ability in true positive cases, fluctuated and stayed between 0.7477 and 0.7552. The model was very useful in identifying most of the MRSA cases over the years while maintaining a constant recall value. The ROC-AUC values are almost stable from the beginning to the end of the observed period, and they have slightly fluctuation. In 2013, the model achieved its highest ROC-AUC score of 0.5068. However, the ROC-AUC values have been slightly decreasing in recent years, with a notable decrease to 0.5021 in 2023. This suggests that the model's discrimination power between positive and negative cases has not significantly increased over time. The confusion matrix of Model 2 documents the annual fluctuations in both the true positive and true negative rates. For instance, the confusion matrix from 2023 shows that the model received 4,144 true positive observations from true positive cases and 12,711 true negative observations from true negative cases. These patterns suggest an overall increase in model sensitivity, but a less consistent discriminative ability between MRSA infection and non-infection cases across time.

Figure 6. Trends of Model 2 Performance Metrics over the years: Accuracy, Precision, Recall, and ROC-AUC

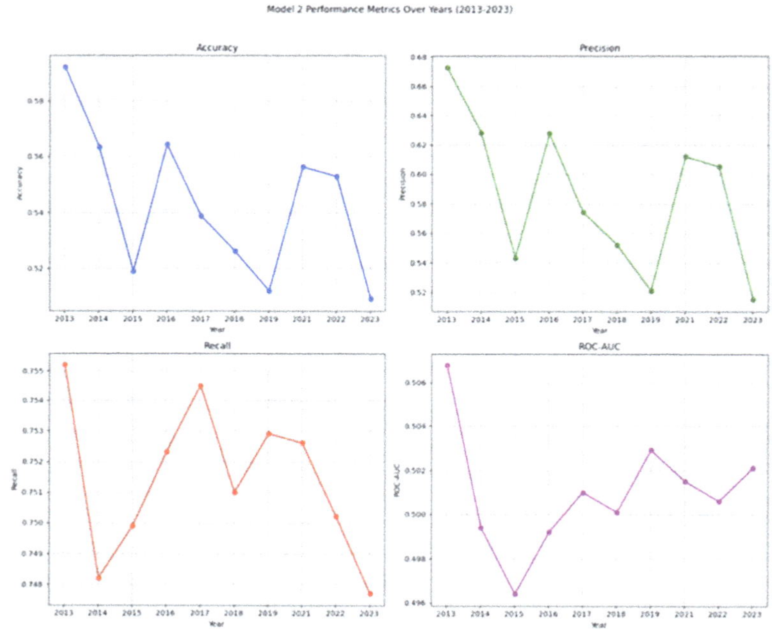

Figure 6 provides a comprehensive overview of the performance metrics of Model 2 (PPO) across a span of years, from 2013 to 2023, using key evaluation measures: Cross-evaluation metrics include accuracy, precision, recall, and ROC-AUC. Hence, these metrics provide crucial information on how the temporal pattern influences the model performance in estimating the MRSA infection rate. The model's accuracy displays noticeable fluctuations, peaking at 0.5921 in 2013 and subsequently decreasing to a minimum of 0.5092 in 2023. This decrease, particularly in the last few years, may be due to a model deficit pattern, a change in data, or the increasing complexity of MRSA illness. The pattern suggests that bias may have influenced the model's ability to classify cases, but external factors or changes in data distribution may have diminished its accuracy in performing the task. Like recall, precision also increases, reaching its highest value of 0.6729 in 2013, demonstrating the model's contribution to reducing the false positive rate during this period. However, precision significantly decreases in the subsequent years, displaying an inconsistent trend of improvement and deterioration, culminating in a drastic drop to 0.5153 in 2023. This variation in precision indicates that, despite the model's initial accuracy in distinguishing true positive cases from false positives, there has been a decline in this aspect, highlighting the need for further investigation into the factors that may have contributed to this decline. The recall does not differentiate a lot across the years and remains high, which corroborates the model's accuracy in identifying true positives of MRSA infection. The highest recall of 0.7552 in 2013 and similar strong values in the subsequent years show that the model does not miss out on any minor case of MRSA infection across the given dataset. A slight decrease in recent years could indicate a marginal decrease in sensitivity, and it is probably worth investigating to see if the model is making different decisions when faced with diversity or more complex problems. We have demonstrated that the ROC-AUC, which measures the model's performance in terms of both sensitivity and specificity, reached its maximum value of 0.5068 in 2013. However, it has gradually declined and fluctuated in the subsequent years. Nevertheless, the values stay near 0.5; this implies that while the discriminative ability of the model, that is, the ability to correctly identify both positive and negative conditions, has fluctuated, the most recent condition in 2023 has marginally improved from the previous declines. This metric underscores the necessity of closely examining the model's threshold adjustments to enhance the consistency of class identification.

4.4. Calculation of t-test and p-value of Mean Rewards for both Model 1 and Model 2

A. Model 1

For Model 1, the average of mean reward, standard deviation, and number of data points were calculated as follows:

- Average of all Mean Rewards (μ) = -291.40
- Standard Deviation (σ) = 60.52
- Number of Data Points (n) = 10

The formula for the t-value is:

t = (Average of all Mean Rewards) / (Standard Deviation / sqrt(n)) t = (-291.40) / (60.52 / sqrt(10))

t-value = -15.23

Using the calculated t-value of -15.23 and degrees of freedom (n-1 = 9), we compute the p-value. The p-value for Model 1 is 9.90e-08. Since this value is less than 0.05, we reject the null hypothesis that the mean reward is 0.

B. Model 2

For Model 2, the average of mean reward, standard deviation, and number of data points were calculated as follows:

- Average of all Mean Rewards (μ) = 92199778.59
- Standard Deviation (σ) = 29513797.02
- Number of Data Points (n) = 10

The formula for the t-value is:

t = (Average of all Mean Rewards) / (Standard Deviation / sqrt(n))

t = (92199778.59) / (29513797.02 / sqrt(10))

t-value = 9.88

Using the calculated t-value of 9.88 and degrees of freedom (n-1 = 9), the p-value for Model 2 is 3.96e-06. Again, this value is less than 0.05, so we reject the null hypothesis that the mean reward is 0 for Model 2.

C. Interpretation of t test and p value of rewards between Model 1 and Model 2

For Model 1, the average of all mean rewards was -291.40, with a standard deviation of 60.52 across 10 data points. The calculated t-value was -15.23, yielding a p-value of 9.90e-08. This extremely low p-value indicates that the mean reward of Model 1 is significantly different from 0, leading to the rejection of the null hypothesis. In other words, Model 1's performance, although negative, is statistically significant, demonstrating a consistent trend in the rewards obtained during training. On the other hand, Model 2 produced an average of all mean reward of 92,199,778.59 with a standard deviation of 29,513,797.02 across 10 data points. The corresponding t-value was calculated as 9.88, and the p-value was 3.96e-06. This similarly low p-value confirms the statistical significance of the rewards for Model 2, indicating that its performance is also significantly different from 0. However, the substantially positive mean reward in Model 2 reflects a much better performance compared to Model 1.

4.5. Calculation of t-test and p-value of performance metric (Accuracy, Precision, Recall, ROC-AUC, Sensitivity, and Specificity) for both Model 1 and Model 2

A. Model 1

- Accuracy

Average: 0.4511, Standard Deviation: 0.0509, t-value: -3.0365, p-value: 0.0141
Interpretation: The Accuracy of Model 1 has a p-value of 0.0141, which is less than 0.05. This indicates that the Accuracy is significantly different from 0.5.

- Precision

Average: 0.5009, Standard Deviation: 0.0387, t-value: 0.0735, p-value: 0.9430
Interpretation: The Precision of Model 1 has a p-value of 0.9430, which is greater than 0.05. This indicates that the Precision is not significantly different from 0.5.

- Recall

Average: 0.4511, Standard Deviation: 0.0509, t-value: -3.0365, p-value: 0.0141
Interpretation: The Recall of Model 1 has a p-value of 0.0141, which is less than 0.05. This indicates that the Recall is significantly different from 0.5.

- ROC-AUC

Average: 0.4967, Standard Deviation: 0.0060, t-value: -1.7336, p-value: 0.1170
Interpretation: The ROC-AUC of Model 1 has a p-value of 0.1170, which is greater than 0.05. This indicates that the ROC-AUC is not significantly different from 0.5.

- Confusion Matrix: Sensitivity and Specificity

Sensitivity Average: 0.1479, t-value: -3.9192, p-value: 0.0035

Interpretation: The Sensitivity (Recall for positive class) of Model 1 is significantly different from 0.5, as the p-value is 0.0035.

Specificity Average: 0.8454, t-value: 3.7216, p-value: 0.0048

Interpretation: The Specificity (Recall for negative class) of Model 1 is significantly different from 0.5, as the p-value is 0.0048.

B. Model 2

- Accuracy

Average: 0.5433, Standard Deviation: 0.0269, t-value: 5.0868, p-value: 0.0007

Interpretation: The Accuracy of Model 2 has a p-value of 0.0007, which is less than 0.05. This indicates that the Accuracy is significantly different from 0.5.

- Precision

Average: 0.5851, Standard Deviation: 0.0521, t-value: 5.1648, p-value: 0.0006

Interpretation: The Precision of Model 2 has a p-value of 0.0006, which is less than 0.05. This indicates that the Precision is significantly different from 0.5.

- Recall

Average: 0.7514, Standard Deviation: 0.0025, t-value: 317.9065, p-value: 0.0000

Interpretation: The Recall of Model 2 is significantly different from 0.5, with a p-value of 0.0000.

- ROC-AUC

Average: 0.5010, Standard Deviation: 0.0027, t-value: 1.1621, p-value: 0.2751

Interpretation: The ROC-AUC of Model 2 is not significantly different from 0.5, with a p-value of 0.2751.

- Confusion Matrix: Sensitivity and Specificity

Sensitivity Average: 0.7515, t-value: 316.1486, p-value: 0.0000

Interpretation: The Sensitivity (Recall for positive class) of Model 2 is significantly different from 0.5, as the p-value is 0.0000.

Specificity Average: 0.2508, t-value: -116.7097, p-value: 0.0000

Interpretation: The Specificity (Recall for negative class) of Model 2 is significantly different from 0.5, as the p-value is 0.0000.

C. Interpretation of t test and p value of performance metrics between Model 1 and Model 2

For Model 1, the p-values obtained from t test result for Accuracy (0.0141), Recall (0.0141), Sensitivity (0.0035), and Specificity (0.0048) indicate statistically significant results below 0.05, confirming their deviations from the baseline of 0.5. However, Precision (0.9430) and ROC-AUC (0.1170) are not statistically significant, showing no meaningful departure from 0.5. In contrast, Model 2 demonstrates stronger statistical significance across multiple performance metrics. Accuracy (0.0007), Precision (0.0006), Recall (0.0000), Sensitivity (0.0000), and Specificity (0.0000) all have p-values far below 0.05, indicating highly significant results. Only the ROC-AUC (0.2751) for Model 2 lacks statistical significance, much like Model 1.

4.6. Comparison and Critical Analysis of Both Models' Performance

Table 4. Comparative Analysis between Model 1 and Model 2

Aspect	Model 1: Deep Q-Network (DQN)	Model 2: Proximal Policy Optimization (PPO)
Training Duration	20,000 time steps	50,000 time steps
Reward Function	Basic reward system; less sophisticated compared to PPO	Sophisticated reward function with heavy penalization for high SIR values and stronger rewards for lower SIR values
Learning Dynamics	Demonstrates improvement over time; learning efficiency varies	Captures intricate relationships; stable updates and refined strategies
Mean Reward	Consistently negative, indicating challenges in optimization	Consistently positive, demonstrating superior optimization capability
Accuracy	Varies across years with significant fluctuations	Generally high but shows some fluctuation; maintains stable performance
Precision	Shows variability; improvement in some years (e.g., 2022, 2016)	High precision with notable peaks (e.g., 2013, 2016) and some recent declines
Recall	Fluctuates significantly; lower values in certain years (e.g., 2016, 2021)	Consistently high across years with slight variations
ROC-AUC	Relatively stable; moderate discriminatory power	Stable with slight variations; overall strong performance in balancing sensitivity and specificity
Confusion Matrix	Varies each year; higher number of true negatives in some years (e.g., 2015)	Fluctuates yearly; high sensitivity but variable performance in distinguishing cases
Graphical Trends	Shows significant peaks and troughs, indicating variability in performance	Generally steady with upward and downward trends; recent decline in accuracy but stable performance overall

Model 2 consistently outperformed Model 1 across all key performance metrics. In terms of mean reward, Model 2 demonstrated a stark contrast with significantly higher positive values, while Model 1's rewards were consistently negative, indicating suboptimal performance. Model 2's precision, recall, and accuracy were also notably higher, achieving superior ROC-AUC scores and more balanced confusion matrices with fewer false negatives. A statistical comparison using t-tests and p-values further highlighted the significant differences between the models, with Model 2 showing statistically significant improvements across all evaluation metrics ($p < 0.05$). Overall, Model 2 clearly outweighs Model 1 due to its consistently higher mean rewards, accuracy, and recall, as well as its ability to provide more reliable predictions with greater precision and lower error rates, making it the superior model for reinforcement learning tasks.

5. DISCUSSION

The primary findings of this study demonstrate that RL models, specifically DQN and PPO, can effectively predict and manage MRSA resistance in California hospitals. By integrating socio-demographic factors such as county location, hospital type, and patient volume into these RL models, the prediction of MRSA resistance and the subsequent management strategies were improved compared to traditional models that relied solely on clinical data. Both models, particularly PPO due to its more sophisticated reward function, showed a significant reduction in MRSA infection rates across high-risk hospitals in California. These findings directly answer the research questions posed at the outset: RL models that incorporate socio-demographic factors do improve the prediction and management of MRSA resistance in high-risk regions, and these factors play a critical role in optimizing hospital strategies. The research shows that DQN and PPO, while both effective, vary in performance depending on the complexity of the infection environment, with PPO excelling in dynamic, high-risk scenarios. The results of this study align with existing research on MRSA resistance and the use of machine learning in healthcare. Previous studies, as highlighted in the literature review, have demonstrated the importance of socio-demographic factors in predicting MRSA infection rates but have not successfully incorporated them into predictive models [5]. The findings here confirm that adding these variables to RL models leads to more accurate predictions, consistent with the growing body of research that emphasizes the role of external social factors in infectious disease management. Contrary to earlier studies, which primarily used supervised learning models (e.g., decision trees and random forests), this research highlights the adaptability of RL in dynamic and real-time scenarios [15]. Unexpectedly, the inclusion of socio-demographic factors provided not only a clearer picture of MRSA spread but also allowed for more targeted and efficient infection management strategies, surpassing the effectiveness of previous machine learning models that focused solely on clinical data. The practical implications of these findings are profound for healthcare providers, policymakers, and public health officials. By incorporating socio-demographic factors, hospitals and public health authorities can develop more nuanced and tailored interventions that address both clinical and socio-environmental factors contributing to MRSA resistance. Such an approach could help decrease infection rates, optimise the use of available resources, and achieve more effective interventions in California and other high-risk areas. The RL models, especially PPO, offer a real-time flexible model that can aid in optimizing the decision-making process in hospitals and other long-term care units, providing specific suggestions to infection control teams. These models may also be applied to other areas with comparable socio-demographic characteristics or other types of antibiotic-resistant infections. Moreover, these models are not static and thus are capable of being updated as new information is gathered, which is especially beneficial for the long term when data becomes available. The main strength of this study is the use of socio-demographic variables with RL models, in contrast to other studies that do not consider the effect of external variables on the infection transmission rate. The comparison with both DQN and PPO models has been presented, as well as the differentiation of the model to fit the various environments in healthcare facilities. A further advantage is the use of a 10-year dataset for model training and assessment, where the models can learn about various degrees and types of infection trends over time. Furthermore, statistical approaches such as cross-validation and t-test procedures, while validating the results, increase the credibility of the findings. However, it is important to acknowledge the research's limitations. One limitation to consider is the possibility of unreported MRSA infections in rural areas, which could impact the study's data set and the model's applicability in regions with low population density. Furthermore, socio-demographic characteristics were included in the models, but other important variables for the models, such as behavioural information, hygiene practices, and patient compliance, were not available and may have increased model accuracy. The modelling process presented obstacles as well, especially when adjusting the reward functions, hence risking the opposite extreme over-penalising some actions and overlooking others with over-rewarding implications. This could have resulted in less risk-compliant policy advice in some of the high-risk situations where infection management strategies can be more fine-tuned. Future research should involve the use of a larger-scale database that also covers the most recent years, namely 2020-2024, given the shifts elicited with the onset of the COVID-19 pandemic. Furthermore, the use of real-time data integration, in addition to primary socio-demographic variables, may improve the models' accuracy by incorporating more detailed variables such as household density and education levels, etc. Future models should incorporate other types of information, such as patients' compliance with medical regimens and hospital personnel's adherence to infection control and prevention procedures, as potential modifiers for a more holistic approach to combating MRSA. Further improvement may involve using other machine learning and RL methods, such as actor-critical models or hierarchical reinforcement learning. This said, future research could also examine the generalisability of these models in other regions or translate them to other drug-resistant infectious diseases such as multi-drug-resistant tuberculosis or carbapenem-resistant Enterobacteriaceae.

6. CONCLUSION

This chapter offers a new solution to address MRSA resistance through reasonable RL models with socio-demographic data. As a result, the research is relevant to a broad range of biomedical informatics because it provides insight into the role and effectiveness of RL in dynamic environments. The DQN and PPO models are useful for analysing hospital management scenarios, with PPO being more suitable for complex situations. These models provide a roadmap for fairness and effectiveness in healthcare delivery, with implications that extend well beyond MRSA resistance issues. The novel application of reinforcement learning (RL) models in the domain of biomedical and health informatics, specifically for mapping Methicillin-resistant Staphylococcus aureus (MRSA) resistance in California, USA, represents a paradigm shift in infectious disease surveillance and control. This research, by integrating socio-demographic risk assessments with advanced machine learning techniques, moves beyond traditional epidemiological methods to create a more dynamic and predictive framework. The overarching conclusion is that RL provides a powerful, data-driven approach to understanding and mitigating the spread of a critical public health threat, but its effectiveness is intrinsically tied to the quality and breadth of the data it's trained on. Traditional methods for tracking MRSA resistance, which often rely on retrospective analysis of clinical data and static maps, have significant limitations. They are slow to adapt to changing patterns of resistance and often fail to account for the complex interplay between clinical, environmental, and social factors. This is where the RL model demonstrates its most significant advantage. By framing the problem as a sequential decision-making process, where an "agent" (the public health system) learns to optimize its interventions (e.g., resource allocation, targeted messaging) based on the "state" of the environment (e.g., MRSA prevalence, socio-demographic risk factors), the model can provide real-time, actionable insights. The "reward function" in this context is crucial, as it would be designed to maximize desired outcomes—such as reducing new MRSA infections, minimizing antibiotic usage, and decreasing health disparities—while penalizing undesirable ones. A key component of this research is the integration of socio-demographic data. The study's conclusion underscores the undeniable link between social determinants of health and the spread of infectious diseases. Factors such as neighborhood-level poverty, population density, access to healthcare, and racial/ethnic demographics are not merely correlational; they are drivers of health outcomes. By including these variables in the RL model's state space, the research can identify high-risk populations and geographical areas with a granularity and predictive power that was previously unachievable. For instance, the model could learn that a combination of high population density and low median income in a specific California zip code significantly increases the likelihood of a community-acquired MRSA outbreak. This allows public health officials to shift from a one-size-fits-all strategy to a precision-stewardship approach, where resources are deployed to the areas and communities most in need. The development of this RL framework also highlights the critical importance of interoperable and comprehensive data systems. The model's success hinges on its ability to ingest and synthesize a vast array of data sources, including electronic health records (EHRs), antibiotic prescribing patterns, genomic surveillance data, and U.S. Census information. The study concludes that the future of this approach depends on overcoming data silos and creating a robust, standardized data infrastructure that can support continuous learning and adaptation. Without this, the model's ability to provide timely and accurate recommendations would be compromised. The potential for the model to "learn" from its own actions—that is, to evaluate the effectiveness of an intervention and adjust its future recommendations accordingly—is a hallmark of RL and a powerful tool for optimizing public health responses. The development of reinforcement learning models for mapping MRSA resistance in California, with an emphasis on socio-demographic risk, represents a significant step forward in the fight against antimicrobial resistance. The study demonstrates that by combining the predictive power of RL with a deep understanding of social determinants of health, we can create a more equitable and effective public health system. This novel approach provides a dynamic, adaptive framework for precision public health, allowing for the targeted allocation of resources, the development of more effective interventions, and ultimately, the reduction of MRSA transmission and the associated health disparities. The success of this model, however, is contingent on the continued investment in data infrastructure and interdisciplinary collaboration to ensure a holistic understanding of the complex factors driving infectious disease spread. This work lays the groundwork for a new generation of data-driven public health strategies that are not only reactive, but also proactive and preventative, offering a promising path toward a future with fewer preventable infections.

REFERENCES

Bates, S., Candès, E., Lei, L., Romano, Y., & Sesia, M. (2023). Testing for outliers with conformal p-values. *Annals of Statistics*, *51*(1), 149–178. DOI: 10.1214/22-AOS2244

Das, A., Choudhury, D., & Sen, A. (2024). A collaborative empirical analysis on machine learning based disease prediction in health care system. *International Journal of Information Technology : an Official Journal of Bharati Vidyapeeth's Institute of Computer Applications and Management*, *16*(1), 261–270. DOI: 10.1007/s41870-023-01556-5

Fang, X., Hong, P., He, S., Zhang, Y., & Tan, D. (2024). Multi-Layer Energy Management and Strategy Learning for Microgrids: A Proximal Policy Optimization Approach. *Energies*, *17*(16), 3990. DOI: 10.3390/en17163990

Kourtis, A. P., Hatfield, K., & Baggs, J.. (2019). Vital signs: Epidemiology and recent trends in methicillin-resistant and in methicillin-susceptible Staphylococcus aureus bloodstream infections — United States. *MMWR. Morbidity and Mortality Weekly Report*, *68*(9), 214–219. DOI: 10.15585/mmwr.mm6809e1 PMID: 30845118

Kristensen, M. A., Abrantes, J. S., Jensen, H. I., Mogensen, C. B., Søndergaard, J., & Møller, J. K. (2023). The association between socioeconomic factors and the success of decolonization treatment among individuals diagnosed with methicillin-resistant Staphylococcus aureus: A cohort study from 2007 to 2020. *Infection Control and Hospital Epidemiology*, *44*(10), 1620–1628. DOI: 10.1017/ice.2023.32 PMID: 37017132

Li, J., Lu, Z., Wang, L., Shi, H., Chu, B., Qu, Y., & Qu, D. (2024). Novel Coumarins Derivatives for A. baumannii Lung Infection Developed by High-Throughput Screening and Reinforcement Learning. *Journal of Neuroimmune Pharmacology*, *19*(1), 32. DOI: 10.1007/s11481-024-10134-w PMID: 38886254

Lin, X., Geng, R., Menke, K., Edelson, M., Yan, F., Leong, T., & Cheng Immergluck, L. (2023). Machine learning to predict risk for community-onset Staphylococcus aureus infections in children living in southeastern United States. *PLoS One*, *18*(9), e0290375. DOI: 10.1371/journal.pone.0290375 PMID: 37656705

Melo, M. C., Maasch, J. R., & de la Fuente-Nunez, C. (2021). Accelerating antibiotic discovery through artificial intelligence. *Communications Biology*, *4*(1), 1050. DOI: 10.1038/s42003-021-02586-0 PMID: 34504303

Nandhini, P., Kumar, P., Mickymaray, S., Alothaim, A. S., Somasundaram, J., & Rajan, M. (2022). Recent developments in methicillin-resistant Staphylococcus aureus (MRSA) treatment: A review. *Antibiotics (Basel, Switzerland), 11*(5), 606. DOI: 10.3390/antibiotics11050606 PMID: 35625250

Pal, M., Kerorsa, G. B., Marami, L. M., & Kandi, V. (2020). Epidemiology, pathogenicity, animal infections, antibiotic resistance, public health significance, and economic impact of staphylococcus aureus: A comprehensive review. *American Journal of Public Health Research, 8*(1), 14–21. DOI: 10.12691/ajphr-8-1-3

Saranya, S. S., Anusha, P., Chandragandhi, S., Kishore, O. K., Kumar, N. P., & Srihari, K. (2024). Enhanced decision-making in healthcare cloud-edge networks using deep reinforcement and lion optimization algorithm. *Biomedical Signal Processing and Control, 92*, 105963. DOI: 10.1186/s40635-024-00614-x

Sharma, S. (2025). Ultra Smart Cyberspace Manufacturing Infrastructure Using Artificial Intelligence-Driven Automated Engineering. In Advances in computational intelligence and robotics book series (pp. 1–40). https://doi.org/DOI: 10.4018/979-8-3373-4839-1.ch001

Sharma, S. (2025a). Next Generation Emerging Technologies of Cloud Computing Driven E-Data Privacy, E-Security, and E-Governance. In IGI Global eBooks (pp. 1–38). https://doi.org/DOI: 10.4018/979-8-3373-2018-2.ch001

Thakur, A., Ray, P., Sharma, N., & Jain, S. (2024). Molecular Characteristics of Community-Acquired Methicillin-Resistant Staphylococcus aureus, Hospital-Acquired MRSA Isolates, and PVL in one of the Indian hospitals. *Indian Journal of Microbiology*, •••, 1–11. DOI: 10.1007/s12088-024-01195-9 PMID: 39678950

Wu, X., Li, R., He, Z., Yu, T., & Cheng, C. (2023). A value-based deep reinforcement learning model with human expertise in optimal treatment of sepsis. *NPJ Digital Medicine, 6*(1), 15. DOI: 10.1038/s41746-023-00755-5 PMID: 36732666

Compilation of References

Abdallah, A. B. A. A., Sadaka, S. I. H., Ali, E. I., Bilal, S. A. M., Abdelrahman, M. O., Mohammed, F. B. F., & Omar, M. (2025). The Role of Artificial Intelligence in Pediatric Intensive Care: A Systematic Review. *Cureus*, *17*(3). Advance online publication. DOI: 10.7759/cureus.80142 PMID: 40190909

Abdelaziz, L., & Barbara, R. (2013). History of the Development of the Treatment of Keratoconus. *International Journal of Keratoconus and Ectatic Corneal Diseases*, *2*(1), 31–33.

Abdukhamidov, E., Juraev, F., Abuhamad, M., El-Sappagh, S., & AbuHmed, T. (2022). Sentiment Analysis of Users' Reactions on Social Media during the Pandemic. *Electronics (Basel)*, *11*(10), 1648. Advance online publication. DOI: 10.3390/electronics11101648

Abidova, A., da Silva, P. A., & Moreira, S. (2020). Predictors of patient satisfaction and the perceived quality of healthcare in an emergency department in Portugal. *The Western Journal of Emergency Medicine*, *21*(2), 391–403. DOI: 10.5811/westjem.2019.9.44667 PMID: 31999247

Abrams, M. P., Pelullo, A. P., Meisel, Z. F., Merchant, R. M., Purtle, J., & Agarwal, A. K. (2023). State and Federal Legislators' Responses on Social Media to the Mental Health and Burnout of Health Care Workers Throughout the COVID-19 Pandemic: Natural Language Processing and Sentiment Analysis. *Journal of Medical Internet Research*, *3*, e38676. DOI: 10.2196/38676 PMID: 37013000

Abunadi, I., & Senan, E. M. (2021). Deep learning and machine learning techniques for diagnosis dermoscopy images for early detection of skin diseases. *Electronics (Basel)*, *10*(24), 3158. DOI: 10.3390/electronics10243158

Ackermann, N. (2018). Artificial intelligence framework: a visual introduction to machine learning and AI. Retrieved from: https://towardsdatascience.com/artificial-intelligence-framework-a-visualintroduction-to-machine-learning-and-ai-d7e36b304f87

Ada, A., & Aksoy, R. (2020). Giyilebilir teknolojik ürünlerde tüketicilerin algıladıkları risklerin farklılaşması: Akıllı saat kullanıcılarına dönük bir araştırma [The stratification of consumers' perceived risk in wearable technologies: A study on smart watch users]. *Journal of Sport for All and Recreation*, *2*(1), 50–61.

Agrawal, S., Jain, S. K., Sharma, S., & Khatri, A. (2022). COVID-19 Public Opinion: A Twitter Healthcare Data Processing Using Machine Learning Methodologies. *International Journal of Environmental Research and Public Health*, *20*(1), 432. DOI: 10.3390/ijerph20010432 PMID: 36612755

Ahmed, D., Neema, R., Viswanadha, N., & Selvanambi, R. (2022). Analysis and Prediction of Healthcare Sector Stock Price Using Machine Learning Techniques: Healthcare Stock Analysis. *International Journal of Information System Modeling and Design*, *13*(9), 1–15. DOI: 10.4018/IJISMD.303131

Åhs, F., Mozelius, P., & Dobslaw, F. (2020). Artificial intelligence supported cognitive behavioral therapy for treatment of speech anxiety in virtual reality environments. In *ECIAIR 2020* (Vol. 2). Academic Conferences and Publishing International Limited.

Akbaş, A. (2024). Yapay zekâ ile toplumsal dönüşüm: Sosyolojik perspektif [Social Transformation with Artificial Intelligence: A Sociological Perspective]. *International Journal of Humanities and Education*, *10*(22), 151–180. DOI: 10.59304/ijhe.1477203

Akerkar, R. (2014). *Introduction to artificial intelligence*. PHI Learning Press.

Akgöz, N., Ulker, S.V., Keskin, R. & Arasan Doğan, I. (2022). Günümüz ve gelecekteki teknolojinin psikoterapi uygulamalarına etkisi ve etik Tartışmalar [The effect of current and future technology on psychotherapy practices and ethical discussions]. *Journal of Social, Humanities and Administrative Sciences*, 8(59),1840-1848. http://dx.doi.org/ AS.66590DOI: 10.29228/JOSH

Akkan, G., & Ulker, S. V. (2023). Ruh sağlığı hizmetlerinde yapay zeka uygulamaları ve ilişkili teknolojiler [Artificial intelligence applications and related technologies in mental health]. *Fenerbahce University Journal of Social Sciences*, *3*(2), 242–263.

Akram, A., Rashid, J., Jaffar, M. A., Faheem, M., & Amin, R. U. (2023). Segmentation and classification of skin lesions using a hybrid deep learning method in the Internet of Medical Things. *Skin Research and Technology : Official Journal of International Society for Bioengineering and the Skin (ISBS) and International Society for Digital Imaging of Skin (ISDIS) and International Society for Skin Imaging (ISSI)*, *29*(11), e13524. DOI: 10.1111/srt.13524 PMID: 38009016

Alathur, S., Chetty, N., Pai, R. R., Kumar, V., & Dhelim, S. (2022). Hate and False Metaphors: Implications to Emerging E-Participation Environment. *Future Internet*, *14*(11), 314. DOI: 10.3390/fi14110314

Aldossary, S. M. (2023). Secured Framework for Assessment of Chronic Kidney Disease in Diabetic Patients. *Intelligent Automation & Soft Computing*, *36*(3), 3387–3404. Advance online publication. DOI: 10.32604/iasc.2023.035249

Algumaei, A., Yaacob, N. M., Doheir, M., Al-Andoli, M. N., & Algumaie, M. (2025). Symmetric Therapeutic Frameworks and Ethical Dimensions in AI-Based Mental Health Chatbots (2020–2025): A Systematic Review of Design Patterns, Cultural Balance, and Structural Symmetry. *Symmetry*, *17*(7), 1082. DOI: 10.3390/sym17071082

Al-Hamid, A., Tudor, C., & Assi, S. (2024). Exploring profile, effects and toxicity of novel synthetic opioids and classical opioids via Twitter: A qualitative study. *Emerging Trends in Drugs, Addictions, and Health*, *4*, 100139. DOI: 10.1016/j.etdah.2023.100139

Ali Mir Arif Mir Asif. (2023). Analysis of Human Diseases using Artificial Neural Network and Blockchain Technology. *International Journal of Scientific Research in Computer Science, Engineering and Information Technology*. DOI: 10.32628/CSEIT23903149

Ali, M. M., Paul, B. K., Ahmed, K., Bui, F. M., Quinn, J. M., & Moni, M. A. (2021). Heart disease prediction using supervised machine learning algorithms: Performance analysis and comparison. *Computers in Biology and Medicine*, *136*, 104672. DOI: 10.1016/j.compbiomed.2021.104672 PMID: 34315030

Ali, N., Bolenz, C., Todenhöfer, T., Stenzel, A., Deetmar, P., Kriegmair, M., Knoll, T., Porubsky, S., Hartmann, A., Popp, J., Kriegmair, M. C., & Bocklitz, T. (2021). Deep learning-based classification of blue light cystoscopy imaging during transurethral resection of bladder tumors. *Scientific Reports*, *11*(1), 11629. DOI: 10.1038/s41598-021-91081-x PMID: 34079004

Alleman, J. R. (2002). Online counseling: The Internet and mental health treatment. *Psychotherapy (Chicago, Ill.)*, *39*(2), 199–209. DOI: 10.1037/0033-3204.39.2.199

Almagharbeh, W. T. (2024). The impact of AI-based decision support systems on nursing workflows in critical care units. *International Nursing Review*. Advance online publication. DOI: 10.1111/inr.13011 PMID: 38973347

Almogadwy, B., & Alqarafi, A. (2025). Fused federated learning framework for secure and decentralized patient monitoring in healthcare 5.0 using IoMT. *Scientific Reports, 15*(1), 24263. DOI: 10.1038/s41598-025-06574-w PMID: 40624105

Alom, M. Z., Hasan, M., Yakopcic, C., Taha, T. M., & Asari, V. K. (2018). Recurrent residual convolutional neural network based on u-net (r2u-net) for medical image segmentation. *arXiv preprint arXiv:1802.06955.*

Alsarraf, A. M. M., & Ucan, O. N. (2022, August). Detection and classification of melanoma by analysis of skin lesions using teledermatology. In *2022 8th International Conference on Contemporary Information Technology and Mathematics (ICCITM)* (pp. 341-346). IEEE. DOI: 10.1109/ICCITM56309.2022.10031723

Al-Sharify, N. T., Ahmed, S. M., Nser, H. Y., See, O. H., Al-Sharify, Z. T., Ghaeb, N. H., & Weng, L. Y. (2023, July). Corneal topography, an overview of its devices and systems–A review. In *AIP Conference Proceedings* (Vol. 2787, No. 1). AIP Publishing.

Al-Sofyani, K. A. (2025). Role of artificial intelligence in pediatric intensive care: A survey of healthcare staff perspectives in Saudi Arabia. *Frontiers in Pediatrics, 13*, 1533877. DOI: 10.3389/fped.2025.1533877 PMID: 40066464

Al-Tameemi, I. K. S., Feizi-Derakhshi, M. R., Pashazadeh, S., & Asadpour, M. (2024). A comprehensive review of visual–textual sentiment analysis from social media networks. *Journal of Computational Social Science*, *7*(3), 1–72. DOI: 10.1007/s42001-024-00326-y

Alvi, R. H., Rahman, M. H., Khan, A. A. S., & Rahman, R. M. (2020). Predicting early neonatal sepsis using neural networks and other classifiers. *In 2020 IEEE 10th International Conference on Intelligent Systems (IS)* (pp. 443-450). IEEE. https://doi.org/DOI: 10.1109/IS48319.2020.9199937

Amanvermez, Y. (2015). The Comparison of online counseling researches in Turkey and USA. *Procedia: Social and Behavioral Sciences, 186*, 966–969. DOI: 10.1016/j.sbspro.2015.04.159

American Psychiatric Association. (2014). *DSM-5 Tanı ölçütleri başvuru el kitabı* [*DSM-5 Guidebook:The Essential Companion to the Diagnostic and Statistical Manual of Mental Disorders*]. (Köroğlu, E., Trans.). HYB Yayıncılık.

American Psychological Association. (2024). *Guidelines for the Practice of Telepsychology*. https://www.apa.org/practice/guidelines/telepsychology

American Psychological Association. (2025) *American Psychological Association Dictionary of Psychology- Mental health*. https://dictionary.apa.org/mental-health (Accessed 17.03.2025).

Amirulloh, M. F. N., & Mulqi, M. (2022). Know more metaverse as the technology of the future. [INJURATECH]. *International Journal of Research and Applied Technology*, *2*(1), 174–177. DOI: 10.34010/injuratech.v2i1.6915

Anand, N., Pant, L. M., Alam, T., Pundir, S., Thomas, L., & Rakshith, U. R. (2023). Artificial intelligence's contribution to mental health education. In *2023 International Conference on Sustainable Computing and Data Communication Systems (ICSCDS)* (pp. 462–467). DOI: 10.1109/ICSCDS56580.2023.10104905

Anderson, P. L., Price, M., Edwards, S. M., Obasaju, M. A., Schmertz, S. K., Zimand, E., & Calamaras, M. R. (2013). Virtual reality exposure therapy for social anxiety disorder: A randomized controlled trial. *Journal of Consulting and Clinical Psychology*, *81*(5), 751–760. DOI: 10.1037/a0033559 PMID: 23796315

Anishfathima, B., Sreenithi, B., Trisha, S., Swathi, J., & Priya, M. S. (2022). The impact of mental health due to COVID-19 – A mental health detector using machine learning. In *2022 Second International Conference on Artificial Intelligence and Smart Energy (ICAIS)* (pp. 248–252). DOI: 10.1109/ICAIS53314.2022.9743009

Anmella, G., Sanabra, M., Prime-Tous, M., Segú, X., Cavero, M., Navinés, R., Mas, A., Olivé, V., Pujol, L., Quesada, S., Pio, C., Villegas, M., Grande, I., Morilla, I., Martínez-Aran, A., Ruiz, V., Vieta, E., & Hidalgo-Mazzei, D. (2023). Vickybot, a chatbot for anxiety-depressive symptoms and work-related burnout. *European Psychiatry : the Journal of the Association of European Psychiatrists*, *66*(S1), S109–S110. DOI: 10.1192/j.eurpsy.2023.301 PMID: 36719325

Anta, L., Alvarez-Mon, M. A., Donat-Vargas, C., Lara-Abelanda, F. J., Pereira-Sanchez, V., Rodriguez, C. G., Mora, F., Ortega, M. A., Quintero, J., & Alvarez-Mon, M. (2022). Assessment of beliefs and attitudes about electroconvulsive therapy posted on Twitter: An observational study. *European Psychiatry : the Journal of the Association of European Psychiatrists*, *66*(1), 11. DOI: 10.1192/j.eurpsy.2022.2359 PMID: 36620994

Anyoha, R. (2017). *Can Machines Think? Blog, special edition on artificial intelligence the history of artificial intelligence*. https://sitn.hms.harvard.edu/flash/2017/history-artificial-intelligence/

Apaydın, Ş. C., & Ersöz, A. R. (2025). Sohbet Robotlarının Akademik Yetersizliği Olan Bireylerin İletişim Deneyimlerine Etkisi [The Effect of Chatbots on the Communication Experiences of Individuals with Academic Disabilities]. *Mevzu–Journal of Social Sciences*, (13), 501–525. DOI: 10.56720/mevzu.1585344

Arafa, M. A., Omar, I., Farhat, K. H., Elshinawy, M., Khan, F., Alkhathami, F. A., Mokhtar, A., Althunayan, A., Rabah, D. M., & Badawy, A. A. (2024). A Comparison of Systematic, Targeted, and Combined Biopsy Using Machine Learning for Prediction of Prostate Cancer Risk: A Multi-Center Study. *Medical Principles and Practice : International Journal of the Kuwait University, Health Science Centre, 33*(5), 491–500. DOI: 10.1159/000540425 PMID: 39047698

Aramberri, J. (2024). Corneal Topography and Tomography. In *Intraocular Lens Calculations* (pp. 265–287). Springer International Publishing.

Arias-de la Torre, J., Vilagut, G., Ronaldson, A., Serrano-Blanco, A., Martín, V., Peters, M., Valderas, J. M., Dregan, A., & Alonso, J. (2021). Prevalence and variability of current depressive disorder in 27 European countries: A population-based study. *The Lancet. Public Health, 6*(10), e729–e738. DOI: 10.1016/S2468-2667(21)00047-5 PMID: 33961802

Arif, D., Ahmad, A., Bakar, M. A., Ihtisham, M. H., & Winberg, S. (2017). Cost effective solution for minimization of medical errors and acquisition of vitals by using autonomous nursing robot. In *Proceedings of the 2017 International Conference on Information System and Data Mining* (pp. 134-138). https://doi.org/DOI: 10.1145/3077584.3077598

Arif, M. S., Mukheimer, A., & Asif, D. (2023). Enhancing the Early Detection of Chronic Kidney Disease: A Robust Machine Learning Model. *Big Data and Cognitive Computing, 7*(3), 144. Advance online publication. DOI: 10.3390/bdcc7030144

Arnal, P. J., Thorey, V., Debellemaniere, E., Ballard, M. E., Bou Hernandez, A., Guillot, A., Jourde, H., Harris, M., Guillard, M., Van Beers, P., Chennaoui, M., & Sauvet, F. (2020). The Dreem Headband compared to polysomnography for electroencephalographic signal acquisition and sleep staging. *Sleep (Basel), 43*(11), 1–13. DOI: 10.1093/sleep/zsaa097 PMID: 32433768

Arora, T., Muhammad-Kamal, H., & Beam, K. (2025). Preserving medical ethics in the era of artificial intelligence: Challenges and opportunities in neonatology. In *Seminars in Perinatology* (p. 152100). WB Saunders. DOI: 10.1016/j.semperi.2025.152100

Artificial Neural Network and Supervised Learning. In (2008). *Soft Computing. Studies in Computational Intelligence* (Vol. 103). Springer.

Asati, M., & Miyachi, T. (2019). A short virtual reality mindfulness meditation training for regaining sustained attention. *arXiv preprint arXiv:1907.04487*.

Asif, A., Majid, M., & Anwar, S. M. (2019). Human stress classification using EEG signals in response to music tracks. *Computers in Biology and Medicine*, *107*, 182–196. DOI: 10.1016/j.compbiomed.2019.02.015 PMID: 30836290

Atalay, E., Özalp, O., & Yıldırım, N. (2021). Advances in the diagnosis and treatment of keratoconus. *Therapeutic Advances in Ophthalmology*, *13*, 25158414211012796.

Atılgan, E., & Uslu, E. (2024). Ruh sağlığı alanında yapay zeka araştırmaları: Bibliyometrik bir değerlendirme [Artificial intelligence research in mental health: A bibliometric evaluation]. *Osmangazi Tip Dergisi*, *46*(4), 627–636. DOI: 10.20515/otd.1435157

Austin, C., Curtin, P., Arora, M., Reichenberg, A., Curtin, A., Iwai-Shimada, M., Wright, R. O., Wright, R. J., Remnelius, K. L., Isaksson, J., Bölte, S., & Nakayama, S. F. (2022). Elemental dynamics in hair accurately predict future autism spectrum disorder diagnosis: An international multi-centre study. *Journal of Clinical Medicine*, *11*(23), 7154. DOI: 10.3390/jcm11237154 PMID: 36498727

Aydogan, H., Bozkurt, F., & Coskun, H. (2015). An assessment of brain electrical activities of students toward teacher's specific emotions. *World Academy of Science, Engineering and Technology, International Journal of Social, Behavioral, Educational, Economic. Business and Industrial Engineering*, *9*(6), 1866–1870.

Badrinarayanan, V., Kendall, A., & Cipolla, R. (2017). Segnet: A deep convolutional encoder-decoder architecture for image segmentation. *IEEE Transactions on Pattern Analysis and Machine Intelligence*, *39*(12), 2481–2495.

Bal, P. K., Mohapatra, S. K., Das, T. K., Srinivasan, K., & Hu, Y. C. (2022). A joint resource allocation, security, with efficient task scheduling in cloud computing using hybrid machine learning techniques. *Sensors (Basel)*, *22*(3), 1242. DOI: 10.3390/s22031242 PMID: 35161987

Bandura, A. (1986). *Social Foundations of Thought and Action: A Social Cognitive Theory*. Prentice - Hall.

Barocas, S., Hardt, M., & Narayanan, A. (2019). *Fairness and Machine Learning*. MIT Press. https://fairmlbook.org/

Barrat, J. (2020). *Yapay Zekâ ve İnsanlık Çağının Sonu Son İcadımız*. Pegasus Yayınları.

Başcıllar, M., Karataş, M., & Güre, M. D. P. (2022). Dijital çağda sosyal algoritmalar yapay zekâ ve sosyal hizmet [Social algorithms in the digital age: artificial intelligence and social work]. *Journal of Social Policy Studies*, *22*(56), 539–565. DOI: 10.21560/spcd.vi.1081060

Baskar, K., Muthuraj, S., Sangeetha, S., Vengatesan, K., Aishwarya, D., & Yuvaraj, P. S. (2023). Framework for Implementation of Smart Driver Assistance System Using Augmented Reality. *Lecture Notes in Electrical Engineering, 1021 LNEE*. DOI: 10.1007/978-981-99-1051-9_15

Bates, D. W., & Syrowatka, A. (2022). Harnessing AI in sepsis care. *Nature Medicine*, *28*(7), 1351–1352. DOI: 10.1038/s41591-022-01878-0 PMID: 35864250

Bates, S., Candès, E., Lei, L., Romano, Y., & Sesia, M. (2023). Testing for outliers with conformal p-values. *Annals of Statistics*, *51*(1), 149–178. DOI: 10.1214/22-AOS2244

Baughman, D. J., Jabbarpour, Y., Westfall, J. M., Jetty, A., Zain, A., Baughman, K., Pollak, B., & Waheed, A. (2022). Comparison of quality performance measures for patients receiving in-person vs telemedicine primary care in a large integrated health system. *JAMA Network Open*, *5*(9), e2233267–e2233267. DOI: 10.1001/jamanetworkopen.2022.33267 PMID: 36156147

Baus, O., & Bouchard, S. (2014). Moving from Virtual Reality Exposure-Based Therapy to Augmented Reality Exposure-Based Therapy: A Review. *Frontiers in Human Neuroscience*, *8*(112), 1–15. DOI: 10.3389/fnhum.2014.00112 PMID: 24624073

Beam, K., Sharma, P., Levy, P., & Beam, A. L. (2024). Artificial intelligence in the neonatal intensive care unit: the time is now. *Journal of Perinatology,* 44(1), 131-135. 5; https://doi.org/DOI: 10.1038/s41372-023-01719-z

Beaumont, E., Dagnall, N., Massey, S., & Irons, C. (2024). Evaluating the impact the Self-Compassion App has on levels of compassion, psychological distress and well-being. *Counselling & Psychotherapy Research*, *00*, 1–11. DOI: 10.1002/capr.12841

Beleza, L. D. O., Ribeiro, L. M., Paula, R. A. P., Guarda, L. E. D. A., Vieira, G. B., & Costa, K. S. F. (2019). Perfil de recién-nacidos de riesgo atendidos por enfermeros en seguimiento ambulatorio: Estudio de cohorte retrospectivo. *Revista Latino-Americana de Enfermagem*, *27*, e3113. DOI: 10.1590/1518-8345.2301.3113 PMID: 30698216

Beltrão, G., Stutz, R., Hornberger, F., Martins, W. A., Tatarinov, D., Alaee-Kerahroodi, M., Lindner, U., Stock, L., Kaiser, E., Goedicke-Fritz, S., Schroeder, U., R, B. S. M., & Zemlin, M. (2022). Contactless radar-based breathing monitoring of premature infants in the neonatal intensive care unit. *Scientific Reports*, *12*(1), 5150. DOI: 10.1038/s41598-022-08836-3 PMID: 35338172

Beluzo, C. E., Silva, E., Alves, L. C., Bresan, R. C., Arruda, N. M., Sovat, R., & Carvalho, T. (2020). Towards neonatal mortality risk classification: A data-driven approach using neonatal, maternal, and social factors. *Informatics in Medicine Unlocked*, *20*, 100398. DOI: 10.1016/j.imu.2020.100398 PMID: 33102685

Bennett, C. C., & Doub, T. W. (2016). Expert systems in mental health care: AI applications in decision-making and consultation. In Luxton, D. D. (Ed.), *Artificial intelligence in behavioral and mental health care* (pp. 27–51). Elsevier Academic Press., DOI: 10.1016/B978-0-12-420248-1.00002-7

Bennion, M. R., Hardy, G. E., Moore, R. K., Kellett, S., & Millings, A. (2020). Usability, acceptability, and effectiveness of web-based conversational agents to facilitate problem solving in older adults: Controlled study. *Journal of Medical Internet Research*, *22*(5), e16794. DOI: 10.2196/16794 PMID: 32384055

Bertels, J., Eelbode, T., Berman, M., Vandermeulen, D., Maes, F., Bisschops, R., & Blaschko, M. B. (2019). Optimizing the dice score and jaccard index for medical image segmentation: Theory and practice. In *Medical Image Computing and Computer Assisted Intervention–MICCAI 2019: 22nd International Conference, Shenzhen, China, October 13–17, 2019* [Springer International Publishing.]. *Proceedings*, *22*(Part II), 92–100.

Bertels, J., Eelbode, T., Berman, M., Vandermeulen, D., Maes, F., Bisschops, R., & Blaschko, M. B. (2019, October). Optimizing the dice score and jaccard index for medical image segmentation: Theory and practice. In *International conference on medical image computing and computer-assisted intervention* (pp. 92-100). Cham: Springer International Publishing.

Bharathi, K. (2024). AI-Powered Vigilance in Neonatal Vital Signs Monitoring for Optimal Health Care. In *Modernizing Maternal Care With Digital Technologies* (pp. 159–182). IGI Global., DOI: 10.4018/979-8-3693-3711-0.ch007

Bhardwaja, P., Ganapathy, K., Pathania, M., Naveen, K. H., Charan, J., Dutta, S., Gadepalli, R., Sriniva, S., Gupta, M. K., Goelj, A. D., Midha, N., Kumar, B., Sharma, M., Sharma, P., Banerjee, M., Mitra, P., & Misra, S. V., V., Subramaniant, G., … Kanchibhotlaz, D. (2021). *An integrative approach to clinical recovery for COVID-19 patients using an Ayurvedic formulation: A multicentric double-blind randomized control trial.* DOI: 10.21203/rs.3.rs-1165680/v1

Bhargavi, K., Vadivelan, N., Kodati, S., Phani Krishna, C. V., & Reddy, K. P. (2022). Automated Skin Disease Detection Using Machine Learning Techniques. In *Innovations in Signal Processing and Embedded Systems* [Singapore: Springer Nature Singapore.]. *Proceedings of ICISPES, 2021*, 169–182.

Bianchi, L., Chessa, F., Angiolini, A., Cercenelli, L., Lodi, S., Bortolani, B., Molinaroli, E., Casablanca, C., Droghetti, M., Gaudiano, C., Mottaran, A., Porreca, A., Golfieri, R., Romagnoli, D., Giunchi, F., Fiorentino, M., Piazza, P., Puliatti, S., Diciotti, S., & Schiavina, R. (2021). The use of augmented reality to guide the intraoperative frozen section during robot-assisted radical prostatectomy. *European Urology, 80*(4), 480–488. DOI: 10.1016/j.eururo.2021.06.020 PMID: 34332759

Bianconi, F., Fravolini, M. L., Pizzoli, S., Palumbo, I., Minestrini, M., Rondini, M., & Palumbo, B. (2021). Comparative evaluation of conventional and deep learning methods for semi-automated segmentation of pulmonary nodules on CT. *Quantitative Imaging in Medicine and Surgery, 11*(7), 3286.

Bilge, Y., Gül, E., & Birçek, N. I. (2020). Bir sosyal fobi vakasında bilişsel davranışçı terapi ve sanal gerçeklik kombinasyonu [Cognitive behavioral therapy and virtual reality combination in a case of social phobia]. *Journal of Cognitive-Behavioral Psychotherapy and Research, 9*(2), 158–165. DOI: 10.5455/JCBPR.61718

Binik, Y. M., Cantor, J., Ochs, E., & Meana, M. (1997). From the couch to the keyboard: Psychotherapy in cyberspace. In Keisler, S. (Ed.), *Culture of the Internet* (pp. 71–100). Lawrence Erlbaum Associates.

Bloom, J. M., Woodward, E. N., Susmaras, T., & Pantalone, D. W. (2012). Use of dialectical behavior therapy in inpatient settings: A systematic review. *Psychiatric Services (Washington, D.C.), 63*(9), 881–888. DOI: 10.1176/appi.ps.201100311 PMID: 22751905

Bond, T. (2017). *Psikolojik Danışmanlıkta Etik ve Yasal Konular* [Standards and Ethics for Counselling in Action]. (Yeşilyaprak, B., Trans.). Nobel Akademik Yayıncılık.

Bora, N., Gutta, S., & Hadaegh, A. (2021). *Using machine learning to predict heart disease* (Doctoral dissertation, California State University San Marcos).

Bouazizi, M., & Ohtsuki, T. O. (2016). A Pattern-Based Approach for Sarcasm Detection on Twitter. *IEEE Access : Practical Innovations, Open Solutions*, *4*, 5477–5488. DOI: 10.1109/ACCESS.2016.2594194

Bouhadana, D., Lu, X. H., Luo, J. W., Assad, A., Deyirmendjian, C., Guennoun, A., Nguyen, D.-D., Kwong, J. C. C., Chughtai, B., Elterman, D. S., Zorn, K. C., Trinh, Q.-D., & Bhojani, N. (2023). Clinical Applications of Machine Learning for Urolithiasis and Benign Prostatic Hyperplasia: A Systematic Review. *Journal of Endourology*, *37*(4), 474–494. DOI: 10.1089/end.2022.0311 PMID: 36266993

Bower, P., & Gilbody, S. (2005). Stepped care in psychological therapies: access, effectiveness and efficiency: narrative literature review. *The British Journal of Psychiatry*, *186*(1), 11–17. DOI: 10.1192/bjp.186.1.11 PMID: 15630118

Brachio, S. S., Gu, W., & Saiman, L. (2023). Next steps for health care-associated infections in the neonatal intensive care unit. *Clinics in Perinatology*, *50*(2), 381–397. DOI: 10.1016/j.clp.2023.02.001 PMID: 37201987

Brandtzeg, P. B., & Folstad, A. (2018). Chatbots: Changing user needs and motivations. *Interactions (New York, N.Y.)*, *25*(5), 38–43. DOI: 10.1145/3236669

Brasher, M., Virodov, A., Raffay, T. M., Bada, H. S., Cunningham, M. D., Bumgardner, C., & Jawdeh, E. G. A. (2024). Predicting extubation readiness in preterm infants utilizing machine learning: A diagnostic utility study. *The Journal of Pediatrics*, *271*, 114043. DOI: 10.1016/j.jpeds.2024.114043 PMID: 38561049

Breiman, L. (2001). Random Forests. *Machine Learning*, *45*(1), 5–32. DOI: 10.1023/A:1010933404324

Broadbent, E. (2017). Interactions with robots: The truths we reveal about ourselves. *Annual Review of Psychology*, *68*(1), 627–652. DOI: 10.1146/annurev-psych-010416-043958 PMID: 27648986

Brødsgaard, A., Pedersen, J. T., Larsen, P., & Weis, J. (2019). Parents' and nurses' experiences of partnership in neonatal intensive care units: A qualitative review and meta-synthesis. *Journal of Clinical Nursing*, *28*(17-18), 3117–3139. DOI: 10.1111/jocn.14920 PMID: 31112337

Bron, A. J. (2001). The architecture of the corneal stroma. *The British Journal of Ophthalmology*, *85*(4), 379–381.

Buchanan, B. G. (2005). A (very) brief history of artificial intelligence. *AI Magazine*, *26*(4), 53–53.

Bui, A. D., Truong, A., Pasricha, N. D., & Indaram, M. (2023). Keratoconus diagnosis and treatment: Recent advances and future directions. *Clinical Ophthalmology (Auckland, N.Z.)*, •••, 2705–2718.

Burns, M. N., Begale, M., Duffecy, J., Gergle, D., Karr, C. J., Giangrande, E., & Mohr, D. C. (2011). Harnessing context sensing to develop a mobile intervention for depression. *Journal of Medical Internet Research, 13*(3), e55. DOI: 10.2196/jmir.1838 PMID: 21840837

Cabrera-Quiros, L., Kommers, D., Wolvers, M. K., Oosterwijk, L., Arents, N., van der Sluijs-Bens, J., Cottaar, E. J. E., Andriessen, P., & van Pul, C. (2021). Prediction of late-onset sepsis in preterm infants using monitoring signals and machine learning. *Critical Care Explorations, 3*(1), e0302. DOI: 10.1097/CCE.0000000000000302 PMID: 33532727

Cacciamani, G. E., Chen, A., Gill, I. S., & Hung, A. J. (2024). Artificial intelligence and urology: Ethical considerations for urologists and patients. *Nature Reviews. Urology, 21*(1), 50–59. DOI: 10.1038/s41585-023-00796-1 PMID: 37524914

Çalışır, Ö. M., & Can, N. (2021). Dijital Ruh Sağlığı Hizmetlerinde Güncel Durum: Üniversite Öğrencilerine Sunulan Hizmetlerle İlgili Bir Derleme [The Current Status of Digital Mental Health Services: A Compilation of Services Offered to University Students]. *Inönü University Journal of the Faculty of Education, 22*(3), 2013–2033. DOI: 10.17679/inuefd.952666

Canbulat, N., & Dursun, A. (2024). Travma sürecinde yeni ve sistemli bir model: Duygu odaklı travma modeli [A new and systematic model in the trauma process: the emotion-focused trauma model]. *Milli Eğitim Dergisi, 53*(242), 1153–1178. DOI: 10.37669/milliegitim.1233140

Canpolat, M. (2021). Psikolojik danışmanlık ve rehberlikte yapay zekâ kullanılabilirliği üzerine bir araştırma [A research on the usability of artificial intelligence in psychological counseling and guidance]. *Milli Eğitim Özel Eğitim ve Rehberlik Dergisi, 1*(1), 1–25.

Cavas-Martínez, F., De la Cruz Sánchez, E., Nieto Martínez, J., Fernández Cañavate, F. J., & Fernández-Pacheco, D. G. (2016). Corneal topography in keratoconus: State of the art. *Eye and Vision (London, England), 3*, 1–12.

Cay, G.. (2021). Baby-Guard: An IoT-based neonatal monitoring system integrated with smart textiles. In *2021 IEEE International Conference on Smart Computing (SMARTCOMP)* (pp. 129-136). IEEE. https://doi.org/DOI: 10.1109/SMARTCOMP52413.2021.00038

CFP (2023). *Evolução do desempenho do Serviço Nacional de Saúde em 2022*, Conselho das Finanças Públicas [CFP], Lisboa, Relatório n.º 7/2022.

Chaari, A., Kallel, I. F., Hammouda, F. B., & Frikha, M. (2023, December). Corneal Endothelial Images Segmentation Using Deep Learning Model. In *2023 IEEE 11th International Conference on Systems and Control (ICSC)* (pp. 855-861). IEEE.

Chaari, A., Kammoun, K., Kallel, I. F., Frikha, M., Kammoun, S., & Feki, J. 2020, September. Performance Evaluation of Various Denoising Filters and segmentation methods for OCT images. In *2020 5th International Conference on Advanced Technologies for Signal and Image Processing (ATSIP)* (pp. 1-6). IEEE.

Chaari, A., Fourati Kallel, I., Kammoun, S., & Frikha, M. (2025). Hybrid Data Augmentation Strategies for Robust Deep Learning Classification of Corneal Topographic MapTopographic Map. *Biomedical Physics & Engineering Express.*

Chaari, A., Kallel, I. F., Daoud, H., Omri, I., Kammoun, S., & Frikha, M. (2024). Automated feature selection for early keratoconus screening optimization. *Biomedical Physics & Engineering Express*, *11*(1), 015039.

Chakraborty, S. (Ed.). (Forthcoming 2025). *Human values, ethics, and dignity in the age of artificial intelligence*. IGI Global.

Chan, C. M. H., Ng, S. L., In, S., Wee, L. H., & Siau, C. S. (2021). Predictors of psychological distress and mental health resource utilization among employees in Malaysia. *International Journal of Environmental Research and Public Health*, *18*(1), 314. DOI: 10.3390/ijerph18010314 PMID: 33406714

Chandra, P., Iqbal, F., Unnikrisnan, M. K., Jayashree, P., Shenoy, P. A., Anburaj, S. E., Rajesh, V., Surulivelrajan, M., & Lewis, L. E. (2023). Neonatal outcomes associated with antimicrobial resistance: a retrospective cross-sectional study. *Journal of Applied Pharmaceutical Science, 13*(5), 081-094. https://doi.org/DOI: 10.7324/JAPS.2023.120166

Chang, T. C., Shkolyar, E., Del Giudice, F., Eminaga, O., Lee, T., Laurie, M., Seufert, C., Jia, X., Mach, K. E., Xing, L., & Liao, J. C. (2023, July 11). Real-time Detection of Bladder Cancer Using Augmented Cystoscopy with Deep Learning: A Pilot Study. *Journal of Endourology*, end.2023.0056. Advance online publication. DOI: 10.1089/end.2023.0056 PMID: 37432899

Chan, S. H., & Shorey, S. (2021). Healthcare professionals' sense of coherence of parental involvement in neonatal intensive care units: A framework synthesis. *Research in Nursing & Health*, *44*(6), 875–890. DOI: 10.1002/nur.22178 PMID: 34414586

Cheah, M. H., Gan, Y. N., Altice, F. L., Wickersham, J. A., Shrestha, R., Salleh, N. A. M., Ng, K. S., Azwa, I., Balakrishnan, V., Kamarulzaman, A., & Ni, Z. (2024). Testing the feasibility and acceptability of using an artificial intelligence chatbot to promote HIV testing and pre-exposure prophylaxis in Malaysia: Mixed methods study. *JMIR Human Factors*, *11*, e52055. DOI: 10.2196/52055 PMID: 38277206

Chen, T., & Guestrin, C. (2016). *XGBoost: A Scalable Tree Boosting System. KDD Conference.*

Chen, Y., Zhang, W., Wang, N., Wang, Y., Wang, C., Wan, H., & Lu, Y. (2020). Thyroid Parameters and Kidney Disorder in Type 2 Diabetes: Results from the MET-AL Study. *Journal of Diabetes Research*, *2020*, 1–11. DOI: 10.1155/2020/8358102 PMID: 32337292

Chng, S. Y., Tern, M. J. W., Lee, Y. S., Cheng, L. T.-E., Kapur, J., Eriksson, J. G., Chong, Y. S., & Savulescu, J. (2025). Ethical considerations in AI for child health and recommendations for child-centered medical AI. *NPJ Digital Medicine*, *8*(1), 152. DOI: 10.1038/s41746-025-01541-1 PMID: 40065130

Chouchana, L., Preta, L.-H., Tisseyre, M., Terrier, B., Treluyer, J.-M., & Montastruc, F. (2021). Kidney disorders as serious adverse drug reactions of remdesivir in coronavirus disease 2019: A retrospective case–noncase study. *Kidney International*, *99*(5), 1235–1236. DOI: 10.1016/j.kint.2021.02.015 PMID: 33647327

Choudhury, A. R., Vanguri, R., Jambawalikar, S. R., & Kumar, P. (2019). Segmentation of brain tumors using DeepLabv3+. In *Brainlesion: Glioma, Multiple Sclerosis, Stroke and Traumatic Brain Injuries: 4th International Workshop, BrainLes 2018, Held in Conjunction with MICCAI 2018, Granada, Spain, September 16, 2018, Revised Selected Papers, Part II 4* (pp. 154-167). Springer International Publishing.

Choudhury, A., & Urena, E. (2022). Artificial intelligence in NICU and PICU: a need for ecological validity, accountability, and human factors. *In Healthcare* (Vol. 10, No. 5, p. 952). MDPI. https://doi.org/DOI: 10.3390/healthcare10050952

Choudhury, A., Li, H., Greene, C., & Perumalla, S. (2018). Humanoid robot-application and influence. *Archives of Clinical and Biomedical Research*, *2*(6), 197–187. DOI: 10.26502/acbr.50170059

Chung-Do, J., Helm, S., Fukuda, M., Alicata, D., Nishimura, S., & Else, I. (2012). Rural mental health: Implications for telepsychiatry in clinical service, workforce development, and organizational capacity. *Telemedicine Journal and e-Health*, *18*(3), 244–246. DOI: 10.1089/tmj.2011.0107 PMID: 22356526

Çınar, F. I., Erpay, F., Yıldırım, E., Küçük, E. Ö., & Demirtaş, A. (2022). Demansta bilişsel aktiviteyi artırıcı yöntemler ve bakımda teknolojinin kullanımı [Interventions to increase cognitive activity in dementia and the use of technology in dementia care]. *Hacettepe University Faculty of Health Sciences Nursing Journal. Nursing Insights*, *9*(3), 308–315. DOI: 10.31125/hunhemsire.1229981

Cirban Ekrem, E., & Daşıkan, Z. (2021). Perinatal dönemde yapay zekâ teknolojisinin kullanımı [Use of Artificial Intelligence Technology in the Perinatal Period]. *Eurasian Journal of Health Technology Assessment*, *5*(2), 147–162. DOI: 10.52148/ehta.980568

Clipper, B., Batcheller, J., Thomaz, A. L., & Rozga, A. (2018). Artificial intelligence and robotics: A nurse leader's primer. *Nurse Leader*, *16*(6), 379–384. DOI: 10.1016/j.mnl.2018.07.015

Cohen, G. E., & Kerr, B. A. (1998). Computer-mediated counseling: An empirical study of a new mental health treatment. *Computers in Human Services*, *15*(4), 13–26. DOI: 10.1300/J407v15n04_02

Colby, K. M. (1981). Modeling a paranoid mind. *Behavioral and Brain Sciences*, *4*(4), 515–560. DOI: 10.1017/S0140525X00000030

Corbett, M. C., Marshall, J., O'Brart, D. P., & Rosen, E. S. (1995). New and future technology in corneal topography. *European journal of Implant and Refractive Surgery*, *7*(6), 371-385.

Corey, G., Corey, M. S., & Callanan, P. (2024). *Issues and ethics in the helping professions*. Brooks/Cole.

Coskun, A. B., Kenner, C., & Elmaoglu, E. (2024). Neonatal Intensive Care Nurses' Perceptions of Artificial Intelligence: A Qualitative Study on Discharge Education and Family Counseling. *The Journal of Perinatal & Neonatal Nursing*, •••, 10–1097. DOI: 10.1097/JPN.0000000000000904 PMID: 39740134

Coşkun, H. (2024). An automatic labeling approach towards multi-class sitting posture classification based on depth-sensor data. *Dicle Üniversitesi Mühendislik Fakültesi Mühendislik Dergisi*, *15*(3), 559–568.

Coskun, H., & Yigit, T. (2018). Classification of normal and extrasystole heart sounds using artificial intelligence methods. In Arabnia, H. R., & Dehkordi, A. A. (Eds.), *Nature-Inspired Intelligent Techniques for Solving Biomedical Engineering Problems* (pp. 146–183). IGI Global. DOI: 10.4018/978-1-5225-4769-3.ch007

Coyle, T. N., Shaver, J. A., & Linehan, M. M. (2018). On the potential for iatrogenic effects of psychiatric crisis services: The example of dialectical behavior therapy for adult women with borderline personality disorder. *Journal of Consulting and Clinical Psychology*, *86*(2), 116–124. DOI: 10.1037/ccp0000275 PMID: 29369662

Crawford, A. Z., Zhang, J., Gokul, A., McGhee, C. N., & Ormonde, S. E. (2020). The enigma of environmental factors in keratoconus. *Asia-Pacific Journal of Ophthalmology*, *9*(6), 549–556.

Cresta, F. B., Orlandin, L. F., & Lucas, M. B. (2022). Clinical Presentation and Evolution of Keratoconus. In *Keratoconus: A Comprehensive Guide to Diagnosis and Treatment* (pp. 3–12). Springer International Publishing.

Croes, E. A., & Antheunis, M. L. (2021, February). 36 Questions to Loving a Chatbot: Are People. In *Chatbot Research and Design: 4th International Workshop, CONVERSATIONS 2020, Virtual Event, November 23–24, 2020, Revised Selected Papers* (Vol. 12604, p. 81). Springer Nature. https://doi.org/DOI: 10.1007/978-3-030-68288-0_6

D'Alfonso, S. (2020). AI in mental health. *Current Opinion in Psychology*, *36*, 112–117. DOI: 10.1016/j.copsyc.2020.04.005 PMID: 32604065

D'Oria, F., Bagaglia, S. A., Del Barrio, J. L. A., Alessio, G., Alio, J. L., & Mazzotta, C. (2024). Refractive surgical correction and treatment of keratoconus. *Survey of Ophthalmology*, *69*(1), 122–139.

Dagoglu, T., & Ovali, F. (2017). Newborn development and environmental factors. Dağoğlu, T., Görak, G. (Ed). Basic Neonatology and Nursing Principles (2nd Edition, pp.759-768). Istanbul: Nobel Medical Bookstores.

Damar, E. (2019). *Çevrimiçi psikolojik danışmaya yönelik psikolojik danışmanların görüşleri: Nitel bir çalışma [Psychological counsellors' views on online psychological counselling: A qualitative study].* [Unpublished master thesis]. *Akdeniz Üniversitesi, Antalya.*

Das, A., Choudhury, D., & Sen, A. (2024). A collaborative empirical analysis on machine learning based disease prediction in health care system. *International Journal of Information Technology : an Official Journal of Bharati Vidyapeeth's Institute of Computer Applications and Management*, *16*(1), 261–270. DOI: 10.1007/s41870-023-01556-5

Daud, M. M., Zaki, W. M. D. W., Hussain, A., & Mutalib, H. A. (2020). Keratoconus detection using the fusion features of anterior and lateral segment photographed images. *IEEE Access : Practical Innovations, Open Solutions*, *8*, 142282–142294.

Day, S. X., & Schneider, P. L. (2002). Psychotherapy using distance technology: A comparison of face-to-face, video, and audio treatment. *Journal of Counseling Psychology*, *49*(4), 499–503. DOI: 10.1037/0022-0167.49.4.499

Degadwala, S., Vyas, D., Mitra, P., Roja, S. S. E., & Mandal, S. K. (2023, December). Methods of Transfer Learning for Multiclass Hair Disease Categorization. In *2023 2nd International Conference on Automation, Computing and Renewable Systems (ICACRS)* (pp. 612-616). IEEE. DOI: 10.1109/ICACRS58579.2023.10404492

del Castillo Torres, G., Roig-Maimó, M. F., Mascaró-Oliver, M., Amengual-Alcover, E., & Mas-Sansó, R. (2022). Understanding How CNNs Recognize Facial Expressions: A Case Study with LIME and CEM. *Sensors (Basel)*, *23*(1), 131. DOI: 10.3390/s23010131 PMID: 36616728

Demaerschalk, B. M., Pines, A., Butterfield, R., Haglin, J. M., Haddad, T. C., Yiannias, J., Colby, C. E., TerKonda, S. P., Ommen, S. R., Bushman, M. S., Lokken, T. G., Blegen, R. N., Hoff, M. D., Coffey, J. D., Anthony, G. S., Zhang, N., Anaya, S., Arbon, J., Berry, N., & Wu, S. (2022). Assessment of clinician diagnostic concordance with video telemedicine in the integrated multispecialty practice at Mayo Clinic during the beginning of the COVID-19 pandemic from March to June 2020. *JAMA Network Open*, *5*(9), e2229958–e2229958. DOI: 10.1001/jamanetworkopen.2022.29958 PMID: 36053531

Demir, A. (2018). Ölümsüzlük ve yapay zekâ bağlamında trans-hümanizm [Trans-humanism in the context of immorality and artifical intelligence]. *AJIT-e: Academic Journal of Information Technology*, *9*(31), 95–104. DOI: 10.5824/1309-1581.2018.1.006.x

Demir, A. E., & Yücedağ, I. (2024). Siber mekânda duygu deneyimleri bağlamında meditasyon uygulamaları [Meditation practices in the context of emotional experiences in cyberspace]. *Anadolu University Journal of Scoial Sciences*, *24*(1), 177–200. DOI: 10.18037/ausbd.1253208

Demir, O. (2019). *"Sürdürülebilir Kalkınma İçin Yapay Zekâ". Yapay Zekâ ve Gelecek* (Telli, G., Ed.). Doğu Kitap Evi.

Denecke, K., Schmid, N., & Nüssli, S. (2022). Implementation of cognitive behavioral therapy in e– mental health apps: Literature review. *Journal of Medical Internet Research*, *24*(3), e27791. DOI: 10.2196/27791 PMID: 35266875

Derin, G., & Öztürk, E. (2020). Yapay zeka psikolojisi ve sanal gerçeklik uygulamaları. [Psychology of artificial intelligence and virtual reality applications] In Öztürk, E. (Ed.), *Siber Psikoloji* [Cyber Psychology]. (pp. 41–47). Türkiye Klinikleri.

Deshmukh, H. K., Parekh, S. J., Sapkal, S. S., & Kamble, P. (2023). MindMap: A review on mental health analysis using ML. In *2023 6th International Conference on Advances in Science and Technology (ICAST)* (pp. 325–329). IEEE. DOI: 10.1109/ICAST59062.2023.10454965

Devalla, S. K., Renukanand, P. K., Sreedhar, B. K., Subramanian, G., Zhang, L., Perera, S., & Girard, M. J. (2018). DRUNET: A dilated-residual U-Net deep learning network to segment optic nerve head tissues in optical coherence tomography images. *Biomedical Optics Express*, *9*(7), 3244–3265.

DeWitt, E. N. (1931). The histopathology of Bowman's membrane. *Transactions of the American Ophthalmological Society*, *29*, 461.

DiSalvo, C. F., Gemperle, F., Forlizzi, J., & Kiesler, S. (2002). All robots are not created equal: the design and perception of humanoid robot heads. In *Proceedings of the 4th conference on Designing interactive systems: processes, practices, methods, and techniques* (pp. 321-326). ACM. DOI: 10.1145/778712.778756

Donker, T., Petrie, K., Proudfoot, J., Clarke, J., Birch, M. R., & Christensen, H. (2013). Smartphones for smarter delivery of mental health programs: A systematic review. *Journal of Medical Internet Research*, *15*(11), e247. DOI: 10.2196/jmir.2791 PMID: 24240579

Donmez, S. (2020). Artificial intelligence and 2025 syndrome in philosophical context. *Journal of Çukurova University Faculty of Theology*, *20*(2), 748–760. DOI: 10.30627/cuilah.690645 0063

Doshi, K., Rehm, G. B., Vadlaputi, P., Lai, Z., Lakshminrusimha, S., Chuah, C. N., & Siefkes, H. M. (2021). A novel system to collect dual pulse oximetry data for critical congenital heart disease screening research. *Journal of Clinical and Translational Science*, *5*(1), e56. DOI: 10.1017/cts.2020.550 PMID: 33948277

Dosovitsky, G., & Bunge, E. L. (2021). Bonding with bot: User feedback on a chatbot for social isolation. *Frontiers in Digital Health*, *3*, 735053. Advance online publication. DOI: 10.3389/fdgth.2021.735053 PMID: 34713203

Dua, H. S., Gomes, J. A., & Singh, A. (1994). Corneal epithelial wound healing. *The British Journal of Ophthalmology*, *78*(5), 401.

Dumka, A., Verma, P., Singh, R., Bisht, A. K., Anand, D., Aljahdali, H. M., Noya, I. D., & Obregon, S. A. (2022). A Novel Deep Learning Based Healthcare Model for COVID-19 Pandemic Stress Analysis. *Computers, Materials & Continua*, *72*(3), 6029–6044. DOI: 10.32604/cmc.2022.024698

Durak, H. Y., & Balıkçı, H. C. (2025). *Yapay Zekâ Sohbet Botu Bağımlılık Ölçeğinin Türkçeye Uyarlanması*. 3 rd International Conference on Trends in Advanced Research, Konya, Turkey

Ediboğlu, G. O. (2023). Yapay zekanın insan zekasına psikoterapötik yaklaşımı [Psychotherapeutic approach of artificial intelligence to human intelligence]. *Çukurova Medical Student Journal, 3*(1), 12-18.

Ediz, C., & Kucuk, S. (2023). An Important Issue in the Neonatal Intensive Care Unit: The Importance of Sound and Light Isolation for Premature Babies. *Turkish Journal of Health Sciences and Research, 6*(3), 77–85. DOI: 10.51536/tusbad.1184972

Edwards, M., McGhee, C. N., & Dean, S. (2001). The genetics of keratoconus. *Clinical & Experimental Ophthalmology, 29*(6), 345–351.

ElGendy, M. S., Moustafa, H., Nafea, H., & Mohammed, W. (2025). A machine learning model based on the Archimedes optimization algorithm for heart disease prediction. *International Journal of Telecommunications, 5*(01), 1–21. DOI: 10.21608/ijt.2025.338194.1067

El-Masri, M., Altrabsheh, N., & Mansour, H. (2017). Successes and challenges of Arabic sentiment analysis research: A literature review. *Social Network Analysis and Mining, 7*(1), 1–22. DOI: 10.1007/s13278-017-0474-x

Elsawy, A., & Abdel-Mottaleb, M. (2022). PIPE-Net: A pyramidal-input-parallel-encoding network for the segmentation of corneal layer interfaces in OCT images. *Computers in Biology and Medicine, 147*, 105595.

Emmelkamp, P. M. (2005). Technological innovations in clinical assessment and psychotherapy. *Psychotherapy and Psychosomatics, 74*(6), 336–343. DOI: 10.1159/000087780 PMID: 16244509

Eryılmaz, H. E. (2023). Yapay zekâ çağında kişisel veri mahremiyeti [Personal Data Privacy in the Age of Artificial Intelligence]. *Journal of Arts and Social Sciences, 1*(2), 6–25.

Esteva, A., Kuprel, B., Novoa, R. A., Ko, J., Swetter, S. M., Blau, H. M., & Thrun, S. (2017). Dermatologist-level classification of skin cancer with deep neural networks. *Nature, 542*(7639), 115–118. DOI: 10.1038/nature21056 PMID: 28117445

Etzioni, A., & Etzioni, O. (2017). Incorporating ethics into artificial intelligence. *The Journal of Ethics, 21*(4), 403–418. DOI: 10.1007/s10892-017-9252-2

Ezawa, I. D., Robinson, N., & Hollon, S. D. (2024). Prevalence increases as treatments improve: An evolutionary perspective on the treatment–prevalence paradox in depression. *Annual Review of Clinical Psychology*, *20*(1), 201–228. DOI: 10.1146/annurev-clinpsy-080822-040442 PMID: 38996078

Fakhoury, M. (2019). Artificial intelligence in psychiatry. *Frontiers in psychiatry: artificial intelligence, precision medicine, and other paradigm shifts*, 1192,119-125.

Fang, X., Hong, P., He, S., Zhang, Y., & Tan, D. (2024). Multi-Layer Energy Management and Strategy Learning for Microgrids: A Proximal Policy Optimization Approach. *Energies*, *17*(16), 3990. DOI: 10.3390/en17163990

Fan, S. (2020). *Önemli sorular yapay zeka yerimizi alacak mı? 21. yüzyıl için bir rehber* [Important questions Will artificial intelligence replace us? A guide for the 21st century]. (Çıgay, I. G., Trans.). Hep Kitap.

Fantaci, B., Calvo, B., & Rodríguez, J. F. (2024). Modeling biological growth of human keratoconus: On the effect of tissue degradation, location and size. *Computers in Biology and Medicine*, *180*, 108976.

Farhan, A. M. Q., & Yang, S. (2023). Automatic lung disease classification from the chest X-ray images using a hybrid deep learning algorithm. *Multimedia Tools and Applications*, *82*(25), 1. DOI: 10.1007/s11042-023-15047-z PMID: 37362647

Farjo, N. P., Mysore, V., & True, R. H. (2023, November). Clinical Practice Guidelines for Virtual Consultations in the Practice of Hair Restoration Surgery: Developed by the International Society of Hair Restoration Surgery Task Force for Guidelines for Virtual Consultations. In *Hair Transplant Forum International* (Vol. 33, No. 6, pp. 197-212). Hair Transplant Forum International.

Feldman, K., & Rohan, A. J. (2022). Data-driven nurse staffing in the neonatal intensive care unit. *MCN. The American Journal of Maternal Child Nursing*, *47*(5), 249–264. DOI: 10.1097/NMC.0000000000000839 PMID: 35960217

Fenstermaker, M., Tomlins, S. A., Singh, K., Wiens, J., & Morgan, T. M. (2020). Development and validation of a deep-learning model to assist with renal cell carcinoma histopathologic interpretation. *Urology*, *144*, 152–157. DOI: 10.1016/j.urology.2020.05.094 PMID: 32711010

Ferhat, S. (2016). Dijital dünyanın gerçekliği, gerçek dünyanın sanallığı bir dijital medya ürünü olarak sanal gerçeklik [Reality of the digital world, virtuality of the real world virtual reality as a digital media product]. *TRT Academy Journal*, *1*(2), 724–746.

Fernandez-Moral, E., Martins, R., Wolf, D., & Rives, P. (2018, June). *A new metric for evaluating semantic segmentation: leveraging global and contour accuracy. In 2018 IEEE intelligent vehicles symposium (iv)*. IEEE.

Ferro, M., Falagario, U. G., Barone, B., Maggi, M., Crocetto, F., Busetto, G. M., Giudice, F., Terracciano, D., Lucarelli, G., Lasorsa, F., Catellani, M., Brescia, A., Mistretta, F. A., Luzzago, S., Piccinelli, M. L., Vartolomei, M. D., Jereczek-Fossa, B. A., Musi, G., Montanari, E., & Tataru, O. S. (2023). Artificial intelligence in the advanced diagnosis of bladder cancer: Comprehensive literature review and future advancement. *Diagnostics (Basel)*, *13*(13), 2308. DOI: 10.3390/diagnostics13132308 PMID: 37443700

Feuerriegel, S., Hartmann, J., Janiesch, C., & Zschech, P. (2023). Generative AI. *Business & Information Systems Engineering*, *66*(1), 111–126. DOI: 10.1007/s12599-023-00834-7

Fiske, A., Henningsen, P., & Buyx, A. (2019). Your robot therapist will see you now: Ethical implications of embodied artificial intelligence in psychiatry, psychology, and psychotherapy. *Journal of Medical Internet Research*, *21*(5), e13216. DOI: 10.2196/13216 PMID: 31094356

Fitzpatrick, K. K., Darcy, A., & Vierhile, M. (2017). Delivering cognitive behavior therapy to young adults with symptoms of depression and anxiety using a fully automated conversational agent (Woebot): A randomized controlled trial. *JMIR Mental Health*, *4*(2), e7785. DOI: 10.2196/mental.7785 PMID: 28588005

Fitzsimmons-Craft, E. E., Chan, W. W., Smith, A. C., Firebaugh, M. L., Fowler, L. A., Topooco, N., DePietro, B., Wilfley, D. E., Taylor, C. B., & Jacobson, N. C. (2022). Effectiveness of a chatbot for eating disorders prevention: A randomized clinical trial. *International Journal of Eating Disorders*, *55*(3), 343–353. DOI: 10.1002/eat.23662 PMID: 35274362

Flannery, B. T., Sandler, H. M., Lal, P., Feldman, M. D., Santa-Rosario, J. C., Pathak, T., Mirtti, T., Farre, X., Correa, R., Chafe, S., Shah, A., Efstathiou, J. A., Hoffman, K., Hallman, M. A., Straza, M., Jordan, R., Pugh, S. L., Feng, F., & Madabhushi, A. (2025). Stress testing deep learning models for prostate cancer detection on biopsies and surgical specimens. *The Journal of Pathology*, *265*(2), 146–157. DOI: 10.1002/path.6373 PMID: 39660731

Fortney, J. C., Pyne, J. M., Turner, E. E., Farris, K. M., Normoyle, T. M., Avery, M. D., Hilty, D. M., & Unützer, J. (2015). Telepsychiatry integration of mental health services into rural primary care settings. *International Review of Psychiatry (Abingdon, England)*, *27*(6), 525–539. DOI: 10.3109/09540261.2015.1085838 PMID: 26634618

Frize, M., Walker, R. C., & Ennett, C. M. (2003). Development of an evidence-based ethical decision-making tool for neonatal intensive care medicine. In Proceedings of the 25th Annual International Conference of the IEEE Engineering in Medicine and Biology Society (IEEE Cat. No. 03CH37439) (Vol. 2, pp. 1260-1263). IEEE. https://doi.org/DOI: 10.1109/IEMBS.2003.1279490

Froń, A., Semianiuk, A., Lazuk, U., Ptaszkowski, K., Siennicka, A., Lemiński, A., Krajewski, W., Szydełko, T., & Małkiewicz, B. (2023). Artificial Intelligence in Urooncology: What We Have and What We Expect. *Cancers (Basel)*, *15*(17), 4282. DOI: 10.3390/cancers15174282 PMID: 37686558

Fulmer, R. (2019). Artificial intelligence and counseling: Four levels of implementation. *Theory & Psychology*, *29*(6), 807–819. DOI: 10.1177/0959354319853045

Galijašević, T., Škarić, M., Podolski, E., Musta, F., Matovinović, M., & Marinko, D. (2024). New breakthroughs in AI chatbots and their potential in mental health services. In *2024 9th International Conference on Smart and Sustainable Technologies (SpliTech)* (pp. 1–4).

Garcia-Marin, Y. F., Alonso-Caneiro, D., Fisher, D., Vincent, S. J., & Collins, M. J. (2023). Patch-based CNN for corneal segmentation of AS-OCT images: Effect of the number of classes and image quality upon performance. *Computers in Biology and Medicine*, *152*, 106342.

Garg, A., Sharma, B., & Khan, R. (2021). Heart disease prediction using machine learning techniques. [). IOP Publishing.]. *IOP Conference Series. Materials Science and Engineering*, *1022*(1), 012046. DOI: 10.1088/1757-899X/1022/1/012046

Gayathri Hegde, M., Shrishti Bekal, M., Prasad, S. S., Shenoy, P. D., & Venugopal, K. R. (2022). Analysis of Secure EHR Storage Methods on Blockchain and Integrating ML to Predict Chronic Kidney Disease. *7th IEEE International Conference on Recent Advances and Innovations in Engineering, ICRAIE 2022 - Proceedings*. DOI: 10.1109/ICRAIE56454.2022.10054247

Geetha, K., Srivani, A., Gunasekaran, S., Ananthi, S., & Sangeetha, S. (2023). Geospatial Data Exploration Using Machine Learning. *Proceedings of the 4th International Conference on Smart Electronics and Communication, ICOSEC 2023*. DOI: 10.1109/ICOSEC58147.2023.10275920

Ghosh, S. (2025). *Mathematical Foundations of Deep Learning*.

Gleason, A., Richter, F., Beller, N., Arivazhagan, N., Feng, R., Holmes, E., Glicksberg, B. S., Morton, S. U., La Vega-Talbott, M., Fields, M., Guttmann, K., Nadkarni, G. N., & Richter, F. (2024). Detection of neurologic changes in critically ill infants using deep learning on video data: A retrospective single center cohort study. *EClinicalMedicine*, *78*, 102919. Advance online publication. DOI: 10.1016/j.eclinm.2024.102919 PMID: 39764545

Gogoi, P., & Valan, J. A. (2024a). Machine learning approaches for predicting and diagnosing chronic kidney disease: Current trends, challenges, solutions, and future directions. *International Urology and Nephrology*, *57*(4), 1245–1268. Advance online publication. DOI: 10.1007/s11255-024-04281-5 PMID: 39560857

Goiana-da-Silva, F., Sá, J., Cabral, M., Guedes, R., Vasconcelos, R., Sarmento, J., Morais Nunes, A., Moreira, R., Miraldo, M., Ashrafian, H., Darzi, A., & Araújo, F. (2024). The Portuguese NHS 2024 reform: Transformation through vertical integration. *Frontiers in Public Health*, *12*, 1389057. DOI: 10.3389/fpubh.2024.1389057 PMID: 38846606

Gokul, A., Vellara, H. R., & Patel, D. V. (2018). Advanced anterior segment imaging in keratoconus: A review. *Clinical & Experimental Ophthalmology*, *46*(2), 122–132.

Go, M. A., MacDonald, K. D., Durand, M., & McEvoy, C. T. (2025). Pulmonary function tests in the neonatal intensive care unit and beyond: A clinical review. *Journal of Perinatology*, •••, 1–12. DOI: 10.1038/s41372-025-02243-y PMID: 40021840

Gordon-Shaag, A., Millodot, M., Shneor, E., & Liu, Y. (2015). The genetic and environmental factors for keratoconus. *BioMed Research International*, *2015*(1), 795738.

Goswami, S., & Sharma, S. (2022). Industry 4.0 enabled molecular imaging using an artificial intelligence technique. *2022 1st International Conference on Computational Science and Technology (ICCST)*, 455–460. https://doi.org/DOI: 10.1109/ICCST55948.2022.10040406

Goswami, S., & Sharma, S. (2023). Deep learning enabled computational design and analysis of effective ligands targeting estrogen receptor beta in breast cancer diagnosis. *2023 IEEE World Conference on Applied Intelligence and Computing*, 45–50. https://doi.org/DOI: 10.1109/AIC57670.2023.10263932

Goswami, S., & Sharma, S. (2024). Artificial intelligence, quantum computing, and cloud computing enabled personalized medicine in next-generation sequencing bioinformatics. *2024 IEEE International Conference on Interdisciplinary Approaches in Computational Technology*, 1–6. https://doi.org/DOI: 10.1109/IATMSI60426.2024.10502533

Goswami, S., Thakur, N., & Singh, P. (2024). Application of deep learning in cytopathology and prostate adenocarcinoma diagnosis. *2024 IEEE International Conference on Interdisciplinary Approaches in Technology and Management for Social Innovation (IATMSI)*, 2, 1–6. https://doi.org/DOI: 10.1109/IATMSI60426.2024.10502565

Graglia, F., Mari, J. L., Baikoff, G., & Sequeira, J. (2007, August). Contour detection of the cornea from OCT radial images. In *2007 29th Annual International Conference of the IEEE Engineering in Medicine and Biology Society* (pp. 5612-5615). IEEE.

Graham, S., Depp, C., Lee, E. E., Nebeker, C., Tu, X., Kim, H. C., & Jeste, D. V. (2019). Artificial intelligence for mental health and mental illnesses: An overview. *Current Psychiatry Reports*, *21*(11), 1–18. DOI: 10.1007/s11920-019-1094-0 PMID: 31701320

Greer, S., Ramo, D., Chang, Y. J., Fu, M., Moskowitz, J., & Haritatos, J. (2019). Use of the chatbot "vivibot" to deliver positive psychology skills and promote well-being among young people after cancer treatment: Randomized controlled feasibility trial. *JMIR mHealth and uHealth*, *7*(10), e15018. DOI: 10.2196/15018 PMID: 31674920

Grubb, A. (2020). Shrunken pore syndrome - a common kidney disorder with high mortality. Diagnosis, prevalence, pathophysiology and treatment options. *Clinical Biochemistry*, *83*, 12–20. DOI: 10.1016/j.clinbiochem.2020.06.002 PMID: 32544475

Grubbs, K. M., Fortney, J. C., Dean, T., Williams, J. S., & Godleski, L. (2015). A comparison of mental health diagnoses treated via interactive video and face to face in the Veterans Healthcare Administration. *Telemedicine Journal and e-Health*, *21*(7), 564–566. DOI: 10.1089/tmj.2014.0152 PMID: 25799233

Grünerbl, A., Muaremi, A., Osmani, V., Bahle, G., Oehler, S., Tröster, G., & Lukowicz, P. (2015). Smartphone-based recognition of states and state changes in bipolar disorder patients. *IEEE Journal of Biomedical and Health Informatics*, *19*(1), 140–148. DOI: 10.1109/JBHI.2014.2343154 PMID: 25073181

Grzybowski, A., & McGhee, C. N. (2013). The early history of keratoconus prior to Nottingham's landmark 1854 treatise on conical cornea: A review. *Clinical & Experimental Optometry*, *96*(2), 140–145.

Gudivaka, R. K., Hussein, L., Aruna, T. M., Bharattej, R. R. V. S. S., & Kumar, P. M. (2024, May). Cloud-based Early Acute Lymphoblastic Leukaemia Detection Using Deep Learning-Based Improved YOLO V4. In *2024 Second International Conference on Data Science and Information System (ICDSIS)* (pp. 1-4). IEEE.

Gujarathi, P., Menon, K., Patel, J., & Halbe, A. (2024). NeuroSafe–Advancing mental health using AI, ML, and blockchain. In *2024 3rd International Conference for Innovation in Technology (INOCON)* (pp. 1–5).

Gulshan, V., Peng, L., Coram, M., Stumpe, M. C., Wu, D., Narayanaswamy, A., Venugopalan, S., Widner, K., Madams, T., Cuadros, J., Kim, R., Raman, R., Nelson, P. C., Mega, J. L., & Webster, D. R. (2016). Development and validation of a deep learning algorithm for detection of diabetic retinopathy in retinal fundus photographs. *Journal of the American Medical Association, 316*(22), 2402–2410. DOI: 10.1001/jama.2016.17216 PMID: 27898976

Gültekin, M. (2022). Yapay Zekânın Ruh Sağlığı Hizmetlerinde Kullanımına İlişkin Fırsatlar ve Sorunlar [The Advantages and Disadvantages of Using Artificial Intelligence in Mental Health Services]. *The Journal of Humanity and Society, 12*(3), 121–158. DOI: 10.12658/M0664

Gümüş, A. E., & Gümüş, M. A. (2020). *Psikolojik danışmada etik ve hukuk* [Ethics and law in psychological counselling]. Vedat Kitapçılık.

Guo, Y., Hao, Z., Zhao, S., Gong, J., & Yang, F. (2020). Artificial intelligence in health care: Bibliometric analysis. *Journal of Medical Internet Research, 22*(7), e18228. DOI: 10.2196/18228 PMID: 32723713

Gupta, S., Kamboj, S., & Bag, S. (2023). Role of Risks in the Development of Responsible Artificial Intelligence in the Digital Healthcare Domain. *Information Systems Frontiers, 25*(6), 2257–2274. DOI: 10.1007/s10796-021-10174-0

Gürlek, Y. (2024). Yapay Zekanın Eğitime Etkileri ve Uygulamaları [The effects and applications of artificial intelligence in education]. *International Journal of New Trends in Education and Social Sciences, 1*(1), 125–132.

Gürlek, Y., Bozkoyun, E., Ulutürk, M., & Zeyrekgündüz, F. (2023). Yapay Zekanın Eğitime Etkileri ve Uygulamaları [The effects and applications of artificial intelligence in education]. *International Journal of Original Educational Research, 1*(1), 25–132.

Gutierrez, J. (2002). Aplicaciones de la relidad virtual en pcilogia clinica. *Aula Medica Psiquiatria, 4*(2), 92–126.

Güzel, Ş., Dömbekci, H. A., & Eren, F. (2022). Yapay zekânın sağlık alanında kullanımı: Nitel bir araştırma [The Use of Artificial Intelligence in the Health Institutions: A Qualitative Research]. *Celal Bayar University Health Sciences Institute Journal, 9*(4), 509–519. DOI: 10.34087/cbusbed.1140122

Hafez Elsayed, Z. E., Melika, S. W., & Mohamed Ads, S. E. (2024). Effect of Mind Mapping with Artificial Intelligence for High Alert Medications on Novice Nurses' Performance at Neonatal Intensive Care Unit. *Assiut Scientific Nursing Journal, 12*(43), 98–107. DOI: 10.21608/asnj.2024.279442.1804

Hailemariam, Y., Yazdinejad, A., Parizi, R. M., Srivastava, G., & Dehghantanha, A. (2020, December). An empirical evaluation of AI deep explainable tools. In 2020 IEEE Globecom Workshops (GC Wkshps (pp. 1-6). IEEE.

Hall, W., & Pesenti, J. (2017). Growing the artificial intelligence industry in the UK. *Department for Digital, Culture, Media & Sport and Department for Business, Energy & Industrial Strategy. Part of the Industrial Strategy UK and the Commonwealth.*

Hardal, M. (2011). *Common ethical violations and ethical action patterns among Turkish mental health professionals and the factors that influence them* [Doctoral dissertation], Istanbul Bilgi Üniversitesi, Istanbul.

Hardy, M., & Harvey, H. (2020). Artificial intelligence in diagnostic imaging: Impact on the radiography profession. *The British Journal of Radiology, 93*(1108), 20190840. DOI: 10.1259/bjr.20190840 PMID: 31821024

Hasan, M., Yasmin, F., Hassan, M. M., Yu, X., Yeasmin, S., Joshi, H., & Islam, S. M. S. (2025). Enhancing stroke disease classification through machine learning models via a novel voting system by feature selection techniques. *PLoS One, 20*(1), e0312914. DOI: 10.1371/journal.pone.0312914 PMID: 39787105

Hasanova, H., Tufail, M., Baek, U.-J., Park, J.-T., & Kim, M.-S. (2022). A novel blockchain-enabled heart disease prediction mechanism using machine learning. *Computers & Electrical Engineering, 101*, 108086. DOI: 10.1016/j.compeleceng.2022.108086

Hashemi, H., Heydarian, S., Hooshmand, E., Saatchi, M., Yekta, A., Aghamirsalim, M., & Khabazkhoob, M. (2020). The prevalence and risk factors for keratoconus: A systematic review and meta-analysis. *Cornea, 39*(2), 263–270.

Hassan, A., Prasad, V. K., Bhattacharya, P., Dutta, P., & Damaševičius, R. (Eds.). (2024). *Federated learning and AI for healthcare 5.0.* IGI Global.

Heerebrand, S. L., Bray, J., Ulbrıch, C., Roberts, R. M., & Edwards, S. (2021). Effectiveness of dialectical behavior therapy skills training group for adults with borderline personality disorder. *Journal of Clinical Psychology, 77*(7), 1573–1590. DOI: 10.1002/jclp.23134 PMID: 33821506

Hegde, M. G., Ruthvika, B., Jain, R. B., Shenoy, P. D., Venugopal, K. R., & Canchi, A. (2025). A Privacy-Preserving Federated Learning Method with Homomorphic Encryption for Chronic Kidney Disease Stage Prediction. *Engineering, Technology & Applied Scientific Research, 15*(4), 26019–26026. DOI: 10.48084/etasr.11928

Helguera-Repetto, A. C., Soto-Ramírez, M. D., Villavicencio-Carrisoza, O., Yong-Mendoza, S., Yong-Mendoza, A., León-Juárez, M., González-y-Merchand, J. A., Zaga-Clavellina, V., & Irles, C. (2020). Neonatal sepsis diagnosis decision-making based on artificial neural networks. *Frontiers in Pediatrics, 8*, 525. DOI: 10.3389/fped.2020.00525 PMID: 33042902

Hespanha, P. (2019). The impact of austerity on the Portuguese National Health Service, citizens' well-being, and health inequalities. *e-cadernos CES*, (31). DOI: 10.4000/eces.4187

He, Y., Yang, L., Zhu, X., Wu, B., Zhang, S., Qian, C., & Tian, T. (2022). Mental health chatbot for young adults with depressive symptoms during the COVID-19 pandemic: Single-blind, three-arm randomized controlled trial. *Journal of Medical Internet Research, 24*(11), e40719. DOI: 10.2196/40719 PMID: 36355633

Hilty, D. M., Ferrer, D. C., Parish, M. B., Johnston, B., Callahan, E. J., & Yellowlees, P. M. (2013). The effectiveness of telemental health: A 2013 review. *Telemedicine Journal and e-Health, 19*(6), 444–454. DOI: 10.1089/tmj.2013.0075 PMID: 23697504

Hintz, S. R., Barnes, P. D., Bulas, D., Slovis, T. L., Finer, N. N., Wrage, L. A., Das, A., Tyson, J. E., Stevenson, D. K., Carlo, W. A., Walsh, M. C., Laptook, A. R., Yoder, B. A., Van Meurs, K. P., Faix, R. G., Rich, W., Newman, N. S., Cheng, H., Heyne, R. J., & Higgins, R. D. (2015). Neuroimaging and neurodevelopmental outcome in extremely preterm infants. *Pediatrics, 135*(1), e32–e42. DOI: 10.1542/peds.2014-0898 PMID: 25554820

Houston, T. K., Cooper, L. A., & Ford, D. E. (2002). Internet support groups for depression: A 1-year prospective cohort study. *The American Journal of Psychiatry, 159*(12), 2062–2068. DOI: 10.1176/appi.ajp.159.12.2062 PMID: 12450957

Hruska, K. A., & Seifert, M. (2013). Pathophysiology of Chronic Kidney Disease Mineral Bone Disorder (CKD-MBD). In *Primer on the Metabolic Bone Diseases and Disorders of Mineral Metabolism* (pp. 632–639). Wiley. DOI: 10.1002/9781118453926.ch77

Hsu, J. F., Chang, Y. F., Cheng, H. J., Yang, C., Lin, C. Y., Chu, S. M., Huang, H. R., Chiang, M. C., Wang, H. C., & Tsai, M. H. (2021). Machine learning approaches to predict in-hospital mortality among neonates with clinically suspected sepsis in the neonatal intensive care unit. *Journal of Personalized Medicine*, *11*(8), 695. DOI: 10.3390/jpm11080695 PMID: 34442338

https://entokey.com/9-optical-coherence-tomography-in-corneal-ectasia/

https://williamseye.com/services/glaucoma-care-treatment/optical-coherence-tomography-scanner-oct/

https://www.indiamart.com/proddetail/specular-microscopy-pachymetry-7322736755.html

https://www.urmc.rochester.edu/eye-institute/lasik/technology/orbscan-corneal-topographer

Huang, S., Lai, X., Ke, L., Li, Y., Wang, H., Zhao, X., Dai, X., & Wang, Y. (2024). AI Technology panic-is AI Dependence Bad for Mental Health? A Cross-Lagged Panel Model and the Mediating Roles of Motivations for AI Use Among Adolescents. *Psychology Research and Behavior Management*, *17*, 1087–1102. DOI: 10.2147/PRBM.S440889 PMID: 38495087

Huang, Y. P., Vadloori, S., Chu, H. C., Kang, E. Y. C., Wu, W. C., Kusaka, S., & Fukushima, Y. (2020). Deep learning models for automated diagnosis of retinopathy of prematurity in preterm infants. *Electronics (Basel)*, *9*(9), 1444. DOI: 10.3390/electronics9091444

Hudlicka, E. (2016). Virtual affective agents and therapeutic games. In Luxton, D. L. (Ed.). In *Artificial Intelligence in Behavioral And Mental Health Care*, (s.s. 81-115), Elsevier Academic Press DOI: 10.1016/B978-0-12-420248-1.00004-0

Hunkin, H. (2022). *The Acceptability and Efficacy of Wearable Devices in Digital Mental Health* [Doctor of Philosophy/Master of Psychology (Clinical)]. The University of Adelaide.

Hunkin, H., King, D. L., & Zajac, I. T. (2019). Wearable devices as adjuncts in the treatment of anxiety-related symptoms: A narrative review of five device modalities and implications for clinical practice. *Clinical Psychology : a Publication of the Division of Clinical Psychology of the American Psychological Association*, *26*(3), 987–1003. DOI: 10.1111/cpsp.12290

Hunkin, H., King, D. L., & Zajac, I. T. (2021). Evaluating the feasibility of a consumer-grade wearable EEG headband to aid assessment of state and trait mindfulness. *Journal of Clinical Psychology*, *77*(11), 2559–2575. DOI: 10.1002/jclp.23189 PMID: 34061998

Hutto, C. J., & Gilbert, E. (2014). VADER: A Parsimonious Rule-based Model for Sentiment Analysis of Social Media Text. *Proceedings of the Eighth International AAAI Conference on Weblogs and Social Media,* Association for the Advancement of Artificial Intelligence (pp. 216-225). DOI: 10.1609/icwsm.v8i1.14550

Illovsky, M. E. (1994). Counseling, artificial intelligence, and expert systems. *Simulation & Gaming*, *25*(1), 88–98. DOI: 10.1177/1046878194251009

Im, J. E., Park, S., Kim, Y. J., Yoon, S. A., & Lee, J. H. (2022). Predicting the need for intubation within 3 hours in the neonatal intensive care unit using a multimodal deep neural network [Preprint]. *Research Square.* https://doi.org/DOI: 10.21203/rs.3.rs-1872902/v1

Inkster, B., Sarda, S., & Subramanian, V. (2018). An empathy-driven, conversational artificial intelligence agent (Wysa) for digital mental well-being: Real-world data evaluation mixedmethods study. *JMIR mHealth and uHealth*, *6*(11), e12106. DOI: 10.2196/12106 PMID: 30470676

Interaxon Inc. (2020). Brain sensing headband: What it measures. https://choosemuse.com/what-it-measures/

Iqbal, F., Chandra, P., Lewis, L. E. S., Acharya, D., Purkayastha, J., Shenoy, P. A., & Patil, A. K. (2024). Application of artificial intelligence to predict the sepsis in neonates admitted in neonatal intensive care unit. *Journal of Neonatal Nursing*, *30*(2), 141–147. DOI: 10.1016/j.jnn.2023.07.016

Ismail, S., Siddiqi, I., & Akram, U. (2018). Localization and classification of heart beats in phonocardiography signals—A comprehensive review. *EURASIP Journal on Advances in Signal Processing*, *2018*(1), 1–27. DOI: 10.1186/s13634-018-0545-9

ISO/IEC 42001:2023 [Internet]. ISO; 2023. https://www.iso.org/standard/81230.html. [Accessed 27 January 2025].

İvelik, H. İ., Alkış, O., Kartal, İ. G., Sevim, M., & Aras, B. (2025). AI-assisted cystoscopy image analysis for detecting urological pathologies: A novel approach. *Grand Journal of Urology*, *5*(2), 37–41. DOI: 10.5505/GJU.2025.94824

Jain, A., Sandhu, R., Singh, G., & Rakhra, M. (2024). The role of AI counselling in journaling for mental health improvement. In *2024 International Conference on Electrical Electronics and Computing Technologies (ICEECT)* (pp. 1–6). DOI: 10.1109/ICEECT61758.2024.10739128

Janbain, A., Farolfi, A., Guenegou-Arnoux, A., Romengas, L., Scharl, S., Fanti, S., ... & Shelan, M. (2024). A machine learning approach for predicting biochemical outcome after PSMA-PET–guided salvage radiotherapy in recurrent prostate cancer after radical prostatectomy: retrospective study. *JMIR cancer*, *10*, e60323.

Jang, W., Choi, Y. S., Kim, J. Y., Yon, D. K., Lee, Y. J., Chung, S. H., Kim, C. Y., Image, A. O., Yeo, S. G., & Lee, J. (2023). Artificial intelligence–driven respiratory distress syndrome prediction for very low birth weight infants: Korean multicenter prospective cohort study. *Journal of Medical Internet Research*, *25*, e47612. DOI: 10.2196/47612 PMID: 37428525

Jibb, L. A., Birnie, K. A., Nathan, P. C., Beran, T. N., Hum, V., Victor, J. C., & Stinson, J. N. (2018). Using the MEDiPORT humanoid robot to reduce procedural pain and distress in children with cancer: A pilot randomized controlled trial. *Pediatric Blood & Cancer*, *65*(9), e27242. DOI: 10.1002/pbc.27242 PMID: 29893482

Jirsova, K. (2017). The cornea, anatomy and function. *Light and specular microscopy of the cornea*, 1-21.

Jobin, A., Ienca, M., & Vayena, E. (2019). The global landscape of AI ethics guidelines. *Nature Machine Intelligence*, *1*(9), 389–399. DOI: 10.1038/s42256-019-0088-2

Jones, R. N. (2014). *Uygulamalı danışmanlık ve yardım becerileri* [Practical counselling and helping skills]. (Sart, G., Trans.). Nobel Akademi Yayıncılık.

Joseph, F. J. J., Nonsiri, S., & Monsakul, A. (2021). Keras and TensorFlow: A hands-on experience. *Advanced deep learning for engineers and scientists: A practical approach*, 85-111.

Kabadayı, F., & Güven, M. (2023). Psikolojik yardım hizmetlerindeki mobil uygulamalarla ilgili bir inceleme. [A Review of Mobile Applications in Psychological Help Services]. *The Journal of Turkish Educational Sciences*, *21*(3), 1660–1689. DOI: 10.37217/tebd.1291285

Kabra, G., & Sangroya, D. (2023, November). Understanding behavioural intention to use telemedicine in healthcare: Insights from medical practitioners. In *AIP Conference Proceedings* (Vol. 2909, No. 1). AIP Publishing.

Kaewkannate, K., & Kim, S. (2016). A comparison of wearable fitness devices. *BMC Public Health*, *16*(1), 1–16. DOI: 10.1186/s12889-016-3059-0 PMID: 27220855

Kafes, A. Y., Çiller, A., & Şakiroğlu, M. (2024). Deprem yaşamış bireylerin travma belirtilerine yönelik sanal gerçeklik destekli müdahale programı: Bir etkililik çalışması [Virtual Reality Supported Intervention Program for Trauma Symptoms of Individuals Who Experienced an Earthquake: An Effectiveness Study]. *Archives Neuropsychiatry*, *61*, 15–23. DOI: 10.29399/npa.28568 PMID: 38496219

Kaliappan, S., Radhika, S., Ravi, D., & Aluvala, S. (2023). A Data-Driven Approach to Improving Neonatal Care through Artificial Intelligence and Clinical Data Integration. In 2023 IEEE International Conference on ICT in Business Industry & Government (ICTBIG) (pp. 1-6). IEEE. https://doi.org/DOI: 10.1109/ICTBIG59752.2023.10456148

Kallel, I. F., Mahfoudhi, O., & Kammoun, S. (2024). Deep learning models based on CNN architecture for early keratoconus detection using corneal topographic maps. *Multimedia Tools and Applications*, *83*(16), 49173–49193.

Kamoji, S., Rozario, S., Almeida, S., Patil, S., Patankar, S., & Pendhari, H. (2024). Mental health prediction using machine learning models and large language model. In *2024 Second International Conference on Inventive Computing and Informatics (ICICI)* (pp. 185–190). DOI: 10.1109/ICICI62254.2024.00040

Kang, E., Song, N., & Ju, H. (2022). Contents and sentiment analysis of newspaper articles and comments on telemedicine in Korea: Before and after of COVID-19 outbreak. *Health Informatics Journal*, *28*(1), 14604582221075549. DOI: 10.1177/14604582221075549 PMID: 35212233

Karabay, M., Kaya, G., Guclu, E., Ogutlu, A., Karabay, O., & Caner, I. (2021). Health care-associated infections in neonatal intensive care unit: Evaluation of the last 6 years. *Turkish Journal of Pediatric Disease*, *15*(2), 87–92. DOI: 10.12956/tchd.597635

Kataru, S., King, K., & Fernando, L. (2024). Machine learning-based early detection and intervention for mental health issues in children. In *2024 IEEE 48th Annual Computers, Software, and Applications Conference (COMPSAC)* (pp. 2001–2007). DOI: 10.1109/COMPSAC61105.2024.00320

Kaushik, E., Jain, E., Gill, K. S., Upadhyay, D., & Devliyal, S. (2024). Optimizing mental health prediction by fine-tuning decision classifier parameters for enhanced accuracy. In *2024 2nd International Conference on Sustainable Computing and Smart Systems (ICSCSS)* (pp. 935–939). DOI: 10.1109/ICSCSS60660.2024.10625480

Kavitha, M., Gnaneswar, G., Dinesh, R., Sai, Y. R., & Suraj, R. S. (2021, January). Heart disease prediction using hybrid machine learning model. In *2021 6th international conference on inventive computation technologies (ICICT)* (pp. 1329-1333). IEEE. DOI: 10.1109/ICICT50816.2021.9358597

Kavitha, V., Suresh, K. T., Vishnu, P. T., & Kumaresan, T. (2025). Forecasting Model Utilization: Converting Knowledge Through Performance. In Ben Ltaifa, M., & Derbali, A. (Eds.), *AI Methods for Environmental Protection and Resource Conservation* (pp. 245–270). IGI Global Scientific Publishing., DOI: 10.4018/979-8-3373-3246-8.ch010

Kavur, A. E., Gezer, N. S., Barış, M., Şahin, Y., Özkan, S., Baydar, B., & Selver, M. A. (2019). Comparison of semi-automatic and deep learning-based automatic methods for liver segmentation in living liver transplant donors. *Diagnostic and Interventional Radiology*, *26*(1), 11.

Kaya, H., Cavusoglu, A., Cakmak, H., Şen, B., & Delen, D. (2016). Supporting the diagnosis process and processes after treatment by using image segmentation and image simulation techniques: Keratoconus example. *Journal of the Faculty of Engineering and Architecture of Gazi University*, *31*(3).

Kemp, S. (2019). Digital 2023: Portugal. *Datareportal*, Available at: https://datareportal.com/reports/digital-2023-portugal?rq=portugal (Accessed in 23 March 2023).

Kerkez, M., & Kaplan, M. (2025). Evaluation of discharge training given by nurses to postpartum mothers to artificial intelligence: An alternative approach to health care. *BMC Nursing*, *24*(1), 296. DOI: 10.1186/s12912-025-02966-5 PMID: 40119346

Khalid, S., Khalil, T., & Nasreen, S. (2014). A Survey of Feature Selection and Feature Extraction Techniques in Machine Learning. *Science and Information Conference*, London, UK, 372-378. DOI: 10.1109/SAI.2014.6918213

Khanam, F. T. Z., Al-Naji, A., Perera, A. G., Gibson, K., & Chahl, J. (2022). Remote vital signs monitoring in neonatal intensive care unit using a digital camera. *International Journal of Biomedical and Biological Engineering*, *16*(10), 138–144.

Khawaja, Z., & Bélisle-Pipon, J. C. (2023). Your robot therapist is not your therapist: Understanding the role of AI-powered mental health chatbots. *Frontiers in Digital Health*, *5*, 1278186. DOI: 10.3389/fdgth.2023.1278186 PMID: 38026836

Khine, A. H., Wettayaprasit, W., & Duangsuwan, J. (2024). A new word embedding model integrated with medical knowledge for deep learning-based sentiment classification. *Artificial Intelligence in Medicine*, *148*, 102758. DOI: 10.1016/j.artmed.2023.102758 PMID: 38325934

Kilicarslan Toruner, E., & Buyukgonenc, L. (2017). Healthy newborn. In *Child Health Basic Nursing Approaches* (pp. 233–290). Göktuğ Publishing.

Kim, J., Ham, W. S., Koo, K. C., Lee, J., Ahn, H. K., Jeong, J. Y., Baek, S. Y., Lee, S. J., & Lee, K. S. (2024). Evaluation of the Diagnostic Efficacy of the AI-Based Software INF-M01 in Detecting Suspicious Areas of Bladder Cancer Using Cystoscopy Images. *Journal of Clinical Medicine*, *13*(23), 7110. DOI: 10.3390/jcm13237110 PMID: 39685568

Kim, M., Lee, S., Kim, S., Heo, J. I., Lee, S., Shin, Y. B., Cho, C.-H., & Jung, D. (2025). Therapeutic potential of social chatbots in alleviating loneliness and social anxiety: Quasi-experimental mixed methods study. *Journal of Medical Internet Research*, *27*, e65589. DOI: 10.2196/65589 PMID: 39808786

Kim, Y. J., Lee, S. H., Park, C. M., & Kim, K. G. (2016). Evaluation of semi-automatic segmentation methods for persistent ground glass nodules on thin-section CT scans. *Healthcare Informatics Research*, *22*(4), 305–315.

Kim, Y., Kim, H., Choi, J., Cho, K., Yoo, D., Lee, Y., Park, S. J., Jeong, M. H., Jeong, S. H., Park, K. Y., Byun, S. Y., Kim, T., Ahn, S. H., Cho, W. H., & Lee, N. (2023). Early prediction of need for invasive mechanical ventilation in the neonatal intensive care unit using artificial intelligence and electronic health records: A clinical study. *BMC Pediatrics*, *23*(1), 525. DOI: 10.1186/s12887-023-04350-1 PMID: 37872515

Kline, T. L., Edwards, M. E., Fetzer, J., Gregory, A. V., Anaam, D., Metzger, A. J., & Erickson, B. J. (2021). Automatic semantic segmentation of kidney cysts in MR images of patients affected by autosomal-dominant polycystic kidney disease. *Abdominal Radiology*, *46*(3), 1053–1061.

Kloonen, R. M., Varisco, G., de Kort, E., Andriessen, P., Niemarkt, H. J., & van Pul, C. (2023). Predicting CPAP failure after less invasive surfactant administration (LISA) in preterm infants by machine learning model on vital parameter data: A pilot study. *Physiological Measurement*, *44*(11), 115005. DOI: 10.1088/1361-6579/ad0ab6 PMID: 37939392

Kong, F., Zou, Y., Li, Z., & Deng, Y. (2024). Advances in portable and wearable acoustic sensing devices for human health monitoring. *Sensors (Basel)*, *24*(16), 5354. DOI: 10.3390/s24165354 PMID: 39205054

Konyalı, A., Naipoğlu, C., Güner, S., Bakkal, I., & Çelik, A. (2025). Psikolojide Yapay Zeka Kullanımı ve Uygulamaları [Use and Applications of Artificial Intelligence in Psychology]. *Journal of Kocaeli Health and Technology University*, *3*(1), 1–17.

Kostekci, Y. E., Bakırarar, B., Okulu, E., Erdeve, O., Atasay, B., & Arsan, S. (2023). An Early Prediction Model for Estimating Bronchopulmonary Dysplasia in Preterm Infants. *Neonatology*, *120*(6), 709–717. DOI: 10.1159/000533299 PMID: 37725910

Kostopoulos, L. (2018). The emerging artificial intelligence wellnesslandscape: Benefits and potential areas of ethical concern. *California Western Law Review*, *55*(1), 235–254.

Kourtis, A. P., Hatfield, K., & Baggs, J.. (2019). Vital signs: Epidemiology and recent trends in methicillin-resistant and in methicillin-susceptible Staphylococcus aureus bloodstream infections — United States. *MMWR. Morbidity and Mortality Weekly Report*, *68*(9), 214–219. DOI: 10.15585/mmwr.mm6809e1 PMID: 30845118

Kretzschmar, K., Tyroll, H., Pavarini, G., Manzini, A., & Singh, I. (2019). Can your phone be your therapist? Young people's ethical perspectives on the use of fully automated conversational agents(chatbots) in mental health support. *Biomedical Informatics Insights*, *11*, 1–9. DOI: 10.1177/1178222619829083 PMID: 30858710

Kristensen, M. A., Abrantes, J. S., Jensen, H. I., Mogensen, C. B., Søndergaard, J., & Møller, J. K. (2023). The association between socioeconomic factors and the success of decolonization treatment among individuals diagnosed with methicillin-resistant Staphylococcus aureus: A cohort study from 2007 to 2020. *Infection Control and Hospital Epidemiology*, *44*(10), 1620–1628. DOI: 10.1017/ice.2023.32 PMID: 37017132

Krittanawong, C., Johnson, K. W., Rosenson, R. S., Wang, Z., Aydar, M., Baber, U., Min, J. K., Tang, W. H. W., Halperin, J. L., & Narayan, S. M. (2019). Deep learning for cardiovascular medicine: A practical primer. *European Heart Journal*, *40*(25), 2058–2073. DOI: 10.1093/eurheartj/ehz056 PMID: 30815669

Krizhevsky, A., Sutskever, I., & Hinton, G. E. Imagenet classification with deep convolutional neural networks. In: Advances in neural information processing systems. 2012; p. 1097-105.

Krysia, W. H., & Marion, J. B. (2018). The challenge for nursıng and healthcare ın the dıgıtal age. *Texto & Contexto-Enfermagem*, 27. https://doi.org/DOI: 10.1590/0104-07072018002018editorial2

Kucuk, S., & Yagmur, B. (2019). Job Stress Factors and Perceived Job Stress Levels of Neonatal Intensive Care Unit Nurses. *The Journal of Academic Social Science, 72*(72), 142–152. DOI: 10.16992/ASOS.13762

Kukreti, M., Sehjpal, S., Tiwari, R., & Sood, K. (Eds.). (Forthcoming 2025). *Driving global health and sustainable development goals with smart technology*. IGI Global.

Kumar, R. (2017). Artificial intelligence—basics. Machine learning and cognition in enterprises: Business intelligence transformed, pp. 33–49. DOI: 10.1007/978-1-4842-3069-5_3

Kumar, V. V., Sahoo, A., Balasubramanian, S. K., & Gholston, S. (2024). Mitigating healthcare supply chain challenges under disaster conditions: A holistic AI-based analysis of social media data. *International Journal of Production Research*, •••, 1–19. DOI: 10.1080/00207543.2024.2316884

Kuruca, Y., Üstüner, M., & Şimşek, I. (2022). Dijital pazarlamada yapay zekâ kullanımı: Sohbet robotu (Chatbot) [Using Artificial Intelligence in Digital Marketing: Chatbot]. *Medya ve Kültür, 2*(1), 88–113.

Kymes, S. M., Walline, J. J., Zadnik, K., & Gordon, M. O.Collaborative Longitudinal Evaluation of Keratoconus (CLEK) Study Group. (2004). Quality of life in keratoconus. *American Journal of Ophthalmology, 138*(4), 527–535.

Langarizadeh, M., Tabatabaei, M. S., Tavakol, K., Naghipour, M., Rostami, A., & Moghbeli, F. (2017). Telemental health care, an effective alternative to conventional mental care: A systematic review. *Acta Informatica Medica, 25*(4), 240. DOI: 10.5455/aim.2017.25.240-246 PMID: 29284913

Lanier, M., Waddell, T. F., Elson, M., Tamul, D. J., Ivory, J. D., & Przybylski, A. (2019). Virtual reality check: Statistical power, reported results, and the validity of research on the psychology of virtual reality and immersive environments. *Computers in Human Behavior, 100*, 70–78. DOI: 10.1016/j.chb.2019.06.015

LaRocca, F., Chiu, S. J., McNabb, R. P., Kuo, A. N., Izatt, J. A., & Farsiu, S. (2011). Robust automatic segmentation of corneal layer boundaries in SDOCT images using graph theory and dynamic programming. *Biomedical Optics Express, 2*(6), 1524–1538.

Latha, C. B. C., & Jeeva, S. C. (2019). Improving the accuracy of the prediction of heart disease risk based on ensemble classification techniques. *Informatics in Medicine Unlocked, 16*, 100203. DOI: 10.1016/j.imu.2019.100203

Lau, Y., Chee, D. G. H., Chow, X. P., Wong, S. H., Cheng, L. J., & Lau, S. T. (2020). Humanoid robot-assisted interventions among children with diabetes: A systematic scoping review. *International Journal of Nursing Studies*, *111*, 103749. DOI: 10.1016/j.ijnurstu.2020.103749 PMID: 32911362

Lazzeri, E., Ronconi, E., Angelotti, M. L., Peired, A., Mazzinghi, B., Becherucci, F., Conti, S., Sansavini, G., Sisti, A., Ravaglia, F., Lombardi, D., Provenzano, A., Manonelles, A., Cruzado, J. M., Giglio, S., Roperto, R. M., Materassi, M., Lasagni, L., & Romagnani, P. (2015). Human Urine-Derived Renal Progenitors for Personalized Modeling of Genetic Kidney Disorders. *Journal of the American Society of Nephrology*, *26*(8), 1961–1974. DOI: 10.1681/ASN.2014010057 PMID: 25568173

Lee, C. K., & Huang, X. Y. (2022). Psychological processes of postpartum mothers with newborns admitted to the intensive care unit. *Asian Nursing Research*, *16*(1), 9–17. DOI: 10.1016/j.anr.2021.12.007 PMID: 34990888

Lee, C. S., Tyring, A. J., Deruyter, N. P., Wu, Y., Rokem, A., & Lee, A. Y. (2017). Deep-learning based, automated segmentation of macular edema in optical coherence tomography. *Biomedical Optics Express*, *8*(7), 3440–3448.

Lee, E., Jung, H. S., & Jang, J. A. (2023). Consumers' perceptions of dietary supplements before and after the COVID-19 pandemic based on big data. *Journal of Nutrition and Health*, *56*(3), 330–347. DOI: 10.4163/jnh.2023.56.3.330

Lei, H., Ashrafi, A., Chang, P., Chang, A., & Lai, W. (2022). Patent ductus arteriosus (PDA) detection in echocardiograms using deep learning. *Intelligence-Based Medicine*, *6*, 100054. DOI: 10.1016/j.ibmed.2022.100054

Leung, L. B., Yoo, C., Chu, K., O'Shea, A., Jackson, N. J., Heyworth, L., & Der-Martirosian, C. (2023). Rates of primary care and integrated mental health telemedicine visits between rural and urban veterans affairs beneficiaries before and after the onset of the COVID-19 pandemic. *JAMA Network Open*, *6*(3), e231864–e231864. DOI: 10.1001/jamanetworkopen.2023.1864 PMID: 36881410

Liang, H. F., Wu, K. M., Weng, C. H., & Hsieh, H. W. (2019). Nurses' views on the potential use of robots in the pediatric unit. *Journal of Pediatric Nursing*, *47*, e58–e64. DOI: 10.1016/j.pedn.2019.04.027 PMID: 31076190

Li, J., Lu, Z., Wang, L., Shi, H., Chu, B., Qu, Y., & Qu, D. (2024). Novel Coumarins Derivatives for A. baumannii Lung Infection Developed by High-Throughput Screening and Reinforcement Learning. *Journal of Neuroimmune Pharmacology*, *19*(1), 32. DOI: 10.1007/s11481-024-10134-w PMID: 38886254

Ling, Z., Zhou, W., Ren, Y., Wang, J., & Guo, L. (2022). Non-contact heart rate monitoring based on millimeter wave radar. *IEEE Access : Practical Innovations, Open Solutions, 10*, 74033–74044. DOI: 10.1109/ACCESS.2022.3190355

Lin, X., Geng, R., Menke, K., Edelson, M., Yan, F., Leong, T., & Cheng Immergluck, L. (2023). Machine learning to predict risk for community-onset Staphylococcus aureus infections in children living in southeastern United States. *PLoS One*, *18*(9), e0290375. DOI: 10.1371/journal.pone.0290375 PMID: 37656705

Liu, Y., Li, D., Guo, Y., Zhou, X., Dong, Y., Guo, Z., . . . Lv, B. (2020, April). Hierarchy-constrained network for corneal tissue segmentation based on anterior segment OCT images. In *2020 IEEE 17th International Symposium on Biomedical Imaging (ISBI)* (pp. 1579-1582). IEEE.

Liu, Y., Pu, H., & Sun, D. W. (2021). Efficient extraction of deep image features using convolutional neural network (CNN) for applications in detecting and analysing complex food matrices. *Trends in Food Science & Technology*, *113*, 193–204.

Li, Y., Wang, M., Wang, L., Cao, Y., Liu, Y., Zhao, Y., Yuan, R., Yang, M., Lu, S., Sun, Z., Zhou, F., Qian, Z., & Kang, H. (2024). Advances in the application of AI robots in critical care: Scoping review. *Journal of Medical Internet Research, 26*, e54095. DOI: 10.2196/54095 PMID: 38801765

Loder, J., & Nicholas, L. (2018). *Confronting Dr Robot: Creating a people-powered future for AI in health*. Nesta.

Long, J., Shelhamer, E., & Darrell, T. (2015). Fully convolutional networks for semantic segmentation. In *Proceedings of the IEEE conference on computer vision and pattern recognition* (pp. 3431-3440).

Lucas, S. E., & Burdon, K. P. (2020). Genetic and environmental risk factors for keratoconus. *Annual Review of Vision Science*, *6*(1), 25–46.

Lum, P. T., Sekar, M., Gan, S. H., Jeyabalan, S., Bonam, S. R., Rani, N. N. I. M., Ku-Mahdzir, K.-M., Seow, L. J., Wu, Y. S., Subramaniyan, V., Fuloria, N. K., & Fuloria, S. (2022). Therapeutic potential of mangiferin against kidney disorders and its mechanism of action: A review. *Saudi Journal of Biological Sciences*, *29*(3), 1530–1542. DOI: 10.1016/j.sjbs.2021.11.016 PMID: 35280538

Lustgarten, S. D., & Elhai, J. D. (2018). Technology use in mental health practice and research: Legal and ethical risks. *Clinical Psychology : a Publication of the Division of Clinical Psychology of the American Psychological Association*, *25*(2), e12234. DOI: 10.1111/cpsp.12234

Luxton, D. D. (2014). Artificial intelligence in psychological practice: Current and future applications and implications. *Professional Psychology, Research and Practice*, *45*(5), 332–339. DOI: 10.1037/a0034559

Maile, H. (2023). *Keratoconus detection and personalised progression modelling using computational methods* (Doctoral dissertation, UCL (University College London)).

Mair, F., & Whitten, P. (2000). Systematic review of studies of patient satisfaction with telemedicine. *BMJ (Clinical Research Ed.)*, *320*(7248), 1517–1520. DOI: 10.1136/bmj.320.7248.1517 PMID: 10834899

Majd, A., AlJasser, M., Mirzaalian, H., Shapiro, J., Hamarneh, G., Lui, H., Santos, L. D. N., Chu, T., & Lee, T. K. (2021). A novel automated approach to rapid and precise in vivo measurement of hair morphometrics using a smartphone. *Skin Research and Technology : Official Journal of International Society for Bioengineering and the Skin (ISBS) and International Society for Digital Imaging of Skin (ISDIS) and International Society for Skin Imaging (ISSI)*, *27*(6), 1128–1134. DOI: 10.1111/srt.13076 PMID: 34251055

Majidi, E., & Manshaee, G. (2024). Effects of virtual reality exposure therapy on state-trait anxiety in individuals with dentophobia. *Current Psychology (New Brunswick, N.J.)*, *43*(3), 2425–2431. DOI: 10.1007/s12144-023-04485-5

Malak, J. S., Zeraati, H., Nayeri, F. S., Safdari, R., & Shahraki, A. D. (2019). Neonatal intensive care decision support systems using artificial intelligence techniques: A systematic review. *Artificial Intelligence Review*, *52*(4), 2685–2704. DOI: 10.1007/s10462-018-9635-1

Manworren, R. C., Horner, S., Joseph, R., Dadar, P., & Kaduwela, N. (2024). Performance evaluation of a supervised machine learning pain classification model developed by neonatal nurses. *Advances in Neonatal Care*, *24*(3), 301–310. DOI: 10.1097/ANC.0000000000001145 PMID: 38775675

Marandi, K., & Shah, H. (2023). Treatment of mental health disorders improved by artificial intelligence. In *2023 3rd International Conference on Advance Computing and Innovative Technologies in Engineering (ICACITE)* (pp. 2569–2573).

Marchionni, P., Scalise, L., Ercoli, I., Palazzi, M. L., & Carnielli, V. P. (2016). Effect of limbs' motion on pulse oximetry in preterm infants. In 2016 IEEE International Symposium on Medical Measurements and Applications (MeMeA) (pp. 1-6). IEEE. https://doi.org/DOI: 10.1109/MeMeA.2016.7533788

Marshall, J. M., Dunstan, D. A., & Bartik, W. (2020). Apps with maps—anxiety and depression mobile apps with evidence-based frameworks: Systematic search of major app stores. *JMIR Mental Health*, *7*(6), e16525. DOI: 10.2196/16525 PMID: 32579127

MARTEL, (2014). Association des optométristes du Québec. Clinique optométrique,

Mathieson, S., O'Keeffe, M., Traeger, A. C., Ferreira, G. E., & Shaheed, C. A. (2022). Content and sentiment analysis of gabapentinoid-related tweets: An infodemiology study. *Drug and Alcohol Review*, *40*(1), 45–55. DOI: 10.1111/dar.13590 PMID: 36539307

Ma, X., Zhang, Q., He, L., Liu, X., Xiao, Y., Hu, J., Cai, S., Cai, H., & Yu, B. (2024). Artificial intelligence application in the diagnosis and treatment of bladder cancer: Advance, challenges, and opportunities. *Frontiers in Oncology*, *14*, 1487676. DOI: 10.3389/fonc.2024.1487676 PMID: 39575423

Mbanuzue, C. E., Hassan, O. E., & Owolabi, F. M. (2024). Real-Time Monitoring of Neonatal Incubator Parameters Via Iot-Integrated Device: Design, Implementation, and Evaluation. *International Journal of Research and Innovation in Applied Science*, *9*(4), 127–143. DOI: 10.51584/IJRIAS.2024.90409

McCarthy, J. (2007a). *What is artificial intelligence*. Computer Science Department, Stanford University. https://trilliumdynamix.com/jmc/whatisai.pdf

McCarthy, J. (2007b). From here to human-level AI. *Artificial Intelligence*, *171*(18), 1174–1182. DOI: 10.1016/j.artint.2007.10.009

McGregor, C. (2013). Big data in neonatal intensive care. *Computer*, *46*(6), 54–59. DOI: 10.1109/MC.2013.157

Meeus, M., Beirnaert, C., Mahieu, L., Laukens, K., Meysman, P., Mulder, A., & Van Laere, D. (2024). Clinical Decision Support for Improved Neonatal Care: The Development of a Machine Learning Model for the Prediction of Late-onset Sepsis and Necrotizing Enterocolitis. *The Journal of Pediatrics*, *266*, 113869. DOI: 10.1016/j.jpeds.2023.113869 PMID: 38065281

Melo, M. C., Maasch, J. R., & de la Fuente-Nunez, C. (2021). Accelerating antibiotic discovery through artificial intelligence. *Communications Biology*, *4*(1), 1050. DOI: 10.1038/s42003-021-02586-0 PMID: 34504303

Menon, V., Rajan, T. M., & Sarkar, S. (2017). Psychotherapeutic applications of mobile phone-based technologies: A systematic review of current research and trends. *Indian Journal of Psychological Medicine*, *39*(1), 4–11. DOI: 10.4103/0253-7176.198956 PMID: 28250552

Meske, C., Bunde, E., Schneider, J., & Gersch, M. (2022). Explainable Artificial Intelligence: Objectives, Stakeholders, and Future Research Opportunities. *Information Systems Management*, *39*(1), 53–63. DOI: 10.1080/10580530.2020.1849465

Mesquita, A. C., Zamarioli, C. M., & de Carvalho, E. C. (2016). The use of robots in nursing care practices: An exploratory descriptive study. *Online Brazilian Journal of Nursing*, *15*(3), 404–413. DOI: 10.17665/1676-4285.20165395

Meyer, J. J., Gokul, A., Vellara, H. R., & McGhee, C. N. (2023). Progression of keratoconus in children and adolescents. *The British Journal of Ophthalmology*, *107*(2), 176–180.

Mihret, E. T. (2020). Robotics and artificial intelligence. *International Journal of Artificial Intelligence and Machine Learning*, *10*(2), 57–78. DOI: 10.4018/IJAIML.2020070104

Miller, D. D., & Brown, E. W. (2018). Artificial intelligence in medical practice: The question to the answer? *The American Journal of Medicine*, *131*(2), 129–133. DOI: 10.1016/j.amjmed.2017.10.035 PMID: 29126825

Ming, Q., & Xiao, X. (2023). Towards accurate medical image segmentation with gradient-optimized dice loss. *IEEE Signal Processing Letters*, *31*, 191–195.

Mishra, A., Singh, A., Singh, A., Chauhan, M., & Kamboj, D. (2024). Analysis of mental health disorders from survey reports using time series-based linear regression. In *2024 2nd International Conference on Networking, Embedded and Wireless Systems (ICNEWS)* (pp. 1–6). DOI: 10.1109/ICNEWS60873.2024.10730817

Mishra, C., & Gupta, D. (2017). Deep machine learning and neural networks: An overview. *IAES Int J Artif Intell.*, *6*(2), 66–73. DOI: 10.11591/ijai.v6.i2.pp66-73

Miskelly, F. (2005). Electronic tracking of patients with dementia and wandering using mobile phone technology. *Age and Ageing*, *34*(5), 497–499. DOI: 10.1093/ageing/afi145 PMID: 16107453

Mohammad, F., Clark, B., Agarwal, R., & Garg, S. (2023). Scaling mental health with advanced analytics utilizing responsible AI: Next generation emotionally smart AI agents. In *2023 Congress in Computer Science, Computer Engineering, & Applied Computing (CSCE)* (pp. 1411–1418).

Mohan, S., Thirumalai, C., & Srivastava, G. (2019). Effective heart disease prediction using hybrid machine learning techniques. *IEEE Access : Practical Innovations, Open Solutions*, *7*, 81542–81554. DOI: 10.1109/ACCESS.2019.2923707

Mokadem, N., Jabeen, F., Treur, J., Taal, H. R., & Roelofsma, P. H. (2024). An adaptive network model for AI-assisted monitoring and management of neonatal respiratory distress. *Cognitive Systems Research*, *86*, 101231. DOI: 10.1016/j.cogsys.2024.101231

Molu, B. (2025). Improving Nursing Students' Learning Outcomes in Neonatal Resuscitation: A Quasi-Experimental Study Comparing AI-Assisted Care Plan Learning With Traditional Instruction. *Journal of Evaluation in Clinical Practice*, *31*(1), e14286. DOI: 10.1111/jep.14286 PMID: 39733257

Monaghan, J., Kim, T., Dol, J., Orovec, A., & Campbell-Yeo, M. (2020). Parents' learning needs and preferences in a neonatal intensive care unit: A desire for enhanced communication and eHealth technology. *Journal of Neonatal Nursing*, *26*(2), 101–105. DOI: 10.1016/j.jnn.2019.09.001

Morgan, S. (2014). Understanding the structural basis of corneal refractive function and its modification via novel therapeutic approaches (Doctoral dissertation, Cardiff University).

Morsünbül, Ü. (2018). Robotlarla Bağlanma ve Cinsellik: Ruh Sağlığı Bakış Açısından Bir Değerlendirme [Attachment and Sex with Robots: An Assessment from Mental Health Perspective]. *Psikiyatride Güncel Yaklasimlar*, *10*(4), 427–439. DOI: 10.18863/pgy.363669

Müller, A. M., Alley, S., Schoeppe, S., & Vandelanotte, C. (2016). The effectiveness of e-& mHealth interventions to promote physical activity and healthy diets in developing countries: A systematic review. *The International Journal of Behavioral Nutrition and Physical Activity*, *13*(1), 109. DOI: 10.1186/s12966-016-0434-2 PMID: 27724911

Munsamy, A. J., Moodley, V. R., Naidoo, P., Mangwarara, T. R., Abdullah, R., Govender, D., & Dlamini, P. (2015). A frequency analysis of cone characteristics for the different stages of keratoconus. *African Vision and Eye Health*, *74*(1), 6.

Murphy, K. P. (2012). *Machine Learning: A Probabilistic Perspective*. MIT Press.

Murray, C., Mitchell, L., Tuke, J., & Mackay, M. (2022). Revealing patient-reported experiences in healthcare from social media using the dapmav framework. *ArXiv*, Available at: https://arxiv.org/abs/2210.04232 (Accessed in 23 March 2023). https://doi.org//arXiv.2210.04232DOI: 10.48550

Murugan, T. W., J., & P., V. (Eds.). (2024). *Artificial intelligence transformations for healthcare applications: Medical diagnosis, treatment, and patient care*. IGI Global.

Mutaguchi, J., Morooka, K., Kobayashi, S., Umehara, A., Miyauchi, S., Kinoshita, F., Inokuchi, J., Oda, Y., Kurazume, R., & Eto, M. (2022). Artificial Intelligence for Segmentation of Bladder Tumor Cystoscopic Images Performed by U-Net with Dilated Convolution. *Journal of Endourology*, *36*(6), 827–834. DOI: 10.1089/end.2021.0483 PMID: 35018828

Mystakidis, S. (2022). Metaverse. *Encyclopedia*, *2*(1), 486–497. DOI: 10.3390/encyclopedia2010031

Nandhini, P., Kumar, P., Mickymaray, S., Alothaim, A. S., Somasundaram, J., & Rajan, M. (2022). Recent developments in methicillin-resistant Staphylococcus aureus (MRSA) treatment: A review. *Antibiotics (Basel, Switzerland)*, *11*(5), 606. DOI: 10.3390/antibiotics11050606 PMID: 35625250

Narin, N. G. (2021). A content analysis of the metaverse articles. *Journal of Metaverse*, *1*(1), 17–24.

Narula, S., Tandon, C., & Tandon, S. (2018). Role of Matrix Metalloproteinases in Degenerative Kidney Disorders. *Current Medicinal Chemistry*, *25*(15), 1805–1816. DOI: 10.2174/0929867325666171205143441 PMID: 29210632

Nasir, M. U., Zubair, M., Ghazal, T. M., Khan, M. F., Ahmad, M., Rahman, A. U., Al Hamadi, H., Khan, M. A., & Mansoor, W. (2022). Kidney Cancer Prediction Empowered with Blockchain Security Using Transfer Learning. *Sensors (Basel)*, *22*(19), 7483. Advance online publication. DOI: 10.3390/s22197483 PMID: 36236584

Naswa, R., Jaiswal, S., Mavila, R., Yuwen, W., Erdly, B., & Si, D. (2024). Assessing empathy in mental health caregivers using conversational AI. In *2024 IEEE 12th International Conference on Healthcare Informatics (ICHI)* (pp. 538–540). DOI: 10.1109/ICHI61247.2024.00079

Neacsiu, A. D., Rizvi, S. L., & Linehan, M. M. (2010). Dialectical behavior therapy skills use as a mediator and outcome of treatment for borderline personality disorder. *Behaviour Research and Therapy*, *48*(9), 832–839. DOI: 10.1016/j.brat.2010.05.017 PMID: 20579633

Niazi, S., Gatzioufas, Z., Doroodgar, F., Findl, O., Baradaran-Rafii, A., Liechty, J., & Moshirfar, M. (2024). Keratoconus: Exploring fundamentals and future perspectives–a comprehensive systematic review. *Therapeutic Advances in Ophthalmology*, *16*, 25158414241232258.

Nieradzik, L., Scheuermann, G., Saur, D., & Gillmann, C. (2021). Effect of the output activation function on the probabilities and errors in medical image segmentation. *arXiv preprint arXiv:2109.00903*.

Nilsson, N. J. (2014). *Principles of artificial intelligence*. Morgan Kaufmann.

Ning, Y., Liu, X., Collins, G. S., Moons, K. G., McCradden, M., Ting, D. S. W., Ong, J. C. L., Goldstein, B. A., Wagner, S. K., Keane, P. A., Topol, E. J., & Liu, N. (2024). An ethics assessment tool for artificial intelligence implementation in healthcare: CARE-AI. *Nature Medicine*, *1-2*(11), 3038–3039. Advance online publication. DOI: 10.1038/s41591-024-03310-1 PMID: 39424948

Nishat, M. M., Faisal, F., Dip, R. R., Shikder, M. F., Ahsan, R., Asif, M. A. A. R., & Hasan Udoy, M. (2020). Performance Investigation of Different Boosting Algorithms in Predicting Chronic Kidney Disease. *2020 2nd International Conference on Sustainable Technologies for Industry 4.0, STI 2020*. DOI: 10.1109/STI50764.2020.9350440

Nishimiya, K., Yin, B., Piao, Z., Ryu, J., Osman, H., Leung, H. M., & Tearney, G. J. (2019). Micro-optical coherence tomography for endothelial cell visualization in the coronary arteries. *JACC: Cardiovascular Imaging*, *12*(9), 1878–1880.

Nomura, T., Kanda, T., Suzuki, T., & Kato, K. (2008). Prediction of human behavior in human—Robot interaction using psychological scales for anxiety and negative attitudes toward robots. *IEEE Transactions on Robotics*, *24*(2), 442–451. DOI: 10.1109/TRO.2007.914004

North, M. M., North, S. M., & Coble, J. R. (1997a). Virtual reality therapy: An effective treatment for psychological disorders. In Riva, G. (Ed.), *Virtual Reality in Neuro-Psycho-Physiology* (pp. 59–65). Ios Press.

North, M. M., North, S. M., & Coble, J. R. (1997b). Virtual reality therapy for fear of flying. *The American Journal of Psychiatry*, *154*(1), 130. DOI: 10.1176/ajp.154.1.130b PMID: 8988975

Nramban Kannan, S. K., Aseervatham, J., Moholkar, K., Palanimuthu, M., Marappan, S., Narendran, M., Sathar, B., & Sengan, S. (2024). A Model for Predicting Chronic Kidney Diseases Based on Medical Data Using Reinforcement Learning. *SN Computer Science*, *5*(4), 353. Advance online publication. DOI: 10.1007/s42979-024-02665-z

Ntoutsi, E., Fafalios, P., Gadiraju, U., Iosifidis, V., Nejdl, W., Vidal, M. E., Ruggieri, S., Turini, F., Papadopoulos, S., Krasanakis, E., Kompatsiaris, I., Kinder-Kurlanda, K., Wagner, C., Karimi, F., Fernandez, M., Alani, H., Berendt, B., Kruegel, T., Heinze, C., & Staab, S. (2020). Bias in data-driven artificial intelligence systems- An introductory survey. *Wiley Interdisciplinary Reviews. Data Mining and Knowledge Discovery*, *10*(3), 1356. DOI: 10.1002/widm.1356

Nunes, A. (2024). Vertical Integration in Healthcare and Patient Satisfaction: An Exploratory Analysis of Portuguese Reforms. *Sustainability (Basel), 16*(3), 1078. DOI: 10.3390/su16031078

Ogamba, M., Gitonga, J., Muriithi, B., Olukuru, J., & Sevilla, J. (2023). Wellness Buddy: An AI mental health chatbot for Kenyan university students. In *2023 First International Conference on the Advancements of Artificial Intelligence in African Context (AAIAC)* (pp. 1–6). DOI: 10.1109/AAIAC60008.2023.10465291

Ogawa, M., Oyama, G., Morito, K., Kobayashi, M., Yamada, Y., Shinkawa, K., Kamo, H., Hatano, T., & Hattori, N. (2022). Can AI make people happy? The effect of AI-based chatbot on smile and speech in Parkinson's disease. *Parkinsonism & Related Disorders, 99*, 43–46. DOI: 10.1016/j.parkreldis.2022.04.018 PMID: 35596975

Oh, K. J., Lee, D., Ko, B., & Choi, H. J. (2017). A chatbot for psychiatric counseling in mental healthcare service based on emotional dialogue analysis and sentence generation. In *2017 18th IEEE international conference on mobile data management (MDM)* (pp. 371-375). IEEE. DOI: 10.1109/MDM.2017.64

Oh, J., Jang, S., Kim, H., & Kim, J. J. (2020). Efficacy of mobile app-based interactive cognitive behavioral therapy using a chatbot for panic disorder. *International Journal of Medical Informatics, 140*, 104171. DOI: 10.1016/j.ijmedinf.2020.104171 PMID: 32446158

Oktay, B., & Oktay, Y. F. (2018). Bir etik ihlal olarak hasta ve terapist arasındaki cinsel ilişkiler [Sexual relations between patient and therapist as an ethical violation]. *SDU Faculty of Arts And Sciences Journal of Social Sciences, 44*, 103–110.

Olano-Espinosa, E., Avila-Tomas, J. F., Minue-Lorenzo, C., Matilla-Pardo, B., Serrano, M. E. S., Martinez-Suberviola, F. J., & Del Cura-González, I. (2022). Effectiveness of a conversational chatbot (Dejal@ bot) for the adult population to quit smoking: Pragmatic, multicenter, controlled, randomized clinical trial in primary care. *JMIR mHealth and uHealth, 10*(6), e34273. DOI: 10.2196/34273 PMID: 35759328

Omarov, B., Narynov, S., & Zhumanov, Z. (2023). Artificial intelligence-enabled chatbots in mental health: A systematic review. *Computers, Materials & Continua, 74*(3), 5105–5122. DOI: 10.32604/cmc.2023.034655

Ordonez, C. (2006). Association rule discovery with the train and test approach for heart disease prediction. *IEEE Transactions on Information Technology in Biomedicine, 10*(2), 334–343. DOI: 10.1109/TITB.2006.864475 PMID: 16617622

Osvin Nancy, V. A., Prabhavathy, P., & Arya, M. S. (2024). Role of artificial intelligence and deep learning in skin disease prediction: A systematic review and meta-analysis. *Annals of Data Science, 11*(6), 2109–2139. DOI: 10.1007/s40745-023-00503-2

Otapo, A. T., Othmani, A., Khodabandelou, G., & Ming, Z. (2024). Prediction and Detection of Terminal Diseases Using Internet of Medical Things: A Review. *arXiv preprint arXiv:2410.00034.*

Özcan, N. (2025). *Benliğin Dijital Dönüşümü, Yapay Zekâ ve Yalnızlık [Digital Transformation of the Self, Artificial Intelligence and Loneliness].* 5th International Artificial Intelligence And Data Science Congress (Icada 2025) Full Papers And Abstracts, İzmir.

Özcan, A., & Fırat, E. H. (2024). Giyilebilir teknoloji kullanımına dair; fırat üniversitesi çalışanlarının akıllı saat alırken ya da kullanırken risk algılarının ölçülmesi [On the use of wearable technology; measurıng the rısk perceptıons of fırat unıversıty employees when buyıng or usıng smart watches]. *International Journal of Communication and Art, 5*(11), 18–44.

Özdoğan, H. K., & Özdemir, N. K. (2023). 21. yüzyılda kariyer psikolojik danışmanlığı ve yapay zeka uygulamaları [21st century career counseling and artificial intelligence Practices]. *Dokuz Eylül University Buca Faculty of Education Journal,* (57), 2127–2152. DOI: 10.53444/deubefd.1326692

Özgür, N. (2023). *Sohbet botları ve yapay zekâ etiği [Chatbots and artificial intelligence ethics].* [Yüksek lisans bitirme projesi], https://core.ac.uk/download/pdf/586376297.pdf

Özkol, I., Doğan, K., & Köseali, G. (2019). EBYS uygulamalarında yapay zekâ destekli chatbot (sohbet robotu) kullanımı [Artificial intelligence supported chatbot usage in ERMS applications]. In Yalçınkaya, B. (Ed.), Ünal, M. A. (Ed.), Yılmaz, B.(Ed.), Özdemirci, F.(Ed.). *Bilgi Yönetimi ve Bilgi Güvenliği*, 229-250.

Ozsezer, G. (2022). The future of artificial intelligence in nursing. *International Journal of Human Sciences, 19*(2), 285–299. https://orcid.org/0000-0003-4352-1124. DOI: 10.14687/jhs.v19i2.6217

Öztürk, K., & Şahin, M. E. (2018). Yapay sinir ağları ve yapay zekaya genel bir bakış [A general view of artificial neural networks and artificial intelligence]. *Takvim-i Vekayi, 6*(2), 25–36.

Öztürk, M. O., & Uluşahin, N. A. (2015). *Ruh sağlığı ve bozuklukları* [Mental health and disorders]. Nobel Tıp Kitabevi.

Pal, M., Kerorsa, G. B., Marami, L. M., & Kandi, V. (2020). Epidemiology, pathogenicity, animal infections, antibiotic resistance, public health significance, and economic impact of staphylococcus aureus: A comprehensive review. *American Journal of Public Health Research*, *8*(1), 14–21. DOI: 10.12691/ajphr-8-1-3

Panda, K., & Mazumder, A. (2024). *KidneyChain: Leveraging Blockchain & Artificial Intelligence for a Streamlined Organ Donation Solution*. DOI: 10.1101/2024.06.08.24308145

Pant, M., Joshi, N., Vidyarthi, A., & Mohan, L. (2024, September). Heart Disease Prediction and Its Important Parameters Analysis Using Machine Learning. In *2024 International Conference on Distributed Systems, Computer Networks and Cybersecurity (ICDSCNC)* (pp. 1-5). IEEE. DOI: 10.1109/ICDSCNC62492.2024.10939364

Pan, Y., Fu, M., Cheng, B., Tao, X., & Guo, J. (2020). Enhanced deep learning assisted convolutional neural network for heart disease prediction on the internet of medical things platform. *IEEE Access : Practical Innovations, Open Solutions*, *8*, 189503–189512. DOI: 10.1109/ACCESS.2020.3026214

Parimala, G., Kayalvizhi, R., & Nithiya, S. (2022). Mental health: Detection & diagnosis. In *2022 International Conference on Computer Communication and Informatics (ICCCI)* (pp. 1–6).

Paris, J. (2015). *Personality disorders over time: Precursors, course, and outcome*. American Psychiatric Publishing.

Park, T., Gu, P., Kim, C. H., Kim, K. T., Chung, K. J., Kim, T. B., Jung, H., Yoon, S. J., & Oh, J. K. (2023). Artificial intelligence in urologic oncology: The actual clinical practice results of IBM Watson for Oncology in South Korea. *Prostate International*, *11*(4), 218–221. DOI: 10.1016/j.prnil.2023.09.001 PMID: 38196551

Paro, M. R., Lambert, W. A., Leclair, N. K., Chakraborty, A. R., Angelo, S., Pesante, B., Stoltz, P., Martin, J. E., Bookland, M. J., & Hersh, D. S. (2022). Family-acquired photographs for the evaluation of pediatric head shape via telemedicine: An analysis of photograph quality. *Neurosurgical Focus*, *52*(6), E11. DOI: 10.3171/2022.3.FOCUS2235 PMID: 35921182

Parsons, T. D., & Rizzo, A. A. (2008). Affective outcomes of virtual reality exposure therapy for anxiety and specific phobias: A meta-analysis. *Journal of Behavior Therapy and Experimental Psychiatry*, *39*(3), 250–261. DOI: 10.1016/j.jbtep.2007.07.007 PMID: 17720136

Patton, J., Dawe, G., Scharver, C., Mussa-Ivaldi, F., & Kenyon, R. (2006). Robotics and virtual reality: A perfect marriage for motor control research and rehabilitation. *Assistive Technology*, *18*(2), 181–195. DOI: 10.1080/10400435.2006.10131917 PMID: 17236477

Pendlebury, G. A., Roman, J., Shrivastava, V., & Yuan, J. (2022). A call to action: Evidence for the military integration of teledermoscopy in a pandemic era. *Dermatopathology (Basel, Switzerland)*, *9*(4), 327–342. DOI: 10.3390/dermatopathology9040039 PMID: 36278540

Persad, E., Jost, K., Honoré, A., Forsberg, D., Coste, K., Olsson, H., Rautiainen, S., & Herlenius, E. (2021). Neonatal sepsis prediction through clinical decision support algorithms: A systematic review. *Acta Paediatrica (Oslo, Norway)*, *110*(12), 3201–3226. DOI: 10.1111/apa.16083 PMID: 34432903

Peuters, C., Maenhout, L., Cardon, G., De Paepe, A., DeSmet, A., Lauwerier, E., Leta, K., & Crombez, G. (2024). A mobile healthy lifestyle intervention to promote mental health in adolescence: A mixed-methods evaluation. *BMC Public Health*, *24*(1), 44. DOI: 10.1186/s12889-023-17260-9 PMID: 38166797

Pine, D. S., Grun, J., Maguire, E. A., Burgess, N., Zarahn, E., Koda, V., Fyer, A., Szeszko, P. R., & Bilder, R. M. (2002). Neurodevelopmental aspects of spatial navigation: A virtual reality fMRI study. *NeuroImage*, *15*(2), 396–406. DOI: 10.1006/nimg.2001.0988 PMID: 11798274

Pinnamaneni, N., & Funderburgh, J. L. (2012). Concise review: Stem cells in the corneal stroma. *Stem Cells (Dayton, Ohio)*, *30*(6), 1059–1063.

Ponthier, L., Ensuque, P., Destere, A., Marquet, P., Labriffe, M., Jacqz-Aigrain, E., & Woillard, J. B. (2022). Optimization of vancomycin initial dose in term and preterm neonates by machine learning. *Pharmaceutical Research*, *39*(10), 2497–2506. DOI: 10.1007/s11095-022-03351-6 PMID: 35918452

Poongodi, J., Kavitha, K., Sathish, S., & Lakshmana Kumar, R. (2025). Hybrid AI-Driven Bio-Inspired Wearable Sensors With Aquasense AI Technology for Multi-modal Health Monitoring and Rehabilitation in Dynamic Environments. *Transactions on Emerging Telecommunications Technologies*, *36*(3), e70081. DOI: 10.1002/ett.70081

Possati, L. M. (2023). Psychoanalyzing artificial intelligence: The case of Replika. *AI & Society*, *38*(4), 1725–1738. DOI: 10.1007/s00146-021-01379-7

Praveen, R., Hemavathi, U., Sathya, R., Abubakkar Siddiq, A., Gokul Sanjay, M., & Gowdish, S. (2024). AI Powered Plant Identification and Plant Disease Classification System. *2024 4th International Conference on Sustainable Expert Systems (ICSES)*, 1610–1616. DOI: 10.1109/ICSES63445.2024.10763167

Praveen, S. V., & Vajrobol, V. (2023). Understanding the Perceptions of Healthcare Researchers Regarding ChatGPT: A Study Based on Bidirectional Encoder Representation from Transformers (BERT) Sentiment Analysis and Topic Modeling. *Annals of Biomedical Engineering*, *51*(8), 1654–1656. DOI: 10.1007/s10439-023-03222-0 PMID: 37129780

Prochaska, J. J., Vogel, E. A., Chieng, A., Kendra, M., Baiocchi, M., Pajarito, S., & Robinson, A. (2021). A therapeutic relational agent for reducing problematic substance use (Woebot): Development and usability study. *Journal of Medical Internet Research*, *23*(3), e24850. DOI: 10.2196/24850 PMID: 33755028

Pulakhandam, W., Rao, V. V., Samudrala, V. K., & Hemnath, R. (2025). Edge AI-Powered Chronic Kidney Disease Prediction: Integrating Dynamic CNN-LSTM Networks and Neuro-Fuzzy Models for Advanced Diagnosis and Monitoring in IoMT-Enabled Healthcare Systems. *International Journal of Engineering Research and Science & Technology*, *21*(1), 115–128.

Puri, V., Priyadarshini, I., Kataria, A., Rani, S., & Min, H. (2025). Privacy-First ML for Chronic Kidney Disease Prediction: Exploring a Decentralized Approach Using Blockchain and IPFS. *IEEE Access : Practical Innovations, Open Solutions*, *13*, 43178–43189. DOI: 10.1109/ACCESS.2025.3548645

Quon, S., Ahani, S., Holsti, L., Lavoie, P. M., & Dumont, G. (2021). Video-Based Respiratory Rate Estimation for Infants in Low Resource Settings. https://doi.org/ DOI: 10.14288/1.0406240

Rabbani, H., Kafieh, R., Kazemian Jahromi, M., Jorjandi, S., Mehri Dehnavi, A., Hajizadeh, F., & Peyman, A. (2016). Obtaining thickness maps of corneal layers using the optimal algorithm for intracorneal layer segmentation. *International Journal of Biomedical Imaging*, *2016*(1), 1420230.

Rabbi, M., Philyaw-Kotov, M., Lee, J., Mansour, A., Dent, L., Wang, X., & Murphy, S. (2017, September). SARA: a mobile app to engage users in health data collection. In *Proceedings of the 2017 ACM International Joint Conference on Pervasive and Ubiquitous Computing and Proceedings of the 2017 ACM International Symposium on Wearable Computers* (pp. 781-789). DOI: 10.1145/3123024.3125611

Rabinowitz, Y. S. (1998). Keratoconus. *Survey of Ophthalmology*, *42*(4), 297–319.

Racine, N., Chow, C., Hamwi, L., Bucsea, O., Cheng, C., Du, H., Fabrizi, L., Jasim, S., Johannsson, L., Jones, L., Laudiano-Dray, M. P., Meek, J., Mistry, N., Shah, V., Stedman, I., Wang, X., & Riddell, R. P. (2024). Health care professionals' and parents' perspectives on the use of AI for pain monitoring in the neonatal intensive care unit: Multisite qualitative study. *JMIR AI, 3*, e51535. DOI: 10.2196/51535 PMID: 38875686

Rahman, E., Sadeghi-Esfahlani, S., Rao, P., Garcia, P., Ioannidis, S., Nosta, J., Rahman, Z., & Webb, W. R. (2025). Skin, scalpel and the silicon chip: A systematic review on the accuracy, bias and data governance of artificial intelligence in dermatology, minimally invasive aesthetics, aesthetic, plastic and reconstructive surgery. *European Journal of Plastic Surgery*, *48*(1), 17. Advance online publication. DOI: 10.1007/s00238-025-02278-6

Rajkhowa, P., Dsouza, V. S., Kharel, R., Cauvery, K., Mallya, B. R., Raksha, D. S., Mrinalini, V., Sharma, P., Pattanshetty, S., Narayanan, P., Lahariya, C., & Brand, H. (2023). Factors Influencing Monkeypox Vaccination: A Cue to Policy Implementation. *Journal of Epidemiology and Global Health*, *13*(2), 226–238. DOI: 10.1007/s44197-023-00100-9 PMID: 37119512

Rajpurkar, P., Chen, E., Banerjee, O., & Topol, E. J. (2022). AI in health and medicine. *Nature Medicine*, *28*(1), 31–38. DOI: 10.1038/s41591-021-01614-0 PMID: 35058619

Rallis, D., Baltogianni, M., Kapetaniou, K., & Giapros, V. (2024). Current Applications of Artificial Intelligence in the Neonatal Intensive Care Unit. *BioMedInformatics*, *4*(2), 1225–1248. DOI: 10.3390/biomedinformatics4020067

Ramasamy, L. K., Khan, F., Joghee, S., Dempere, J., & Garg, P. (2024). Forecast of students' mental health combining an artificial intelligence technique and fuzzy inference system. In *2024 International Conference on Automation and Computation (AUTOCOM)* (pp. 85–90). DOI: 10.1109/AUTOCOM60220.2024.10486194

Rathenau, S., Sousa, D., Vaz, A., & Geller, S. (2021). The effect of attitudes toward online therapy and the difficulties perceived in online therapeutic presence. *Journal of Psychotherapy Integration*. Advance online publication. DOI: 10.1037/int0000266

Ravirahul, B. M., Balaji, V. R., Balaji, K. R., Gowtham, S., & Surya, S. (2021). Mind wave controlled assistive robot. In *2021 7th International Conference on Advanced Computing and Communication Systems (ICACCS)* (Vol. 1, pp. 1507-1509). IEEE DOI: 10.1109/ICACCS51430.2021.9441684

Ray, A., Bhardwaj, A., Malik, Y. K., Singh, S., & Gupta, R. (2022). Artificial intelligence and Psychiatry: An overview. *Asian Journal of Psychiatry*, *70*, 103021. DOI: 10.1016/j.ajp.2022.103021 PMID: 35219978

Reed, M., Huang, J., Graetz, I., Muelly, E., Millman, A., & Lee, C. (2021). Treatment and follow-up care associated with patient-scheduled primary care telemedicine and in-person visits in a large integrated health system. *JAMA Network Open*, *4*(11), e2132793–e2132793. DOI: 10.1001/jamanetworkopen.2021.32793 PMID: 34783828

Rezk, N. G., Alshathri, S., Sayed, A., & Hemdan, E. E.-D. (2025). Explainable AI for Chronic Kidney Disease Prediction in Medical IoT: Integrating GANs and Few-Shot Learning. *Bioengineering (Basel, Switzerland)*, *12*(4), 356. DOI: 10.3390/bioengineering12040356 PMID: 40281716

Ricciardi, C., Edmunds, K. J., Recenti, M., Sigurdsson, S., Gudnason, V., Carraro, U., & Gargiulo, P. (2020). Assessing cardiovascular risks from a mid-thigh CT image: A tree-based machine learning approach using radiodensitometric distributions. *Scientific Reports*, *10*(1), 2863. DOI: 10.1038/s41598-020-59873-9 PMID: 32071412

Rich, C., Ponsler, B., Holroyd, A., & Sidner, C. L. (2010). Recognizing engagement in human-robot interaction. In *2010 5th ACM/IEEE International Conference on Human-Robot Interaction (HRI) (pp. 375-382)*. IEEE.

Richards, D., & Viganó, N. (2013). Online counseling: A narrative and critical review of the literature. *Journal of Clinical Psychology*, *69*(9), 994–1011. DOI: 10.1002/jclp.21974 PMID: 23630010

Rigby, M., Magrabi, F., Scott, P., Doupi, P., Hypponen, H., & Ammenwerth, E. (2016). Steps in moving evidence-based health informatics from theory to practice. *Healthcare Informatics Research*, *22*(4), 255–260. DOI: 10.4258/hir.2016.22.4.255 PMID: 27895956

Rio-Cristobal, A., & Martin, R. (2014). Corneal assessment technologies: Current status. *Survey of Ophthalmology*, *59*(6), 599–614.

Riva, G., Di Lernia, D., & Sajno, E. (2021). Virtual reality therapy in the metaverse: Merging VR for the outside with VR for the inside. *Annual Review of Cybertherapy and Telemedicine*, *19*, 3–8.

Robert, N. (2019). How artificial intelligence is changing nursing. *Nursing Management*, *50*(9), 30–39. DOI: 10.1097/01.NUMA.0000578988.56622.21 PMID: 31425440

Romano, D. M. (2005). Virtual reality therapy. *Developmental Medicine and Child Neurology, 47*(9), 580–580. DOI: 10.1111/j.1469-8749.2005.tb01206.x PMID: 16138662

Ronneberger, O., Fischer, P., & Brox, T. (2015, October). U-net: Convolutional networks for biomedical image segmentation. In *International Conference on Medical image computing and computer-assisted intervention* (pp. 234-241). Cham: Springer international publishing.

Roscigno, G., Quintavalle, C., Biondi-Zoccai, G., De Micco, F., Frati, G., Affinito, A., Nuzzo, S., Condorelli, G., & Briguori, C. (2021). Urinary Dickkopf-3 and Contrast-Associated Kidney Damage. *Journal of the American College of Cardiology, 77*(21), 2667–2676. Advance online publication. DOI: 10.1016/j.jacc.2021.03.330 PMID: 34045024

Rossin, G., Zorzi, F., Ongaro, L., Piasentin, A., Vedovo, F., Liguori, G., Zucchi, A., Simonato, A., Bartoletti, R., Trombetta, C., Pavan, N., & Claps, F. (2023). Artificial Intelligence in Bladder Cancer Diagnosis: Current Applications and Future Perspectives. *BioMedInformatics, 3*(1), 104–114. DOI: 10.3390/biomedinformatics3010008

Roy, M., & Protity, A. T. (2022). Hair and scalp disease detection using machine learning and image processing. *arXiv preprint arXiv:2301.00122.*

Roy, A. G., Conjeti, S., Karri, S. P. K., Sheet, D., Katouzian, A., Wachinger, C., & Navab, N. (2017). ReLayNet: Retinal layer and fluid segmentation of macular optical coherence tomography using fully convolutional networks. *Biomedical Optics Express, 8*(8), 3627–3642.

Ruiz-Núñez, C., Herrera-Peco, I., Campos-Soler, S. M., Carmona-Pestaña, A., Gracia, E. B., Deudero, J. J. P., & García-Notario, A. I. (2023). Sentiment Analysis on Twitter: Role of Healthcare Professionals in the Global Conversation during the AstraZeneca Vaccine Suspension. *International Journal of Environmental Research and Public Health, 20*(3), 2225. DOI: 10.3390/ijerph20032225 PMID: 36767591

Safıya, P. A., & Saleena, B. (2024). Designing a hybrid stack ensemble model to enhance sepsis classification using data triangulation approach. *Results in Engineering, 103748.* Advance online publication. DOI: 10.1016/j.rineng.2024.103748

Sah, R., Titiyal, J. S., & Sharma, N. (2022). Treatment & Management of Keratoconus: New Clinical Pathways. *Ophthalmology and Vision Care, 2*(2).

Saha, S., Pagnozzi, A., Bourgeat, P., George, J. M., Bradford, D., Colditz, P. B., Boyd, R. N., Rose, S. E., Jurgen Fripp, J., & Pannek, K. (2020). Predicting motor outcome in preterm infants from very early brain diffusion MRI using a deep learning convolutional neural network (CNN) model. *NeuroImage*, *215*, 116807. DOI: 10.1016/j.neuroimage.2020.116807 PMID: 32278897

Şahin, A. R., Doğan, K., & Sivri, S. (2020). *Sağlık Bilimlerinde Yapay Zeka* [Artificial Intelligence in Health Sciences]. Akademisyen Kitabevi. DOI: 10.37609/akya.786

Şahin, M. (2024). Afetlerde krize müdahale: Kahramanmaraş Depremi'nde aile ve sosyal hizmetler bakanlığının çalışmaları [Crisis intervention in disasters: the work of the ministry of family and social services in the Kahramanmaraş Earthquake]. *International Journal of Social Work Research*, *4*(2), 17–50. DOI: 10.57114/jswrpub.1257945

Sahoo, S., Sachdeva, D., Yumnam, S., Shah, R., Mehra, A., & Grover, S. (2022). Play Therapy via Telemedicine in a Child with Sudden-onset Emotional Disorder During the COVID-19 Lockdown Period: A Case Report. *Innovations in Clinical Neuroscience*, *19*(10-12), 40. PMID: 36591545

Salamanca-Sanabria, A., Richards, D., & Timulak, L. (2019). Adapting an internet-delivered intervention for depression for a Colombian college student population: An illustration of an integrative empirical approach. *Internet Interventions : the Application of Information Technology in Mental and Behavioural Health*, *15*, 76–86. DOI: 10.1016/j.invent.2018.11.005 PMID: 30740313

Saleem, M., & Afzal, H. (2024). A review of mental health analysis through social media using machine learning and deep learning approaches. In *2024 International Conference on Engineering & Computing Technologies (ICECT)* (pp. 1–7). DOI: 10.1109/ICECT61618.2024.10581373

Salekin, M. S., Mouton, P. R., Zamzmi, G., Patel, R., Goldgof, D., Kneusel, M., Elkins, S. L., Murray, E., Coughlin, M. E., Maguire, D., Ho, T., & Sun, Y. (2021). Future roles of artificial intelligence in early pain management of newborns. *Paediatric and Neonatal Pain*, *3*(3), 134–145. DOI: 10.1002/pne2.12060 PMID: 35547946

Salinas, M. P., Sepúlveda, J., Hidalgo, L., Peirano, D., Morel, M., Uribe, P., Rotemberg, V., Briones, J., Mery, D., & Navarrete-Dechent, C. (2024). A systematic review and meta-analysis of artificial intelligence versus clinicians for skin cancer diagnosis. *NPJ Digital Medicine*, *7*(1), 62. Advance online publication. DOI: 10.1038/s41746-024-01103-x PMID: 38454007

Salvi, M., Acharya, U. R., Molinari, F., & Meiburger, K. M. (2021). The impact of pre-and post-image processing techniques on deep learning frameworks: A comprehensive review for digital pathology image analysis. *Computers in Biology and Medicine, 128,* 104129. DOI: 10.1016/j.compbiomed.2020.104129 PMID: 33254082

Sampath, S., Prasad, M. L., Hussain, M. M., Parameswari, R., Anil Kumar, D., & Reddy, P. C. S. (2023). Ensemble Nonlinear Machine Learning Model for Chronic Kidney Diseases Prediction. *2023 IEEE 3rd Mysore Sub Section International Conference (MysuruCon)*, 1–6. DOI: 10.1109/MysuruCon59703.2023.10397049

Sanchez-Vives, M. V., & Slater, M. (2005). From presence to consciousness through virtual reality. *Nature Reviews. Neuroscience, 6*(4), 332–339. DOI: 10.1038/nrn1651 PMID: 15803164

Sangeetha, S., Suganya, P., Shanthini, S., Murthy, G. N. K., & Sathya, R. (2023). Crime Rate Prediction and Prevention: Unleashing the Power of Deep Learning. *Proceedings of the 4th International Conference on Smart Electronics and Communication, ICOSEC 2023.* DOI: 10.1109/ICOSEC58147.2023.10276012

Santos, V. A. D., Schmetterer, L., Stegmann, H., Pfister, M., Messner, A., Schmidinger, G., & Werkmeister, R. M. (2019). CorneaNet: Fast segmentation of cornea OCT scans of healthy and keratoconic eyes using deep learning. *Biomedical Optics Express, 10*(2), 622–641.

Sapkota, R. P., Valli, E., Dear, B. F., Titov, N., & Hadjistavropoulos, H. D. (2024). Satisfaction, engagement, and outcomes in internet-delivered cognitive behaviour therapy adapted for people of diverse ethnocultural groups: An observational trial with benchmarking. *Frontiers in Psychiatry, 15,* 1270543. DOI: 10.3389/fpsyt.2024.1270543 PMID: 38501087

Saraiva, M., Alfaiate, C., Gomes, L. P., Correia, A. R., & Jorge, F. (2023). The Perception of quality and the performance in primary health Care of central Alentejo–Portugal. *Cogent Business & Management, 10*(1), 2208423. DOI: 10.1080/23311975.2023.2208423

Saranya, S. S., Anusha, P., Chandragandhi, S., Kishore, O. K., Kumar, N. P., & Srihari, K. (2024). Enhanced decision-making in healthcare cloud-edge networks using deep reinforcement and lion optimization algorithm. *Biomedical Signal Processing and Control, 92,* 105963. DOI: 10.1186/s40635-024-00614-x

Sarıkaya Karabudak, S., & Ergün, S. (2018). Neonatal diseases and nursing care. In Conk, Z., Başbakkal, Z., Yılmaz, H. B., & Bolışık, B. (Eds.), *Pediatric Nursing, 2.*

Savaş, B. Ç. (2024). Yapay zekâya bağımlılık ölçeğinin Türkçe'ye uyarlanması: Geçerlik ve güvenirlik çalışması [Adaptation of the Dependence to Artificial Intelligence Scale into Turkish: Validity and Reliability Study]. *Journal of Sport and Recreation for All*, *6*(3), 306–315. DOI: 10.56639/jsar.1509301

Saxena, S., Saxena, S., Tahilramani, N., & Charanarur, P. (2025). Blockchain enhanced smart healthcare management for chronic diseases. *Discover Computing*, *28*(1), 112. DOI: 10.1007/s10791-025-09574-6

Sayar, K. (2011). *Terapi kültürel bir eleştiri* [Therapy is a cultural criticism]. Timaş Yayınları.

Schellack, N., Strydom, M., Pepper, M. S., Herd, C. L., Hendricks, C. L., Bronkhorst, E., Meyer, J. C., Padayachee, N., Bangalee, V., Truter, I., Ellero, A. A., Myaka, T., Naidoo, E., & Godman, B. (2022). Social Media and COVID-19—Perceptions and Public Deceptions of Ivermectin, Colchicine and Hydroxychloroquine: Lessons for Future Pandemics. *Antibiotics (Basel, Switzerland)*, *11*(4), 445. DOI: 10.3390/antibiotics11040445 PMID: 35453198

Scholten, M. R., Kelders, S. M., & Van Gemert-Pijnen, J. E. (2017). Self-guided web-based interventions: Scoping review on user needs and the potential of embodied conversational agents to address them. *Journal of Medical Internet Research*, *19*(11), e383. DOI: 10.2196/jmir.7351 PMID: 29146567

Schouten, J. S., Kalden, M. A., van Twist, E., Reiss, I. K., Gommers, D. A., van Genderen, M. E., & Taal, H. R. (2024). From bytes to bedside: A systematic review on the use and readiness of artificial intelligence in the neonatal and pediatric intensive care unit. *Intensive Care Medicine*, *50*(11), 1767–1777. DOI: 10.1007/s00134-024-07629-8 PMID: 39264415

Schulze, N., Reuter, S. C., Kuchler, I., Reinke, B., Hinkelmann, L., Stöckigt, S., Siemoneit, H., & Tonn, P. (2019). Differences in attitudes toward online interventions in psychiatry and psychotherapy between health care professionals and nonprofessionals: A survey. *Telemedicine Journal and e-Health*, *25*(10), 926–932. Advance online publication. DOI: 10.1089/tmj.2018.0225 PMID: 30412450

Seitz, B., Behrens, A., & Langenbucher, A. (1997). Corneal topography. *Current Opinion in Ophthalmology*, *8*(4), 8–24.

Seligman, M. E., & Csikszentmihalyi, M. (2000). Positive psychology: An introduction, *American Psychological Association*, 55(1), 5-14. https://doi.org/DOI: 10.1037//0003-066X.55.1.5

Şencan Karakuş, B. (2021). Psikoterapide mobil uygulama kullanımının etik kurallar çerçevesinde ele alınması [Considering the use of mobile application in psychotherapy within the framework of ethics]. *Life Skills Journal of Psychology*, *5*(10), 133–140. DOI: 10.31461/ybpd.1019155

Senthil, G. A., Prabha, R., Latha, K., & Sridevi, S. (2025). A Block Chain-Enabled Novel Intelligent System Analysis for Medical Image Processing of Kidney Stone Prediction Using Deep Learning Techniques and Augmented Reality. In *Blockchain-Enabled Solutions for the Pharmaceutical Industry* (pp. 335–353). Wiley., DOI: 10.1002/9781394287970.ch16

Sergueeva, K., & Shaw, N. (2017). Improving healthcare with wearables: overcoming the barriers to adoption. In *HCI in Business, Government and Organizations. Interacting with Information Systems: 4th International Conference, HCIBGO 2017, Held as Part of HCI International 2017, Vancouver, BC, Canada, July 9-14, 2017, Proceedings, Part I 4* (pp. 209-223). Springer International Publishing. **https://doi .org/**DOI: 10.1007/978-3-319-58481-2_17

Shah, D., Patel, S., & Bharti, S. K. (2020). Heart disease prediction using machine learning techniques. *SN Computer Science*, *1*(6), 345. DOI: 10.1007/s42979-020-00365-y

Shah, L. B. I., Torres, S., Kannusamy, P., Chng, C. M. L., He, H. G., & Klainin-Yobas, P. (2015). Efficacy of the virtual reality-based stress management program on stress-related variables in people with mood disorders: The feasibility study. *Archives of Psychiatric Nursing*, *29*(1), 6–13. DOI: 10.1016/j.apnu.2014.09.003 PMID: 25634868

Shaik, M. A., Sreeja, R., Zainab, S., Sowmya, P. S., Akshay, T., & Sindhu, S. (2023, March). Improving accuracy of heart disease prediction through machine learning algorithms. In *2023 International Conference on Innovative Data Communication Technologies and Application (ICIDCA)* (pp. 41-46). IEEE. DOI: 10.1109/ICIDCA56705.2023.10100244

Shajari, S., Kuruvinashetti, K., Komeili, A., & Sundararaj, U. (2023). The emergence of AI-based wearable sensors for digital health technology: A review. *Sensors (Basel)*, *23*(23), 9498. DOI: 10.3390/s23239498 PMID: 38067871

Shane, A. L., Sánchez, P. J., & Stoll, B. J. (2017). Neonatal sepsis. *Lancet*, *390*(10104), 1770–1780. DOI: 10.1016/S0140-6736(17)31002-4 PMID: 28434651

Sharif, M. S., Raj Theeng Tamang, M., Fu, C. H. Y., Baker, A., Alzahrani, A. I., Alalwan, N. (2023). An Innovative Random-Forest-Based Model to Assess the Health Impacts of Regular Commuting Using Non-Invasive Wearable Sensors. *Sensors* (Basel, Switzerland), 23(6), 3274. 4. https://doi.org/DOI: 10.3390/s23063274

Sharma, S. (2025). Ultra Smart Cyberspace Manufacturing Infrastructure Using Artificial Intelligence-Driven Automated Engineering. In Advances in computational intelligence and robotics book series (pp. 1–40). https://doi.org/DOI: 10.4018/979-8-3373-4839-1.ch001

Sharma, S. (2025a). Next Generation Emerging Technologies of Cloud Computing Driven E-Data Privacy, E-Security, and E-Governance. In IGI Global eBooks (pp. 1–38). https://doi.org/DOI: 10.4018/979-8-3373-2018-2.ch001

Shi, Y., Payeur, P., Frize, M., & Bariciak, E. (2020, June). Thermal and rgb-d imaging for necrotizing enterocolitis detection. In 2020 IEEE International Symposium on Medical Measurements and Applications (MeMeA) (pp. 1-6). IEEE. https://doi.org/DOI: 10.1109/MeMeA49120.2020.9137344

Shin, D., & Park, Y. J. (2019). Role of fairness, accountability, and transparency in algorithmic affordance. *Computers in Human Behavior*, *98*, 277–284. DOI: 10.1016/j.chb.2019.04.019

Shroff, R. (2019). *Artificial Intelligence Explained in Simple Terms*. Retrieved from https://medium.com/mytake/artificial-intelligence-explained-in-simple-englishpart-1-2-1b28c1f762cf

Shruthi, K., & Poornima, A. S. (2023). Medical Data Asset Management and an Approach for Disease Prediction using Blockchain and Machine Learning. *International Journal of Engineering Trends and Technology*, *71*(4), 491–514. Advance online publication. DOI: 10.14445/22315381/IJETT-V71I4P242

Shukla, A. K. (2023). Computer vision and AI-integrated IoT technologies in the medical. *Neural Networks*, *1*, 1–1.

Shyamala Devi, M., Aruna, R., Almufti, S., Punitha, P., & Lakshmana Kumar, R. (2024). Bone feature quantization and systematized attention gate UNet-based deep learning framework for bone fracture classification. *Intelligent Data Analysis*, *29*(2), 513–538. DOI: 10.3233/IDA-240431

Siddals, S., Coxon, A., & Torous, J. (2024). " It just happened to be the perfect thing": Real-life experiences of generative AI chatbots for mental health. *npj Mental Health Res* 3, 48. https://doi.org/DOI: 10.1038/s44184-024-00097-4

Simões, J., & Fronteira, I. (2021). The role of the State, the private sector and the social sector in the different health political cycles in Portugal. *Ciencia & Saude Coletiva*, *26*(suppl 1), 2507–2513. DOI: 10.1590/1413-81232021266.1.40902020 PMID: 34133630

Simon, G., Ren, Q., Kervick, G. N., & Parel, J. M. (1993). Optics of the corneal epithelium. *Journal of Refractive Surgery (Thorofare, N.J.)*, *9*(1), 42–50.

Singh, A., & Kakkar, R. (2025). Optimizing Chronic Kidney Disease Prediction Through Advanced Data Imputation and Clustering. *2025 Fourth International Conference on Smart Technologies, Communication and Robotics (STCR)*, 1–7. DOI: 10.1109/STCR62650.2025.11020378

Singh, O. P. (2019). Chatbots in psychiatry: Can treatment gap be lessened for psychiatric disorders in India. *Indian Journal of Psychiatry*, *61*(3), 225–227. DOI: 10.4103/0019-5545.258323 PMID: 31142896

Singh, P., Nagori, A., Lodha, R., & Sethi, T. (2022). Early prediction of hypothermia in pediatric intensive care units using machine learning. *Frontiers in Physiology*, *13*, 921884. DOI: 10.3389/fphys.2022.921884 PMID: 36171970

Singh, R. B., Koh, S., Sharma, N., Woreta, F. A., Hafezi, F., Dua, H. S., & Jhanji, V. (2024). Keratoconus. *Nature Reviews. Disease Primers*, *10*(1), 81.

Sitaraman, S. R., Alagarsundaram, P., & Kumar, V. (2024). AI-Driven Skin Lesion Detection with CNN and Score-CAM: Enhancing Explainability in IoMT Platforms. *Indo-American Journal of Pharma and Bio Sciences*, *22*(4), 1–13.

Sivaparthipan, C. B., Muthu, B. A., Fathima, G., Kumar, P. M., Alazab, M., & Díaz, V. G. (2022). Blockchain Assisted Disease Identification of COVID-19 Patients with the Help of IDA-DNN Classifier. *Wireless Personal Communications*, *126*(3), 2597–2620. Advance online publication. DOI: 10.1007/s11277-022-09831-7 PMID: 35789579

Skandha, S. S., Agarwal, M., Utkarsh, K., Gupta, S. K., Koppula, V. K., & Suri, J. S. (2022). A novel genetic algorithm-based approach for compression and acceleration of deep learning convolution neural network: An application in computer tomography lung cancer data. *Neural Computing & Applications*, *34*(23), 20915–20937. DOI: 10.1007/s00521-022-07567-w

Solanki, A., Vardhan, A., Jharwal, A., & Kumar, N. (2023, July). Heart Diseases Prediction Using Machine Learning. In *2023 14th International Conference on Computing Communication and Networking Technologies (ICCCNT)* (pp. 1-6). IEEE. DOI: 10.1109/ICCCNT56998.2023.10307839

Solomonides, A. E., Koski, E., Atabaki, S. M., Weinberg, S., McGreevey, J. D.III, Kannry, J. L., Petersen, C., & Lehmann, C. U. (2022). Defining AMIA's artificial intelligence principles. *Journal of the American Medical Informatics Association : JAMIA*, *29*(4), 585–591. DOI: 10.1093/jamia/ocac006 PMID: 35190824

Song, W., Jung, S. Y., Baek, H., Choi, C. W., Jung, Y. H., & Yoo, S. (2020). A predictive model based on machine learning for the early detection of late-onset neonatal sepsis: Development and observational study. *JMIR Medical Informatics*, *8*(7), e15965. DOI: 10.2196/15965 PMID: 32735230

So, R., Emura, N., Okazaki, K., Takeda, S., Sunami, T., Kitagawa, K., Takebayashi, Y., & Furukawa, T. A. (2024). Guided versus unguided chatbot-delivered cognitive behavioral intervention for individuals with moderate-risk and problem gambling: A randomized controlled trial (GAMBOT2 study). *Addictive Behaviors*, *149*, 107889. DOI: 10.1016/j.addbeh.2023.107889 PMID: 37857043

Sorrentino, G., Thekkan, K. R., Genna, C., Aite, L., Ragni, A., Bevilacqua, F., Dall'Oglio, I., Roberti, M., Tiozzo, E., & Gawronski, O. (2025). The implementation and impact of narrative diaries in neonatal intensive care units: A scoping review. *Nursing in Critical Care*, *30*(2), e13281. DOI: 10.1111/nicc.13281 PMID: 40000364

Sree, P. K., Prasad, M., Pbv, R. R., Ramana, C. V., Murty, P. T. S., Mallesh, A. S., & Raju, P. J. R. S. (2023). A comprehensive analysis on risk prediction of heart disease using machine learning models. *International Journal on Recent and Innovation Trends in Computing and Communication*, *11*(11s), 605–610. DOI: 10.17762/ijritcc.v11i11s.8295

Stedman, I., Racine, N., Wang, X., Fitzgerald, M., Fabrizi, L., Jones, L., Shah, V., Cheng, C., & Riddell, R. P. (2023) Artificial Intelligence for NICU Pain Assessment: Ethical, Legal and Social Implications. *Legal and Social Implications*. http://dx.doi.org/DOI: 10.2139/ssrn.4336962

Steele, T. M., Fabinyi, D. C., Couper, T. A., & Loughnan, M. S. (2008). Prevalence of Orbscan II corneal abnormalities in relatives of patients with keratoconus. *Clinical & Experimental Ophthalmology*, *36*(9), 824–830.

Stofle, G. S. (2001). *Choosing an online therapist: A step-by-step guide to finding professional help on the web*. White Hat Communications.

Stoll, J., Müller, J. A., & Trachsel, M. (2020). Ethical issues in online psychotherapy: A narrative review. *Frontiers in Psychiatry*, *10*, 993. DOI: 10.3389/fpsyt.2019.00993 PMID: 32116819

Sturrock, G. D., Sherrard, E. S., & Rice, N. S. (1978). Specular microscopy of the corneal endothelium. *The British Journal of Ophthalmology*, *62*(12), 809–814.

Sucala, M., Schnur, J. B., Brackman, E. H., Constantino, M. J., & Montgomery, G. H. (2013). Clinicians' attitudes toward therapeutic alliance in E-therapy. *The Journal of General Psychology*, *140*(4), 282–293. DOI: 10.1080/00221309.2013.830590 PMID: 24837821

Suiçmez, Ç., Kahraman, H. T., Suiçmez, A., Yılmaz, C., & Balcı, F. (2023). Detection of melanoma with hybrid learning method by removing hair from dermoscopic images using image processing techniques and wavelet transform. *Biomedical Signal Processing and Control*, *84*, 104729. DOI: 10.1016/j.bspc.2023.104729

Sullivan, B. A., Beam, K., Vesoulis, Z. A., Aziz, K. B., Husain, A. N., Knake, L. A., Moreira, A., Hooven, T. A., Weiss, E. M., Carr, N. R., El-Ferzli, G. T., Patel, R. M., Simek, K. A., Hernandez, A. J., Barry, J. S., & McAdams, R. M. (2024). Transforming neonatal care with artificial intelligence: Challenges, ethical consideration, and opportunities. *Journal of Perinatology*, *44*(1), 1–11. DOI: 10.1038/s41372-023-01848-5 PMID: 38097685

Sumathi, M., & Raja, S. P. (2025). Explainable Artificial Intelligence-Based Diseases Diagnosis From Unstructured Clinical Data and Decision Making Using Blockchain Technologies. *International Journal of Interactive Multimedia and Artificial Intelligence, 9*(3), 40. DOI: 10.9781/ijimai.2025.02.003

Sunshine, I. L., Kysh, L., & Lakshmanan, A. (2023). Mobile applications to support parents in the transition from neonatal intensive care unit to home: A narrative review. *mHealth*, *9*, 27. DOI: 10.21037/mhealth-23-10 PMID: 37492120

Supriya, M., & Chattu, V. K. (2021). A review of artificial intelligence, big data, and blockchain technology applications in medicine and global health. In *Big Data and Cognitive Computing* (Vol. 5, Issue 3). DOI: 10.3390/bdcc5030041

Ta-Johnson, V., Boatfeld, C., Wang, X., DeCero, E., Krupica, I., Rasof, S., Motzer, A., & Pedryc, W. (2022). Assessing the topics and motivating factors behind human-social chatbot interactions: Thematic analysis of user experiences. *JMIR Human Factors*, *9*(4), e38876. DOI: 10.2196/38876 PMID: 36190745

Tang, X., Yang, X., Yuan, J., Yang, J., Jin, Q., Zhang, H., Zhao, L., & Guo, W. (2024). Call for Decision Support for Electrocardiographic Alarm Administration Among Neonatal Intensive Care Unit Staff: Multicenter, Cross-Sectional Survey. *Journal of Medical Internet Research*, *26*, e60944. DOI: 10.2196/60944 PMID: 39705688

Tan, H. (2014). *Psikolojik yardım ilişkileri* [*Psychological help relationships*]. Nobel Yayınevi.

Tarricone, F., Brunetti, A., Buongiorno, D., Altini, N., Bevilacqua, V., Del Vecchio, A., & Petrillo, F. (2021). Intelligent neonatal sepsis early diagnosis system for very low birth weight infants. *Applied Sciences (Basel, Switzerland)*, *11*(1), 404. DOI: 10.3390/app11010404

Ta, V., Griffith, C., Boatfield, C., Wang, X., Civitello, M., Bader, H., & Loggarakis, A. (2020). User experiences of social support from companion chatbots in everyday contexts: Thematic analysis. *Journal of Medical Internet Research*, *22*(3), e16235. DOI: 10.2196/16235 PMID: 32141837

Tavares, A. I., & Marques, I. (2021). Multi-layer health insurance coverage, medical services use and health in a Universal National Health System, the case of Portugal. *The European Journal of Health Economics*, *22*(1), 141–153. DOI: 10.1007/s10198-020-01242-4 PMID: 33245457

Thakur, A., Ray, P., Sharma, N., & Jain, S. (2024). Molecular Characteristics of Community-Acquired Methicillin-Resistant Staphylococcus aureus, Hospital-Acquired MRSA Isolates, and PVL in one of the Indian hospitals. *Indian Journal of Microbiology*, •••, 1–11. DOI: 10.1007/s12088-024-01195-9 PMID: 39678950

Thakur, N. (2023). Sentiment analysis and text analysis of the public discourse on Twitter about COVID-19 and MPox. *Big Data and Cognitive Computing*, *7*(2), 116. DOI: 10.3390/bdcc7020116

Thamil Selvi, C. P., Vinoth Kumar, S., Rajab Asaad, R., Punitha, P., & Lakshmana Kumar, R. (2024). An integrative framework for brain tumor segmentation and classification using NeuraClassNet. *Intelligent Data Analysis*, *29*(2), 435–458. DOI: 10.3233/IDA-230112

Thunström, A. O., Carlsen, H. K., Ali, L., Larson, T., Hellström, A., & Steingrimsson, S. (2024). Usability Comparison Among Healthy Participants of an Anthropomorphic Digital Human and a Text-Based Chatbot as a Responder to Questions on Mental Health: Randomized Controlled Trial. *JMIR Human Factors*, *11*(1), e54581. DOI: 10.2196/54581 PMID: 38683664

Topçu, S. Y., Semerci, R., Kostak, M. A., Güray, Ö., Sert, S., & Yavuz, G. (2023). The effect of an interactive robot on children's post-operative anxiety, mobilization, and parents' satisfaction; randomized controlled study. *Journal of Pediatric Nursing*, *68*, e50–e57. DOI: 10.1016/j.pedn.2022.11.009 PMID: 36437131

Torab-Miandoab, A., Samad-Soltani, T., Jodati, A., & Rezaei-Hachesu, P. (2023). Interoperability of heterogeneous health information systems: A systematic literature review. *BMC Medical Informatics and Decision Making*, *23*(1), 18. DOI: 10.1186/s12911-023-02115-5 PMID: 36694161

Tuft, S. J., & Coster, D. J. (1990). The corneal endothelium. *Eye*, *4*(3), 389–424. https://www.oscarwylee.com.au/glasses/eye/cornea

Ugucu, G., Celebioglu, A., & Isbir, G. G. (2024). Supporting the neurodevelopment of premature infants in the neonatal intensive care unit: Creating a healing environment. *Adnan Menderes University Journal of Faculty of Health Sciences*, *8*(2), 192–208. DOI: 10.46237/amusbfd.1278780

UlHussna., I. I., Trisha, I., Ritun, I. J., & Alam, M. G. R. (2021). COVID-19 impact on students' mental health: Explainable AI and classifiers. In *2021 International Conference on Decision Aid Sciences and Application (DASA)* (pp. 847–851).

Ulrich, S., Gantenbein, A. R., Zuber, V., Von Wyl, A., Kowatsch, T., & Künzli, H. (2024). Development and evaluation of a smartphone-based chatbot coach to facilitate a balanced lifestyle in individuals with headaches (BalanceUP App): Randomized controlled trial. *Journal of Medical Internet Research*, *26*, e50132. DOI: 10.2196/50132 PMID: 38265863

Unal, A. S., & Avci, A. (2024). Artificial intelligence in pediatric nursing. Mediterranean. *Journal of Nursing (Luton, England)*, *3*(1), 36–43. DOI: 10.59398/ahd.1346089

United Nations Children's Fund. (2021). Policy guidance on AI for children 2.0. UNICEF. https://www.unicef.org/innocenti/reports/policy-guidance-ai-children

United Nations General Assembly. (2015). Transforming our world: The 2030 agenda for sustainable development (Resolution 70/1). https://sdgs.un.org/goals

Urban, G., Feil, N., Csuka, E., Hashemi, K., Ekelem, C., Choi, F., Mesinkovska, N. A., & Baldi, P. (2021). Combining deep learning with optical coherence tomography imaging to determine scalp hair and follicle counts. *Lasers in Surgery and Medicine*, *53*(1), 171–178. DOI: 10.1002/lsm.23324 PMID: 32960994

Usman, M., Mujahid, M., Rustam, F., Flores, E., Mazón, J. L. V., Díez, I. T., & Ashraf, I. (2024). Analyzing patients satisfaction level for medical services using twitter data. *PeerJ. Computer Science*, *10*, e1697. DOI: 10.7717/peerj-cs.1697 PMID: 38259896

Üzümcü, E., Akın, B., Nergiz, H., Inözü, M., & Çelikcan, U. (2018). Anksiyete bozukluklarında sanal gerçeklik [Virtual Reality for Anxiety Disorders]. *Psikiyatride Güncel Yaklasimlar*, *10*(1), 99–117. DOI: 10.18863/pgy.336593

Vahia, I. V., Ng, B., Camacho, A., Cardenas, V., Cherner, M., Depp, C. A., Palmer, B. W., Jeste, D. P., & Agha, Z. (2015). Telepsychiatry for neurocognitive testing in older rural Latino adults. *The American Journal of Geriatric Psychiatry*, *23*(7), 666–670. DOI: 10.1016/j.jagp.2014.08.006 PMID: 25708655

Vaidyam, A., Wisniewski, H., Halamka, J., Kashavan, M., & Torous, J. (2019). Chatbots and conversational agents in mental health: A review of the psychiatric landscape. *Canadian Journal of Psychiatry*, *64*(7), 456–464. DOI: 10.1177/0706743719828977 PMID: 30897957

Valmaggia, L. R., Latif, L., Kempton, M. J., & Rus-Calafell, M. (2016). Virtual reality in the psychological treatment for mental health problems: An systematic review of recent evidence. *Psychiatry Research*, *236*, 189–195. DOI: 10.1016/j.psychres.2016.01.015 PMID: 26795129

van Assen, M., Lee, S. J., & De Cecco, C. N. (2020). Artificial intelligence from A to Z: From neural network to legal framework. *European Journal of Radiology*, *129*, 109083. DOI: 10.1016/j.ejrad.2020.109083 PMID: 32526670

van der Wijst, J., Belge, H., Bindels, R. J. M., & Devuyst, O. (2019). Learning Physiology from Inherited Kidney Disorders. *Physiological Reviews*, *99*(3), 1575–1653. DOI: 10.1152/physrev.00008.2018 PMID: 31215303

van Loenen, I., Scholten, W., Muntingh, A., Smit, J., & Batelaan, N. (2022). The effectiveness of virtual reality exposure–based cognitive behavioral therapy for severe anxiety disorders, obsessive-compulsive disorder, and posttraumatic stress disorder: Meta-analysis. *Journal of Medical Internet Research*, *24*(2), e26736. DOI: 10.2196/26736 PMID: 35142632

Van Rossum, G. (2007, June). Python programming language. In *USENIX annual technical conference* (Vol. 41, No. 1, pp. 1-36).

Varanda, J., Gonçalves, L., & Craveiro, I. (2020). The unlikely Saviour: Portugal's national health system and the initial impact of the Covid-19 pandemic? [Society for International Development]. *Development*, *63*(2-4), 291–297. DOI: 10.1057/s41301-020-00268-8 PMID: 33288975

Venkatasubramanian, K., Ranalli, T. M., Kirupaharan, P., Solanki, D., & Mankodiya, K. (2023). Understanding the challenges nurses encounter with monitoring technologies in a NICU. *International Journal of Human-Computer Interaction*, *40*(23), 8142–8165. DOI: 10.1080/10447318.2023.2278297

Vereschagin, M., Wang, A. Y., Richardson, C. G., Xie, H., Munthali, R. J., Hudec, K. L., Leung, C., Wojcik, K. D., Munro, L., Halli, P., Kessler, R. C., & Vigo, D. V. (2024). Effectiveness of the Minder mobile mental health and substance use intervention for university students: Randomized controlled trial. *Journal of Medical Internet Research*, *26*, e54287. DOI: 10.2196/54287 PMID: 38536225

Vieira, S., Pinaya, W. H., & Mechelli, A. (2017). Using deep learning to investigate the neuroimaging correlates of psychiatric and neurological disorders: Methods and applications. *Neuroscience and Biobehavioral Reviews*, *74*, 58–75. DOI: 10.1016/j.neubiorev.2017.01.002 PMID: 28087243

Vimala, B. B., Srinivasan, S., Mathivanan, S. K., Muthukumaran, V., Babu, J. C., Herencsar, N., & Vilcekova, L. (2023). Image noise removal in ultrasound breast images based on a hybrid deep learning technique. *Sensors (Basel)*, *23*(3), 1167. DOI: 10.3390/s23031167 PMID: 36772207

Visin, F., Ciccone, M., Romero, A., Kastner, K., Cho, K., Bengio, Y., & Courville, A. (2016). Reseg: A recurrent neural network-based model for semantic segmentation. In *Proceedings of the IEEE conference on computer vision and pattern recognition workshops* (pp. 41-48).

Voinescu, A., Petrini, K., Stanton Fraser, D., Lazarovicz, R. A., Papavă, I., Fodor, L. A., & David, D. (2023). The effectiveness of a virtual reality attention task to predict depression and anxiety in comparison with current clinical measures. *Virtual Reality (Waltham Cross)*, *27*(1), 119–140. DOI: 10.1007/s10055-021-00520-7

Wang, Y., Xiong, M., & Olya, H. (2020) Toward an understanding of responsible artificial intelligence practices. In: Bui, T.X., (ed.) Proceedings of the 53rd Hawaii International Conference on System Sciences. Hawaii International Conference on System Sciences (HICSS 2020), 07-10 Jan 2020, Maui, Hawaii, USA. Hawaii International Conference on System Sciences (HICSS), s. 4962-4971. DOI: 10.24251/HICSS.2020.610

Wang, L. Y., Wang, L. Y., Sung, M. I., Lin, I. C., Liu, C. F., & Chen, C. J. (2024). Implementing Explainable Machine Learning Models for Practical Prediction of Early Neonatal Hypoglycemia. *Diagnostics (Basel)*, *14*(14), 1571. DOI: 10.3390/diagnostics14141571 PMID: 39061708

Wang, M. (2024). *Corneal Topography: A Guide for Clinical Application in Wavefront Era*. CRC Press.

Weiss, S. L., Fitzgerald, J. C., Balamuth, F., Alpern, E. R., Lavelle, J., Chilutti, M., Grundmeier, R., Nadkarni, V., & Thomas, N. J. (2014). Delayed antimicrobial therapy increases mortality and organ dysfunction duration in pediatric sepsis. *Critical Care Medicine*, *42*(11), 2409–2417. DOI: 10.1097/CCM.0000000000000509 PMID: 25148597

Wei, Y., Xiao, H., Shi, H., Jie, Z., Feng, J., & Huang, T. S. (2018). Revisiting dilated convolution: A simple approach for weakly-and semi-supervised semantic segmentation. In *Proceedings of the IEEE conference on computer vision and pattern recognition* (pp. 7268-7277).

Weizenbaum, J. (1966). ELIZA—A computer program for the study of natural language communication between man and machine. *Communications of the ACM*, *9*(1), 36–45. DOI: 10.1145/365153.365168

WHO (2007). *Assessment of Osteoporosis at the Primary Health Care Level: Technical Report.*

WHO. (2022) Strengthening Mental Health Promotion (Fact sheet). Geneva, World Health Organization https://www.who.int/news-room/fact sheets/detail/mental-health-strengthening-our-response (Accessed 17.03.2025)

WHO. (World Health Organization). (2022). SDG Target 3.2: End preventable deaths of newborns and children under 5 years of age in 2021. https://www.who.int/data/gho/data/themes/theme-details/GHO/child-health

Wilson, S. E., & Hong, J. W. (2000). Bowman's layer structure and function: Critical or dispensable to corneal function? A hypothesis. *Cornea*, *19*(4), 417–420.

World Health Organization (WHO). (2024). https://www.who.int/news/item/18-01-2024-who-releases-ai-ethics-and-governance-guidance-for-large-multi-modal-models (Retrieved: 15.07.2025)

Wu, E., Hadjiiski, L. M., Samala, R. K., Chan, H. P., Cha, K. H., Richter, C., Cohan, R. H., Caoili, E. M., Paramagul, C., Alva, A., & Weizer, A. Z. (2019). Deep Learning Approach for Assessment of Bladder Cancer Treatment Response. *Tomography : a Journal for Imaging Research*, *5*(1), 201–208. DOI: 10.18383/j.tom.2018.00036 PMID: 30854458

Wu, Q., Xu, G., Wei, F., Kuang, J., Qin, P., Li, Z., & Zhang, S. (2022). Supine infant pose estimation via single depth image. *IEEE Transactions on Instrumentation and Measurement*, *71*, 1–11. DOI: 10.1109/TIM.2022.3178693

Wu, S., Chen, X., Pan, J., Dong, W., Diao, X., Zhang, R., Zhang, Y., Zhang, Y., Qian, G., Chen, H., Lin, H., Xu, S., Chen, Z., Zhou, X., Mei, H., Wu, C., Lv, Q., Yuan, B., Chen, Z., & Lin, T. (2022). An Artificial Intelligence System for the Detection of Bladder Cancer via Cystoscopy: A Multicenter Diagnostic Study. *Journal of the National Cancer Institute, 114*(2), 220–227. DOI: 10.1093/jnci/djab179 PMID: 34473310

Wu, X., Li, R., He, Z., Yu, T., & Cheng, C. (2023). A value-based deep reinforcement learning model with human expertise in optimal treatment of sepsis. *NPJ Digital Medicine, 6*(1), 15. DOI: 10.1038/s41746-023-00755-5 PMID: 36732666

Xie, T., & Pentina, I. (2022). "Attachment theory as a framework to understand relationships with social chatbots: a case study of Replika", *Proceedings of the 55th Hawaii International Conference on System Sciences*. 2046-2055. DOI: 10.24251/HICSS.2022.258

Xie, T., Pentina, I., & Hancock, T. (2023). Friend, mentor, lover: Does chatbot engagement lead to psychological dependence? *Journal of Service Management, 34*(4), 806–828. DOI: 10.1108/JOSM-02-2022-0072

Yalcin, N., Kasikci, M., Celik, H. T., Allegaert, K., Demirkan, K., Yigit, S., & Yurdakok, M. (2022). An Artificial ıntelligence approach to support detection of neonatal adverse drug reactions based on severity and probability scores: A new risk score as web-tool. *Children (Basel, Switzerland), 9*(12), 1826. DOI: 10.3390/children9121826 PMID: 36553270

Yalcin, N., Kasikci, M., Celik, H. T., Demirkan, K., Yigit, S., & Yurdakok, M. (2023). Development and validation of machine learning-based clinical decision support tool for identifying malnutrition in NICU patients. *Scientific Reports, 13*(1), 5227. DOI: 10.1038/s41598-023-32570-z PMID: 36997630

Yang, P., Zhao, G., & Zeng, P. (2019). Phishing website detection based on multi-dimensional features driven by deep learning. *IEEE Access : Practical Innovations, Open Solutions, 7*, 15196–15209. DOI: 10.1109/ACCESS.2019.2892066

Yasukawa, S., Tanaka, T., Yamane, K., Kano, R., Sakata, M., Noma, H., Furukawa, T. A., & Kishimoto, T. (2024). A chatbot to improve adherence to internet-based cognitive–behavioural therapy among workers with subthreshold depression: A randomised controlled trial. *BMJ Mental Health, 27*(1), 1–7. DOI: 10.1136/bmjment-2023-300881 PMID: 38199786

Yavrutürk, A. R. (2025). Psikolojik danışmanlık uygulamalarında teknolojinin kullanımı [Use of technology in counseling practices]. *İstanbul Aydın Üniversitesi Eğitim Fakültesi Dergisi, 11*(1), 5-6.

Yeh, P. L., Kuo, W. C., Tseng, B. L., & Sung, Y. H. (2025). Does the AI-driven Chatbot Work? Effectiveness of the Woebot app in reducing anxiety and depression in group counseling courses and student acceptance of technological aids. *Current Psychology (New Brunswick, N.J.)*, *44*(9), 1–13. DOI: 10.1007/s12144-025-07359-0

Yeung, M., Sala, E., Schönlieb, C. B., & Rundo, L. (2022). Unified focal loss: Generalising dice and cross entropy-based losses to handle class imbalanced medical image segmentation. *Computerized Medical Imaging and Graphics*, *95*, 102026.

Yigit, D., & Acikgoz, A. (2024). Evaluation of comfort behavior levels of newborn by artificial intelligence techniques. *The Journal of Perinatal & Neonatal Nursing*, *38*(3), E38–E45. DOI: 10.1097/JPN.0000000000000768 PMID: 37773591

Yılmaz, A., & Kaya, U. (2021). *Derin öğrenme* [Deep Learning]. Kodlab.

Yin, L., Zhang, C., & Cui, Z. (2020). Experimental research on real-time acquisition and monitoring of wearable EEG based on TGAM module. *Computer Communications*, *151*, 76–85. DOI: 10.1016/j.comcom.2019.12.055

Yoo, J. W., Koo, K. C., Chung, B. H., Baek, S. Y., Lee, S. J., Park, K. H., & Lee, K. S. (2022). Deep learning diagnostics for bladder tumor identification and grade prediction using RGB method. *Scientific Reports*, *12*(1), 17699. DOI: 10.1038/s41598-022-22797-7 PMID: 36271252

Yorulmaz, O., Sapmaz-Yurtsever, S., Gökdag, C., Kaçar-Basaran, S., Göcek-Yorulmaz, E., Yalçin, M., & Görgü-Akçay, N. S. (2018). The future of pychotherapy in Turkey: Predictions for the next 10 years. *The Journal of Nervous and Mental Disease*, *206*(5), 332–339. DOI: 10.1097/NMD.0000000000000797 PMID: 29498955

Younisse, R., Ghnemat, R., & Al Saraireh, J. (2023). Fine-tuning U-net for medical image segmentation based on activation function, optimizer and pooling layer. *International Journal of Electrical & Computer Engineering (2088-8708), 13*(5).

Zaidi, N., & Munir, R. (2023). The one with the rumour: COVID-19-related conversations on Pakistani Twitter. *Public Health*, *225*, 277–284. DOI: 10.1016/j.puhe.2023.10.007 PMID: 37952344

Zea-Vera, A., & Ochoa, T. J. (2015). Challenges in the diagnosis and management of neonatal sepsis. *Journal of Tropical Pediatrics*, *61*(1), 1–13. DOI: 10.1093/tropej/fmu079 PMID: 25604489

Zeng, Y., Yu, D., Song, X., Wang, Q., Pan, L., Lu, H., & Wang, W. (2024). Camera-based cardiorespiratory monitoring of preterm infants in nicu. *IEEE Transactions on Instrumentation and Measurement*, *73*, 1–13. Advance online publication. DOI: 10.1109/TIM.2024.3395314

Zeren, Ş. G., & Bulut, E. (2018). Çevrimiçi psikolojik danışmada etik ve standartlar: Bir model önerisi [Ethics and Standards for Online Counseling: A Model Proposal]. *Turkish Psychological Counseling and Guidance Journal*, *8*(49), 63–80.

Zhang, G., Xie, Q., Wang, C., Xu, J., Liu, G., & Su, C. (2024). Intelligent alert system for predicting invasive mechanical ventilation needs via noninvasive parameters: Employing an integrated machine learning method with integration of multicenter databases. *Medical & Biological Engineering & Computing*, *62*(11), 3445–3458. DOI: 10.1007/s11517-024-03143-7 PMID: 38861056

Zhang, J., Xie, Y., Wang, Y., & Xia, Y. (2020). Inter-slice context residual learning for 3D medical image segmentation. *IEEE Transactions on Medical Imaging*, *40*(2), 661–672.

Zhang, Q., Cui, Z., Niu, X., Geng, S., & Qiao, Y. (2017). Image segmentation with pyramid dilated convolution based on ResNet and U-Net. In *Neural Information Processing: 24th International Conference, ICONIP 2017, Guangzhou, China, November 14-18, 2017* [Springer International Publishing.]. *Proceedings*, *24*(Part II), 364–372.

Zhang, S., Yan, Z., Sapkota, S., Zhao, S., & Ooi, W. T. (2021). Moment-to-moment continuous attention fluctuation monitoring through consumer-grade EEG device. *Sensors (Basel)*, *21*(10), 3419. DOI: 10.3390/s21103419 PMID: 34069027

Zhao, H., Cao, J., Xie, J., Liao, W. H., Lei, Y., Cao, H., Qu, Q., & Bowen, C. (2023). Wearable sensors and features for diagnosis of neurodegenerative diseases: A systematic review. *Digital Health*, *9*, 1–22. DOI: 10.1177/20552076231173569 PMID: 37214662

Zhou, X., Liang, H., & Zhang, Y. (2023). Psychological Therapy with AI: An Overview of Chatbot Applications. *Frontiers in Psychology*, *14*, 112345.

Zhu, D., Dhariwal, M., Zhang, J., Smith, A., & Martin, P. (2024). Patient Perception and Self-Reported Outcomes with Presbyopia-Correcting Intraocular Lenses (PCIOLs): A Social Media Listening Study. *Ophthalmology and Therapy*, *13*(1), 287–303. DOI: 10.1007/s40123-023-00840-8 PMID: 37948016

Zim, M. K. I., & Kaur, U. (2023). Mental health detection and anticipation analysis using deep learning. In *2023 International Conference on Computer Communication and Informatics (ICCCI)* (pp. 1–6). DOI: 10.1109/ICCCI56745.2023.10128581

Zoccali, C., Mallamaci, F., Halimi, J.-M., Rossignol, P., Sarafidis, P., De Caterina, R., Giugliano, R., & Zannad, F. (2024). Chronic cardiovascular–kidney disorder: A new conceptual framework. *Nature Reviews. Nephrology*, *20*(4), 201–202. DOI: 10.1038/s41581-023-00789-8 PMID: 37968510

Zuo, Q., Chen, S., & Wang, Z. (2021). R2AU-Net: Attention recurrent residual convolutional neural network for multimodal medical image segmentation. *Security and Communication Networks*, *2021*(1), 6625688.

About the Contributors

Hüseyin Coşkun received his bachelor's, master's and doctorate degrees from Süleyman Demirel University (SDU), Department of Computer Engineering. He is currently working as an Assistant Professor at Kütahya University of Health Sciences. He is the head of the department of Medical Informatics at the graduate education institute. His research interests include machine learning, audio processing, computer vision, quality control, biomedical signals, mobile programming.

***

Gopu A P is an accomplished academician and researcher with over 14 years of experience in teaching and research. He is currently an Assistant Professor at Velalar College of Engineering and Technology, Erode. His expertise lies in Network Security, Deep Learning, and Cloud Computing. With a Ph.D. from Anna University, Chennai, his research focuses on next-generation secure data transmission solutions, leveraging Improved CGAN and Federated Learning with PPGAN.

Poovendran Alagarsundaram has extensive experience in Data from DBMS, RDBMS, NoSQL and Big data technologies such as Apache Spark, Airflow, Kafka, DBT, and various streaming and API solutions. His areas of focus include Cloud, IoT, and AWS Data Technologies. Additionally, he is a certified AWS Solution Architect Associate and AWS Data Specialist.

Avinash Bhagat is serving as Associate Professor in in School of Computer Applications, Lovely Professional University, Punjab, INDIA has a vast experience of more than 22 years in the field of academics, research and administration. Dr. Avinash Bhagat has been awarded with his Doctorate degree from Lovely Professional University, Punjab in 2021 in the field of Wireless Sensor Networks. His areas of interest include Wireless Sensor Networks, Adhoc Networks, Mobile computing, Machine Learning etc. A number of research papers authored and coauthored, published in International or National journals of repute and conference proceedings comes under his credits. He has edited 4 books and 38 book chapters. He has guided more than 1000 PG and UG projects during his service period. He is also completed the certifications like Microsoft Certified System Administrator, Microsoft Certified System Engineer and Microsoft Certified Professional.

Chinmoy Bharadwaj holds a B.Tech in Computer Science and Engineering, a M.Tech in Computer Science and Engineering, and a Ph.D. With over 10 years and 9 months of teaching experience at the Masters and Bachelors levels in Computer Applications, he has developed expertise in several key areas, including cloud security, edge computing, network security, wireless sensor networks, the Internet of Things, artificial intelligence, and machine learning. His extensive teaching experience and research focus allow him to bring cutting-edge knowledge to his students and contribute to the advancement of these rapidly evolving fields.

Sippee Bharadwaj is an assistant professor in the Department of Business Analytics, specialising in Electronics and Communication Engineering. She holds a PhD in Speech Signal Processing and has over seven years of academic research experience in the fields of electronics and communication engineering. Her work is characterized by a strong foundation in scientific inquiry and a commitment to excellence in interdisciplinary research. She has been actively involved in high-impact, science-driven ventures and has significantly contributed to the advancement of research initiatives across multiple institutions. A proactive leader and collaborative team member, she continues to support the development of innovative methodologies in speech processing and data analytics, with publications in peer-reviewed journals and active participation in academic conferences.

Abir Chaari graduated with a Master's degree in computer science from the University of Sfax in Tunisia (Tunisia, 2015). She is member of the MIRACL Laboratory (Multimedia, Information systems and Advanced Computing Laboratory). Her research interests include audiovisual document and knowledge representation.

Nila A Chotai has a progressive record in the academic domain with over 20 years of experience in teaching at the higher education sector and distinguished record of publications in Academic Journals and she has a strong philosophy of teaching, and knowledge of many different methods to motivate students to develop their expertise in specific areas. Dr. Nila's extensive research contributions include over 25 research papers published in renowned national and international journals, as well as contributions to edited books. She actively engages with the academic community by serving as a Track Chair. She is a Guest Editor for Scopus Journal

Empirical Economics letter. She is also a reviewer of IGI Global publications. She has authored a book in Marketing Management.

Rishita Das is a graduate student and researcher specializing in data analytics and machine learning. Her work focuses on biological data analysis and AI-driven healthcare solutions. She is interested in explainable AI, medical diagnostics, and smart systems. She is passionate about leveraging data-driven approaches to solve real-world problems.

Sureshkumar G. is currently working as Assistant Professor in the department of Computer Science, Pondicherry University. He is having more than 12 years of experience in teaching and researching. He has completed his Masters in Computer science and engineering from college of engineering Guindy of Anna University in the year 2006. He has completed his PhD. in Computer science and engineering in the year 2014. He has published his research works in international journals and conferences.

Kalyan Gattupalli has a Masters in Computer Applications from University of Madras in 2007 have diversified experience in the world of Cloud and CRM including but not limited to Azure Cloud, Micrsoft Dynamcis CE, Salesforce CRM . I have been working as a computer systems analyst with some federal deprtments in Canada and with financial institiutions over the past decade. I work as a Independet contractor providing the services in the name of Yash Tek Inc and Sunny Information Technology Services Inc .

Venkata Surya Bhavana Harish has a wealth of experience in the field of data engineering, with roles ranging from Senior Data Platform Engineer at Under Armour to Software Engineer, Data Ingestion Lead at Asurion in Nashville. Prior to these positions, He served as a Senior Technical Engineer at Informatica in Austin and gained experience as an Energy Market Analyst Intern at Austin Energy.

Halil İbrahim İvelik is an Assistant Professor in the Department of Urology at Kütahya Health Sciences University, Turkey (since 2025). He completed his medical education and urology specialization in Turkey. His academic interests include uro-oncology, reconstructive urology, minimally invasive surgical techniques, and functional urology. He has also taken part in studies involving the use of artificial intelligence in urology. Dr. İvelik has published in national and international journals and contributes to the education of medical students and residents.

Shahnazeer C K has 9 years of experience as an Assistant Professor in various Engineering Colleges in Kerala and 4 years of experience in Industry.

She is a research scholar in Computer Science and Engineering, at Pondicherry University Karaikal Campus, Puducherry, India. Her qualifications include B.Tech in Information Technology from Government Engineering College Sreekrishnapuram Palakkad Kerala, India in 2006 and M.Tech in Information Technology from Anna University Coimbatore Tamil Nadu, India in 2010. Her research interests include Computational Intelligence and Cloud computing.

Imen Kallel is a research member at ESSE (Advanced Electronic Systems and Sustainable Energy), ENET'COM –Tunisia. Research interests include image processing, digital watermarking and data hiding, multimedia authentication, human machine interaction (HMI), computer vision and environmental health and agriculture.

Emine Buse Kurnaz graduated from Kütahya Health Sciences University, Department of Nursing in 2024. She started her master's degree at Kütahya Health Sciences University, Graduate Institute, Department of Child Health and Disease Nursing in 2024. She also works as a nurse in the hospital Kütahya Health Sciences University, Graduate Education Institute, Department of Nursing, Kütahya, Türkiye, 0009-0008-3473-6602, ebuse.kurnaz@ogr.ksbu.edu.tr, 05458391605

Ajay Shriram Kushwaha is a Professor & Research Guide at Sharda School of Engineering & Technology (SUSET), Sharda University, Greater Noida since June 2023. With over 15 years of academic and research experience, he has worked in esteemed state & private universities like RTM, Gondwana, LPU, Jain University. He has successfully guided 2 PhD scholars and currently co-guiding 3 scholars from Jain (Deemed-to-be-University) & Lovely Professional University. His research areas include Networking, Software Engineering, Cyber Security & Forensics, with a focus on Blockchain, IoT & Cloud implementation. He holds 4 patents, with 1 patent under final grant communication. He is a life-time member of Indian Science Congress and IAENG (Hongkong) and is a member of IAENG societies for AI, Computer Science, Data Mining & Software Engineering. He serves as an Editor, Guest Editor, and reviewer for 12+ Scopus, UGC listed or Peer Reviewed International Journals. He has published over 37 research papers in SCOPUS/UGC Listed/Peer Reviewed Journals and co-authored 7 books & news magazine articles. He has conducted 40+ Refresher Courses, FDPs, Seminars, Webinars, Workshops, and Technical Sessions across the country on e-content development, pedagogy, and innovative content creation & assessment techniques. He also conducts sessions on Cyber Security, Ethical Hacking, and related domains. He has completed several MOOC courses from platforms like LinkedIn Learning, Coursera, Alison, Udemy, and Basis Technology. Contributing to open learning, he creates content for YouTube and social media.

Harikumar Nagarajan has a wealth of extensive IT experience as IT architect as well as full stack software developer, specializing in software development across web, mobile, on-premise, and cloud platforms, as well as data science. His expertise lies in Java and JEE frameworks, object retaliation mapping frameworks and handling relational and non relational databases on multi cloud platforms. Also his specialization involves the architecture and design of Microservices development utilizing Docker and Kubernetes on AWS and Azure cloud platforms.

Surendar Rama Sitaraman is currently an AI Frameworks Engineer at Intel Corporation, where he contributes to the development and optimization of AI frameworks, driving innovation in AI and machine learning technologies. Prior to rejoining Intel, Surendar served as a Staff Engineer at Samsung Austin R&D Center (SARC), Advanced Computing Lab (ACL), contributing to the development and optimization of software solutions for Samsung's flagship devices.

Célia M. Q. Ramos holds a PhD in Quantitative Methods Applied to Economics and Management from Faculty of Economics, University of Algarve, obtained her Master in Electrical and Computers Engineering from the Higher Technical Institute, Lisbon University, and is graduated in Computer Engineering from the University of Coimbra, Portugal. She is Coordinator Professor with Habilitation at School for Management, Hospitality and Tourism, also in the UALG, where she lectures mainly Information Systems. Current research interests includes, information systems, data analytics, electronic tourism, business intelligence, digital marketing, panel data models. Has published in the fields of information systems, marketing and tourism, She is reviewer of several scientific journals. At the level of applied research, she has participated in several funded projects. Researcher at the Centre for Tourism, Sustainability and Well-being (CinTurs). Email: cmramos@ualg.pt. ORCID ID: 0000-0002-3413-4897

Faika Şanal Karahan received her bachelor's degree from Konya Necmettin Erbakan University, Department of Foreign Languages Education, Department of English Language Teaching, Türkiye. She received her master's and doctorate degrees from Konya Necmettin Erbakan University, Department of Educational Sciences, Department of Guidance and Psychological Counselling, Türkiye. Since 2017, she has still been a faculty member at Uşak University, Faculty of Education, Department of Guidance and Psychological Counselling as a lecturer and a researcher. Her research interests are acceptance and commitment therapy, short-term solution-focused approach, solution-focused thinking, acceptance, value, compassion, positive psychology, trauma-focused psychological counseling, crisis intervention, preventive guidance and counselling.

V. Santhi has received her Ph.D. in Computer Science and Engineering from VIT University, Vellore, India. She has pursued her M.Tech. in Computer Science and Engineering from Pondicherry University, Puducherry. She has received her B.E. in Computer Science and Engineering from Bharathidasan University, Trichy, India. Currently she is working as Associate Professor in the School of Computing Science and Engineering, VIT University, Vellore, India. She has authored many national and international journal papers and one book. She is currently in the process of editing two books. Also, she has published many chapters in different books published by International publishers. She is senior member of IEEE and she is holding membership in many professional bodies like CSI, ISTE, IACSIT, IEEE and IAENG. Her areas of research include Image Processing, Digital Signal Processing, Digital Watermarking, Data Compression and Computational Intelligence.

Emel Sezici graduated from Zonguldak Karaelmas University, Department of Nursing in 2003. She completed her master's degree at Zonguldak Karaelmas University and her doctorate at Marmara University, Institute of Health Sciences, Department of Child Health and Disease Nursing. She currently continues her academic duties as an associate professor at Kütahya Health Sciences University, Faculty of Health Sciences, Department of Child Health and Disease Nursing. Her academic research interests include newborn health, pain management in children and general child health; she has numerous scientific articles and book chapters in these areas. Kütahya Health Sciences University, Faculty of Health Sciences, Department of Nursing, Department of Child Health and Disease Nursing, Kütahya, Turkey, 0000-0002-6325-6607, emel.sezici@ksbu.edu.tr, 05064980691

Sachin Sharma is currently working as a Professor at Amity School of Engineering and Technology, Amity University, Punjab, Mohali, India since January 2025. He also worked as Associate Dean of International Affairs and Professor, Department of Computer Science and Engineering at Graphic Era Deemed to be University, Dehradun, Uttarakhand, India from February, 2018 to January 2025. He has experience of 15+ years in industry and academia. He is also Co-founder and Chief Technology officer (CTO) of IntelliNexus LLC, Arkansas, USA based company. He also worked as a Senior Systems Engineer at Belkin International, Inc., Irvine, California, USA. He received his Philosophy of Doctorate (Ph.D.) degree in Engineering Science and Systems specialization in Systems Engineering from University of Arkansas at Little Rock, USA with 4.0 out 4.0 GPA and M.S. degree in Systems engineering from University of Arkansas at Little Rock with 4.0

out 4.0 GPA. Dr. Sharma has authored/coauthored over 300+ publications in the form of books, patents, and papers in refereed journals and conference proceedings. He holds 100+ US, Indian and international patents in the area of IoT, wireless communication.

Sureshkumar T. is a Professor currently affiliated with AVS Engineering College,Salem. He holds a Ph.D. in Information and Communication Engineering from Anna University, an M.E. in Computer Science Engineering, and an MBA in HR. His research interests include web data mining, document clustering, and intelligent information retrieval, and he has published several papers in reputed journals.

Kavitha V is a dedicated academician and researcher in the field of Image Processing. She obtained her Ph.D. from Anna University in 2020, specializing in Image Processing. Dr. Kavitha V is currently affiliated with Velalar College of Engineering and Technology, Thindal, Erode, Tamil Nadu, India. Her research interests include cloud computing, software engineering, and emerging technologies in the field of information and communication engineering.

Latha Jothi V is a Professor and Head at Velalar College of Engineering and Technology, Erode - 638012. Published around in 20 international Journals, presented around 35 papers in National and International Conferences, attended around 50 Workshops, Seminars, FDPs etc. Also delivered around 10 lectures in Data Mining, Data Structures, Design and Analysis of Algorithms, Big Data Analytics, Biometrics, Machine Learning, Deep Learning etc. in reputed institutions. Organized around 15 Workshops, Seminars, FDPs, Conferences etc. Also completed 10 courses in SWAYAM-NPTEL with 4 Gold and 3 Silver and recognized by NPTEL as NPTEL Discipline Star and NPTEL Domain Scholar. Also authored books on the titles Object Oriented Programming, Cyber Forensics, Software Project Management and Human Computer Interaction

Deniz Yigit, graduated from Dumlupınar University, Department of Nursing in 2013. She completed her master's degree at Dumlupınar University, Institute of Health Sciences, Department of Child Health and Disease Nursing. She received her PhD degree from Eskişehir Osmangazi University, Institute of Health Sciences, Department of Child Health and Disease Nursing in 2022. She started her academic career in 2013 and currently serves as an Assistant Professor at Kütahya Health Sciences University. Her academic interests include newborn health and artificial intelligence-based applications; she has numerous national and international publications, scientific articles and registered patents in these fields. Kütahya Health Sciences University, Faculty of Health Sciences, Department of Nursing, Department of Child Health and Disease Nursing, Kütahya, Turkey, 0000-0001-5627-7963, deniz.yigit@ksbu.edu.tr, 05428092848

Index

A

Accuracy 2, 3, 4, 5, 6, 8, 9, 13, 19, 20, 21, 22, 26, 27, 29, 30, 31, 34, 35, 37, 38, 39, 41, 42, 43, 50, 52, 53, 54, 55, 56, 57, 58, 59, 60, 61, 62, 64, 68, 98, 99, 138, 139, 140, 142, 148, 166, 171, 172, 173, 174, 178, 179, 181, 183, 185, 187, 194, 202, 204, 205, 207, 208, 209, 212, 213, 214, 216, 217, 220, 223, 233, 234, 236, 238, 243, 244, 245, 247, 248, 249, 250, 251, 258, 261, 262, 265, 266, 268, 270, 271, 272, 273, 276, 282, 291, 292, 296, 298, 299, 300, 301, 302, 303, 304, 308, 310, 311, 312, 313, 314, 315, 316, 318, 320, 321, 322, 323, 324, 325, 326, 362, 369, 371, 372, 373, 375, 378, 379, 380, 381, 382, 383, 385, 386, 387, 388, 389

American Psychological Association 79, 109, 118, 120, 126

Artificial Intelligence 2, 3, 28, 31, 35, 40, 66, 67, 68, 69, 71, 72, 73, 74, 75, 76, 77, 78, 79, 80, 81, 82, 83, 84, 86, 95, 96, 97, 98, 99, 100, 101, 103, 106, 108, 109, 110, 111, 112, 113, 114, 115, 116, 117, 118, 119, 120, 121, 122, 123, 124, 125, 126, 127, 129, 131, 132, 133, 134, 135, 136, 137, 138, 139, 140, 141, 142, 143, 144, 145, 146, 147, 148, 149, 151, 153, 154, 155, 156, 157, 158, 159, 160, 161, 162, 163, 165, 166, 167, 168, 170, 173, 177, 178, 181, 183, 184, 187, 188, 189, 190, 191, 194, 229, 230, 231, 232, 233, 234, 235, 239, 251, 257, 258, 259, 262, 287, 289, 330, 357, 392, 393

AUROC 3, 4, 13, 22, 23, 24, 26, 27, 28, 31, 299, 300

B

behavioral patterns 230, 235

Biomedical informatics 119, 362, 368, 390

Bladder Cancer 165, 166, 170, 175, 177, 178, 179, 180, 181, 183, 188, 189, 190, 191

Blockchain 234, 258, 261, 262, 263, 264, 265, 266, 267, 268, 269, 270, 271, 272, 273, 274, 275, 276, 281, 282, 283, 285, 286, 287, 288, 289, 290

Bone Mineral Density 293, 294, 298, 300, 301, 303, 305, 306, 328, 330

C

CBAM 33, 34, 35, 36, 43, 50, 51, 52, 54, 56, 58, 59, 60, 61, 62, 63, 64

ChatGPT 81, 85, 94, 100, 131, 340, 358

class imbalance 33, 34, 35, 36, 43, 46, 47, 48, 50, 56, 58, 60, 61, 62, 64, 212, 213, 242, 249, 312, 316, 318, 324, 325, 326

Cornea 193, 194, 195, 196, 197, 198, 199, 200, 202, 203, 204, 205, 208, 212, 216, 219, 224, 227, 228

Corneal Layers 193, 194, 205, 206, 209, 210, 216, 218, 219, 220, 226

Cystoscopy 166, 169, 170, 171, 172, 173, 175, 177, 178, 179, 180, 185, 188, 189, 190, 191

D

Data 2, 3, 4, 5, 6, 7, 8, 9, 10, 12, 13, 16, 25, 27, 28, 30, 31, 32, 33, 34, 36, 37, 38, 40, 41, 42, 43, 44, 45, 46, 47, 48, 49, 50, 51, 52, 53, 55, 56, 60, 61, 62, 63, 64, 67, 68, 69, 74, 76, 77, 81, 84, 91, 92, 94, 95, 98, 99, 100, 101, 103, 104, 105, 107, 115, 118, 122, 123, 124, 131, 134, 135, 136, 137, 139, 140, 141, 142, 143, 144, 145, 146, 148, 151, 152, 153, 154, 155, 156, 157, 159, 162, 163, 165, 166, 167, 168, 169, 170, 171, 172, 173, 174, 175, 176, 177, 179, 180, 181, 182, 183, 184, 185, 186, 187, 194, 204,

208, 209, 211, 212, 218, 220, 222, 230, 231, 232, 234, 235, 236, 237, 238, 239, 241, 242, 243, 244, 245, 246, 249, 250, 251, 252, 253, 254, 257, 262, 263, 264, 265, 266, 267, 268, 269, 270, 271, 272, 273, 274, 275, 276, 277, 278, 279, 281, 282, 283, 284, 285, 286, 287, 289, 290, 291, 292, 296, 297, 298, 299, 300, 301, 302, 303, 304, 305, 306, 307, 308, 310, 314, 320, 321, 322, 325, 326, 327, 328, 329, 330, 337, 338, 339, 341, 342, 343, 344, 345, 353, 354, 355, 357, 359, 362, 363, 364, 365, 366, 368, 369, 370, 371, 380, 381, 382, 383, 384, 385, 388, 389, 390, 391, 393
decentralized model 55, 267, 281
Deep Learning 4, 5, 6, 28, 29, 30, 31, 33, 34, 35, 36, 37, 38, 39, 40, 42, 43, 48, 55, 56, 58, 64, 65, 66, 67, 69, 70, 75, 76, 83, 98, 99, 101, 107, 129, 130, 136, 154, 155, 156, 159, 167, 170, 171, 175, 177, 181, 185, 187, 188, 189, 191, 193, 194, 205, 206, 208, 209, 210, 217, 218, 219, 220, 221, 222, 223, 224, 227, 234, 235, 237, 244, 245, 259, 260, 262, 266, 271, 272, 288, 289, 290, 302, 304, 330, 338, 340, 344, 356, 357
Deep Q-Network 361, 363, 370, 371, 374, 387
Disease Prediction 2, 3, 4, 5, 6, 7, 21, 22, 29, 30, 31, 37, 67, 262, 274, 286, 288, 289, 290, 291, 292, 392

E

EfficientNet-B3 33, 34, 43, 44, 45, 48, 49, 50, 52, 54, 56, 58, 59, 60, 61, 62, 63, 64
ELIZA 73, 80, 83, 86, 94, 95, 107, 129
Ensemble Learning 3, 311, 314, 326
Ethical Issues 10, 99, 101, 104, 105, 127, 145, 147, 149, 183, 237

F

Feature Selection 4, 6, 8, 10, 12, 13, 14, 20, 22, 29, 31, 222, 265, 272, 302, 307, 357

G

GAN-based augmentation 36, 50, 56, 60, 61, 62

H

Hair disease diagnosis 33, 45, 56, 58, 61, 64
Healthcare 2, 3, 4, 5, 6, 7, 10, 27, 28, 31, 35, 36, 41, 42, 48, 56, 60, 67, 82, 86, 90, 96, 97, 98, 99, 101, 106, 116, 122, 126, 131, 134, 135, 136, 137, 139, 141, 142, 143, 144, 145, 146, 148, 149, 151, 152, 153, 156, 158, 159, 163, 166, 167, 168, 169, 182, 184, 185, 186, 225, 230, 231, 232, 234, 236, 237, 238, 239, 251, 252, 253, 254, 255, 258, 259, 262, 263, 264, 265, 267, 268, 269, 270, 271, 272, 273, 276, 281, 282, 283, 285, 288, 290, 291, 292, 293, 294, 295, 296, 297, 300, 304, 311, 325, 329, 333, 334, 335, 336, 338, 339, 340, 341, 353, 354, 355, 356, 357, 358, 362, 363, 364, 365, 366, 367, 368, 369, 388, 389, 390, 391, 393
Health Service 137, 333, 334, 345, 352, 353, 354, 356
Heart Disease 2, 3, 4, 5, 6, 7, 11, 12, 13, 14, 15, 16, 17, 18, 19, 21, 22, 23, 26, 27, 29, 30, 31, 32, 153, 276, 286
Heart failure 1, 2, 3, 5, 7, 8, 9, 10, 13

I

Image Analysis 35, 36, 38, 40, 43, 44, 54, 69, 142, 165, 166, 171, 177, 178, 179, 180, 189, 218
Infant 135, 139, 140, 144, 148, 162
IoT 43, 45, 69, 144, 148, 152, 157, 261, 262, 263, 264, 265, 267, 268, 269,

272, 274, 276, 281, 282, 283, 288, 290

K

Keratoconus 193, 194, 195, 196, 197, 198, 199, 200, 201, 202, 203, 204, 205, 208, 210, 212, 214, 216, 219, 220, 221, 222, 223, 224, 225, 226, 227

M

Machine Learning 2, 3, 4, 5, 6, 7, 9, 10, 13, 14, 18, 19, 21, 22, 25, 27, 28, 29, 30, 31, 32, 34, 37, 38, 40, 41, 65, 68, 72, 75, 76, 77, 82, 83, 84, 101, 107, 108, 110, 119, 121, 136, 142, 152, 155, 156, 157, 158, 160, 162, 163, 166, 167, 168, 169, 170, 174, 177, 182, 184, 186, 187, 188, 190, 229, 230, 232, 233, 234, 235, 236, 239, 241, 242, 250, 257, 258, 259, 263, 265, 270, 271, 272, 273, 282, 285, 286, 288, 289, 290, 291, 292, 296, 297, 298, 299, 300, 302, 303, 304, 307, 308, 309, 325, 326, 327, 328, 329, 330, 331, 333, 338, 355, 357, 362, 368, 388, 389, 390, 392

Mental Health 40, 41, 67, 71, 72, 73, 74, 75, 79, 80, 82, 83, 85, 86, 87, 90, 94, 95, 97, 98, 100, 101, 103, 104, 105, 106, 107, 108, 109, 110, 112, 113, 114, 115, 116, 117, 118, 119, 120, 121, 123, 124, 127, 128, 129, 130, 131, 132, 229, 230, 231, 232, 233, 234, 235, 236, 237, 238, 239, 240, 241, 242, 243, 245, 246, 247, 249, 250, 251, 252, 253, 254, 255, 256, 257, 258, 259, 260, 340, 355

MRSA resistance 361, 362, 363, 365, 366, 367, 368, 369, 370, 371, 373, 374, 388, 389, 390, 391

N

natural language processing 77, 82, 136, 168, 169, 172, 175, 230, 231, 253, 337, 341, 355

Neonatal 133, 134, 135, 137, 140, 143, 144, 145, 147, 148, 149, 151, 152, 153, 154, 155, 156, 157, 158, 159, 160, 161, 162, 163, 290

Neonatal Intensive Care Unit 133, 134, 137, 145, 151, 152, 153, 154, 155, 156, 158, 159, 161

Non-Invasive Screening 291

O

OCT Image 194, 205, 207, 208, 209, 219, 220

Osteoporosis 291, 292, 293, 294, 295, 296, 297, 298, 299, 300, 301, 302, 303, 304, 305, 306, 307, 311, 312, 313, 314, 316, 320, 321, 322, 323, 324, 325, 326, 327, 328, 329, 330, 331

P

prevention 2, 42, 82, 115, 137, 142, 149, 230, 253, 280, 288, 296, 297, 305, 334, 362, 363, 365, 390

Proximal Policy Optimization 372, 375, 387, 392

Psychotherapy 73, 79, 80, 81, 87, 93, 95, 96, 105, 106, 108, 110, 111, 113, 115, 124, 126, 127, 131

Public Health 109, 112, 119, 124, 132, 235, 262, 266, 283, 295, 326, 329, 333, 355, 356, 358, 359, 362, 363, 364, 365, 366, 367, 369, 389, 390, 391, 393

R

Random Forest 3, 4, 5, 6, 9, 12, 20, 21, 22, 28, 38, 40, 243, 290, 291, 298, 299, 300, 301, 302, 303, 311, 314, 315, 316, 318, 319, 320, 321, 322, 323, 324, 325, 326

Reinforcement learning 168, 185, 287, 361, 362, 363, 368, 369, 370, 375, 377, 378, 388, 390, 391, 392, 393

Residual Connections 37, 194, 208, 210, 214, 215, 217, 220

S

Semantic Segmentation 193, 194, 206, 210, 220, 223, 225, 227, 228
Sentiment Analysis 169, 238, 333, 336, 337, 338, 339, 341, 342, 344, 353, 354, 355, 356, 357, 358, 359
Social Media 73, 107, 167, 231, 235, 237, 252, 253, 259, 333, 336, 337, 338, 340, 341, 343, 344, 345, 347, 348, 349, 352, 353, 354, 355, 356, 357, 358, 359
Socio-demographic risk 361, 363, 364, 365, 390, 391
Specificity 3, 4, 5, 6, 9, 13, 26, 27, 32, 37, 41, 173, 176, 178, 179, 180, 187, 246, 247, 252, 271, 299, 302, 303, 380, 383, 385, 386, 387
supervisor learning 267, 274

T

Technology 1, 4, 27, 30, 33, 37, 41, 42, 65, 66, 67, 68, 69, 72, 73, 75, 78, 81, 84, 87, 88, 89, 91, 92, 95, 97, 101, 105, 106, 107, 108, 109, 112, 113, 114, 118, 119, 120, 121, 123, 124, 125, 130, 131, 133, 134, 136, 145, 148, 149, 158, 167, 168, 171, 202, 208, 222, 224, 225, 229, 233, 236, 237, 238, 239, 240, 252, 254, 255, 257, 258, 262, 263, 264, 265, 268, 270, 282, 283, 285, 286, 288, 289, 291, 330, 334, 355, 363, 392
telemedicine 33, 34, 35, 36, 39, 40, 41, 42, 43, 48, 55, 56, 58, 59, 63, 64, 65, 66, 67, 68, 112, 116, 117, 120, 125, 126, 253, 339, 357
text analysis 230, 231, 359
Thallium Stress Test 13, 27, 32
Therapist 73, 81, 82, 83, 93, 94, 96, 105, 106, 107, 115, 119, 123, 127
treatment 2, 26, 37, 39, 40, 41, 68, 72, 73, 80, 81, 82, 83, 84, 88, 90, 93, 94, 96, 97, 98, 99, 100, 104, 107, 108, 113, 115, 116, 118, 122, 127, 129, 132, 133, 135, 136, 137, 138, 139, 140, 141, 143, 144, 148, 149, 163, 165, 166, 168, 170, 174, 175, 176, 181, 183, 184, 185, 190, 191, 195, 203, 204, 205, 221, 222, 223, 224, 227, 230, 231, 232, 234, 237, 239, 255, 256, 259, 264, 266, 267, 270, 276, 277, 281, 283, 286, 297, 304, 326, 363, 364, 367, 368, 392, 393

U

UNet 38, 69, 194, 206, 207, 208, 210, 214, 217, 219, 220

V

virtual mental health assistants 230

W

World Health Organization 79, 106, 129, 130, 162, 293, 294, 295, 305

X

XGBoost 6, 243, 267, 291, 298, 303, 311, 312, 313, 314, 316, 317, 318, 319, 320, 321, 322, 323, 324, 325, 326, 327, 331

www.ingramcontent.com/pod-product-compliance
Lightning Source LLC
LaVergne TN
LVHW062332300926
849161LV00007B/1665